Nanoparticles and Nanocarriers Based Pharmaceutical Formulations

Edited by

Akhlesh K. Jain

Institute of Pharmaceutical Sciences
Guru Ghasidas University, Koni
Bilaspur, CG- 495009
India

&

Keerti Mishra

Institute of Pharmaceutical Sciences
Guru Ghasidas University, Koni
Bilaspur, CG- 495009
India

Nanoparticles and Nanocarriers Based Pharmaceutical Formulations

Editors: Akhlesh K. Jain and Keerti Mishra

ISBN (Online): 978-981-5049-78-7

ISBN (Print): 978-981-5049-79-4

ISBN (Paperback): 978-981-5049-80-0

First published in 2022.

need for a court order if at any point you breach any terms of this License Agreement. In no event will any delay or failure by Bentham Science Publishers in enforcing your compliance with this License Agreement constitute a waiver of any of its rights.

3. You acknowledge that you have read this License Agreement, and agree to be bound by its terms and conditions. To the extent that any other terms and conditions presented on any website of Bentham Science Publishers conflict with, or are inconsistent with, the terms and conditions set out in this License Agreement, you acknowledge that the terms and conditions set out in this License Agreement shall prevail.

Bentham Science Publishers Pte. Ltd.
80 Robinson Road #02-00
Singapore 068898
Singapore
Email: **subscriptions@benthamscience.net**

BENTHAM
SCIENCE

CONTENTS

PREFACE

Researchers working in pharmaceutical research have been interested in changing existing medication delivery systems for decades. Pharmaceutical industry research faces an unclear future due to the vast spread of numerous scientific disciplines and skill sets, such as polymer science, biotechnology, genetics, and molecular pharmaceutics. Higher clinical development costs, along with a lower rate of drug discovery and clinical success, result in a lower flow of new chemical entities (NCE) in research development.

The development of analytical tools and the ability to quantify particle size on a nanometre scale has shifted research in particulate drug delivery systems from the micro to the nanoscale. Nanocarriers are assisting in overcoming obstacles in conventional drug delivery due to their adaptability in targeting tissues, accessing deep molecular targets, and managing drug release.

The current book is an attempt to describe the global scientific community's research on this topic. Nanoparticulate drug delivery devices are difficult to develop and have been equipped with vivacious changes. The goal of this book is to explore current developments and upcoming technology in the field of nanoparticulate drug delivery systems.

We hope that the current multiauthored book on nanoparticles and nanocarriers will help and improve readers' understanding of the various types of nanocarrier-based formulations that are either existing or in development. We also hope that persons working in academic, industrial, and scientific fields concerned with pharmaceutical medication delivery would find the book useful. The book is organised so that each chapter covers a distinct topic of research that can be followed without referring to previous chapters.

To go with the flow, we have initiated this book with chapter one, which introduces readers to nanoparticles and nanocarriers. The chapter outlines the introduction of nanoparticles and nanocarriers, within which it describes their classification, including polymeric nanoparticles, metal nanoparticles, magnetic nanoparticles, inorganic nanocarriers, dendrimers, vesicular carriers, micelles and a lot more, along with their synthesis techniques and applications. Overall, this chapter is a comprehensive compilation of available information on recent advances in the field of nanomedicine through an elucidation of nanoparticles and nanocarriers systems. Second chapter focuses on various polymers and techniques engaged with the advancement of polymer-based nanoparticles and their applications in therapeutic intervention. Third chapter highlights the specific and targeted nanoparticles and the use of various nanocarriers for the targeted delivery of drugs in various diseases, along with their opportunities and challenges in targeted delivery. Chapter four mainly focuses on the role and benefits of nanocarriers in drug-targeting and nanocarriers as a prominent system for targeting and delivering drugs to achieve maximum effects with improved therapeutic response. Fifth chapter presents the state of various nanocarriers in the form of nanoparticles and nanodevices applications in medical diagnosis and disease treatments providing essential insights and recent progress on the exciting biomedical applications of nanoparticles, including bioimaging of biological environments, and their role as a critical tool for the early detection of many diseases.

Chapter six focuses on the targeting potential of nanocarriers for the effective treatment of *H. Pylori.* Seventh chapter covers various merits and demerits of gastro-retentive nanocarriers, including some gastro-retentive strategies and their applications in the therapy of various illnesses. In chapter eight, an overview of the recent developments in nanoparticle formulations for cancer treatment is presented with a comprehensive outlook of the clinical studies and utilization in different prevalent cancers affecting the brain, lung, breast, colon, cervix, and prostate.

Chapter nine outlines the recent development in the area of nanoemulsion as a delivery system with respect to topical drug delivery can be studied. In chapter ten, a deep discussion about the micro/nano-sized lipid-based carriers can be studied. In continuation with chapter tenth, chapter eleven represents the various aspects of the liposomes which further relates to the growing advances and interest in the nanotechnology field. Chapter twelve contains a brief knowledge about structural components and integrity concerning the advanced method of niosome preparation and characterization techniques. Recent examples for different applications are also included in the chapter for therapy/diagnostic purposes based on the route of administration and disease state.

Chapter thirteen emphasizes the advantages, limitations, source, isolation, loading methodology, characterization parameters, and clinical applications, and future potential of resealed erythrocytes. Chapter fourteen summarizes the recent development of therapeutic gene delivery approaches for the effective management of ocular diseases and their use in ophthalmology. The last chapter highlights the green approach to synthesize nanoparticles using microorganisms, enzymes or plant extracts as an alternative to chemical synthesis and their further application in the delivery of herbal drugs process preferably green.

We would like to thank Bentham Science Publishers for inviting us to put this book together and for being patient with us throughout the long development process. Their encouragement and guidance were vital in ensuring the book's completion.

We would also like to extend our sincere gratitude to all of the authors who have taken time out of their busy schedules to be a part of this book and authored fantastic chapters that have brought depth and value to it. Their prompt contributions are greatly appreciated.

Akhlesh K. Jain
Institute of Pharmaceutical Sciences
Guru Ghasidas University, Koni
Bilaspur, CG- 495009
India

&

Keerti Mishra
Institute of Pharmaceutical Sciences
Guru Ghasidas University, Koni
Bilaspur, CG- 495009
India

List of Contributors

Abhimanyu Dev	Department of Pharmaceutical Sciences and Technology, Birla Institute of Technology, Mesra, Ranchi-835215, Jharkhand, India
Aditi Pradhan	Department of Pharmaceutical Sciences and Technology, Birla Institute of Technology, Mesra, Ranchi-835215, Jharkhand, India
Akhlesh K. Jain	School of Pharmaceutical Sciences, Guru Ghasidas Central University, Bilaspur-495009 (C.G.), India
Amber Vyas	University Institute of Pharmacy, Pt. Ravishankar Shukla University, Raipur, C.G, India
Amit Kumar Jain	Department of Pharmaceutics, Faculty of Pharmacy, B. R. Nahata College of Pharmacy, Mandsaur University, Mandsaur M.P. 458001, India
Atul Tripathi	People's Institute of Pharmacy & Research Centre, Bhopal, (M.P.), India
Ashish K. Parashar	Chameli Devi Institute of Pharmacy, Indore-452020, (M.P.), India
Aseem Setia	Department of Pharmaceutics, ISF College of Pharmacy, Moga, Punjab, 142001, India
Atul Chaudhary	Department of Pharmaceutics, ISF College of Pharmacy, Moga, Punjab, 142001, India
Awesh Yadav	Department of Pharmaceutics, National Institute of Pharmaceutical Education and Research, Raebareli, India
Balaga Venkata Krishna Rao	Department of Pharmaceutical Sciences and Technology, Birla Institute of Technology, Mesra, Ranchi-835215, Jharkhand, India
Balak Das Kurmi	ISF College of Pharmacy, Moga-142001, Punjab, India
Bhavisha Patel	School of Pharmacy, Parul University, Vadodara, Gujarat, India
Bina Gidwani	Columbia Institute of Pharmacy, Raipur (C.G.), India
Dilpreet Singh	ISF College of Pharmacy, Moga-142001, Punjab, India
G.D. Gupta	ISF College of Pharmacy, Moga-142001, Punjab, India
Gautam Singhvi	Department of Pharmacy, Birla Institute of Technology and Science (BITS), Pilani, Rajasthan, India
Kesavan Karthikeyan	Department of Pharmacy, Guru Ghasidas Vishwavidyalaya (A Central University), Bilaspur, Chhattisgarh, India
Krishna Yadav	Raipur Institute of Pharmaceutical Education and Research (RIPER), Sarona, Raipur-492010, (C.G.), India
Kuldeep Rajpoot	Department of Pharmacy, Guru Ghasidas Vishwavidyalaya (A Central University), Bilaspur (C.G.)-495009, India
Manu Singhai	Department of Pharmaceutics, ISF College of Pharmacy, Moga, Punjab, 142001, India
Monika Kaurav	KIET School of Pharmacy, Ghaziabad-201206, (U.P.), India
Neha Gahlot	Department of Pharmaceutics, Faculty of Pharmacy, B. R. Nahata College of Pharmacy, Mandsaur University, Mandsaur M.P. 458001, India

Nivedita Gautam	Department of Pharmacy, Guru Ghasidas Vishwavidyalaya (A Central University), Bilaspur, Chhattisgarh, India
Olivia Parra-Marín	Departamento de Biología Molecular y Biotecnología, Instituto de Investigaciones Biomédicas, Universidad Nacional Autónoma de México, Ciudad Universitaria, 04510, Ciudad de México, Mexico
Parasuraman Mohan	Department of Pharmacy, Guru Ghasidas Vishwavidyalaya (A Central University), Bilaspur, Chhattisgarh, India
Prem N. Gupta	CSIR-Indian Institute of Integrative Medicine, Canal Road, Jammu-180001, India
Preeti Patel	ISF College of Pharmacy, Moga-142001, Punjab, India
Priya Namdeo	University Institute of Pharmacy, Pt. Ravishankar Shukla University, Raipur (C.G.), India
Ranendra N. Saha	Department of Pharmacy, Birla Institute of Technology and Science (BITS), Pilani, Rajasthan, India
Ravindra Kumar Pandey	Columbia Institute of Pharmacy, Raipur (C.G.), India
Sakshi Tiwari	University Institute of Pharmacy, Pt. Ravishankar Shukla University, Raipur (C.G.), India
Saroj Dangi Rajpoot	Mahatma Gandhi Homoeopathic Medical College, Rani Durgavati Vishwavidyalaya, Jabalpur, M.P. 482001, India
Selvasankar Murugesan	Mother and Child Health Department, SIDRA Medicine, Doha, Qatar
Sneha Singh	Department of Bio-Engineering, Birla Institute of Technology, Mesra, Ranchi-835215, Jharkhand, India
Shiv Shankar Shukla	Columbia Institute of Pharmacy, Raipur (C.G.), India
Shyam S. Pancholi	Shree S.K. Patel College of Pharmaceutical Education and Research, Ganpat University, 384012, Mahesana, Gujarat, India
Sunil K. Jain	Department of Pharmacy, Guru Ghasidas Vishwavidyalaya (A Central University), Bilaspur (C.G.) 495 009, India
Suresh Thareja	Department of Pharmaceutical Sciences, Natural Products Central University of Punjab, Bathinda, 151001, Punjab, India
Tejashree Waghule	Department of Pharmacy, Birla Institute of Technology and Science (BITS), Pilani, Rajasthan, India
Umesh Gupta	Department of Pharmacy, Central University of Rajasthan, Ajmer, Rajasthan 305801, India
Unnati Batra	Department of Pharmacy, Birla Institute of Technology and Science (BITS), Pilani, Rajasthan, India
Varsha Sahu	University Institute of Pharmacy, Pt. Ravishankar Shukla University, Raipur (C.G), India
Veenu Joshi	Center of Basic Science, Pt. Ravishankar Shukla University, Raipur (C.G.), India
Vikas Kumar Jain	Department of Chemistry, Government Engineering College, Raipur, C.G, India

Vishal Jain University Institute of Pharmacy, Pt. Ravishankar Shukla University, Raipur (C.G.), India

Vivek Shrivastava School of Pharmacy, Parul University, Vadodara, Gujarat, India

CHAPTER 1

Introduction to Nanoparticles and Nanocarriers

Amit Kumar Jain[1,*] and **Neha Gahlot**[1]

[1] *Department of Pharmaceutics, Faculty of Pharmacy, B. R. Nahata College of Pharmacy, Mandsaur University, Mandsaur M.P. 458001, India*

Abstract: This chapter outlines the introduction of nanoparticles and nanocarriers, within which it delineates their classification into various categories of polymeric nanoparticles, metal nanoparticles, magnetic nanoparticles, inorganic nanocarriers, dendrimers, vesicular carriers, micelles, and a lot more, their synthesis techniques such as physical, chemical and biological, and their application in the medical sector. The chapter also focuses on various challenges faced by these nanocarrier systems in nanomedicine as well as their advantages over conventional drug delivery. Overall, this chapter is a comprehensive compilation of available information on recent advances in the field of nanomedicine through an elucidation of nanoparticles and nanocarrier systems. During the last decade, surplus new nano-based strategies for improved drug delivery and nanocarriers centered therapeutic approaches have been adopted for oral drug delivery, pulmonary drug delivery, cutaneous drug delivery, drug delivery into the brain, for cardiovascular diseases, intracellular targeting, gene delivery, protein delivery, insulin delivery, anticancer targeting and many more. Currently, nanoparticle-integrated diagnosis and imaging have been in abundant use seeing an urgent need for early detection and diagnosis of various lethal diseases.

Keywords: Anticancer drugs, Antidiabetic, Biomedical imaging, Brain drug delivery, Carbon nanotubes, Dendrimers, Ellipsometers, Encapsulation, Ethosomes, Gene delivery, Hybrid nanocarriers, Inorganic nanocarriers, Lipid carriers, Liposomes, Magnetic nanoparticles, Metal nanoparticles, Nano-composites, Nanovaccines, Quantum dots, Vesicular carriers.

INTRODUCTION

In recent years, a plethora of innovations based on nanotechnology has been introduced in the market through various sectors such as medicine, cosmetics, biotechnology, and the pharmaceutical industry. These innovations have improved the quality of life linked with human health perspectives through

* **Corresponding author Amit Kumar Jain:** Department of Pharmaceutics, Faculty of Pharmacy, B. R. Nahata College of Pharmacy, Mandsaur University, Mandsaur M.P. 458001, India; Tel: +919501846476; E-mail: director.brncop@meu.edu.in

Akhlesh K. Jain & Keerti Mishra (Eds.)

various developments in drug delivery through nanotechnology. Nanotechnology deals with substances at a nanometer scale that is the size equal to one billionth of something (range 10-1000 nm). This chapter focuses on the latest trends in nanotechnological research and nanomedicine through a comprehensive overview of nanoparticles and nanocarriers in drug delivery and other developments in the pharmaceutical sector. The whole system leads to the prevention, treatment, and diagnosis of diseases through various smart formulations or theragnostic. Many existing systems for the administration and release of drugs and therapeutics have been converted into nanotechnology-based systems for the delivery of genes, proteins, and cells for oral, pulmonary, and topical delivery of drugs and therapeutics for therapeutic effect. In addition, various diagnostic and imaging techniques based on nanotechnology have evolved for economic and rapid detection of diseases.

Overview of Nanoparticles (NPs)

Recent research in nanoscience and the application of nanotechnology in medicine has raised high expectations that technologies using nanosystems in medicine will make great strides in disease prognosis and treatment [1]. Nanotechnology is a relatively new advance in scientific research, but its basic concepts have been around for a long time. A Nobel prize-winning physicist Richerd P. Fineman introduced the term nanotechnology in his lecture at a meeting organized by the American Physical Society in December 1959. In 1974, a professor at the Tokyo University of Science described the term nanotechnology as a system encompassing dimensions in an ultra-fine range. In short, nanotechnology can best be defined as creating or manipulating materials on a nanometric scale. The class of particles in this very fine dimension is defined as nanoparticles and can be obtained by size reduction or clustering [2].

The unique properties of nanoparticles have a spectrum of uses that normally do not exist in particles of greater size (> 500 nm) or their bulk equivalents. Nanoparticles below 100 nm in size are widely used in medicine (targeted drug delivery, imaging, and personalized medicine), except for solid lipid nanoparticles, which are larger than 100 nm in diameter and have different physicochemical properties [3]. Nanoparticle applications in a variety of disciplines necessitate a low-cost, simplified method of producing high-quality shaped nanoparticles. In recent years, so many synthesis approaches have been employed or improved in an attempt to optimize physicochemical attributes and lower production costs [4].

Structure, Morphology, and Size Analysis

To understand the properties and performance of nanoparticles, a thorough study of size, shape, and surface structure is necessary which can be accomplished by morphological characterization by use of different techniques of microscopy such as transmission electron microscopy, scanning electron microscopy, scanning transmission electron microscopy, optical microscopy, and scanning probe microscopy. Diffraction techniques such as X-Ray diffraction of powder, small-angle X-ray scattering, electron diffraction, and small-angle neutron scattering are used to investigate the atomic and molecular structure of crystals [5, 6]. A widespread range of techniques can be used for the assessment of NPs size including Transmission electron microscopy, Scanning electron microscopy, Atomic Force Microscopy, X-Ray Diffraction, and Dynamic light dispersion. While the first four give a better estimate of size than the Dynamic light dispersion, only the zeta potential size analyzer/DLS can estimate NPs size at extremely low dimensions. The NTA model allows the size distribution of nanoparticles in a fluid medium with diameters between 10 and 1000 nm to be analyzed and visualized by comparing the Brownian motion rate with the size of the NPs [7]. AFM is used to measure the surface roughness of nanoparticles [8].

Electron Microscopy

TEM and SEM are widely used in various research areas to observe particles under high magnification. When an electron beam drops on the surface of the specimen in a TEM, the microscope measures the changes in the electron beam scattered within the test specimen. However, in SEM, electron beams drop on the specimen surface and scan it in a raster scan pattern; here, the electrons will interact only with the specimen surface, containing the information only about the specimen surface. Based on how the SEM image is formed, the image has a distinct three-dimensional (3D) appearance and is useful for analyzing the surface morphology of the target sample. Electrons scattered at very high angles are used in Z-contrast annular-dark-field (ADF) imaging in scanning transmission electron microscopy (STEM).

Optical Microscopy

The mechanism involved in the optical microscope particle size analysis is based on the 1000-fold resolution of particles in the sub-micron range at a wavelength of 2000-8000 A° of light rays [5].

Diffraction Techniques

The morphology of nanoparticles can be described using XRD powders, small-angle X-ray scattering (SAXS), small-angle neutron scattering (SANS), and electron diffraction (ED). The atomic and molecular structure of a crystal is determined by XRD, wherein the crystal structure deflects incident X-rays in different directions [6].

Optical Characterization

To collect data on nanoparticles' properties like absorption, reflectivity, luminescence, and phosphorescence, several optical characterization techniques are being used. Various color NPs, especially semiconductor NPs and metallic NPs are well known and are widely used in imaging systems due to their optical properties. Photoluminescence, the use of UV spectrophotometer, and the use of ellipsometers are important for the assessment of the optical properties of NPs. The information on absorption and reflection values of NPS gives an understanding of the basic principle of each application of these NPs [7, 8].

Physicochemical Properties of Nanoparticles

Nanoparticles exhibit size-related properties that are very different from those seen in particles the size of a micrometer or bulk substances. Nanoparticles exist in a variety of forms: spheres, flakes, rods, tubes, fibers, cords, and random variants that can have all of these forms. Nanoparticles can also be embedded in many polymer matrices, such as silicone rubbers, polystyrene, polycarbonate, nylon, polyamide, polyethylene forming nanocomposites. These nanocomposites show advanced optical, electrical, magnetic, and dielectric properties compared to microparticle-reinforced polymers [9]

Electrical Properties

The most important property of metal is its electrical conductivity, which can be used in a variety of applications. Each metal has a unique and distinct characteristic. Metal properties generally change when their size is reduced to the nanometre scale, such as the transition from a semiconductor to a ferromagnetic property, a shift in absorption (Plasmon Absorption), and the use of nanometre-size metal in thermoelectric material uses. Depending on the temperature, the bulk metal has a different electrical conductivity. When the size of the metal is reduced to the nanometre scale, this behavior is no longer in effect. The electrical conductivity of metal nanoparticles varies depending on their size. Because of this variation, the metal can be used for a variety of applications by varying its size. When the electrical conductivity is less than the critical value, it is proportional to the size of the nanoparticles. When the electrical conductivity is greater than the critical value, increasing the particle size does not affect the electrical conductivity [10].

Mechanical Properties

Nanoparticle mechanical features such as hardening, elastic modulus, adhesion, friction, and movement differ from microparticles and bulk materials. Comprehending some fundamental mechanical properties such as hardness and elastic modulus of nanoparticles will greatly help to design the particles properly and to evaluate their roles and mechanisms in specific applications. Nanoindentation is used to determine particle hardness. Because of AFM measurements of particle deformation, the elastic modulus of nanoparticles has rapidly evolved. Adhesion and friction are of great significance in the design and delivery of nanoparticles and nanofabrication. During the last 10 years, many researchers have been interested in characterizing the adhesion and friction behavior of nanoparticles. Atomic force microscope is currently a powerful instrument for measuring the adhesion and friction between nanoparticles and solid surfaces. Various forces, including gravitational (buoyancy) forces, surface forces, viscous flow forces, and Brownian motion forces, cause nanoparticles to move in different ways in the media. However, due to the small particle size that prevents the use of the most common imaging techniques, the experiments to directly monitor the movement of nanoparticles are limited. High-resolution measurements of the motion of single nanoparticles have been made using a variety of methods. The first method is particle tracking using fluorescence. The second method is TEM wherein the observations are capable of providing quite detailed data on the motion of particles and overall knowledge of NP's role in distinct utilization. The main applications of nanoparticles include lubricant additives, nanomanufacturing, and nanoparticle reinforced composite coating [11].

Magnetic Properties

Magnetic nanoparticles have sparked a lot of interest since their properties typically differ significantly from those of bulk materials, allowing them to be exploited to create new materials and gadgets. The nature of nanoparticles depends on the external magnetic field. When an external magnet is present, the nanoparticles become magnetic but revert to a non-magnetic state when the external magnet is withdrawn. Nanoparticles of several different ferromagnetic and ferrimagnetic materials are utilized in modern technology. Magnetic nanoparticles are used in magnetic data storage, suspensions of magnetic nanoparticles (ferrofluid), magnetic beads, magnetic resonance imaging, drug targeting, *etc*. In bioseparation technology, magnetic beads with sizes in the micrometer range are often used. Bulk magnetic materials are usually split up into domains with different magnetization directions. In ferromagnetic and ferri-magnetic materials this is due to a lowering of the energy of the magnetostatic field. In antiferromagnetic materials, it can be explained by nucleation of antiferromagnetic clusters with different sublattice magnetization directions when the material is cooled through the Neel temperature. Across a domain wall, separating two domains with different magnetization directions, the spins gradually change their direction. The width of a domain wall is determined by the exchange interaction and the magnetic anisotropy constant. Magnetic anisotropy is a very important parameter for magnetic materials. Materials with a large anisotropy can be used as permanent magnets, whereas so-called soft magnetic materials with a small magnetic anisotropy are used in, for example, as transformers, for magnetic shielding and magnetic sensors. A considerable portion of the atoms in nanoparticles is found on the surface. Because of the low symmetry around the surface atoms, they may contribute a significant amount of magnetic anisotropy, referred to as surface anisotropy. Single domain superparamagnetic NPs have a magnetic moment that is aligned with the applied field. Due to the quick reversal of the magnetic moment, ferromagnetic NPs will maintain a net magnetization in the absence of an external field, whereas superparamagnetic NPs would not. The zero-field-cooled (ZFC) and field-cooled (FC) magnetization curves are two typical methods for characterizing magnetic nanoparticles. After cooling the sample in zero magnetic fields, magnetization measurements are carried out. The magnetism is then monitored as a function of temperature during the heating process using a smaller field. The magnetization of a sample is measured as a function of temperature during heating in the same applied magnetic field in an FC magnetization curve [12, 13].

Thermal Properties

Nanofluids are utilized for commercial cooling because their huge surface area allows for increased heat transmission. Particles less than 20 nm in diameter have 20% of their atoms on their surface, making them immediately ready for thermal action. Metal nanoparticles have a higher thermal conductivity than solid fluids, which is a well-known phenomenon. For instance, at ambient temperature copper has 700 times higher thermal conductivity than water and 3000 times higher than motor oil. The thermal conductivity of oxides such as aluminum oxide (Al_2O_3) is higher than that of water. As a result, the thermal conductivities of fluids containing suspended solid particles or nanofluids are projected to be much higher than those of conventional heat transfer fluids. Nanofluids are made by dispersing solid particles on the nanometric scale in a liquid such as water, ethylene glycol, or oils. Ceramic particles, pure metallic particles, and carbon nanotubes are three types of nanoparticles that are commonly used in various combinations with liquids to obtain various nano liquids. The advantage of employing nanoparticles is their mobility, which is due to their small size and can result in micro-convection of fluid and hence improved heat transmission. Micro-convection and improved heat transmission may also increase dispersion, allowing for faster heating of the fluid. Because the particles are tiny, they weigh less and have a lower risk of sedimenting. This reduced sedimentation can solve one of the suspensions' key limitations, particle settling, and make nanofluids more stable. The improvement of conductivity was discovered to be dependent on particle size as well as particle concentration. In general, with decreasing particle size, an increase in enhancement is observed [14, 15].

Classification of Nanoparticles

Based on Dimensions

One-D, Two-D, and Three-D nanoparticles are the three types of nanoparticles (Fig. **1.1**). For decades, one-dimensional system (thin film or fabricated surfaces) has been used. Thin films (1-100 nm) or monolayers, with a variety of technical applications, including chemical and biological sensors, data storage systems, magneto-optic and optical devices, and fiber-optic systems, are currently commonly used. Carbon nanotubes, for example, are two-dimensional nanoparticles with two dimensions on the nanometre scale. 3D nanomaterials are three-dimensional nanoparticles that are nano in all three dimensions. Dendrimers, Quantum Dots, and Fullerenes are all examples of nanomaterials [16].

Based on Structural Composition and Morphology

NPs can be made up of a single constituent material or a combination of several (Fig. **1.1**). Pure single-composition materials may be easily manufactured using a variety of processes, but NPs observed in nature are often agglomerations of materials with varied compositions. In hybrid nanoparticles, three primary types of chemical ordering define how the atoms of the elements are ordered within the same nanoparticle. The order of mixed NPs might be random or ordered. Ordered nanoalloys relate to ordered arrangements of two distinct atoms, whereas randomly mixed alloys correspond to solid solutions. A shell of one type of atom surrounds a core of another type of atom in core-shell NPs. The segregation of materials within the core or shell is caused by a variety of thermodynamic concerns. Multi-shell (or "onion-like") NPs are a subset of the core-shell category. The shells of these NPs alternate A–B–A, or A–B–C in the case of ternary NPs. Janus (or "dumbbell-like") NPs are a term used in the literature to describe layered NPs. They are made up of two different types of NPs (A and B) that share a common interface. These NPs tend to lower the number of bonds that exist between components A and B. The phase separation is aided by this heterojunction arrangement. Other complicated topologies of NPs, such as multicore–shell structures in which the cores can exhibit either 'dumbbell-like' or 'onion-like' structures, are becoming more popular as the demand for multifunctional NPs grows [1].

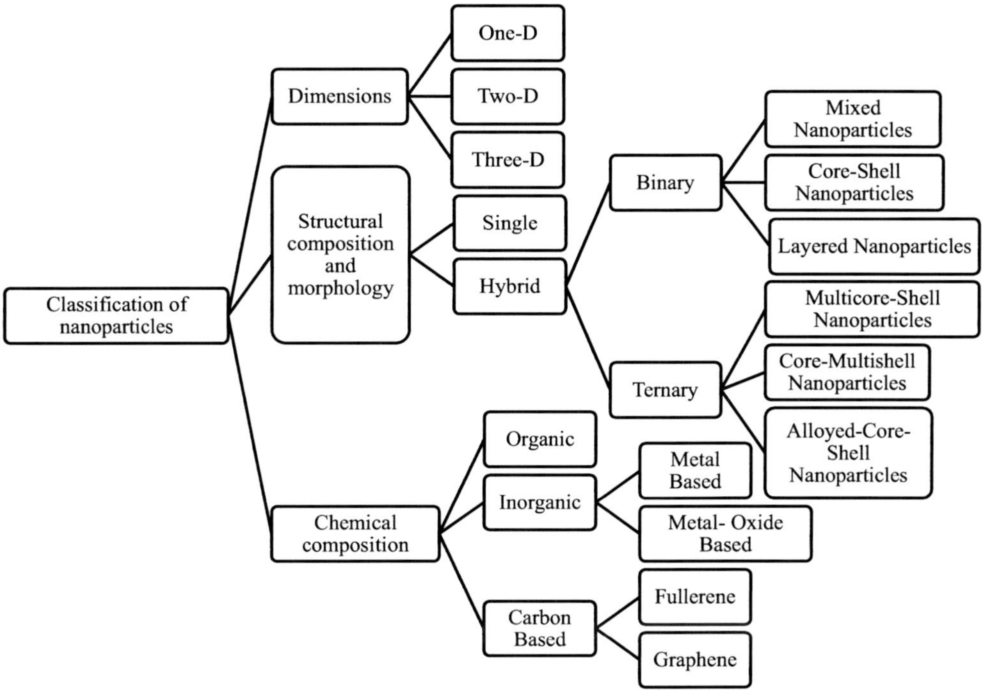

Fig. (1.1). Classification of nanoparticles.

Based on Chemical Compositions

Organic nanoparticles, inorganic nanoparticles, and carbon-based nanoparticles are the most common types (Fig. **1.1**). Organic nanoparticles or polymers include dendrimers, micelles, liposomes, and ferritin, among others. Non-carbon nanoparticles or inorganic nanoparticles are made up of metal or metal oxides. Metal-based nanoparticles are nanoparticles that are synthesized from metals using destructive or constructive processes. Nanoparticles of almost all metals can be synthesized. Aluminum (Al), cadmium (Cd), cobalt (Co), copper (Cu), gold (Au), iron (Fe), lead (Pb), silver (Ag), and zinc are the most widely employed metals for nanoparticle synthesis (Zn). Metal oxide-based nanoparticles are synthesized to change the properties of their respective metal-based nanoparticles. For example, iron nanoparticles (Fe) quickly oxidize to iron oxide (Fe_2O_3) in the presence of oxygen at ambient temperature, increasing their reactivity. Nanoparticles of metal oxide are also produced for increased activity and efficiency. Those nanoparticles that are entirely comprised of carbon are known as carbon nanoparticles. They can be categorized into fullerenes, graphene, carbon nanotubes (CNT), carbon nanofibers, and carbon black and sometimes activated carbon in nanosize [17].

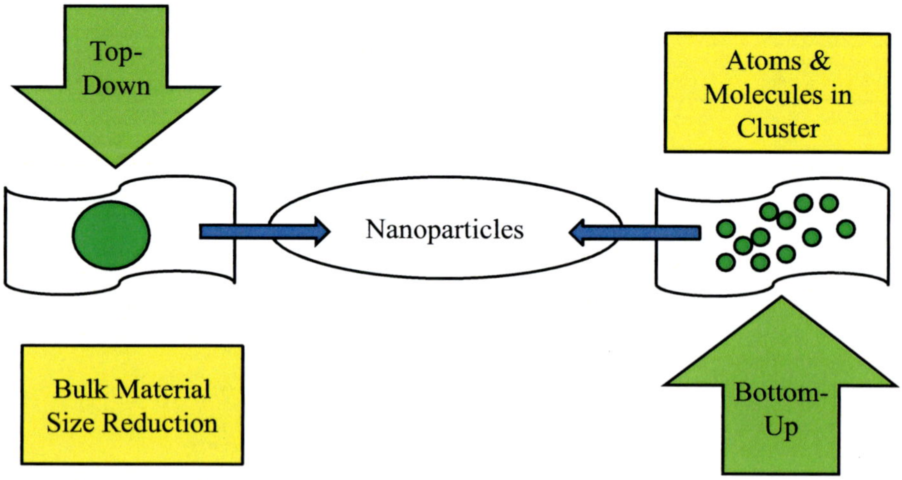

Fig. (1.2). Methods of synthesis.

Methods of Synthesis

A variety of materials, including proteins, polysaccharides, and synthetic polymers, can be used to produce nanoparticles. Various methods for the production of different nanoparticles have been developed with infinite applications through the decades (Table **1.1**). The two basic approaches for the formulation of nanoparticles are the top-down and bottom-up approaches

(Fig. **1.2**). Grinding, lithography, and repetitive wrecking are the methods that take the top-down approach. The particle size and structure are not well controlled by this approach and thus it is not used mostly by scientists. Whereas the methods involving the Bottom-up approach are mostly used for nanoparticles synthesis because this approach is based on framing a nanoparticle by clustering material at the atomic or molecular level [17, 18].

Table 1.1. Methods of Synthesis [17, 19 - 22].

S. No.	Types of Nanoparticles	Methods of Synthesis	Mechanism
1.	Polymeric Nanoparticles	Solvent evaporation	Emulsions formulated in volatile solvents of polymers. Here the emulsion can be converted into a suspension of nanoparticles by evaporation of the polymer-solvent and dispersed in the continuous phase of the emulsion.
		Salting-out	Nanoparticle emulsions are usually formulated with polymer solvents that are completely miscible with water, resulting in the emulsification of polymer solutions in the aqueous phase without the need for high shear forces but high salt or sucrose concentrations are required for a strong salting-out effect in the aqueous phase.
		Nanoprecipitation	In this method, polymer deposition occurs by replacing a water-soluble semi-polar solvent with a lipophilic solution. The rapid dispersion of the solvent in the non-solvent phase lowers the interfacial tension between the two phases, increases the surface area, and forms small droplets of organic solvent.
		Dialysis	The Polymer is dissolved in an organic solvent and placed inside a dialysis tube. The inside membrane displacement of the solvent is followed by a progressive polymer aggregation due to a loss of solubility and the formation of homogeneous nanoparticles suspensions.
		Supercritical fluid technology	In this process, the solute dissolves in the SCF to form a solution and expands rapidly through an orifice or capillary nozzle. A high degree of supersaturation, combined with a rapid drop in pressure during expansion, results in uniform nucleation to form well-dispersed particles.
		Emulsion polymerization	In this method, polymeric nanoparticles of typically 100 nm in size are formed containing many polymer chains

(Table 1) cont.....

S. No.	Types of Nanoparticles	Methods of Synthesis	Mechanism
2.	Lipid-based Nanoparticles	High-Pressure Homogenization	Based on shear because of heavy turbulence.
		Solvent Emulsification Evaporation Method	Emulsification (or diffusion) of the globules and their subsequent evaporation result in deposition into particles.
		Solvent Emulsification Diffusion Method	This method includes emulsifying globules and vaporizing them, leading to particle precipitation.
		Membrane contractor	Here the lipid phase is forced to form tiny droplets through the porous membrane.
		Phase Inversion Techniques	Transitional emulsion spontaneously reversed from o/w to w/o with temperature rise.
		Coacervation Technique	In this method when the pH of a micelle solution of an alkaline fatty acid salt is lowered by acidification (coacervation solution) in the presence of a polymer stabilizer, proton exchange occurs which leads to lipid deposition (coacervation).
		Gas-Assisted Melting Atomisation	The lipid or protein/lipid mixture is placed in a thermostatically controlled mixing chamber (CM) and dissolved in supercritical carbon dioxide under defined conditions of temperature and pressure. The lipid-saturated liquid is then pushed out of the nozzle through a valve at the bottom of the chamber to produce nanoparticles.

(Table 1) cont.....

S. No.	Types of Nanoparticles	Methods of Synthesis	Mechanism
3.	Inorganic Nanoparticles	Precipitation of Salts in Aqueous Medium	This process involves the precipitation of salts by oxidation or co-precipitation in an aqueous environment.
		Hydrothermal Synthesis	This process uses water as a solvent to increase the solubility of precursors by exploiting conditions of temperature and pressure and accelerating the reaction.
		Polyol Process	This process leads to nanoparticles formation due to the decline of dissolved metal salts concentration in polyol at high temperatures.
		Decomposition in Organic Media	The thermal decomposition of metallic compounds in organic solvents with high boiling points is involved in this process.
		Laser Pyrolysis	Here, a laser heats a diluted mix of precursors to decompose and triggers the nucleation of particles into nanoparticles.
		Spray pyrolysis	A solution of salts is sprayed into a series of reactors, which evaporate the aerosol droplets. The particles are then further dried and processed at high temperatures.
		Sol-Gel	It is a wet chemical process in which a chemical solution serves as the initial stage in an integrated system of individual particles.
		Spinning	The spin method should be used to synthesize nanoparticles in a reactor with a spinning disc so that atoms or molecules are melted and fused for drying together.
4.	Hybrid Nanoparticles	Inorganic–inorganic	Hybrid nanoparticles are made up of two or more different components, typically inorganic components like metal ions, salts, sulfides, metal clusters or particles, non-metallic elements, and their derivatives, *etc*.
		Organic-inorganic	Hybrid nanoparticles are made up of two or more components, typically inorganic components like metal ions, metal clusters or particles, salts, oxides, sulfides, *etc*., and organic components like organic groups or molecules, ligands, biomolecules, pharmaceutical substances, polymers, *etc*.
5.	Bio-inspired Nanoparticles	Microorganisms mediated synthesis of nanoparticles	Nanoparticles synthesis by Bacteria.
			Nanoparticles synthesis by Virus.
			Nanoparticles synthesis by Fungus.
		Plants mediated synthesis of nanoparticles	These nanoparticles are biosynthesized using leaf extract or other plant components
		Human cell line mediated synthesis of nanoparticles	Intracellularly, certain metal nanoparticles are produced in *in-vitro* conditions that resemble their natural cellular environment.

Overview on Nanocarriers

Nanocarriers are colloidal nanoparticles broadly utilized for the transportation of a drug substance or any other agents to a specific site in the body. Since the nanocarriers are used for therapeutic application, therefore, the size of the nanocarriers has to be less than 200 nm as the diameter of microcapillaries that are present in the body lies nearly 200 nm. Nanocarriers are generally inactive and safe thus providing good biocompatibility with the human body. These nanocarriers offer good bio consistency because they are generally considered to be safe. The nanocarriers with the sustained release of the drug have a long-term circulation period overcoming the endosome–lysosome mechanism [23]. Presently nanocarriers are widely considered to address the emerging need to improve drug treatment to treat various diseases. Nanotechnology incorporates systems engineering that works on the molecular scale. Such systems are characterized by a wide range of physical, physical, and electrical properties that attract sectors ranging from science to nanomedicine as one of the most effective research tools, using nano-technology in specialized medical interventions for prevention, diagnosis, and disease treatment [24].

Classification

According to the high surface-to-volume ratio, nanocarriers are classified into three major categories as organic nanocarriers, inorganic nanocarriers, and hybrid nanocarriers (Table **1.2**).

Table 1.2. Classification of Nanocarriers [24 - 26].

<table>
<tr><th>Category</th><th>Nanocarrier</th><th colspan="3">Vesicular/Non-vesicular/Polymeric Nanocarrier</th><th>Biodegradable/
Non- biodegradable</th></tr>
<tr><td rowspan="7">Organic</td><td rowspan="3">Liposomes</td><td colspan="3">Vesicular</td><td rowspan="3">Biodegradable</td></tr>
<tr><td rowspan="2">Multilamellar vesicles</td><td colspan="2">Unilamellar vesicles</td></tr>
<tr><td>Small unilamellar vesicles</td><td>Large unilamellar vesicles</td></tr>
<tr><td>Solid-lipid nanoparticles</td><td colspan="3">Non- vesicular</td><td>Biodegradable</td></tr>
<tr><td>Dendrimer</td><td colspan="3">Polymeric nanocarrier</td><td>Biodegradable</td></tr>
<tr><td>Micelles</td><td colspan="3">Polymeric nanocarrier</td><td>Both</td></tr>
<tr><td>Polymeric nanoparticles</td><td colspan="3">Polymeric nanocarrier</td><td>Both</td></tr>
</table>

(Table 2) cont.....

Category	Nanocarrier	Vesicular/Non-vesicular/Polymeric Nanocarrier	Biodegradable/ Non- biodegradable
Inorganic	Carbon nanotubes	Non- vesicular	Both
	Magnetic nanoparticles	Non- vesicular	Both
	Quantum dots	Non- vesicular	Both
	Mesoporous silica nanoparticles	Non- vesicular	Both

Liposomes

Liposomes are vesicular nanocarriers used to deliver the therapeutic agent to a specific site. Liposome's vesicles consist of an aqueous core enclosed in the lipid bilayer (Fig. **1.3**). These vesicular nanocarriers act as an agent to transport active hydrophilic and lipophilic drug molecules to a specific area. These are the most clinically established vesicular nanocarrier for the delivery of biologically active agents. They are synthetic composites made from amphiphilic phospholipids and their size can vary from 50 nm to 300 nm. Liposomes may also be classified into two main groups according to their size and number of layers: (1) the multilamellar vesicles (MLV) and (2) the unilamellar vesicles. Unilamellar vesicles are further divided into two categories: (1) large unilamellar vesicles and small unilamellar vesicles. The vesicle contains an aqueous core with one phospholipid bilayer in unilameleous liposomes. The vesicles of multilamellar liposomes have an onion-like structure. Liposomes have several structural and non-structural components of which phospholipids are the major structural component of liposomal membranes and cholesterol can be incorporated into phospholipid membranes. Liposomes are completely biodegradable, flexible, non-toxic, biocompatible, and non-immunogenic for both systemic and non-systemic use. Liposomes can trap hydrophobic and hydrophilic compounds, prevent degradation of the trapped drug, and release the trapped drug at specific targets. Therefore, liposomes are widely used as carriers of many drug molecules in the pharmaceutical industry. A summarized detail of liposomes is presented in Table **1.3**.

Solid- Lipid Nanoparticle

Solid lipid nanoparticles (SLNs) are colloidal dispersions typically spherical with a diameter of 50 to 1000 nm. The main components of SLNs include a mixture of lipids usually in solid state at room temperature, emulsifiers and, the active ingredient (API) in an appropriate solvent system. SLNs drug loading and release depend on the crystalline condition and lipid melting behavior. All properties of lipid nanoparticles are enhanced by surface modification like increased pharmacokinetic tolerability, occlusive complex formation, improved stability profile, and chemical absorption. Because SLN is dispersed in aqueous or superficial solutions, it is suitable for intravenous administration. Because nanoparticles are absorbed by phagocytosis, surface modifications often reduce phagocytosis. Often, particle size, bio index, and charge analysis can be measured with dynamic light dissemination (DLS) and quasi-scattering elasticity (QELS). The size and qualitative properties of nano-particles may also be measured by nuclear magnetic resonance (NMR). Microscopy is an advanced technology that offers direct control of nanoparticles. The best way to assess SLNs size, surface morphology, stability, and time structural change is by microscopy SEM & TEM. The surface distribution of surfactant molecules is often estimated, and only the organic structure is confirmed by X-ray photoelectron spectroscopy (XPS) for the adsorption of SLNs and positively charged nanoparticles. SLN entrapment is often measured using centrifugation or microcentrifugation techniques. Samples are centrifuged at high speed so that the number of free compounds can be determined by UV-Visible spectroscopy or high-performance liquid chromatography [26].

Table 1.3. Liposome summary chart [27, 28].

Characterization Parameter	Visual Appearance	Depending on composition and particle size, the liposome suspension can range from translucent to milky.
	Size distribution	The dynamic light dispersion is usually used to measure the size distribution.
	Lamellarity	Electron microscopy or spectroscopic techniques measure the lamellarity of liposomes.
	Stability	The stability of liposomes is a complex problem, consisting of physical, chemical, and biological stability. Physical stability mainly indicates the size constancy and lipid to active ingredient ratio. Biological stability includes stability after interaction with plasma proteins.
	Entrapped volume	The captured volume of a liposome population (phospholipids of μL/mg) can often be determined by measuring the total amount of solution encased within the liposome.
	Surface charge	For the assessment of charges, free-flow electrophoresis and zeta potential measurement are methods used. The surface load on the vesicles is due to the mobility of the lipo-splitting in a suitable buffer.

(Table 3) cont.....

Method of preparation	Mechanical dispersion method	a) Sonication.
		b) French pressure cell: extrusion.
		c) Freeze-thawed liposomes.
		d) Lipid film hydration by handshaking, non-hand.
		e) Shaking or freeze-drying.
		f) Micro-emulsification.
		g) Membrane extrusion.
	Solvent dispersion method.	a) Ether injection (solvent vaporization)
		b) Ethanol injection
		c) Reverse phase evaporation method
	Detergent removal method	a) Dialysis
		b) Gel-permeation chromatography
Marketed Formulations	AmBisome®	Contains Amphotericin B for fungal infection
	Caelyx®	Contains doxorubicin for ovarian cancer

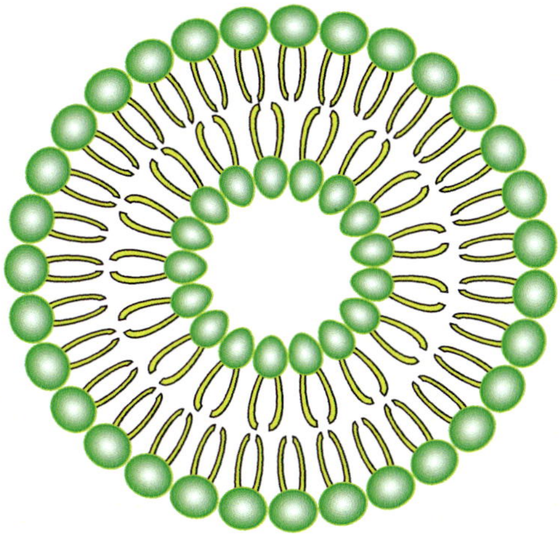

Fig. (1.3). Structure of liposome.

Dendrimers

Dendrimers are radially symmetric nanoscale molecules, consisting of tree-like branches, with a well-defined, unified, and monodispersed structure (Fig. **1.4**). Dendrimers are small, homogeneous particles with dimensions ranging from 1 to 10 nanometres. Dendrimers have unique properties that make them intriguing candidates for a variety of applications. Drugs can be contained inside the macromolecule interior and employed to offer regulated release from the inner core owing to their globular shapes and the presence of internal cavities. The three primary sites for drug entrapment in the dendrimer architecture are (i) void spaces (by molecular entrapment), (ii) branching points (by hydrogen bonding), and (iii) outer surface groups (by charge-charge interactions). The drug's high absorption is limited by the dendrimer's small size, but due to its branching structure, the drug can be charged on the scaffold's outer surface *via* covalent or electrostatic interactions. With increasing dendrimer synthesis, dendritic macromolecules tend to grow linearly in diameter and become more spherical. As a result, dendrimers have emerged as a promising delivery vehicle for investigating the effects of polymer size, charge, and composition on biologically important properties like lipid bilayer interactions, cytotoxicity, internalization, blood plasma retention time, biodistribution, and filtration. Polyamide amines (PAMAM), polypropyleneimines (PPI), and dendrimers generated from biomolecules such as amino acids, modified polysaccharides, nitrogenous bases, and polyester dendrimers are all examples of dendrimers [29, 30].

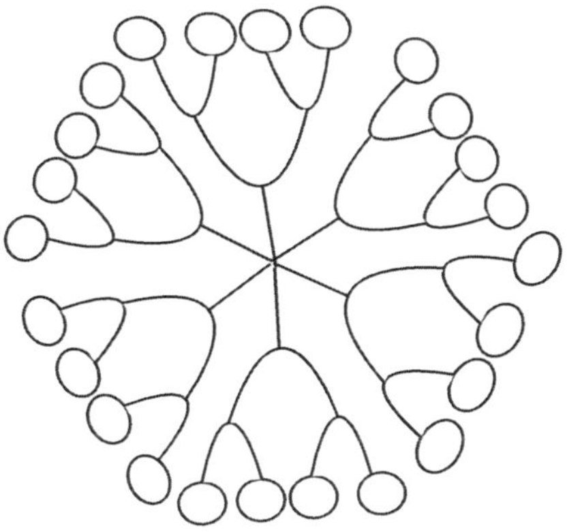

Fig. (1.4). Structure of dendrimer.

Micelles

Self-alligated nanostructures formed by aqueous amphiphilic block polymers are polymeric mice (Fig. **1.5**). Micelles are formed in an aqueous solution when the copolymer block concentration, a critical aggregation concentration (CAC), or a critical concentration in the micelle is achieved (CMC). In CAC or CMC, the hydrophobic segments of the block polymer combine to form a vesicular micellar structure or core layer with minimal contact with water molecules. The size of polymer micelles usually ranges from 20 nm to 100 nm, and usually, the inner core of the micelles is formed by hydrophobic interactions within hydrophobic block copolymers. The hydrophilic blocks of the copolymers create the outer shell of polymeric micelles, which play a critical role in *in-vivo* behavior, particularly in terms of steric stability and cell interaction. PM offers great potential as a drug delivery system for hydrophobic compounds with low bioavailability due to the unique structure of the shell core. They can be developed to entrap nanoscale pharmaceuticals or bioactive agents, such as therapeutic proteins and DNA, and trigger their release at the target site [24, 31, 32].

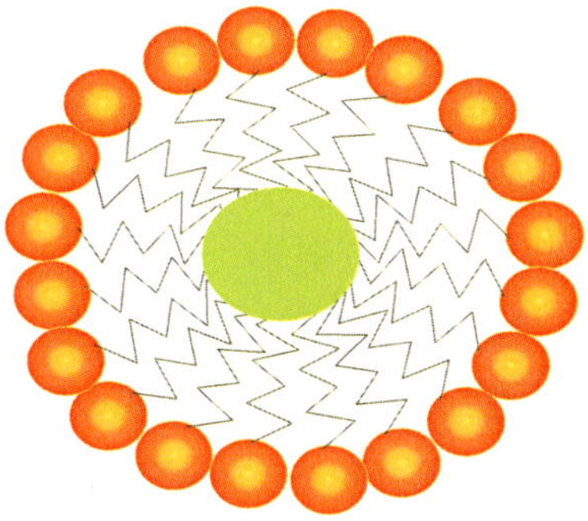

Fig. (1.5). Structure of Micelle.

Carbon Nanotubes

Carbon nanotubes (CNTs) are carbon allotropes with a cylindrical nanostructure. Carbon nanotubes are large cylindrical molecules composed of a hexagonal arrangement of carbon atoms with sp2-hybrids (the C-C distance is about 1.4). CNT walls are made by overlaying one or more layers of graphene foil, single-walled carbon nanotubes (SWCNTs) by wrapping the foil, and multi-walls (MWCNT) by wrapping several films. . The size, shape, and surface properties of single-walled nanotubes (SWNTs), multi-walled nanotubes (MWNTS), and C60 fullerenes make them attractive as therapeutic media. CNTs can be used as medicinal nanocarriers in cancer therapy and other medicinal areas, while allowing long drug release, without causing healthy tissue toxicity. There are three forms of immobilization of an active ingredient on carbon nanocarriers. Encapsulation of the active ingredient in carbon nanotubes, chemisorption on the surface (*via* electrostatic bond, hydrophobic bond, hydrogen bond), or binding of the active substance to the space between the nanotubes and functional carbon nanotubes [33].

Magnetic Nanocarriers

Magnetic nanoparticles (MNPs) typically range in size from 1 to 100 nm and are composed of discrete superparamagnetic nano metallic compounds having magnetic components such as iron, nickel, cobalt, and chromium. MNPs are usually synthesized using materials containing iron oxide compounds and metal nanoparticles. These are small MNPs with a large surface area that help transport a large number of DNA fragments, drugs, and modified compounds. Targeting of therapeutic MNP conjugates to diseased tissues can be achieved through passive or active mechanisms, depending on the size and chemical composition of the surface. The main advantage of magnetic NPs (organic or inorganic) is that they can be: (i) visualized (superparamagnetic NPs are used for MRI), (ii) induced or supported by a magnetic field and (iii) Heating in a magnetic field causes drug release or hyperthermia/tissue ablation. It is important to note that the latter ability is not limited to magnetic NPs but also applies to other particles capable of absorbing near-infrared, microwaves, and ultrasound. Magnetic nanoparticles or compounds are attractive for drug delivery because of their ability to respond to external stimuli through magnetic fields. This allows you to control the release of the drug in space, time, and in controlled doses. Nanocarriers can passively reach the tumor medium either through a leaky vascular medium or through the use of aggressive selective ligands [24, 34 - 36].

Quantum Dot

Quantum dots (QDs) are nanometer-sized semiconductor crystals, typically in the range of 1 to 10 nanometers. Quantum dots are made up of tiny pieces of metal. Quantum dots can be shaped and coated with different biomaterials. QDs have unique optical properties that make them potential candidates as carriers for biological applications and luminous nano-probes. Different techniques like dissolution, dispersion, adsorption, and coupling can be adopted for loading drugs into quantum dots. QD drug carriers can enhance efficacy, reduce drug reaction side effects, and increase the therapeutic index. An ideal QD nano preparation for drugs should have the following characteristics: (1) should not react with the drug, (2) high absorption capacity and encapsulation efficiency, (3) correct manufacturing and purification processes, (4) low toxicity and good biocompatibility, (5) several degrees of strength and mechanically stable; desired particle size and shape (6) longer residence time *in vivo*. Currently, the main nanoparticles of anti-cancer drugs commonly used in pharmaceuticals are liposomes, chitosan, silica nanoparticles, and polymer nanoparticles. Quantum dots have unique optical properties due to their size and quantum effects. When the particle size is nanoscale, quantum confinement effect, size effect, dielectric confinement effect, macroscopic quantum tunneling effect, and surface effect occur. As a result, quantum dots exhibit many optical properties and have a very broad prospect for their use in fluorescent biological probes and functional materials. Thus, quantum dots will have a big impact on the sustainable development of life sciences [37, 38].

Mesoporous Silica Nanoparticles

Mesoporous silica nanoparticles (MSN) live up to their expectations as they provide controlled release and targeted delivery of a wide range of drug molecules with unique mesoporous structures that maintain a high level of chemical stability, surface functionality, and biocompatibility (Fig. **1.6**). Mesoporous nanoparticles have a dense framework with a porous structure and a large surface area so that different functional groups can be linked to direct the remaining active ingredients to specific sites. Chemically, MSN has a honeycomb structure and an active surface. Thanks to the active surface, functionalization changes the surface properties and binds to therapeutic molecules. Because of their low toxicity and high elasticity, mesoporous silica nanoparticles are used inefficient and controlled drug delivery systems. The mesoporous form of silica has unique properties, especially in the loading and subsequent releases of therapeutic substances. The mesoporous particle can be synthesized by simple sol-gel or spray-drying techniques. Synthetic strategies must satisfy two conditions for biomedical applications: (1) controlled nucleation and growth rate of MSNs for uniform sizes of 30-300 nm, and (2) the non-adhesive nature of MSNs during the work process. Mesoporous silica is also used as a coating material. The MSN density can be increased in two ways: gold coating of the MSN pores on gold nanoparticles and the MSN surface [39, 40].

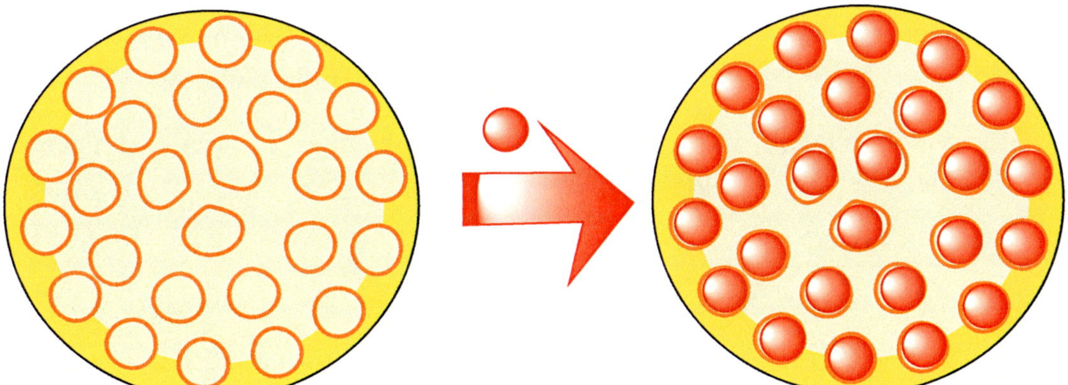

Fig. (1.6). Drug entrapment in mesoporous silica nanoparticles.

Advantages Over Conventional Drug Delivery

The pharmaceutical and therapeutic properties of conventional medicines are improved by the nanocarriers as drug delivery systems. The incorporation of medicines molecules into nanocarriers can protect medication from degradation as well as allow for controlled release and targeting. Nanocarriers can pass the biological membranes and operate on a cellular level because of their small dimensions. Compared with the traditionally used form of drugs, nanocarrier-drug conjugates are more effective and selective. By accumulating drugs at target sites, it can decrease toxicity and other adverse side effects in normal tissue. As a result, the doses of drugs required are lower.

Challenges Faced by these Systems in Nanomedicine

While several nanoparticles are currently developed and assessed in a preclinical context, only a few nanoparticles are available in the market. This is due to numerous drawbacks and limitations in nanoparticulate drug delivery systems. Some of them are caused by problems with scaling. The small size and large area of the targeting system of nanoparticles may lead to aggregation and difficult physical processing. Cell-phagocytic conjugates can be phagocytic, while cytotoxic effects can result from their intracellular deterioration. Other problems include low capacity for drug charging, low efficiency of loading, and poor capacity for carrier management. In addition, technological methods are lacking, leading to the approvable quality of nanodevices. Due to several functional groups on the nanoparticle surface, the drug can only be attached to the carrier in a stoichiometrical relation. Oxidative stress and inflammation are often explained by the toxic mechanisms of different nanoparticles in different cell types. Cells can contain nanoparticles up to 10 nm in diameter that stimulates chronic inflammatory responses and tissue fibrosis. Another problem is the lack of distribution knowledge and the unpredictability of drug suppliers. Therapeutic carriers involving nanoparticles, which respond to subtle changes in the local cellular environment, have the potential to solve many of today's drug-related problems, which have limitations and drawbacks [41, 42].

APPLICATIONS

The field of nanotechnology is expected to revolutionize manufacturing and have a significant impact on the life sciences, especially in the drug delivery, diagnosis, and production of nutrients and biomaterials. Nanotechnology developments have recently been made with the development of several systems for diagnostic and therapeutic procedures. Nanoparticle systems hold promising applications such as gene therapy, molecular imaging, anti-inflammatory therapy, anticancer therapy, antiviral therapy, phototherapy, and polymer delivery across various physiological barriers. In addition, the combination of diagnostic and therapeutic production of unique nano- or microparticles for theragnostic purposes has a great potential for the delivery of image-guided drugs and customized treatment modalities (Table **1.4**) [6, 15, 16, 43, 44].

Table 1.4. Applications of nanoparticles and nanocarriers [6, 15, 16, 29, 32 - 34, 39, 43, 44].

S.No.	Drug/Therapeutics	Particle class	Indication
1.	Gd^{3+} metal ion	Nanoparticle	MRI
2.	CdSe-ZnS	Quantum dot	Optical imaging
3.	131I-labelled HPMA copolymers	Nanoparticles	Theranostic in Tumor
4.	TiO_2, ZnO, $BiVO_4$	Nanoparticles	Antimicrobials
5.	Gold	Nanoparticles	laser photothermal therapy of cancer
6.	Silver	Nanoparticles	Wound dressings
7.	Thioflavins	Nanoparticles	Alzheimer's disease
8.	Gold	Liposomes	Neurodegenerative diseases
9.	HIV-1 Tat protein	Solid- lipid nanoparticle	AIDS
10.	Flurbiprofen and Ibuprofen	Nanoparticle	inhibited inflammatory responses after surgical trauma
11.	Paclitaxel, Cisplatin, Carboplatin, Folic acid, Methotrexate	Carbon nanotubes	cancer
12.	Efavirenz	Dendrimer	HIV
13.	Insulin	Liposome	Diabetes
14.	Vincristine sulfate	Liposome	Cancer
15.	Porphyrins	Dendrimer	Photodynamic therapy
16.	Cetuximab, Doxorubicin, Erotinib	Magnetic nanoparticles	Lung cancer
17.	Doxorubicin and Cisplatin	Mesoporous silica nanocarrier	Hepatocellular carcinoma
18.	Paclitaxel	Polymeric micelles	Human ovarian carcinoma
19.	Doxorubicin	Polymeric micelles	Kaposi's Carcinoma

CONCLUSION

Nanoparticles are colloidal solid particles with a size range of 1–1000 nm. In the areas of drug delivery, gene delivery, and diagnostics, NPs became extremely well-known. This chapter outlines the different types and methods of preparation and characterization of NPs and emphasizes the nanoparticles class for many diagnostic and treatment applications. This also summarises different nanocarriers which are being used in drug delivery with their advantages over conventional drug delivery and challenges faced by these systems in nanomedicine showing future prospectus in these areas.

CONSENT FOR PUBLICATION

Not applicable.

CONFLICT OF INTEREST

The authors declare no conflict of interest, financial or otherwise.

ACKNOWLEDGEMENT

Declared none.

REFERENCES

[1] de Jong WH, Borm PJ. Drug delivery and nanoparticles: Applications and hazards. Int J Nanomedicine 2008; 3(2): 133-49. [http://dx.doi.org/10.2147/IJN.S596] [PMID: 18686775]

[2] Benelmekki M. An introduction to nanoparticles and nanotechnology. Designing Hybrid Nanoparticles. Morgan & Claypool Publishers 2015.

[3] Singh AK. Introduction to nanoparticles and nanotoxicology.Engineered Nanoparticles: Structure, Properties, and Mechanisms of Toxicity. Properties, and Mechanisms of Toxicity 2016; pp. 1-8.

[4] Horikoshi SA, Serpone NI. Introduction to nanoparticles. Microwaves in nanoparticle synthesis: Fundamentals and applications. 2013; pp. 1-24. [http://dx.doi.org/10.1002/9783527648122.ch1]

[5] Mayeen A, Shaji LK, Nair AK, Kalarikkal N. Morphological characterization of nanomaterials. Characterization of Nanomaterials. Woodhead Publishing 2018; pp. 335-64. [http://dx.doi.org/10.1016/B978-0-08-101973-3.00012-2]

[6] Mohanraj VJ, Chen Y. Nanoparticles-a review. Trop J Pharm Res 2006; 5(1): 561-73.

[7] Afolalu SA, Soetan SB, Ongbali SO, Abioye AA, Oni AS. Morphological characterization and physio-chemical properties of nanoparticle-review. IOP Conference Series: Materials Science and Engineering. IOP Publishing 2019; 640: p. (1)012065. [http://dx.doi.org/10.1088/1757-899X/640/1/012065]

[8] Kröner A, Hirsch T. Current trends in the optical characterization of two-dimensional carbon nanomaterials. Front Chem 2020; 7: 927. [http://dx.doi.org/10.3389/fchem.2019.00927] [PMID: 32047734]

[9] Khosla A. Nanoparticle-doped electrically-conducting polymers for flexible nano-micro systems. Electrochem Soc Interface 2012; 21(3-4): 67-70. [http://dx.doi.org/10.1149/2.F04123-4if]

[10] Yuliza E, Murniati R, Rajak A, Abdullah M. Effect of particle size on the electrical conductivity of metallic particles. In 2014 International Conference on Advances in Education Technology (ICAET-14). 2015 Jan; Atlantis Press. 2015. [http://dx.doi.org/10.2991/icaet-14.2014.37]

[11] Guo D, Xie G, Luo J. Mechanical properties of nanoparticles: Basics and applications. J Phys D Appl Phys 2014; 47(1): 013001. [http://dx.doi.org/10.1088/0022-3727/47/1/013001]

[12] Tronc E, Prene P, Jolivet JP, *et al.* Magnetic behaviour of γ-Fe2O3 nanoparticles by mössbauer spectroscopy and magnetic measurements. Hyperfine Interact 1995; 95(1): 129-48. [http://dx.doi.org/10.1007/BF02146310]

[13] Akbarzadeh A, Samiei M, Davaran S. Magnetic nanoparticles: Preparation, physical properties, and applications in biomedicine. Nanoscale Res Lett 2012; 7(1): 144.
[http://dx.doi.org/10.1186/1556-276X-7-144] [PMID: 22348683]

[14] Das SK, Choi SUS, Patel HE. Heat transfer in nanofluids—a review. Heat Transf Eng 2006; 27(10): 3-19.
[http://dx.doi.org/10.1080/01457630600904593]

[15] Khan I, Saeed K, Khan I. Nanoparticles: Properties, applications and toxicities. Arab J Chem 2019; 12(7): 908-31.
[http://dx.doi.org/10.1016/j.arabjc.2017.05.011]

[16] Bhatia S. Nanoparticles types, classification, characterization, fabrication methods, and drug delivery applications. Natural polymer drug delivery systems. Cham: Springer 2016; pp. 33-93.
[http://dx.doi.org/10.1007/978-3-319-41129-3_2]

[17] Ealia SA, Saravanakumar MP. A review on the classification, characterization, synthesis of nanoparticles and their application. IOP Conference Series: Materials Science and Engineering. IOP Publishing 2017; 263: p. (3)032019.

[18] Cele T. Preparation of nanoparticles.Engineered nanomaterials-Health and safety. 2020.
[http://dx.doi.org/10.5772/intechopen.90771]

[19] Rao JP, Geckeler KE. Polymer nanoparticles: Preparation techniques and size-control parameters. Prog Polym Sci 2011; 36(7): 887-913.
[http://dx.doi.org/10.1016/j.progpolymsci.2011.01.001]

[20] Ganesan P, Narayanasamy D. Lipid nanoparticles: Different preparation techniques, characterization, hurdles, and strategies for the production of solid lipid nanoparticles and nanostructured lipid carriers for oral drug delivery. Sustain Chem Pharm 2017; 6: 37-56.
[http://dx.doi.org/10.1016/j.scp.2017.07.002]

[21] Salas G, Costo R, Morales MP. Synthesis of inorganic nanoparticles. Frontiers of Nanoscience 2012; 4: 35-79.
[http://dx.doi.org/10.1016/B978-0-12-415769-9.00002-9]

[22] Velusamy P, Kumar GV, Jeyanthi V, Das J, Pachaiappan R. Bio-inspired green nanoparticles: Synthesis, mechanism, and antibacterial application. Toxicol Res 2016; 32(2): 95-102.
[http://dx.doi.org/10.5487/TR.2016.32.2.095] [PMID: 27123159]

[23] Chamundeeswari M, Jeslin J, Verma ML. Nanocarriers for drug delivery applications. Environ Chem Lett 2019; 17(2): 849-65.
[http://dx.doi.org/10.1007/s10311-018-00841-1]

[24] Farah HF. Nanocarriers as delivery systems for therapeutic agents. Int J Pharm Sci Res 2019; 10(8): 3487-507.

[25] Allen TM, Cullis PR. Drug delivery systems: Entering the mainstream. Science 2004; 303(5665): 1818-22.
[http://dx.doi.org/10.1126/science.1095833] [PMID: 15031496]

[26] Duan Y, Dhar A, Patel C, *et al.* A brief review on solid lipid nanoparticles: Part and parcel of contemporary drug delivery systems. RSC Advances 2020; 10(45): 26777-91.
[http://dx.doi.org/10.1039/D0RA03491F] [PMID: 35515778]

[27] Akbarzadeh A, Rezaei-Sadabady R, Davaran S, *et al.* Liposome: Classification, preparation, and applications. Nanoscale Res Lett 2013; 8(1): 102.
[http://dx.doi.org/10.1186/1556-276X-8-102] [PMID: 23432972]

[28] Anwekar H, Patel S, Singhai AK. Liposome- as drug carriers. International Journal of Pharmacy & Life Sciences 2011; 2(7)

[29] Abbasi E, Aval SF, Akbarzadeh A, *et al.* Dendrimers: Synthesis, applications, and properties.

Nanoscale Res Lett 2014; 9(1): 247.
[http://dx.doi.org/10.1186/1556-276X-9-247] [PMID: 24994950]

[30] Chauhan A. Dendrimers for drug delivery. Molecules 2018; 23(4): 938.
[http://dx.doi.org/10.3390/molecules23040938] [PMID: 29670005]

[31] Xu W, Ling P, Zhang T. Polymeric micelles, a promising drug delivery system to enhance bioavailability of poorly water-soluble drugs. J Drug Deliv 2013; 2013: 1-15.
[http://dx.doi.org/10.1155/2013/340315] [PMID: 23936656]

[32] Batrakova EV, Bronich TK, Vetro JA, Kabanov AV. Polymer micelles as drug carriers.Nanoparticulates as drug carriers. 2006; pp. 57-93.
[http://dx.doi.org/10.1142/9781860949074_0005]

[33] Kushwaha SKS, Ghoshal S, Rai AK, Singh S. Carbon nanotubes as a novel drug delivery system for anticancer therapy: A review. Braz J Pharm Sci 2013; 49(4): 629-43.
[http://dx.doi.org/10.1590/S1984-82502013000400002]

[34] Sadhasivam J, Sugumaran A. Magnetic nanocarriers: Emerging tool for the effective targeted treatment of lung cancer. J Drug Deliv Sci Technol 2020; 55: 101493.
[http://dx.doi.org/10.1016/j.jddst.2019.101493]

[35] Kudr J, Haddad Y, Richtera L, *et al.* Magnetic nanoparticles: From design and synthesis to real world applications. Nanomaterials (Basel) 2017; 7(9): 243.
[http://dx.doi.org/10.3390/nano7090243] [PMID: 28850089]

[36] Dobson J. Magnetic nanoparticles for drug delivery. Drug Dev Res 2006; 67(1): 55-60.
[http://dx.doi.org/10.1002/ddr.20067]

[37] Dey NS, Rao MB. Quantum dot: Novel carrier for drug delivery. Int J Res Pharm Biomed Sci 2011; 2(2): 448-58.

[38] Zhao MX, Zhu BJ. The research and applications of quantum dots as nano-carriers for targeted drug delivery and cancer therapy. Nanoscale Res Lett 2016; 11(1): 207.
[http://dx.doi.org/10.1186/s11671-016-1394-9] [PMID: 27090658]

[39] Wu SH, Hung Y, Mou CY. Mesoporous silica nanoparticles as nanocarriers. Chem Commun (Camb) 2011; 47(36): 9972-85.
[http://dx.doi.org/10.1039/c1cc11760b] [PMID: 21716992]

[40] Bharti C, Gulati N, Nagaich U, Pal AK. Mesoporous silica nanoparticles in target drug delivery system: A review. Int J Pharm Investig 2015; 5(3): 124-33.
[http://dx.doi.org/10.4103/2230-973X.160844] [PMID: 26258053]

[41] Wilczewska AZ, Niemirowicz K, Markiewicz KH, Car H. Nanoparticles as drug delivery systems. Pharmacol Rep 2012; 64(5): 1020-37.
[http://dx.doi.org/10.1016/S1734-1140(12)70901-5] [PMID: 23238461]

[42] Prabhakar P, Banerjee M. Nanotechnology in drug delivery system: Challenges and opportunities. Journal of Pharmaceutical Sciences and Research 2020; 12(4): 492-8.

[43] Baetke SC, Lammers T, Kiessling F. Applications of nanoparticles for diagnosis and therapy of cancer. Br J Radiol 2015; 88(1054): 20150207.
[http://dx.doi.org/10.1259/bjr.20150207] [PMID: 25969868]

[44] Murthy SK. Nanoparticles in modern medicine: State of the art and future challenges. Int J Nanomedicine 2007; 2(2): 129-41.
[PMID: 17722542]

CHAPTER 2

Polymeric Nanoparticles as Drug Delivery System: Basic Concepts and Applications

Sakshi Tiwari[1], Bina Gidwani[2], Priya Namdeo[1], Atul Tripathi[4], Ravindra Kumar Pandey[2], Shiv Shankar Shukla[2], Veenu Joshi[3], Vishal Jain[1], Vikas Kumar Jain[5] and **Amber Vyas[1,*]**

[1] *University Institute of Pharmacy, Pt. Ravishankar Shukla University, Raipur (C.G.), India*

[2] *Columbia Institute of Pharmacy, Raipur (C.G.), India*

[3] *Center of Basic Science, Pt. Ravishankar Shukla University, Raipur (C.G.), India*

[4] *People's Institute of Pharmacy & Research Centre, Bhopal, (M.P.), India*

[5] *Department of Chemistry, Government Engineering College, Raipur, C.G, India*

Abstract: Delivering drugs through various delivery systems into the body for successful treatment of diseases is most entrancing deeds for the pharmaceutical analyst. Conventional drug delivery systems have various hindrances like loss of medication and poor bioavailability of drugs. Polymer-based nanocarriers such as polymeric nanoparticles upgrade bioavailability of drug, delivery of drug to specific site and improve solubility of drugs. They are widely explored as controlled, precise, sustained and continuous release systems for drug delivery and are easily incorporated and appropriate for practically all parts of nanomedicines and bring new trust in field of drug conveyance by redesigning drug viability and diminishing drug toxicity. This chapter mainly focuses on polymers and techniques engaged with advancement of polymer-based nanoparticles and their applications in therapeutic intervention.

Keywords: Bioavailability, Controlled release, Diagnosis, Dispersion, Drug delivery system, Drug efficacy, Drug toxicity, Diffusion, Polymeric nanoparticles, Macromolecules, Natural polymers, Nanoprecipitation, Interfacial polymerization, Synthetic polymers, Targeted drug delivery, Potent drug delivery, Polymerization, Sustained release, Treatment, Solvent evaporation.

INTRODUCTION

The intricacy of specific diseases and the related toxicity of certain therapies progressively request novel courses for drug conveyance [1]. In the mid of the twentieth century, Paul Ehrlich conjectured the concept of "Magic bullet" that has

* **Corresponding author Amber Vyas**: University Institute of Pharmacy, Pt. Ravishankar Shukla University, Raipur (C.G); Tel: 9926807999; E-mail: **ambervyas@gmail.com**

the capacity to target drugs with a high particularity and gave rise to advancement and improvement of nanoparticles (NPs) [2]. These novel carriers are characterized as particles range in size from 10–1000 nm and offer several advantages over conventional dosage forms such as improving the medication bioavailability by expanding their absorption or by working with their passage through the biologic films [3]. Nanoparticles can be integrated from lipids, proteins, carbohydrates, just as a few natural and synthetic polymers [4].

There are five fundamental sorts of nanoparticle frameworks for drug conveyance: dendrimers, liposomes, micelles, polymeric nanoparticles, and nanocrystals. In the course of recent many years, there has been significant interest in creating biodegradable nanoparticles (NPs) as successful medication conveyance gadgets. Different polymers are utilized for drug conveyance exploration because they viably convey medication towards an objective spot, also in this way limiting the side effects, incrementing the restorative advantages [5]. The significant objective in designing such devices is to obtain pharmacologically dynamic specialist control arrival to the particular location of activity at the restoratively ideal frequency. The critical goal in planning such gadgets is to acquire controlled arrival of pharmacologically powerful specialists to the specific site of movement at the therapeutically ideal rate and portion routine. The improvements in the nanotechnology field have created unique nanocarriers especially, polymeric nanoparticles, either nanospheres or nanocapsules, may prompt improved bioavailability profiles for well-established drug molecules and also to convey drugs for helpful purposes. The aim of medication conveyance is the controlled release of medications to their site of activity and diminishing medication dose and at the same time limiting the undesirable effects [6]. In the recent couple of years, polymeric nanoparticles (PNPs) attained uncommon significance considering development of drug delivery systems because of the capacity to encapsulate and secure substances just as to present explicit usefulness through surface modifications, polymer-based medication conveyance frameworks are the focal point of extraordinary clinical and scientific interest. Polymeric nanoparticles will in general be more steady than different transporters, like liposomes and micelles, and their conveyance properties can be changed by controlling the design, composition, chemical and physical properties of the polymer [7]. The chapter primarily emphases on polymeric nanoparticles and their applications in therapeutic interventions.

POLYMERIC NANOPARTICLES

Nanoparticles for pharmaceutical purposes are solid colloidal particles of macromolecular materials within active material, dissolved or attached resulting in ranging size from 1 to 1000 nm (1 μm) [8]. They are ideally comprised of polymers acquired from natural, synthetic and semisynthetic basis which might be biodegradable or nonbiodegradable where the drug is entangled to a nanoparticle framework. In the previous many years, polymeric nanoparticles have arisen as a generally encouraging and reasonable innovation stage for targeted and controlled medication conveyance [9]. Appropriate information on the polymers is of most extreme significance because they are vital part in the medication conveyance framework for the therapy of different diseases like malignancy, neurodegenerative disorders, cardiovascular issues, and so forth [10]. The covalent association of macromolecular monomers into straight or extended chain is known as polymers. They are framed with at least two functional groups [11]. Nanoparticles, nanospheres or nanocapsules can be obtained contingent on the method of preparation [12]. Into the intended organ and cells, PNPs adequately convey medications and genetic materials as well as proteins. Their aim particularity and utilization in form of savvy polymer with decreased incidental properties expanded its development and utilization in treatment of certain diseases such as malignancy, which is no more a nightmare because of emergence of polymeric nanoparticles [8].

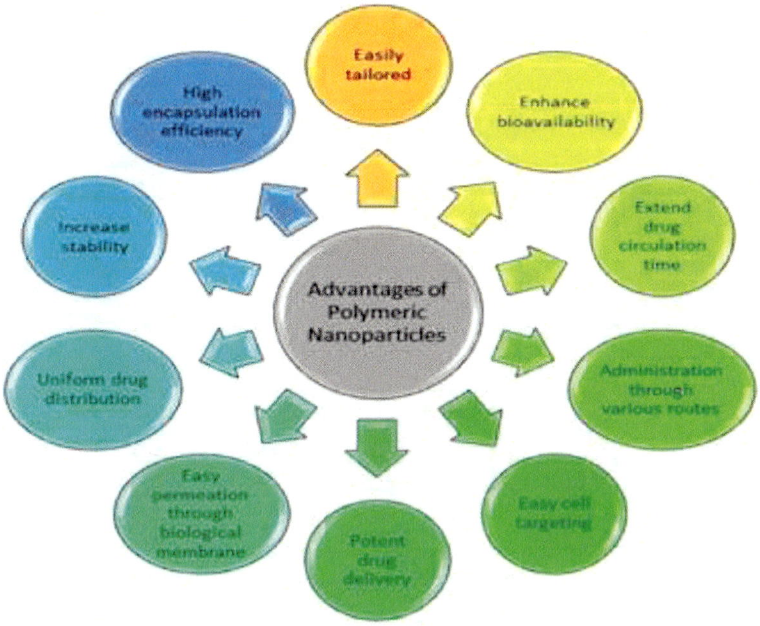

Fig. (2.1). Advantages of polymeric nanoparticles.

Types of Polymeric Nanoparticles

Polymeric nanoparticles are a united term which can be used for any polymeric arrangements but they are classified into two major types, which are Nanospheres and Nanocapsules [13, 14].

1. Nanospheres: It is strong mass of network polymers in which medication molecules are adsorbed at the mass surface or caught inside the circle place.

2. Nanocapsules: They have vesicular structure which act as drug reservoir. Retained drugs are saved in a fluid or non-watery fluid center set in the vesicle depression which was encased by the cemented polymeric shell.

Advantages of Polymeric Nanoparticles

In utilization as a medication conveyance framework, PNPs have following benefits and represented in Fig. **(2.1)** [7, 12, 15, 16]:

1. They can be easily tailored and controlled.

2. Upsurge bioavailability of inadequately water-dissolvable drugs.

3. Extending medication dissemination time within body.

4. Ligands like surface functional gatherings are allowed in huge number due to larger surface region.

5. Effectively focus on cells into modest vessels is assisted with the help of smaller size.

6. Oral, nasal, parenteral, intra ocular courses are available for administration.

7. Have longer clearance time as compared to the conventional nanoparticles.

8. Higher concentration of drug is delivered to intended location.

9. Effectively and efficiently upsurges the stability of volatile drugs by multitude techniques.

10. High drug encapsulation efficiency.

11. The untimely delivery or degradation of drugs prior reaching intended destination is shielded by encapsulation of drug into polymeric lattice.

12. The communication of dynamic substance with the organic objective can especially expanded by surface modification.

13. Provide high thermodynamic stability and permeation through different natural hindrances to the system.

14. Act as transporter for various biologically dynamic particles like monoclonal antibodies, nucleic acids.

15. Effortlessly joined into different exercises like tissue engineering, identified with drug conveyance.

16. Provide targeted medication conveyance, especially desirable as per as malignancy therapy is considered and minimize the adverse effects of anticancer drugs which are highly toxic in nature.

17. Significant upgrading in efficiency and effectiveness of oral and intravenous means of administration.

18. Deprived of chemical reaction, drug loading capacity can be easily increased.

19. On targeted site of action, uniform drug distribution is achieved.

20. Stability of acid-labile preparations are achieved.

Disadvantages of Polymeric Nanoparticles

In spite of various advantages, these polymeric nanoparticles have some disadvantages [7, 12, 15, 16]:

1. Manufacturing of these NPs is troublesome, costly and require modern instruments.

2. Small particle size followed by large surface area makes physical handling of NPs difficult due to particle- particle aggregation.

3. Termination of treatment likewise becomes troublesome if there should be an occurrence of crisis.

4. PVA causes toxicity when used in preparation as a detergent.

Ideal Characteristics of Polymeric Nanoparticles

Features of ideal polymeric nanoparticles are as follows [7, 8, 17]:

1. Easy to synthesize and characterize

2. Scalable and cost-effective

3. Biocompatible

4. Non- toxic

5. Evade reticuloendothelial system

6. Ought to have prolonged circulation time in regards of systemic delivery

7. Biodegradable

8. Water soluble

9. Ought to be 100nm in diameter for ideal CNS delivery

10. Neutral or negatively charged NPs are optimal for local delivery

11. Amenable to robust surface modification

12. Stability in blood is important characteristic

13. Non immunogenic in nature

14. Be pervaded in a little viscous and hyperosmolar solution

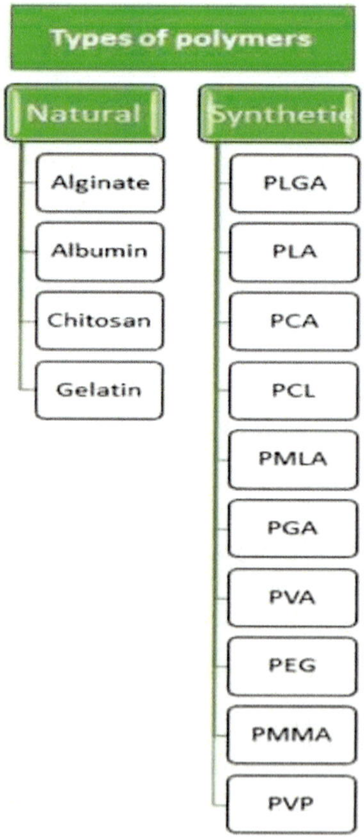

Fig. (2.2). Types for polymeric nanoparticles.

Types of Polymers used for Carrier System

Two significant kinds of polymers based on source of origin which are utilized for polymeric nanoparticles are- natural polymers and synthetic polymers. Not any other class more than this classification is favored of required qualities till now [8, 9, 13, 14, 18 - 20]. Types of polymers are illustrated in Fig. **(2.2)**.

The frequently applied natural polymers in designing PNPs are as follows:

Alginate (AG): Alginate is a biodegradable natural polymer and is highly emerging zone of attention. It is water soluble linear polysaccharide, essentially copolymer of connected β-D mannuronate and α-l-glucoronate which can be utilized as hydrogels, microparticle, nanoparticles, furthermore. By and large, AG NPs are created with techniques such as ionic gelation, emulsion, covalent cross-connecting, complexation technique, and self-assembly strategy, from which ionic gelation and complexation techniques are generally utilized technique for AG nanoparticles. They are controllable, pH-sensitive and utilized way to conveyance specific medications such anticancer medication and so forth [8, 14].

Albumin (AL): These are the naturally occurring protein molecules with exceptional properties to be utilized in various nanomaterials and of course empowers in polymeric nanoparticles. It shows some encouraging attributes like high stability, biodegradability and non-antigenicity. Albumin nanoparticles enjoy tremendous benefits due to which they can be utilized for the designing of nanoparticles. AL NPs are stimuli- sensitive normally and bioactive substances exceptionally and have upgraded drug transporter exercises which can include a huge range of medications. They convey assortment of medications which are generally metal based, hydrophobic, so forth and profoundly flexible [8, 14].

Chitosan (CH): It is deacetylated chitin derived carbohydrate- based natural polymer obtained generally through insects or marine organisms. It is exceptionally demanded polymer in numerous different fields because it is one among the profoundly bountiful natural polymer, can be effectively prepared into shifted structures in a designated drug conveyance framework and is biocompatible and biodegradable too. It has huge job in field of pharmaceutical and biomedicals. In acidic solution it is freely soluble but at pH above 6.5 it had poor solubility. Most of the time CH NPs are framed from consolidating a tripolyphosphate polyanion with chitosan in the presence of consistent blending and utilized as medication conveyance, ant malignant action, gene therapy, and so on [9, 14].

Gelatin (GL): It involves basic and acidic both functional groups and is normally water soluble in nature. In arrangements at low temperature, it shapes a triple stranded helical structure. It Gelatin is acquired through primary and compound collagen- I deprivation and classified on this basis as Gelatin A acquired through acid hydrolysis and Gelatin B through alkaline hydrolysis with isoelectric point of 9.0 and 5.0, respectively. Slow drug release is attained from gelatin nanoparticles because of polymer erosion. The nanoparticle arranged utilizing gelatin do not have unfavorable responses when presented in human body as they are biocompatible polymers [9, 14].

Likewise, a wide assortment of synthetic polymers can be utilized for advancement and designing of polymeric nanoparticles but they ought to be biocompatible and biodegradable with non-antigenic and non-poisonous profile as per Food and Drug Administration. These are as follows:

Poly (lactide co-glycolides) (PLGA): PLGA is a synthetic polymer which is synthesized by ring opening co-polymerization of cyclic dimers (1, 4-dioxane-2,5-diones) of glycolic acid and lactic acid. The main benefit of using PLGA is that it promptly goes through hydrolysis inside the body and this is the reason it slowly and in time dependent manner releases variety of drugs, proteins and peptides from PLGA based systems. Numerous investigations demonstrated their utilization as delivery systems such as nanoparticles, microcapsules, microspheres and so forth because they are biocompatible, biodegradable and causes nearby cell responses and wide assortment solvent solubility. They also have significant disadvantages most importantly the need to utilize a stabilizer which isn't generally biocompatible, to stabilize nanoparticles also, to acquire uniform and small diameter. PLGA nanoparticles are at high risk by the reticulo-endothelial system of liver and spleen that eliminate these from blood dissemination and lessen the residence time of NPs definitely in circulation system consequently keeping away from the conveyance of nanoparticles to the target organs or tumors tissues [9, 14].

Poly (lactic acid) (PLA): It is non- toxic and hydrophobic in nature with biodegradable and biocompatible properties. Because of hydrophobicity this is suitable considering hybrid lipid polymer nanoparticles. It can be utilized as advanced control drug conveyance framework because it displays huge sum of mechanical strength [9, 14].

Polycyanoacrylates: These polymers are adhesive and important as per industrial use. They consolidate fast relieving and high strength and are broadly used to secure an assorted scope of substrate surfaces together with naturally determined substances. These polymers are utilized widely in creation of exemplified colloidal nanoparticles for designated medication conveyance frameworks, especially helpful as therapy in malignant growths because of their biocompatibility. Cyanoacrylate monomers go through incredibly quick polymerization within the sight of reactant measures of anionic initiators or tertiary amines and phosphines like certain covalent bases. Most of the time these nanoparticles are prepared by emulsion polymerization, interfacial polymerization and nanoprecipitation for drug conveyance and nano formulation. Sometimes these polymers animate and harm CNS by some poisonous item which is produced from esterase corruption in biological fluid [14, 21].

Polycaprolactone (PCL): Polycaprolactone is synthetic semicrystalline biodegradable linear polyester produced by ring opening polymerization of ε-caprolactone, which is derived from fossil carbon using catalyst such as stannous octanoate and degraded by lipases and esterase under physiological conditions by hydrolysis. As compared to polylactide it has attributable more slow corruption and this is the reason, it is particularly fascinating for development of implantable devices. PCL nanoparticles get ready generally by nanoprecipitation technique or either by solvent displacement or solvent evaporation technique. PCL is regularly blended in with starch to get a decent biodegradable material at a low cost. An assortment of medications has been embodied inside PCL beads for controlled delivery and targeted drug conveyance [9].

Poly (malic acid) (PMLA): It is a truly appropriate polymer for building proficient delivery system. The polymer and its subsidiaries have been utilized to treat brain and breast tumor in mouse models as amalgation of nanoparticles for drug delivery. After long incubation time, cell toxicity was reported by methylated PMLA because of released method causing harmful impact. New esters acquired by incomplete or complete esterification of PMLA with ethanol or 1- butanol were reported in various literatures, which are relied upon to show less cytotoxicity, utilized for controlled medication conveyance and drug encapsulation [22].

Poly (glutamic acid) (PGA): It is made out of synthetic amalgamation of D- and L- glutamic acid units normally alluded as α- PGA which is biocompatible and aqueous- dissolvable polymer. It can be effectively degraded *in vivo* into glutamic acid deposits. The utilization and properties of thin polymer rely upon its molecular weight and polydispersity which is necessarily controlled in between amalgamation. To frame NPs, medications are epitomized in network of polymer and widely utilized in drug supported delivery [8, 23, 24].

Poly (methyl methacrylate) (PMMA): In the previous many years, poly (methyl methacrylate) (PMMA) has been broadly concentrated among a wide scope of polymeric materials. It is biocompatible and biostable materials, and has effectively been utilized in bone-imperfection rebuilding and in numerous ways.

PMMA-based NPs show significant attributes like very narrow size appropriation and great mechanical soundness. Such NPs don't show huge poisonous impacts since they don't change primary natural highlights like practicality, cell development and metabolic action, as of late exhibited in both tumor and foundational microorganisms. Additionally, PMMA-based NPs by way of medication conveyance vector has extraordinary potential because of chance in creating pH-and thermo-responsive NPs and nanocomposites [8, 25, 26].

Poly (N-vinyl pyrrolidone) (PVP): PVP has long history of pharmaceutical applications. They are also known as polyvidone or povidone and have magnificent binding features and solubility. It is biodegradable, biocompatible, water soluble polymer. It is novel amphiphilic derivative of its monomer N-vinylpyrrolidone. It is hydrophilic polymer consist of only one polymeric fragment and one hydrophobic fragment thus provide stabilizing effect in suspensions including emulsions. It is widely utilized in pharmaceutical, cosmeceuticals, food sectors and in biomedical applications because of it is non-toxic and biocompatible polymer. PVP based particles are prepared mostly by spray dried method and supercritical fluid technique. This polymer is chemically inert, temperature resistant, pH stable and colorless. It has wide applications in development of drug delivery systems, topical administration, gene delivery [8, 27, 28].

Poly (vinyl alcohol) (PVA): PVA is generally hydrophilic uncharged polymer. It has been broadly utilized as a transporter polymer in drug conveyance devices, like sustained release particles and hydrogels. Sometimes it is also used as a surfactant for formulation of polymeric drug carriers and mucoadhesive nanoparticles by the nanoprecipitation or emulsion strategies [8, 29, 30].

Poly (ethylene glycol) (PEG): It is non- biodegradable and non-ionic polyester with molecular weight ranges from 300–100,000 Da. Polymerization technique is utilized to prepare this polymer with ethylene glycol monomer. They are excreted unchanged in kidney, which is one of the major disadvantages of utilizing this polymer but due to their hydrophilic nature, fortunately it does not accumulate in tissues. Beside this, due to hydrophilicity, keep nanoparticles stabilized, especially, in aqueous media. It also prevents particles aggregation during production and storage caused due to stearic hindrance. It also increases solubility of polymer in various solvents. Adding to the advantages, it is not promptly recognized as foreign body by immune system because it suppresses opsonization. Another benefit of this polymer is that it doesn't include ionic moiety and in this manner no issue happens with DNA like charged molecules [8, 31].

MECHANISM OF DRUG RELEASE FROM POLYMERIC NANOPARTICLES

For polymer nanoparticle, drug- release conduct is a significant factor which is straightforwardly related to drug stability and therapeutic outcomes. A decent comprehension of the mechanisms of drug release is required for control of time and rate of drug release from polymeric nanoparticles. It is similarly significant as the drug-polymer formulation in sustained conveyance of medication. It is accounted that the nature of medication delivery system decides the release profile of drugs from polymer nanoparticles. There are five potential methods for drug release [8, 9, 32]:

a. desorption of drug bound to the surface
b. diffusion through the nanoparticle matrix
c. diffusion through the polymer wall of nanocapsules
d. nanoparticle matrix erosion
e. a combined erosion–diffusion process

On account of a polymer nanoparticle matrix, the medication is consistently distributed in the delivery system and the release happens by diffusion or disintegration of the matrix. So, diffusion and biodegradation supervise the method of drug release. Drug release mechanisms from PNPs through diffusion involve various steps represented in Fig. **(2.3)**.

Usually, "burst release" from PNPs are primarily noticed. Normally, drug release rate depends upon:

- Solubility of matrix material
- Diffusion through matrix material
- Biodegradation of matrix material
- Drug loading efficiency of nanoparticle
- Size of nanoparticle

Also, polymer matrices choice can adjust the mechanism of release of drug and its drug loading capacity. Sample and Separate (SS), Continuous flow (CF), and Dialysis membrane (DM) methods are three methods which are utilized for *in vitro* drug release study determination of PNPs. It is troublesome to compare all assortments of testing strategies, thus, Weng *et.al.* (2020) proposed novel sample and separate (SS) method which offer superior analytical technique and development of *in vitro-in vivo* correlation of PNPs [33].

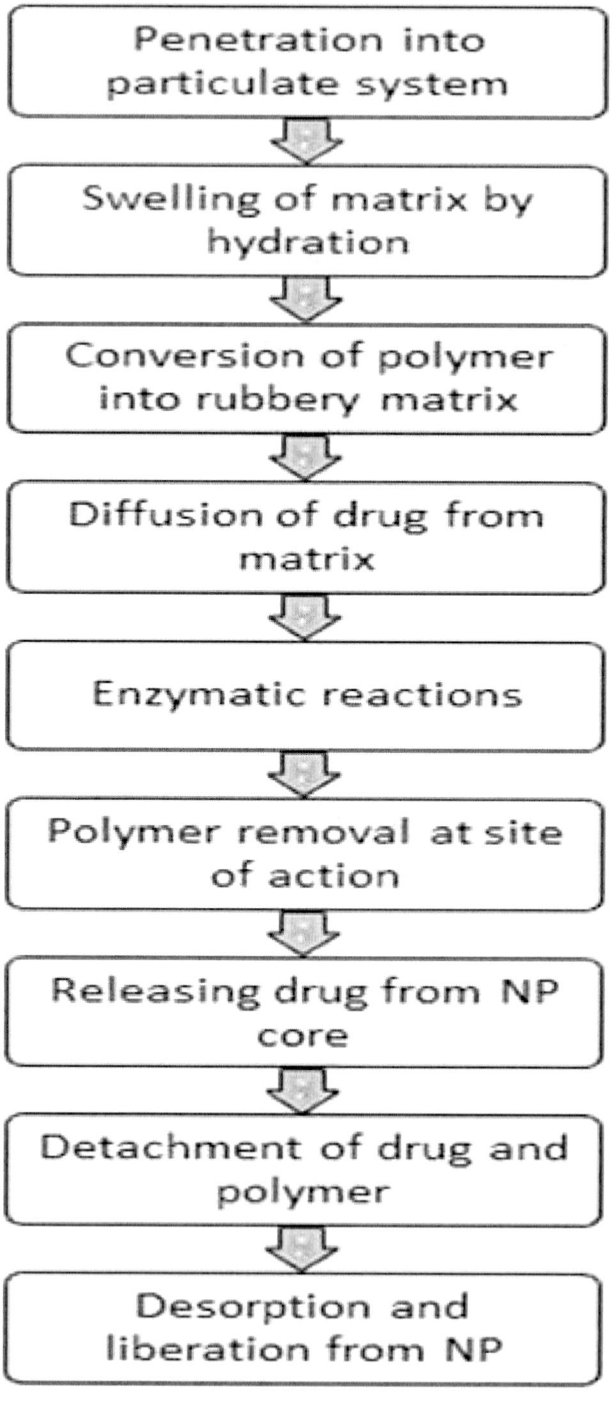

Fig. (2.3). Steps of drug release through diffusion from polymeric nanoparticles.

METHODS OF PREPARATION OF POLYMERIC NANOPARTICLES

Method of preparation of PNPs play essential part in attaining the desired properties. Selection of preparation method is as important as selection of drug and polymer because it chooses the utilization and application of these NPs. They can be appropriately formed either from pre-existed polymers or by direct monomeric polymerization [14, 16]. Method of preparation of PNPs are as follows and illustrated in Fig. **(2.4)**:

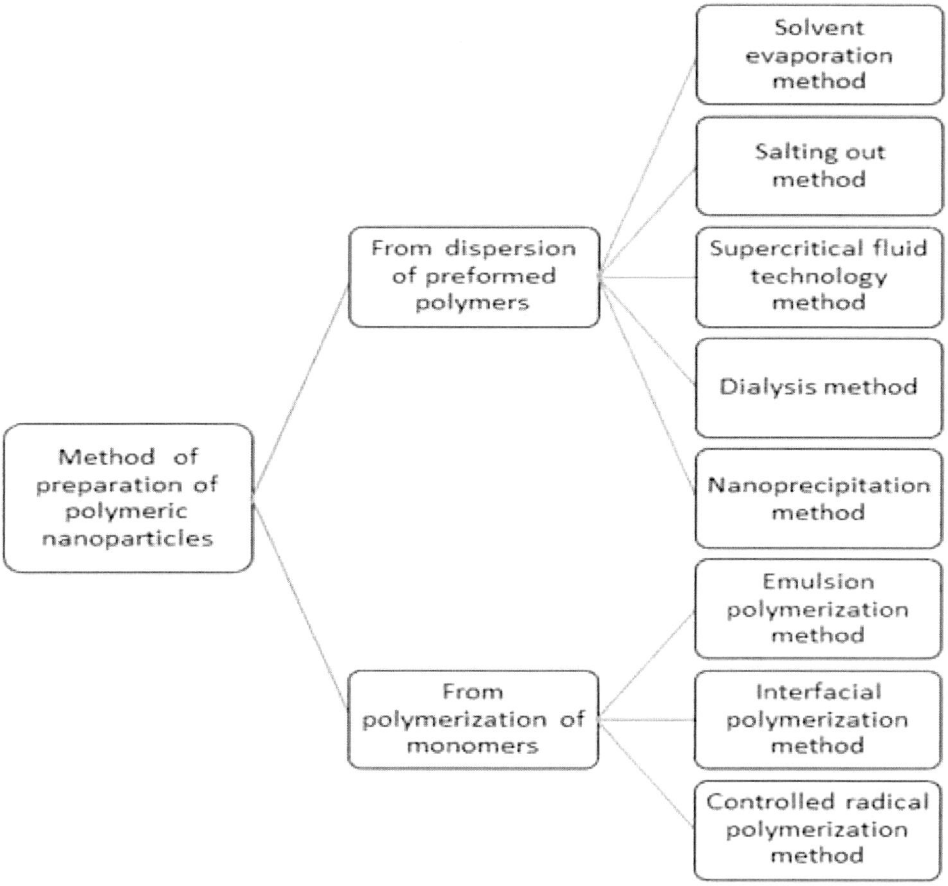

Fig. (2.4). Methods of preparation of polymeric nanoparticles.

Pre-existed Polymer Dispersion Method

Solvent Evaporation Method

Solvent evaporation by dispersion of polymer ensues to be first and common practice for development of PNPs. In this technique, organic solvents such as chloroform, dichloromethane were used but due to toxicity and safety, ethyl acetate is preferably chosen thus, medication is dissolved and dispersed into that solvent. Polymers like PLA, PLGA, PCL *etc*. were also dissolved in the same solution.at that point, organic stage containing drugs and polymers put on to fluid stage. The organic stage and watery stage are blended with high velocity homogenization and brings about the development of a steady emulsion, which is changed over to nanoparticle suspension. The evaporation of dissolvable and ultracentrifugation happens followed by washing off surfactants with distilled water to get the cemented NPs. Lastly, lyophilization of product finishes the process [34, 35].

Salting Out Method

It is the modification of emulsification process which depends upon partition of a water miscible dissolvable from fluid arrangement by means of a salting-out effect. Initially, drug and polymer are disintegrated dissolvable such as acetone, which is water miscible organic solvent. At that point, the subsequent arrangement framed is blended in with the watery part of the solution already containing salting-out specialist and consequently form emulsion. Subsequently, the surfactant containing organic stage is blended with the watery arrangement that contained salting- out specialist like magnesium chloride, calcium chloride, magnesium acetate, sucrose *etc*. to prevent the compatible mixability of watery and organic stages bringing about the development of an emulsion and the stabilizer such as polyvinylpyrrolidone or hydroxyethylcellulose, *etc*, by constant mixing. Exactly, emulsion dilution converse salting- out effect and brings about the precipitation of polymer prompting development of nanoparticles [36].

Supercritical Fluid Technology Method

Supercritical fluid technology is created as an environment secure technique for the production of PNP which utilizes environmentally agreeable solvents in which drug and polymer are dissolved to produce PNPs without any organic solvent and with high purity [37, 38]. Considering development of PNPs by utilizing supercritical fluids, two strategies have been created:

Rapid Expansion Of Supercritical Solution (RESS)

where blend of drug and polymer with the assistance of supercritical fluid is changed over into solution and serious level of supersaturation joined by the quick growth of the arrangement prompts the homogeneous nucleation and finely scattered particles of both micrometer and nanometer sized are obtained.

Rapid Expansion of Supercritical Solution into Liquid Solvent (RESOLV)

is a modest and noteworthy alteration to RESS where micro scaled particles are acquired rather than nano scaled particles. To defeat this drawback of RESS, RESOLV is developed, which evidently smothers the particle growth, making it conceivable to get essentially nanosized particles.

Dialysis Method

In this method drug and polymers are broken down into aqueous mixable organic dissolvable and set in core of a dialysis film. The movement of organic stage by diffusion into the aqueous stage inside the film is trailed by the advanced accumulation of polymer because of a loss of solubility and the development of homogeneous suspensions of nanoparticles. This technique is like nanoprecipitation and offers a basic and powerful technique for the arrangement of PNPs [39].

Nanoprecipitation Method

This technique was proposed by Fessi. Sometimes it is also known as solvent displacement or interfacial deposition method. This technique desired drugs and polymers which are broken up in organic solvents of aqueous mixable nature. In this solution, stabilizer containing aqueous phase is supplemented with continuous blending and because of abetment in the interfacial strain, the of organic dissolvable disperse very rapidly into the aqueous stage to form NPs. This technique is mainly based on encapsulation due to interfacial disposition because showing displacement of water miscible semi polar solvent [40].

Monomer Polymerization Method

Emulsion Polymerization Method

It is the most popular, quickest and versatile strategy utilized for NPs arrangement and polymer production from monomers. The most advantageous point in this method is the utilization of water as a dispersion medium in polymerization process for safety and excellent heat removal control. Based on utilization of continuous phase, this method can be ordered into two classification *i.e.*, use of an organic continuous phase, which mainly involves the dispersion of monomer into an emulsion or inverse microemulsion, or into a material in which the monomer isn't dissolvable. Aforementioned procedure has become less important, in light of a fact that, it requires toxic organic dissolvable, surfactants, monomers and initiators. Later, as a result, diluents such as cyclohexane, n-pentane and toluene are used as the organic continuous stage for production of PNPs. Another category is use of aqueous continuous phase, in which the surfactants and emulsifiers are not needed and monomer is usually disintegrated in aqueous solution which acts as continuous phase. This is a kind of surfactant free emulsion polymerization which is conducted without adding an emulsifier. The utilization of ionizable co- monomers support the adjustment of PNPs in such polymerization framework [41, 42].

Interfacial Polymerization Method

It is one of the grounded techniques utilized for the preparation of polymer nanoparticles. It includes reaction at the interface of two liquids happens due to the step polymerization of two responsive monomer, which are dissolved separately in continuous phase and dispersed phase. Interfacial cross-linking reactions are utilized to orchestrate nanometer sized hollow polymer particles. Nanocapsules containing oil were acquired through polymerization of monomers at the oil/water interface of an extremely fine oil-in-water micro emulsion. Significant surface formed at the oil droplet during emulsification was accepted to provide stage for interfacial polymerization of the monomer. Nanocapsule formation takes place with the help of acetone like aprotic solvent and protic solvents like ethanol, n-butanol and isopropanol were utilized for arrangement of nanospheres. On the other hand, water-containing nanocapsules can be acquired by the interfacial polymerization of monomers in water-in-oil micro emulsions [43].

Controlled Radical Polymerization Method

The essential limits of radical polymerization incorporate the absence of authority over the molar mass, the molar mass distribution, the end functionalities and the macromolecular engineering. The constraints brought about quick radical–radical termination reactions. The new development of some supposed controlled radical polymerization (CRP) measures unlocked another region utilizing an old polymerization method. The main elements adding into aforementioned pattern of CRP measure are expanded ecological bother and keen development of drug including clinical implementations of hydrophilic polymers. To control the attributes of polymers explicitly in emulsion polymerization method, modern revolutionary techniques are applied for molar mass, dissemination, engineering and capacity. Execution of CRP in the modernly significant aqueous dispersed systems, bringing about the development of PNPs with exact molecule size which is critical for succeeding business accomplishment of CRP [44, 45].

APPLICATIONS OF POLYMERIC NANOPARTICLES

Polymeric nanoparticles have wide range of applications in various field due to their biocompatibility and biodegradability and varied properties. They acknowledge drug release process more accessible in comparison to other nano formulations. Some of the applications are discussed below and represented in Fig. (**2.5**):

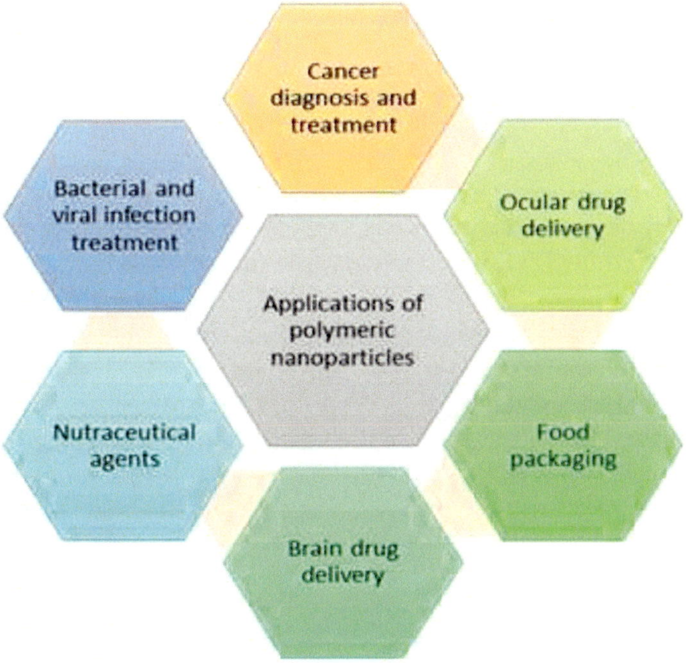

Fig. (2.5). Applications of polymeric nanoparticles.

Cancer Imaging And Diagnosis

Crucial target of developing nanoparticles as drug delivery system in oncology is for effective conduct of cancer and its early determination and recognition. Recent investigations focus on theranostic agents which incorporate both therapeutic and diagnostic goals. In this manner, PNPPs have arisen because of their ability to improve imaging of cancer cells. A portion of polymeric nanoparticle systems for cancer imaging and diagnosis are as follows:

Gold Based Polymeric Nanoparticles (Au NPs): Due to their versatility Au NPs are utmost vital investigation zone for diagnosis and imaging techniques. They provide high resolution and low toxicity. In computed tomography (CT). Au NPs have generated great interest because they are non-toxic and more efficient. Numerous researchers Zaki *et al.* (2014), Lin *et al.* (2017), Wang *et al.* (2012)

have investigated the PNPs constituted metallic NPs and concluded that these systems provide high-contrast properties and in radiotherapy, survival time improvement. It also helps to take images from organelles [46 - 48].

Gadolinium Based Polymeric Nanoparticles (Gd NPs): One of the most useful imaging techniques for cancer diagnosis is Magnetic resonance imaging (MRI) which helps to obtain three-dimensional high-resolution images. Because of low molecular weight gadolinium- based materials can be easily eliminated from the kidney of organisms and this is the reason they are utilized widely instead of various contrast agents. Many researchers Liu *et al.* (2011), Esser *et al.* (2016), Hu *et al.* (2017) have investigated and synthesized Gd NPs to enhance permeability, retention effect and imaging time in cancer cells [49 - 51].

Perfluorocarbons Polymeric Nanoparticles (PFC NPs): Their molecular structure resembles to alkanes but in PFCs all hydrogen atoms are replaced by fluorine. They are utilized in diagnosis of cancer. For medical applications, these new and fascinating properties can be helpful. They can be utilized further to develop Nuclear magnetic resonance for imaging effect of strong constructions situated normally in bone designs which generally limit MRI measures for fluorine signals. PFCs have high hydrophobicity so their solubility is serious issue associated with their utilization but exploration in this area has upgrade their biodistribution [52 - 55].

Cancer Treatment

The significant goal of PNPs in cancer treatment is to transport anticancer agents just into the cancerous tissues and specifically work on their viability and lessen harmfulness. Various well known synthetic and natural polymers are utilized to frame PNPs for cancer treatment. Much of the time, PNPs are comprised of thick networks. As of now, albumin is broadly utilized for the development of NPs as DDS because of its inherent attributes. Albumin-based NPs directly target tumoral cells [56, 57]. The utilization of these PNPs can give enhancements in therapy of malignancy by investigating novel courses for certain medications. Ahmed *et al.* proposed an option for surface altered PNPs for an improvement of doxorubicin oral bioavailability and concluded that NPs would do well to exercises and higher bioavailability contrasted with oral medications [58]. Various instances regarding utilization about PNPs for concrete oncologic disease Table are compiled in Table **2.1**.

Cirpanli *et al.* (2011) examined action of camptothecin-stacked cyclodextrin NPs for brain tumors in a rat glioma model and concluded that camptothecin-staked amphiphilic cyclodextrin nano systems is a successful nanocarrier and showed an improvement of the endurance time [59]. Guo *et al.* created paclitaxel-containing

PEG- PLGA NPs and showed higher tumor development restraint contrasted with paclitaxel-NPs alone and Taxol. Numerous researchers have investigated different PNP systems for the brain tumors included in Table **2.1** [60 - 62].

Table 2.1. Summary of applications of polymeric nanoparticles in cancer diagnosis and treatment.

S. No.	Polymer	Drug	Application	Ref.
1.	PEG-PCL	-	Cancer diagnosis *via* CT by utilization of Au NPs.	[46]
2.	PLGA	-	Au NPs coated with silica and fluorinated and embedded in PLGA NPs is used for cancer diagnosis.	[48]
3.	PLA-PEG	-	Gd NP used for detection of hepatocellular carcinoma in early stage.	[49]
4.	PGMA	-	Agent for MRI for cancer diagnosis.	[50]
5.	PEGMEM and TFEM	-	For enhanced NMR effect and passive targeting for tumor imaging.	[52]
6.	PLGGA-PVA	-	For advanced ultrasound imaging.	[53]
7.	Albumin	-	For enhanced EPR effect in tumors.	[56]
8.	PCL-PEG	Camptothecin	For effective utilization in treatment of glioma.	[59]
9.	PLGA-PEG	Paclitaxel	For effective utilization in treatment of glioma.	[60]
10.	PCLLA-PEG	Doxorubicin	For effective utilization in treatment of breast cancer.	[64]
11.	Gal-pD-TPGS	Docetaxel	For effective utilization in treatment of liver cancer.	[60]
12.	PEI-PLA	Paclitaxel	For effective utilization in treatment of lung cancer.	[65]

Perhaps the most pervasive cancer in women is breast cancer with absence of effective treatment. The utilization of PNPs have open an entryway for successful therapy of this kind of malignant growth. Various investigations in addition to this series is included in Table **2.1** [63].

Liver cancer has turn out to be successive disease nowadays and their medication causes harmfulness. Demonstration by Zhu *et al.* (2016) combined galactosamine and polydopamine copolymer and concluded that it remarkably hinders the cell proliferation [64].

Lung cancer is likewise perhaps the most common. Hu *et al.* (2017) investigated adequacy about paclitaxel-stacked PNPs joined with circadian chrono modulated chemotherapy and uncovered promising anticancer action contrasted with paclitaxel shown by developed nano system. Jin *et al.* (2018) examined the utilization of keen PEG-inferred PNPs to co-deliver paclitaxel and SiRNA against enduring genes in the lung cancer and uncovered that the nanoparticulate formulation introduced not so much toxic but rather more anti proliferation impact of paclitaxel [51, 65].

Ocular Drug Delivery

The major challenge in ocular drug delivery is presence of various barriers that limit the entry of drug molecule and short residence time of delivery system in ocular mucosa due to rapid clearance of eye. Therefore, PNPs have been emerged as an effective nanocarrier for ocular delivery because of its properties such as biodegradability and mucoadhesive. Many researchers have investigated promising applications of PNPs in ocular delivery. Duxfield *et al.* (2015) have developed the cationic PNPs of gatifloxacin to improve its ocular bioavailability and revealed that the developed system showed prolonged antimicrobial effect for gatifloxacin. In present investigation by Mittal *et al.* (2019), PNPs framed with chitosan and gum of flax seeds loaded with timolol maleate, developed for ocular delivery were found to reduce the intra ocular pressure as compared with conventional eye drops for prolonged time in rabbits and suggested a promising role of PNPs in treatment of glaucoma [66, 67].

Vaginal Disease Treatment

Vaginal route by passes the hepatic first-pass metabolism and give local and systemic effect which is beneficial for treatment of sexually transmitted disease or infections. Vagina produces abundant mucus which restrict sustained and targeted action of conventional drug delivery. Therefore, PNPs are utilized as sustained and targeted framework because of their adhesive property and easy penetration to vaginal mucosa. Gatti *et al.* (2019) developed Ascorbic acid loaded chitosan based PNPs for effective treatment of cervical cancer. In another investigation by Das *et al.* (2013) on sexual transmission of HIV in women, efavirenz loaded PLGA based PNPs is found to be effective drug delivery nano system. For treatment of vaginal bacterial infection in 2017, Akbari *et al.* had developed the ovomucin based ciprofloxacin stacked PNPs and concluded that the system was effective nanocarrier for broad- spectrum antibiotics [68 - 70].

Central Nervous System (CNS) Drug Deliver

Benefits of PNPs for CNS delivery of various drug is more prevailing as compared to other nanocarriers which makes it an effective choice for CNS medication conveyance. Shah *et al.* (2021), Rabiee *et al.* (2020). Mahmoud *et al.* (2020) has investigated the effective role of PNPs in drug delivery for glioma. Wong *et al.* (2019) investigated the PNPs-mediated treatment for Alzheimer's disease [71 - 74].

Cardiovascular Disorders

In treatment of cardiovascular diseases, PNPs can be used as effective nanocarriers. Kim *et al.* (2014) developed lipid polymer hybrid NPs for atherosclerosis and revealed the effective utilization of PNP translocation in atherosclerotic endothelial layer in an *in vivo* rabbit model [75].

Bacterial and Viral Infections

PNPs have shown wide applications in bacterial infections against planktonic and biofilm forming bacteria. Correa *et al.* (2021). Ucak *et al.* (2020) investigated the antibacterial effect of teicoplanin-containing PLGA nanoparticles. Durak *et al.* (2020) studied the effects of caffeic acid and juglone PLGA NPs known for their antibacterial activities. Vrouvaki *et al.* (2020) developed Pistacia lentiscus L. var. chia essential oil PLA nanoparticles encapsulating the against Gram-positive and Gram-negative bacteria. From all the studies, it was concluded that all the PNPs can be utilized for antimicrobial activities safely as nanocarriers [76 - 78].

Antidotes

Antidote molecules are delivered *via* blood brain barrier with PNPs. Ghosh *et al.* (2009) examined the PLGA NPs in which quercetin is encapsulated for treatment of oxidative damage in cells of brain induced by arsenic. Hu *et al.* (2012) developed NPs to determine therapeutic potential for mercury overdose, stacked with thiamin rich aptamer and framed with PEG copolymer and PLGA. Likewise, for arsenic toxicity, Yadav *et al.* (2012) framed chitosan NPs stacked with curcumin and demonstrated 10 times enhancement in antioxidant capacity of curcumin [48, 79, 80].

Nutraceutical Agents

Nutraceuticals are referred as pharma food which helps to prevent pathologic conditions and used as a complement to the diet for health improvement. PNPs are developed for improvement of hydrophobic molecules solubility, enhancing nutraceutical bioavailability and minimizing its side effects in systemic circulation. For reduction of intra ocular pressure, Niazvand *et al.* (2017) developed resveratrol and quercetin stacked PEG modified chitosan NPs and revealed the increase in solubility and permeation and decrease in intra ocular pressure in Albino rabbit cornea [81].

Food Packaging

Adriotis *et al.* (2021) studied citrus essential oils and come up with an idea of their potential applications in food packaging. Researchers have developed the

D-limonene stacked cross-linked PNP of methyl methacrylate and Triethylene Glycol Dimethacrylate copolymers. The investigation revealed the overall performance of these PNPs based on their synthesis and antimicrobial potency. It was concluded that, in food packaging, these NPs with enhanced antimicrobial activity forms self-sterilized surfaces [7].

PATENTS ON POLYMERIC NANOPARTICLES

From the last few decades, application of polymer nanoparticles is widely spread in several fields and in treatment of various dreadful diseases. However, some of the patents have been generated for their utilization in drug delivery [82]. A list of patents is summarized in Table **2.2**.

Table 2.2. Patents related to Polymeric Nanoparticles for drug delivery.

S. No.	Patent No.	Title of Patent	Inventors	Year of Publication
1.	US9557332B2	Glucose-sensitive nanoparticle for cancer diagnosis and therapy	Kuen Yong, Lee Jang, Wook Lee	2017
2.	US9555011B2	Formulation of active agent loaded activated PLGA nanoparticles for targeted cancer nano-therapeutics	Arthur R, Braden Jamboor, K. Vishwanatha	2017
3.	US9415011B1	Treating liver cancer and inhibition of metastasis with nanoparticles targeting chemokine receptor type-4 (CXCR4)	Yun- Ching Chen, Jia- Yu Liu, Dong- Yu Gao	2016
4.	US9351933B2	Therapeutic nanoparticle that includes an active agent or therapeutic agent, *e.g.* vinorelbine or vincristine or pharmaceutically acceptable salts thereof, and one, two, or three biocompatible polymers	Stephen E. Zale, Greg Troiano, Mir Mukkaram Ali, Jeff Hrkach James Wright	2016
5.	US9173841B2	Polymer nanoparticle injection formulation composition containing rapamycin with improved water solubility, preparation method thereof, and anticancer composition for combined use with radiotherapy	Hye Won Kang, Min Hyo Seo, Sa Won Lee, Bong Oh Kim, Eun Kyung Choi, Seong Yun Jeong, Ha Na Woo	2015

(Table 2) cont.....

S. No.	Patent No.	Title of Patent	Inventors	Year of Publication
6.	US9149544B2	Bioconjugation of calcium phosphosilicate nanoparticles for selective targeting of cells *in vivo*.	Thomas T. Morgan, Brian M. Barth, James H. Adair, Rahul Sharma, Mark Kester, Sriram S. Shanmugavelandy, Jill P. Smith, Erhan I. Altinoglu, Gail L. Matters, James M. Kaiser, Christopher McGovern	2015
7.	US20130209566 A1	Nanoparticle composition and methods to make and use the same	Monica Jablonski, Mallika Palamoor	2013

CONCLUSION

Nanotechnology is a silver lining for ameliorating drug delivery and pharmaceutical research. Amid these, PNPs are acquiring outrageous consideration because of their biocompatibility, biodegradability and adaptability. Also, they have created another way to accomplish drug conveyance, medication focusing, site explicit medication in new found illness and enhance solubility of existing inadequately solvent medication. PNPs have immense assortment of effective and safe polymers. They viably load the drug and focus on particular site, in this way, declining adverse effects. Many of them set foot in market though numerous in middle of clinical preliminaries.

FUTURE PROSPECTS

The persistent research on polymeric nanoparticle will boost the identification, therapeutics and prohibition of dangerous disorders, sickness and infections. They can be utilized as probable theranostic with minimal aftereffects for malignancy therapy. They will help to overcome the hindrances in conventional drug delivery systems to enhance patient compliance. Research should be focused on developing an easy scaling up technique and simple, proficient, direct manufacturing technique. Although, counting in numerous advancements, there are certain limitations like explication from animal examination to genuine clinical achievement antiquatedly restricted and need to be studied. To upgrade the security of PNPs regarding human and environment, definite regulatory guidelines ought to be constituted. The cooperative examination did amid every logical region will support the present status of the utilization of PNPs and will be converted into proficient and secure medicines and will eventually upgrade treatment and patient consistence.

CONSENT FOR PUBLICATION

Not applicable.

CONFLICT OF INTEREST

The authors declare no conflict of interest, financial or otherwise.

ACKNOWLEDGEMENTS

The authors acknowledge the Department of Science and Technology, New Delhi, India (DST /INSPIRE Fellowship/2019/IF190329 and DST/ NM/NT/2018/20) for providing financial assistance for successful completion of this work.

REFERENCES

[1] Colson YL, Grinstaff MW. Biologically responsive polymeric nanoparticles for drug delivery. Adv Mater 2012; 24(28): 3878-86.
[http://dx.doi.org/10.1002/adma.201200420] [PMID: 22988558]

[2] Begines B, Ortiz T, Pérez-Aranda M, *et al.* Polymeric nanoparticles for drug delivery: Recent developments and future prospects. Nanomaterials (Basel) 2020; 10(7): 1403.
[http://dx.doi.org/10.3390/nano10071403] [PMID: 32707641]

[3] Masood F. Polymeric nanoparticles for targeted drug delivery system for cancer therapy. Mater Sci Eng C 2016; 60: 569-78.
[http://dx.doi.org/10.1016/j.msec.2015.11.067] [PMID: 26706565]

[4] Kulkarni SA, Feng SS. Effects of particle size and surface modification on cellular uptake and biodistribution of polymeric nanoparticles for drug delivery. Pharm Res 2013; 30(10): 2512-22.
[http://dx.doi.org/10.1007/s11095-012-0958-3] [PMID: 23314933]

[5] Han N, Pang L, Xu J, Hyun H, Park J, Yeo Y. Development of surface-variable polymeric nanoparticles for drug delivery to tumors. Mol Pharm 2017; 14(5): 1538-47.
[http://dx.doi.org/10.1021/acs.molpharmaceut.7b00050] [PMID: 28368124]

[6] Mirza Z, Karim S. Nanoparticles-based drug delivery and gene therapy for breast cancer: Recent advancements and future challenges. Elsevier Ltd 2021; Vol. 69.
[http://dx.doi.org/10.1016/j.semcancer.2019.10.020]

[7] Andriotis EG, Papi RM, Paraskevopoulou A, Achilias DS. Synthesis of d-limonene loaded polymeric nanoparticles with enhanced antimicrobial properties for potential application in food packaging. Nanomaterials (Basel) 2021; 11(1): 191.
[http://dx.doi.org/10.3390/nano11010191] [PMID: 33451168]

[8] Jawahar N, Meyyanathan SN. Polymeric nanoparticles for drug delivery and targeting: A comprehensive review. Int J Health Allied Sci 2012; 1(4): 217-23.
[http://dx.doi.org/10.4103/2278-344X.107832]

[9] Kumari A, Yadav SK, Yadav SC. Biodegradable polymeric nanoparticles based drug delivery systems. Colloids Surf B Biointerfaces 2010; 75(1): 1-18.
[http://dx.doi.org/10.1016/j.colsurfb.2009.09.001] [PMID: 19782542]

[10] Patel T, Zhou J, Piepmeier JM, Saltzman WM. Polymeric nanoparticles for drug delivery to the central nervous system. Adv Drug Deliv Rev 2012; 64(7): 701-5.
[http://dx.doi.org/10.1016/j.addr.2011.12.006] [PMID: 22210134]

[11] Fonte P, Reis S, Sarmento B. Facts and evidences on the lyophilization of polymeric nanoparticles for

drug delivery. J Control Release 2016; 225: 75-86.
[http://dx.doi.org/10.1016/j.jconrel.2016.01.034] [PMID: 26805517]

[12] Ghalehkhondabi V, Soleymani M, Fazlali A. Folate-targeted nanomicelles containing silibinin as an active drug delivery system for liver cancer therapy. J Drug Deliv Sci Technol 2021; 61: 102157.
[http://dx.doi.org/10.1016/j.jddst.2020.102157]

[13] Locatelli E, Comes Franchini M. Biodegradable PLGA-b-PEG polymeric nanoparticles: Synthesis, properties, and nanomedical applications as drug delivery system. J Nanopart Res 2012; 14(12): 1316.
[http://dx.doi.org/10.1007/s11051-012-1316-4]

[14] Sur S, Rathore A, Dave V, Reddy KR, Chouhan RS, Sadhu V. Recent developments in functionalized polymer nanoparticles for efficient drug delivery system. Nano-Structures & Nano-Objects 2019; 20: 100397.
[http://dx.doi.org/10.1016/j.nanoso.2019.100397]

[15] El-Say KM, El-Sawy HS. Polymeric nanoparticles: Promising platform for drug delivery. Int J Pharm 2017; 528(1-2): 675-91.
[http://dx.doi.org/10.1016/j.ijpharm.2017.06.052] [PMID: 28629982]

[16] Nagavarma BVN, Yadav HKS, Ayaz A, Vasudha LS, Shivakumar HG. Different techniques for preparation of polymeric nanoparticles- A review. Asian J Pharm Clin Res 2012; 5: 16-23.

[17] Hans M, Lowman A. A dual-responsive mesoporous silica nanoparticle for tumor-triggered targeting drug deliverys for drug delivery and targeting. Curr Opin Solid State Mater Sci 2002; 6: 319-27.
[http://dx.doi.org/10.1016/S1359-0286(02)00117-1]

[18] Rani R, Dilbaghi N, Dhingra D, Kumar S. Optimization and evaluation of bioactive drug-loaded polymeric nanoparticles for drug delivery. Int J Biol Macromol 2015; 78: 173-9.
[http://dx.doi.org/10.1016/j.ijbiomac.2015.03.070] [PMID: 25881957]

[19] Swetledge S, Jung JP, Carter R, Sabliov C. Distribution of polymeric nanoparticles in the eye: Implications in ocular disease therapy. J Nanobiotechnology 2021; 19(1): 10.
[http://dx.doi.org/10.1186/s12951-020-00745-9] [PMID: 33413421]

[20] Gagliardi A, Giuliano E, Venkateswararao E, *et al.* Biodegradable polymeric nanoparticles for drug delivery to solid tumors. Front Pharmacol 2021; 12: 601626.
[http://dx.doi.org/10.3389/fphar.2021.601626] [PMID: 33613290]

[21] Melinda Molnar R, Bodnar M, Hartmann JF, Borbely J. Preparation and characterization of poly(acrylic acid)-based nanoparticles. Colloid Polym Sci 2009; 287(6): 739-44.
[http://dx.doi.org/10.1007/s00396-009-2033-0]

[22] Lanz-Landázuri A, Portilla-Arias J, Martínez de Ilarduya A, *et al.* Nanoparticles of esterified polymalic acid for controlled anticancer drug release. Macromol Biosci 2014; 14(9): 1325-36.
[http://dx.doi.org/10.1002/mabi.201400124] [PMID: 24902676]

[23] Manocha B, Margaritis A. Production and characterization of γ-polyglutamic acid nanoparticles for controlled anticancer drug release. Crit Rev Biotechnol 2008; 28(2): 83-99.
[http://dx.doi.org/10.1080/07388550802107483] [PMID: 18568849]

[24] Lai P, Daear W, Löbenberg R, Prenner EJ. Overview of the preparation of organic polymeric nanoparticles for drug delivery based on gelatine, chitosan, poly(d,l-lactide-co-glycolic acid) and polyalkylcyanoacrylate. Colloids Surf B Biointerfaces 2014; 118: 154-63.
[http://dx.doi.org/10.1016/j.colsurfb.2014.03.017] [PMID: 24769392]

[25] Dhana lekshmi UM, Poovi G, Kishore N, Reddy PN. *in vitro* characterization and *in vivo* toxicity study of repaglinide loaded poly (methyl methacrylate) nanoparticles. Int J Pharm 2010; 396(1-2): 194-203.
[http://dx.doi.org/10.1016/j.ijpharm.2010.06.023] [PMID: 20600729]

[26] Papa S, Ferrari R, De Paola M, *et al.* Polymeric nanoparticle system to target activated microglia/macrophages in spinal cord injury. J Control Release 2014; 174: 15-26.

[http://dx.doi.org/10.1016/j.jconrel.2013.11.001] [PMID: 24225226]

[27] Kuskov AN, Kulikov PP, Goryachaya AV, *et al.* Amphiphilic poly-N-vinylpyrrolidone nanoparticles as carriers for non-steroidal, anti-inflammatory drugs: *In vitro* cytotoxicity and *in vivo* acute toxicity study. Nanomedicine 2017; 13(3): 1021-30.
[http://dx.doi.org/10.1016/j.nano.2016.11.006] [PMID: 27884639]

[28] Franco P, De Marco I. The use of poly(N-vinyl pyrrolidone) in the delivery of drugs: A review. Polymers (Basel) 2020; 12(5): 1114.
[http://dx.doi.org/10.3390/polym12051114] [PMID: 32414187]

[29] Matijašić G, Gretić M, Vinčić J, Poropat A, Cuculić L, Rahelić T. Design and 3D printing of multi-compartmental PVA capsules for drug delivery. J Drug Deliv Sci Technol 2019; 52: 677-86.
[http://dx.doi.org/10.1016/j.jddst.2019.05.037]

[30] Yang M, Lai SK, Yu T, *et al.* Nanoparticle penetration of human cervicovaginal mucus: The effect of polyvinyl alcohol. J Control Release 2014; 192: 202-8.
[http://dx.doi.org/10.1016/j.jconrel.2014.07.045] [PMID: 25090196]

[31] Wenger Y, Schneider RJ II, Reddy GR, Kopelman R, Jolliet O, Philbert MA. Tissue distribution and pharmacokinetics of stable polyacrylamide nanoparticles following intravenous injection in the rat. Toxicol Appl Pharmacol 2011; 251(3): 181-90.
[http://dx.doi.org/10.1016/j.taap.2010.11.017] [PMID: 21134391]

[32] Kamaly N, Yameen B, Wu J, Farokhzad OC. Degradable controlled-release polymers and polymeric nanoparticles: Mechanisms of controlling drug release. Chem Rev 2016; 116(4): 2602-63.
[http://dx.doi.org/10.1021/acs.chemrev.5b00346] [PMID: 26854975]

[33] Weng J, Tong HHY, Chow SF. *in vitro* release study of the polymeric drug nanoparticles: Development and validation of a novel method. Pharmaceutics 2020; 12(8): 732.
[http://dx.doi.org/10.3390/pharmaceutics12080732] [PMID: 32759786]

[34] Pinto Reis C, Neufeld RJ, Ribeiro AJ, Veiga F, Nanoencapsulation I. Methods for preparation of drug-loaded polymeric nanoparticles. Nanomedicine Nanotechnology. Biol Med 2006; 2: 8-21.
[http://dx.doi.org/10.1016/j.nano.2005.12.003]

[35] Rao JP, Geckeler KE. Polymer nanoparticles: Preparation techniques and size-control parameters. Prog Polym Sci 2011; 36(7): 887-913.
[http://dx.doi.org/10.1016/j.progpolymsci.2011.01.001]

[36] Jung T, Kamm W, Breitenbach A, Kaiserling E, Xiao JX, Kissel T. Biodegradable nanoparticles for oral delivery of peptides: Is there a role for polymers to affect mucosal uptake? Eur J Pharm Biopharm 2000; 50(1): 147-60.
[http://dx.doi.org/10.1016/S0939-6411(00)00084-9] [PMID: 10840198]

[37] York P. Strategies for particle design using supercritical fluid technologies. Pharm Sci Technol Today 1999; 2(11): 430-40.
[http://dx.doi.org/10.1016/S1461-5347(99)00209-6] [PMID: 10542389]

[38] Kawashima Y. Nanoparticulate systems for improved drug delivery. Adv Drug Deliv Rev 2001; 47(1): 1-2.
[http://dx.doi.org/10.1016/S0169-409X(00)00117-4] [PMID: 11251241]

[39] Fessi H, Puisieux F, Devissaguet JP, Ammoury N, Benita S. Nanocapsule formation by interfacial polymer deposition following solvent displacement. Int J Pharm 1989; 55(1): R1-4.
[http://dx.doi.org/10.1016/0378-5173(89)90281-0]

[40] Quintanar-Guerrero D, Allémann E, Fessi H, Doelker E. Preparation techniques and mechanisms of formation of biodegradable nanoparticles from preformed polymers. Drug Dev Ind Pharm 1998; 24(12): 1113-28.
[http://dx.doi.org/10.3109/03639049809108571] [PMID: 9876569]

[41] Ekman B, Sjöholm I. Improved stability of proteins immobilized in microparticles prepared by a

modified emulsion polymerization technique. J Pharm Sci 1978; 67(5): 693-6. [http://dx.doi.org/10.1002/jps.2600670533] [PMID: 417171]

[42] Lowe PJ, Temple CS. Calcitonin and insulin in isobutylcyanoacrylate nanocapsules: Protection against proteases and effect on intestinal absorption in rats. J Pharm Pharmacol 2011; 46(7): 547-52. [http://dx.doi.org/10.1111/j.2042-7158.1994.tb03854.x] [PMID: 7996380]

[43] Karode SK, Kulkarni SS, Suresh AK, Mashelkar RA. New insights into kinetics and thermodynamics of interfacial polymerization. Chem Eng Sci 1998; 53(15): 2649-63. [http://dx.doi.org/10.1016/S0009-2509(98)00083-9]

[44] Matyjaszewski K, Xia J. Atom transfer radical polymerization. Chem Rev 2001; 101(9): 2921-90. [http://dx.doi.org/10.1021/cr940534g] [PMID: 11749397]

[45] Nakamura T, Okubo M, Okubo M. Mechanistic investigation of particle size effects in TEMPO-mediated radical polymerization of styrene in aqueous miniemulsion. Macromolecules 2007; 40(24): 8663-72. [http://dx.doi.org/10.1021/ma0712403]

[46] Al Zaki A, Joh D, Cheng Z, *et al.* Gold-loaded polymeric micelles for computed tomography-guided radiation therapy treatment and radiosensitization. ACS Nano 2014; 8(1): 104-12. [http://dx.doi.org/10.1021/nn405701q] [PMID: 24377302]

[47] Lin W, Zhang X, Qian L, Yao N, Pan Y, Zhang L. Doxorubicin-loaded unimolecular micelle-stabilized gold nanoparticles as a theranostic nanoplatform for tumor-targeted chemotherapy and computed tomography imaging. Biomacromolecules 2017; 18(12): 3869-80. [http://dx.doi.org/10.1021/acs.biomac.7b00810] [PMID: 29032674]

[48] Wang LV, Hu S. Photoacoustic tomography: *In vivo* imaging from organelles to organs. Science (80-) 2012; 335: 1458-62. [http://dx.doi.org/10.1126/science.1216210]

[49] Liu Y, Chen Z, Liu C, Yu D, Lu Z, Zhang N. Gadolinium-loaded polymeric nanoparticles modified with Anti-VEGF as multifunctional MRI contrast agents for the diagnosis of liver cancer. Biomaterials 2011; 32(22): 5167-76. [http://dx.doi.org/10.1016/j.biomaterials.2011.03.077] [PMID: 21521627]

[50] Esser L, Truong NP, Karagoz B, *et al.* Gadolinium-functionalized nanoparticles for application as magnetic resonance imaging contrast agents *via* polymerization-induced self-assembly. Polym Chem 2016; 7(47): 7325-37. [http://dx.doi.org/10.1039/C6PY01797E]

[51] Hu J, Fu S, Peng Q, *et al.* Paclitaxel-loaded polymeric nanoparticles combined with chronomodulated chemotherapy on lung cancer: *In vitro* and *in vivo* evaluation. Int J Pharm 2017; 516(1-2): 313-22. [http://dx.doi.org/10.1016/j.ijpharm.2016.11.047] [PMID: 27884713]

[52] Wallat JD, Czapar AE, Wang C, *et al.* Optical and magnetic resonance imaging using fluorous colloidal nanoparticles. Biomacromolecules 2017; 18(1): 103-12. [http://dx.doi.org/10.1021/acs.biomac.6b01389] [PMID: 27992176]

[53] Pisani E, Tsapis N, Paris J, Nicolas V, Cattel L, Fattal E. Polymeric nano/microcapsules of liquid perfluorocarbons for ultrasonic imaging: Physical characterization. Langmuir 2006; 22(9): 4397-402. [http://dx.doi.org/10.1021/la0601455] [PMID: 16618193]

[54] Giraudeau C, Flament J, Marty B, *et al.* A new paradigm for high-sensitivity ^{19}F magnetic resonance imaging of perfluorooctylbromide. Magn Reson Med 2010; 63(4): 1119-24. [http://dx.doi.org/10.1002/mrm.22269] [PMID: 20373415]

[55] Diou O, Fattal E, Delplace V, *et al.* RGD decoration of PEGylated polyester nanocapsules of perfluorooctyl bromide for tumor imaging: Influence of pre or post-functionalization on capsule morphology. Eur J Pharm Biopharm 2014; 87(1): 170-7. [http://dx.doi.org/10.1016/j.ejpb.2013.12.003] [PMID: 24333400]

[56] Jiang Y, Wong S, Chen F, Chang T, Lu H, Stenzel MH. Influencing selectivity to cancer cells with mixed nanoparticles prepared from albumin–polymer conjugates and block copolymers. Bioconjug Chem 2017; 28(4): 979-85.
[http://dx.doi.org/10.1021/acs.bioconjchem.6b00698] [PMID: 28263565]

[57] Kratz F. Albumin as a drug carrier: Design of prodrugs, drug conjugates and nanoparticles. J Control Release 2008; 132(3): 171-83.
[http://dx.doi.org/10.1016/j.jconrel.2008.05.010] [PMID: 18582981]

[58] Ahmed A, Sarwar S, Hu Y, *et al.* Surface-modified polymeric nanoparticles for drug delivery to cancer cells. Expert Opin Drug Deliv 2021; 18(1): 1-24.
[http://dx.doi.org/10.1080/17425247.2020.1822321] [PMID: 32905714]

[59] Çırpanlı Y, Allard E, Passirani C, *et al.* Antitumoral activity of camptothecin-loaded nanoparticles in 9L rat glioma model. Int J Pharm 2011; 403(1-2): 201-6.
[http://dx.doi.org/10.1016/j.ijpharm.2010.10.015] [PMID: 20951783]

[60] Guo J, Gao X, Su L, *et al.* Aptamer-functionalized PEG–PLGA nanoparticles for enhanced anti-glioma drug delivery. Biomaterials 2011; 32(31): 8010-20.
[http://dx.doi.org/10.1016/j.biomaterials.2011.07.004] [PMID: 21788069]

[61] Maksimenko O, Malinovskaya J, Shipulo E, *et al.* Doxorubicin-loaded PLGA nanoparticles for the chemotherapy of glioblastoma: Towards the pharmaceutical development. Int J Pharm 2019; 572: 118733.
[http://dx.doi.org/10.1016/j.ijpharm.2019.118733] [PMID: 31689481]

[62] Hekmatara T, Bernreuther C, Khalansky AS, *et al.* Efficient systemic therapy of rat glioblastoma by nanoparticle-bound doxorubicin is due to antiangiogenic effects. Clin Neuropathol 2009; 28(5): 153-64.
[http://dx.doi.org/10.5414/NPP28153] [PMID: 19537130]

[63] Khanna V, Kalscheuer S, Kirtane A, Zhang W, Panyam J. Perlecan-targeted nanoparticles for drug delivery to triple-negative breast cancer. Future Drug Discov 2019; 1(1): FDD8.
[http://dx.doi.org/10.4155/fdd-2019-0005] [PMID: 31448368]

[64] Zhu H, Bandara R, Conibear TCR, *et al.* Pseudomonas aeruginosa with lasI quorum-sensing deficiency during corneal infection. Invest Ophthalmol Vis Sci 2004; 45(6): 1897-903.
[http://dx.doi.org/10.1167/iovs.03-0980] [PMID: 15161855]

[65] Jin M, Jin G, Kang L, Chen L, Gao Z, Huang W. Smart polymeric nanoparticles with pH-responsive and PEG-detachable properties for co-delivering paclitaxel and survivin siRNA to enhance antitumor outcomes. Int J Nanomedicine 2018; 13: 2405-26.
[http://dx.doi.org/10.2147/IJN.S161426] [PMID: 29719390]

[66] Duxfield L, Sultana R, Wang R, *et al.* Development of gatifloxacin-loaded cationic polymeric nanoparticles for ocular drug delivery. Pharm Dev Technol 2016; 21(2): 172-9.
[http://dx.doi.org/10.3109/10837450.2015.1091839] [PMID: 26794936]

[67] Mittal N, Kaur G. Investigations on polymeric nanoparticles for ocular delivery. Adv Polym Technol 2019; 2019: 1-14.
[http://dx.doi.org/10.1155/2019/1316249]

[68] Gatti THH, Eloy JO, Ferreira LMB, *et al.* Insulin-loaded polymeric mucoadhesive nanoparticles: Development, characterization and cytotoxicity evaluation. Braz J Pharm Sci 2018; 54(1): 1-10.
[http://dx.doi.org/10.1590/s2175-97902018000117314]

[69] das Neves J, Nunes R, Machado A, Sarmento B. Polymer-based nanocarriers for vaginal drug delivery. Adv Drug Deliv Rev 2015; 92: 53-70.
[http://dx.doi.org/10.1016/j.addr.2014.12.004] [PMID: 25550217]

[70] Akbari A, Wu J. Ovomucin nanoparticles: Promising carriers for mucosal delivery of drugs and bioactive compounds. Drug Deliv Transl Res 2017; 7(4): 598-607.

[http://dx.doi.org/10.1007/s13346-017-0406-3] [PMID: 28717995]

[71] Shah B, Khunt D, Misra M. Comparative evaluation of intranasally delivered quetiapine loaded mucoadhesive microemulsion and polymeric nanoparticles for brain targeting: Pharmacokinetic and gamma scintigraphy studies. Future Journal of Pharmaceutical Sciences 2021; 7(1): 6. [http://dx.doi.org/10.1186/s43094-020-00156-5]

[72] Rabiee N, Ahmadi S, Afshari R, *et al.* Polymeric nanoparticles for nasal drug delivery to the brain: Relevance to Alzheimer's disease. Adv Ther (Weinh) 2021; 4(3): 2000076. [http://dx.doi.org/10.1002/adtp.202000076]

[73] Mahmoud BS, AlAmri AH, McConville C. Polymeric nanoparticles for the treatment of malignant gliomas. Cancers (Basel) 2020; 12(1): 175. [http://dx.doi.org/10.3390/cancers12010175] [PMID: 31936740]

[74] Wong K, Riaz M, Xie Y, *et al.* Review of current strategies for delivering Alzheimer's disease drugs across the blood-brain barrier. Int J Mol Sci 2019; 20(2): 381. [http://dx.doi.org/10.3390/ijms20020381] [PMID: 30658419]

[75] Kim Y, Lobatto ME, Kawahara T, *et al.* Probing nanoparticle translocation across the permeable endothelium in experimental atherosclerosis. Proc Natl Acad Sci USA 2014; 111(3): 1078-83. [http://dx.doi.org/10.1073/pnas.1322725111] [PMID: 24395808]

[76] Aguilera-Correa JJ, Esteban J, Vallet-Regí M. Inorganic and polymeric nanoparticles for human viral and bacterial infections prevention and treatment. Nanomaterials (Basel) 2021; 11(1): 137. [http://dx.doi.org/10.3390/nano11010137] [PMID: 33435597]

[77] Ucak S, Sudagidan M, Borsa BA, Mansuroglu B, Ozalp VC. Inhibitory effects of aptamer targeted teicoplanin encapsulated PLGA nanoparticles for Staphylococcus aureus strains. World J Microbiol Biotechnol 2020; 36(5): 69. [http://dx.doi.org/10.1007/s11274-020-02845-y] [PMID: 32333113]

[78] Vrouvaki I, Koutra E, Kornaros M, Avgoustakis K, Lamari FN, Hatziantoniou S. Polymeric nanoparticles of Pistacia lentiscus var. Chia essential oil for cutaneous applications. Pharmaceutics 2020; 12(4): 353. [http://dx.doi.org/10.3390/pharmaceutics12040353] [PMID: 32295134]

[79] Ghosh A, Mandal AK, Sarkar S, Panda S, Das N. Nanoencapsulation of quercetin enhances its dietary efficacy in combating arsenic-induced oxidative damage in liver and brain of rats. Life Sci 2009; 84(3-4): 75-80. [http://dx.doi.org/10.1016/j.lfs.2008.11.001] [PMID: 19036345]

[80] Yadav A, Lomash V, Samim M, Flora SJS. Curcumin encapsulated in chitosan nanoparticles: A novel strategy for the treatment of arsenic toxicity. Chem Biol Interact 2012; 199(1): 49-61. [http://dx.doi.org/10.1016/j.cbi.2012.05.011] [PMID: 22704994]

[81] Niazvand F, Khorsandi L, Abbaspour M, Orazizadeh M, Varaa N, Maghzi M, *et al.* Curcumin-loaded poly lactic-co-glycolic acid nanoparticles effects on mono-iodoacetate -induced osteoarthritis in rats. Vet Res Forum an Int Q J 2017; 8: 155-61.

[82] Pandey P, Dureja H. Recent patents on polymeric nanoparticles for cancer therapy. Recent Pat Nanotechnol 2018; 12(2): 155-69. [http://dx.doi.org/10.2174/1872210512666180327120648] [PMID: 29589551]

CHAPTER 3

An Overview on Nanoparticulate Drug Delivery System for its Specific and Targeted Effects in Various Diseases

Balaga Venkata Krishna Rao[1], **Aditi Pradhan**[1], **Sneha Singh**[2] and **Abhimanyu Dev**[1,*]

[1] *Department of Pharmaceutical Sciences and Technology, Birla Institute of Technology, Mesra, Ranchi-835215, Jharkhand, India*

[2] *Department of Bio-Engineering, Birla Institute of Technology, Mesra, Ranchi-835215, Jharkhand, India*

Abstract: In modern-day medicine, nanoparticles and nanocarriers are rapidly evolving fields in therapeutics and are the building blocks of nanomedicine, which emphasize the use of nanoscale particles that have a wide array of functions from working as a diagnostic tool to the screening, monitoring, and controlling of various diseases to the delivery of drugs at specific targets in a controlled manner. With the advancement in technologies, it is proven that nanoparticles have a greater potential in wide biomedical applications. Due to their ability to bind with both hydrophobic and lyophilic substances, lower particle size, higher carrier capacity, nanoparticles serve as a favorable platform for specific and targeted drug delivery in disease treatment. Nanoformulations can improve the safety, pharmacokinetic characteristics, and bioavailability of administered drugs, and can improve the therapeutic effect when compared with conventional therapies. Besides, nanoparticles may also be effective in delivering nucleotides, vaccines, and recombinant proteins. Several varieties of nanoparticles are available: different metal and polymeric nanoparticles like gold/silver nanoparticles and micelles, dendrimers. Carbon-derived nanoparticles like quantum dots, carbon tubes, and many other nano assemblies. Numerous nanocarriers, nanoparticle-based drug delivery systems, and drug targeting systems are either developed or under development. In this chapter, we will emphasize mainly the specific and targeted nanoparticles and the use of various nanocarriers for the targeted delivery of drugs in various diseases. The opportunities and challenges of using nanoparticles/nanocarriers in targeted delivery along with its clinical applications are also discussed here.

Keywords: Autoimmune disorder, Cancer, Drug delivery, Infectious diseases, Nanoparticles, Polymers pulmonary diseases.

* **Corresponding author Abhimanyu Dev:** Department of Pharmaceutical Sciences & Technology, Birla Institute of Technology, Mesra, Ranchi-835215, India; Tel: 9955165915; E-mail: **abhimanyudev@bitmesra.ac.in**

Akhlesh K. Jain & Keerti Mishra (Eds.)

INTRODUCTION

For decades, pharmaceutical research is concentrated on modifying delivery systems. Tremendous advancements in technology and incorporation of multidisciplinary research faculties like polymer science, physics, biotechnology, genetics, molecular science and their use in the research and development setup have led to the development of newer technologies. Due to the advent of analytical techniques and our growing ability to measure particles in the nanoscale, the focus of current research is shifted from micro to nanoscale. The prefix *'nano'* word has been derived from the Greek word *'dwarf'*. The word nano has attained a lot of significance in recent days due to the existing materials as they exhibit unusual physical and chemical properties that change significantly when their size is reduced to nano levels. Nanoscience refers to the study of particles on an ultra-small scale, while the use of these small atomic particles for industrial applications is defined by the term nanotechnology [1].

There's plenty of room at the bottom were the words by Noble laureate, theoretical physicist Richard Phillips Feynman who envisioned the technology at the molecular level way back in 1959 and inspired the Japanese professor and scientist Norio Taniguchi, at the University of Tokyo, Japan in 1974 when he first referred to the materials in nanometre and was the first to use the word nanotechnology. A nanometre (nm) is 10^{-9}, which is one-billionth of a meter or around one-thousandth of a micrometer. Nanotechnology is the new key in the field of science and technology and if properly exploited to its full potential, would benefit different aspects of mankind for the better.

Nanoparticles (NPs) with their small size, have unique properties that have wide applications and greater potential to benefit wide areas in research. NPs along with nanodevices that form the basis of nanomedicine can be used for treatment, diagnosis, monitoring, and controlling various diseases including cancer. Exploiting nanotechnology has led to the surfacing of various nano particulates which are currently under use as drug delivery systems, often referred to as nanoparticulate drug-delivery systems (NPDDSs). The use of these NPs is also arising from newer challenges in the fields of ethical, safety, and regulatory aspects which need extensive research and revision wherever needed. Some issues need to be resolved, but still, it shows how intense and broad this area is and can be in the future and depicts why the nanoscale-based drug delivery strategies are making a significant impact in the global pharmaceuticals [2].

The need for NPs is increasing rapidly. The research in the pharmaceutical industry is heading towards uncertain ways with a decline in the flow of incoming new chemical entities and drug discovery process coupled with higher rates of clinical failure and clinical development cost. The main problems of the conventional delivery include issues related to but not limited to solubility, permeability, drug release profile, and bioavailability. However, by the application of nanotechnology-driven delivery systems, all these problems could be overcome [1].

Developing nanoscale distribution systems is a rapidly growing and most advanced technology in the field of NP applications.The potential advantage of using NPs is their ability to modify the physicochemical properties of drugs. Drugs with fewer side effects, enhanced biodistribution, and lower toxicity could be developed along with a convenient administration route. NPs are engineered particles that can deliver a drug at a particular (target) site in a controlled manner for a prolonged period. The main aim of these NPs is to develop a safer and effective therapeutic delivery system that can subsequently lead to targeted therapy in disease treatment [3].

The concept of NPs may have become a part of the discussion from the mid-twentieth century but its existence in the natural biological systems as the functional component of living cells cannot be ignored. Various natural NPs exist in nature ranging from organisms like viruses, bacteria, fungi, yeasts, and algae to the components like amino acids, carbohydrates, lipids, and proteins which not only act as a building block of the body but also help in the regular functioning of the body.

SPECIFIC & TARGETED NANOPARTICLES

Nanotechnology in medicine or widely termed nanomedicine comprises mainly two things nanodevices and nanomaterials. Nanodevices contain nanoscale robots, smart pills, microarrays, and other microscopic devices. Nanomaterials are classified as nanocrystalline and nanostructured, while the former contains nanocrystals (carrier-free drug particles), the latter is again classified based upon its core composition into polymer-based NPs, non-polymer based and lipid-based NPs. Polymer-based NPs include micelles, drug conjugates, protein NPs, nanogels, dendrimers, and nanoparticles. Non-polymeric NPs include carbon dots, carbon nanotubes, quantum dots, silica-based NPs, nanodiamonds, and metallic nanoparticles. Lipid-based NPs comprise liposomes, exosomes, and solid lipid nanoparticles. Apart from these main classes of NPs used, various modifications have been done to these existing materials to obtain newer carrier molecules [2]. Further, various nanomedicine used in the biomedical applications are depicted in Fig. **(3.1)**.

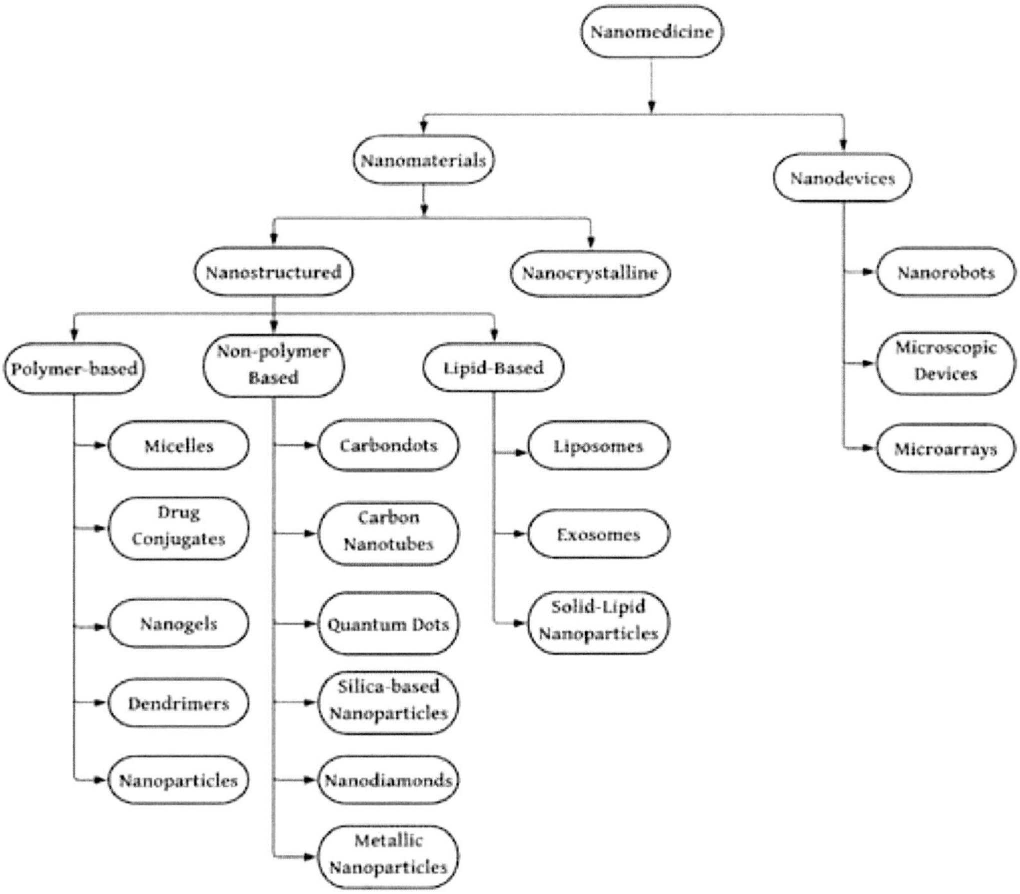

Fig. (3.1). Various nanomedicines used in biomedical applications.

Nanocarriers can be easily administered by any of the routes by virtue of their small size but depending upon the therapeutic payload, and other physiochemical characters the route can be modified. The most commonly employed route for delivery of therapeutic NPs includes oral, transdermal, intravenous, inhalation administration. The oral route is the most preferred and common route of delivery with higher patient acceptability. The oral route also comes up with numerous limitations like degradation of protein and peptides by gastric environment and proteolytic enzymes, poor absorption, and solubility which could be simply overcome with the use of NPs. NPs allow (i) delivery of poorly water-soluble drugs, (ii) transport across the epithelial barrier, (iii) delivery at a specific site and (iv) release of the drug in a controlled manner [4]. The largest organ in the human body, the skin, provides a large surface area for dermal/transdermal delivery of drugs. Liposomes, electrosomes, ethosomes, noisomes, transferosomes, dendrimers, nanoemulsions, and polymeric nanoparticles are the most commonly used nanocarriers for transdermal delivery. To further increase permeability, various modifications are done to integral structures and composition of liposomes to obtain newer carriers like ethosomes, and transferosomes [5].

NPs can be administered through various routes including intravenous (IV), intraperitoneally (IP), and intra-articular injection. The major advantage of intravenous administration is the rapid onset of action, complete bioavailability and distribution, and most suitable for drugs exhibiting poor gastrointestinal (GI) absorption and associated problems. Often, NPs given through IV route are advantageous but come with problems like opsonization or macrophage uptake and rapid clearance, which can be avoided by the use of micellar complexes and nanoemulsions [6]. High surface area and vascularization with rapid absorption are some of the numerous advantages of the inhalation route. Drugs administered through this route often evade the first-pass metabolism reducing dosing rates. This also allows systemic and local delivery of drugs even delivering efficiently to the brain avoiding blood brain barrier (BBB). Numerous antibiotics, chemotherapeutics, proteins and peptides, and even vaccines (as dry powders) can be administered through the pulmonary route. Drugs coated with NPs will pass through the oropharynx and get deposited into the lungs from where drugs will be released in sustained form achieving better distribution in the systemic circulation [7].

Polymer-Based Nanoparticles

Micelles

Polymeric micelles are one of the attractive carriers for water-insoluble drugs. These are formed by the self-assembly of amphiphilic polymers. The critical micelle concentration (CMC) is the most important parameter in defining the stability of the micelles as polymeric concentrations above CMC are said to make micelles stable while micelles get disassembled at lower polymeric concentrations (concentration below CMC) [8]. The size is usually between 10-200 nm. Amphiphilic di-block copolymers (*e.g.*, PEG and Polystyrene), triblock copolymers (*e.g.*, poloxamers) are generally used for micelle preparation. The micelles have numerous advantages over traditional delivery vehicles like small size, enhanced permeation, and retention (EPR) effect, stabilizing water-insoluble drugs, versatile loading capacity making them the obvious vehicles for targeted tumor therapy [9].

Drug Conjugates

Polymeric Drug Conjugates (PDCs) are a result of the conjugation of a polymer to a drug molecule. This concept of PDCs was first introduced by Helmut Ringsdorf in 1975 [10]. The water-soluble polymer PEG is mainly used for the majority of PDCs preparation. Apart from PEG, the recent focus is shifted to natural polymers like dextran (DEX) and polysialic acid (PSA) to combat problems like polymer toxicity and biodegradability. In general, the PDCs as delivery agents offer several advantages including higher payload capacity, improved drug solubility, enhanced stability and efficacy, optimized biodistribution, and site-specific delivery of drugs in a controlled manner. PDCs have wide applications in cancer including diabetes and arthritis [11 - 13].

Nanogels

Nanogels are three-dimensional hydrogels with a diameter of less than 100 nm in size. These are prepared by either chemical/physical crosslinking of the polymers. The crosslinking ensures higher water content and physical integrity [14]. The swelling capacity can be attributed to the presence of polymers; hydrophilic polymers can show hydration up to 90% whereas only 5-10% hydration is exhibited by lipophilic polymers [15]. Nanogels as a delivery agent have numerous advantages like small size, ease of preparation, biocompatibility, decreased toxicity, and drug leakage. Moreover, various modifications can be made to make nanogels stimuli-responsive like pH, temperature, and photoresponsive. These delivery agents have wide applications and are used in the diagnosis and treatment of diseases like cancer, wound healing, arthritis, CNS associated disorders. Among all, they can carry therapeutics like proteins, peptides, nucleic acids, and macromolecules like oligonucleotides [16].

Dendrimers

Dendrimers are hyperbranched polymeric structures with a central core and extending dendrons similar to that of a tree. The name “dendrimers” have been derived from two Greek words “dendron” and “meros” meaning tree and part, respectively. The most commonly used dendrimers are poly (propylene imine) (PPI), carbosilane, glycodendrimer, poly (amido amine) (PAMAM), and peptide dendrimer. The dendrimer has three significant parts: the central core, hyperbranched repeating layers, and multivalent external surface. Dendrimers have advantages like (a) the ability to interact with a large number of compounds which improves their solubility, (b) higher structural and chemical integrity, (c) targeting ability which increases specificity, (d) higher penetration into cells owing to a smaller size, (e) controllable synthesizing and degradation. It also has limitations like (a) higher production cost, (b) improved quality control tests to ensure dendrimer quality and safety. It has wide applications in various bacterial infections, viral, infectious, and neglected tropical diseases [17, 18].

Nanoparticles

Polymeric nanoparticles provide an alternative way for the delivery of therapeutics owing to certain features like biocompatibility, non-toxicity, and non-immunogenicity. The polymers in NPs can be of synthetic or natural origin. To overcome the problems of immunogenicity and toxicity recent focus has shifted to the use of natural polymers like alginate, chitosan, gelatine, and albumin [19]. The ideal size of the NPs is around 5-200 nm while a smaller size implies that it can easily penetrate the capillaries. Also, these NPs have a large surface area where surface functional groups like ligands can be displayed. Some of the general methods employed for the preparation of NPs include nanoprecipitation, polymerization, solvent evaporation, dialysis, and salting out. Depending upon their composition, these can be classified as nanospheres and nanocapsules. In nanospheres, the therapeutic agent is uniformly dispersed within the matrix while a polymeric film encloses the therapeutic payload in nanocapsules. Furthermore, the addition of specific recognition ligands can increase their specificity in target tissues [20]. Various polymeric nanoparticles are depicted in Fig. **(3.2)**.

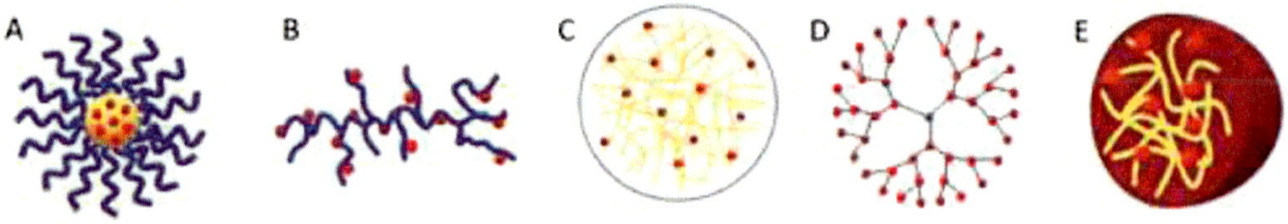

Fig. (3.2). Various polymeric nanocarriers; (A) Micelle, (B) Drug-conjugate, (C) Nanogels, (D) Dendrimer, (E) Nanoparticle.

Non-Polymer Based Nanoparticles

Carbon Dots

Carbon dots (C-dots) are carbon-based, zero-dimensional nanocarriers with a size of less than 10nm. These were accidentally discovered in 2004 while studying single-walled carbon nanotubes (SWCNTs) using gel electrophoresis [21]. These have spherical-shaped, amorphous, or nanocrystalline cores with predominant sp^2 hybridization. C-dots have a spherical structure with a well-ordered surface containing -OH, -COOH, and $-NH_2$ groups, but predominantly depend upon the fabrication technique employed and precursors used. Initially, C-dots were prepared from natural carbon sources but in recent days synthetic carbon probes are used [22]. Currently, there are two types of carbon dots present: Graphene carbon dots (G-Q-dots) and amorphous carbon dots (A-C-dots). C-dots have advantages like small size, biocompatible nature, lower toxicity, and simple functionalization. Poor stability and the inability to maintain certain properties for a prolonged period are some of the limitations of C-dots. C-dots have wide applications in targeted and gene delivery, tumor targeting, diagnostic imaging, and monitoring of cellular trafficking [23].

Carbon Nanotubes

Carbon nanotubes (CNTs) are tubular structures, obtained by wrapping sheets of graphene into a cylinder. These are around 0.3-3.0 nm in diameter and around 100nm in length [24]. These can be classified as single-walled carbon nanotubes (SWCNTs) and multi-walled carbon nanotubes (MWCNTs). The SWCNTs are simple graphene cylinders with smaller diameters while the MWCNTs are the complex dwelling of graphene cylinders that offers endohedral loading space [25]. Depending upon the arrangement of graphene tubes in MWCNTs, they can be classified into two types: (a) parchment-type: where graphene tubes are rolled up around themselves and (b) Russian-doll type: where a single graphene tube encloses several other graphene tubes in its hollow core. These are mainly prepared by either of the three techniques. These include chemical vapor deposition (CVD), electric arc discharge, and laser ablation. The CNTs have higher payload capacity when compared to other spherical NPs of similar sizes, and can penetrate the cell by endocytosis, phagocytosis, or passive diffusion. These exhibit a higher aspect ratio, higher payload capacity, biocompatibility, and ease of functionalization which allowed them as a promising nanocarrier for various diseases including cancer [26 - 28].

Quantum Dots

Quantum dots (QDs), are nanomaterials with a diameter in the size range of 2-10 nm. These are also known as semiconductor nanocrystals, and can be classified according to their structure as core-type QDs, Core-shell QDs, and alloyed QDs [29]. Based upon its size, there are large QDs (5-6 nm in diameter) and small QDs (2-3 nm in diameter). QDs can also be classified based on materials used for their creation as (a) semiconductor QDs made up of inorganic heavy metals and non-metals like cadmium, zinc sulphide, and selenium, (b) carbon-based QDs made up of carbon [30]. QDs made up of carbon are also termed Carbon dots. QDs contains a central core and a peripheral shell to stabilize the core which also acts as a carrier for various biomolecules like peptides, proteins, and DNA. They have wide biomedical applications including biomedical imaging, drug-delivery, analytical imaging, as biosensors in the detection of cancers. QDs are recently gaining popularity owing to their smaller size, higher photostability, and biocompatibility which makes them ideal for the delivery of therapeutic agents [31, 32].

Silica-Based Nanoparticles

Silica is considered "Generally Considered as Safe" (GRAS) by USFDA, and colloidal silica (Aerosil®) has been used for decades as an excipient in tablet manufacturing. There are various silica-based NPs currently being used in various biomedical applications including non-porous silica, amorphous silica, microporous crystalline titanosilicates, zeolites, and mesoporous silica [33]. The presence of special characteristics like adjustable pore size, large pore volume, and surface area, biocompatibility, and rigid structure make mesoporous silica nanoparticles (MSNs) a promising nanocarrier. Moreover, it has surfaces that can be functionalized aiding in drug loading and targeted release. The common strategies employed for loading therapeutic payload to MSNs include melting process, solvent-based methods, and supercritical CO_2 techniques. MSNs has wide applications in delivering drugs in cancer. Drugs like Paclitaxel delivered using lipid bilayer coated MSNs enhanced solubility, exhibiting prolonged release and cytotoxicity in case of breast cancer while Gold Nano shell MSNs containing Sorafenib improved cancer suppression in case of hepatic tumors [34, 35].

Nanodiamonds

Nanodiamonds (NDs) are carbon allotropes and the latest edition to the carbon nano family. There are three major steps in NDs production *i.e.*, synthesis, processing, and modification. The commonly employed methods using carbon precursors for synthesizing NDs include chemical vapor deposition (CVD), detonation, laser ablation, high-pressure high temperature (HPHT), ultrasound cavitation, and chlorination of carbon, *etc.* [36]. NDs obtained cannot be directly used for the biomedical application so, post-synthesis processing needs to be done which includes steps like purification, de-aggregation, and fractionation. Finally, the modification includes doping and surface functionalization. Various biomolecules like peptides, amino acids, polymers, and even genetic materials like siRNA and DNA are added to the surface. NDs owing to properties like biocompatibility, stability, and functionalization capacity has emerged as a novel nanocarrier for delivering drugs [37, 38].

Metallic Nanoparticles

Metal nanoparticles used in biomedical applications are mainly composed of gold, silver, nickel, cobalt, and iron and their respective oxides (such as dioxide, ferrite, and magnetite). Their size is usually between 10 and 100 nm [39]. Gold nanoparticles (AuNP) are the most studied metal nanoparticles due to their unique optical and local surface plasmon resonance (LSPR) activity, especially in cancer diagnosis and treatment. AuNPs are comprised of a central core containing gold encircled by an organic ligand, around 20 nm in size, and can be synthesized using numerous methods. Among, metallic magnetic NPs, super-paramagnetic iron oxide nanoparticles (SPIONs) are the most popular magnetic nanoparticles (MNPs). SPIONs are widely used as contrast in Magnetic resonance imaging. Metallic nanoparticles can be prepared by numerous methods and can be modified with various functional groups including therapeutic agents, bioactive like proteins, peptides, and DNA. These as a carrier exhibit various advantages over other nanocarriers and have wide biomedical applications in imaging, biosensing, and drug delivery [40 - 42]. Fig. **(3.3)** depictes various metallic and non-polymeric based nanoparticles.

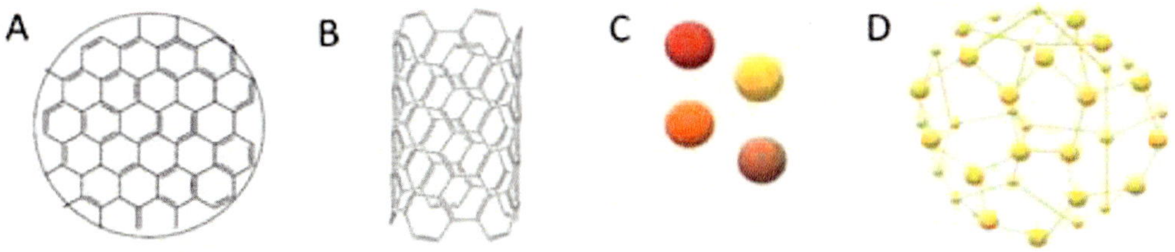

Fig. (3.3). Various Non-Polymeric nanocarriers; (A) Carbon dot, (B) Carbon Nanotube, (C) Quantum Dots, (D) Gold (Mettalic) nanoparticles.

Lipid-Based Nanoparticles

Liposomes

Liposomes are spherical-shaped lipid-based vesicular systems comprising hydrophilic hollow-core enclosed by a lipid bilayer. These are usually prepared by the hydration of dry phospholipids [43]. Depending upon the number of bilayers, they can be classified as small unilamellar, large unilamellar, and multilamellar. Unilamellar vesicles consist of a single lipid bilayer, whereas multilamellar comprises several lipid bilayers separated by a hydrophilic core [44]. These structural characteristics help them to carry both hydrophilic drugs (in central core) and lipophilic drugs (in between the lipid bilayer) and also help in releasing drugs directly to the cytoplasm due to the interaction of the outer lipid core with the natural cell membrane. Liposomes can be employed for the delivery of peptides, genes, small molecules, and even monoclonal antibodies. Moreover, to improve targeted delivery and biological circulation time, its surface structure can be modified by either using PEG or coating with other suitable polymers [45]. Liposomes have wide applications in cancer diagnostics and therapy and brain-targeted drug delivery [44].

Exosomes

Exosomes are homogenous vesicles usually derived from membranes of different origins and can be classified based upon their source as cardiosomes (exosomes derived from cardiomyocytes), ectosomes (secreted by neutrophils or monocytes), and prostasomes (secreted by human prostate glands) [46]. The exosome subpopulation can be further classified as exomeres (35 nm), small exosomes (60-80 nm), and large exosomes (90-120 nm) based on their size. Lipids aids in maintaining exosome rigid, which includes sphingomyelin and monosialotetra-hexosylganglioside (GM1). While the lipid bilayer comprises cholesterol and diacylglycerol. The exosomes have different functions due to their different origins. They act as a medium for the exchange of materials between cells, help in intercellular communication, and present antigens in various diseases including cancer, and contribute to the immune system [47]. As they represent the physiological changes of cells and tissues (their derived source) they can act as a biomarker and as a delivery vehicle [48, 49].

Solid-Lipid Nanoparticles (SLN)

Solid-Lipid Nanoparticles (SLN) is a novel nanosized drug delivery system. These comprise a lipid core that is solid at ambient temperature, stabilized by surfactant enclosing active ingredient in the solid lipid matrix. Their size can vary between 100-200 nm depending upon the fabrication method employed [50]. Surfactants improve their stability profile while lipophilic nature helps in improved solubility and enhanced permeation. The drug in the matrix assures prolonged release and protection from the unfavorable environment. SLN comes with numerous advantages like higher payload capacity, entrapping both lipophilic and hydrophilic drugs, making them the obvious carrier molecules [51, 52]. Furthermore, their surfaces can be loaded with molecules like antibodies, pH-sensitive polymers, and magnetic nanoparticles to modulate drug targeting and sensitive stimuli drug delivery [53, 54]. Unlike traditional delivery forms, these carriers exhibit easy GI transit surpassing problems like chemical instability, poor solubility, low permeability, and the first-pass metabolism making them a superior choice over conventional forms [55, 56]. Various lipid-based nanoparticles are depicted in Fig. **(3.4)**.

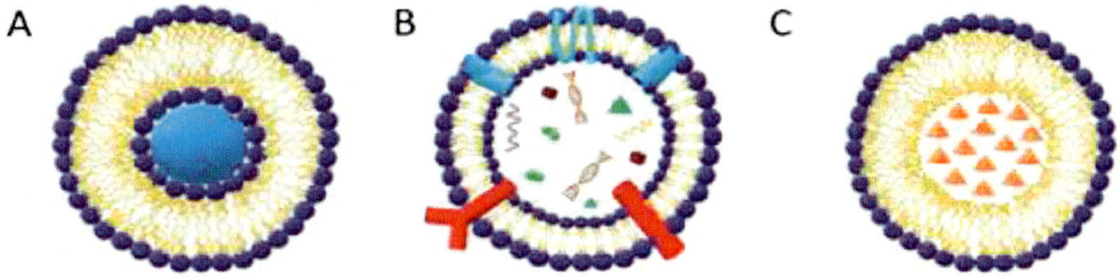

Fig. (3.4). Various Lipid based nanoparticles; (A) Liposome, (B) Exosome, (C) Solid-Lipid Nanoparticle (SLNPs).

Drug Nanocrystals

Nanocrystals are carrier-free nanoparticles, with a crystalline structure and a few hundred nanometres in size. Nanocrystal formulations are an important tool for improving solubility, bioavailability, and other pharmacokinetic parameters of poorly water-soluble drugs [57]. Nanocrystals are synthesized by top-down or bottom-up techniques, and the top-down approach of processing larger crystals is a commonly used manufacturing method. Reduction in size to nanometres significantly enhances its surface area improving solubility & bioavailability profile. This characteristic property helps drug compounds, mainly BCS class II drugs, and BCS class IV drugs (with poor solubility and poor permeability). Fast dissolution and rapid drug absorption are some of the numerous advantages offered by nanocrystals. Furthermore, by modifying the nanocrystal surface, targeted & prolonged release can also be achieved [57, 58].

APPLICATIONS OF TARGETED THERAPEUTIC NANOPARTICLES

A plethora of NPs have been developed over the past few decades and their potential applications in disease diagnosing and therapy have been widely studied. The main objectives of targeted therapeutic NPs are to deliver the therapeutic agents at the desired site. The NPs should also retain in the physiological system for a prolonged time, evading immune cells, releasing medicaments into targeted cells/tissues for efficient targeting. The majority of routinely used nanoformulations in clinical use are for cancer. Furthermore, NPs are also used for diseases of cardiovascular, infectious, neurodegenerative, autoimmune, and pulmonary disorders [2, 59]. Some of the European Medicines Agency (EMA) and Food and Drug Administration (FDA) approved NPs are depicted in Fig. **(3.5)**

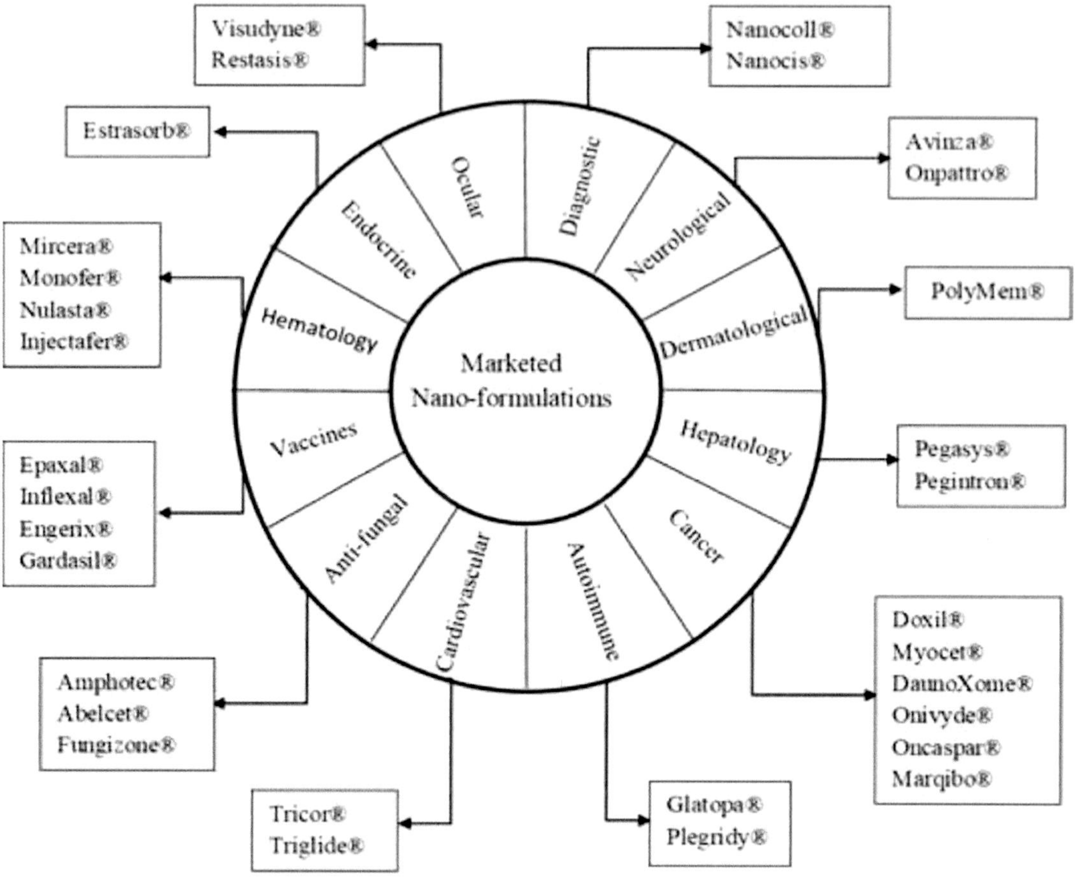

Fig. (3.5). Schematic representation of various marketed nanomedicines.

Autoimmne and Immunodeficient Disorders

A healthy immune system defends the body against diseases and infection but if it malfunctions, then our immune system starts attacking our healthy cells leading to a wide range of diseases commonly referred to as auto-immune diseases. Auto-immune diseases can affect any part of the body and even turn life-threatening. There are more than 80 auto-immune diseases reported such as rheumatoid arthritis, multiple sclerosis, systematic lupus erythematosus, ankylosing spondylitis, AIDS including type 1 diabetes [60]. These diseases may originate from any part or organ related to the immune system such as bone marrow, thymus, spleen, appendix, and lymph nodes. Based on the location of the autoimmune attack, these can be classified into systemic or tissue/organ-specific and pathogenesis can be initiated by multiple factors. Some of them include heredity, hormonal influence, environmental factors, and lifestyle changes [61]. Although there are numerous autoimmune diseases; However, rheumatoid arthritis (RA) and acquired immunodeficiency syndrome (AIDS) are two important immune and immunodeficiency disorders, respectively, which can be treated using nanoparticulate drug delivery systems.

Rheumatoid Arthritis (RA) is a chronic inflammatory disorder affecting mainly the joints in the body including those in the feet and hand. Despite its unknown cause, the bone and cartilage destruction are due to possible interactions between various immune mediators. Although new treatment therapies can improve quality of life still systematic adverse effects may arise due to repetitive long-term usage of medicaments [62]. Some of the conventional therapies used for the treatment of RA are briefly enlisted in Table **3.1**. The nanoparticulate system can acts as a promising carrier for therapeutic agents as they can deliver the drug at the target site evading systemic side effects. Convectional liposome containing methotrexate prepared using egg phosphatidylcholine; cholesterol and dicetylphosphate in a molecular ratio of 5:5:1 are used in the treatment of RA by enhancing retention time of drug [63].

Table 3.1. Convectional drugs used for the treatment of RA.

Drug	Class/Group	Main Indication	Adverse Effect	Ref.
Celecoxib	COXIB	Rheumatic diseases, pain relief	Severe skin and cardiovascular reactions	64
Etodolac	NSAID	Joint diseases, acute pain	Nausea, agranulocytosis, abdominal pain	65
Indomethacin		Ankylosing spondylitis, rheumatic arthritis, pain, swelling, stiffness, and tendonitis.	Gastrointestinal disturbances, dizziness, vertigo, ringing ear, irritation of the rectum	66
Meloxicam		Rheumatoid arthritis, osteoarthritis	Gastrointestinal effects, bloating, diarrhea, nervousness, dizziness	67
Nabumetone		Rheumatic and joint diseases	Abdominal pain, constipation, edema	68
Naproxen		Rheumatoid arthritis, fever, gout, and menstrual cramps	Heartburn, nausea, dizziness, constipation	69
Methoxetrate	DMARDs	Cancer, autoimmune disease	Abdominal discomfort, nausea, fatigue	66
Sulfasalazine		Rheumatoid arthritis, Crohn's disease, ulcerative colitis	Macrocytosis, abdominal discomfort	66

NSAID: Non-steroidal anti-inflammatory drug; COXIB: COX-2 selective NSAID; DMARDs: Disease-modifying anti-rheumatic drugs.

Acquired immune deficiency syndrome (AIDS) is a chronic disease caused by the human immunodeficiency virus (HIV). HIV affects the immune system, destroying and impairing the function of immune cells making the individual immune deficient. Immunodeficiency can make an affected individual susceptible to a large number of infections including some cancers. Highly active antiretroviral treatment (HAART) is the most significant clinical therapy for AIDS which involves the use of at least three anti-HIV drugs in combination [70]. To improve cellular uptake and limit the systematic side effects, the current focus is shifted towards the use of polymeric and liposomal nanoparticles [71]. For instance, higher uptake in HIV-infected macrophages is observed when compared to uninfected cells when efavirenz loaded poly(propylene imine) dendrimers are used [72]. Other examples of nanoparticle formulations for AIDS are summarized in Table **3.2**.

Table 3.2. Therapeutic nanoparticle drug formulations for the treatment of AIDS disease.

Nanostructure	Nanoparticle	Conjugated Drug	Ref.
Polymeric Nanoparticles	Poly(hexylcyanoacrylate) nanoparticles	Zidovudine	73
	Poly (isohexyl cyanate) nanoparticles		74
	Poly(ethylene oxide)-poly (propylene oxide) polymeric micelles	Efavirenz	75
	PPI dendrimer		76
	PLGA nanoparticles	Ritonavir, Lopinavir, Efavirenz	77, 78
	Poly(epsilon-caprolactone)	Saquinavir	79
Liposome	Mannosylated and galactosylated liposomes	Stavudine	80

Table 3.3. Nanomedicine-based applications for autoimmune disease treatments.

Autoimmune Diseases	Drug/Agent	Nano Formulation	Composition	Potential Mechanism	Ref.
Rheumatoid arthritis	siRNA	Liposome	-	Suppress inflammatory cytokine	81
Rheumatoid arthritis	Methotrexate		Cholesterol and Egg phosphatidylcholine	Enhance retention time	63
Systemic lupus erythematosus	Glucocorticoids		Soybean phosphatidylcholine and cholesterol	Target accumulation of the drug	82

(Table 3) cont.....

Autoimmune Diseases	Drug/Agent	Nano Formulation	Composition	Potential Mechanism	Ref.
Multiple sclerosis	Myelin	Polymeric Nanoparticles	Poly (lactic-c- -glycolic acid)	immunosuppression by downregulation of Th1 and Th17 cytokines,	83
Multiple sclerosis	IFN β		PEGylated IFN β	Reduce relapse rate	84
Crohn's disease	Certolizumab pegol		-	Neutralize TNF α	85
Multiple sclerosis	DNA peptide		-	Produce anti-inflammatory cytokines	86
Rheumatoid arthritis	PEG	Nanoparticles	Gold	Inhibiting the activity of the angiogenic factor, reducing inflammation and macrophage infiltration	87, 88, 89
Experimental autoimmune encephalomyelitis	PEG MOG35–55 AhR ligand	Nanoparticles	Gold	Induce tolerogenic APCs	90, 91
Rheumatoid arthritis	Decoy oligodeoxynucleotides	Nanorods	Gold	Reduce the production of TNF a and IL-6	92
Scleroderma	Plasmid DNA	Gemini surfactant-based nanoparticle	-	Enhance cutaneous IFN γ levels	93, 94
Collagen type II-induced arthritis	Methotrexate	Nanosheet	BPNs/Chitosan/PRP	Photoablation-induced cell death	95

Cardiovascular Disease

The cardiovascular system (CVS) consists of the heart and blood vessels play a vital role in circulating blood, nutrients, and other components throughout the body. Dysfunction of this system may lead to various diseases known as cardiovascular diseases (CVDs) [96]. CVDs includes disease like myocardial infarction, atherosclerosis and may also affect vascular systems of the brain, kidney, and peripheral tissues. CVDs are still the leading causes of death globally despite many treatment strategies.

Current treatment strategies for CVDs are practiced at three different levels. At the first-level, health status of a susceptible individual is monitored and possible risk factors (smoking, diet, mental health, and pollution) which may agitate CVDs are prevented. At the second level, risk factors (hypertension, dyslipidemia, and diabetes) linked to the disease are modified. At the final level, the CVD progression is prevented and controlled using medicaments [97]. Recent focus is shifted towards the use of nanoparticle-based formulations and to increase the bioavailability and enhanced retention in the targeted tissue for effective treatment.

Therapeutic molecules, peptides, and genes loaded gold NPs containing ethylene glycol, heparin, and hyaluronan citrate have shown improved conductivity in the cardiac patch. Improved antibacterial activity in heart valves was observed when silver NPs were prepared using similar components. Similarly, PEGylated liposomes containing cytokines and growth factors are used as a vehicle for site-specific targeting within the heart post-myocardial infarction (MI) [98]. Cardiac tissue regeneration was observed post-MI when Pluronic F-127 was used as a functionalized ligand [99]. Various nanoparticle formulations in various proportions and dimensions are used in CVDs treatment, theranostic, and as biosensors including tissue engineering which are briefly discussed in Table **3.4** [100].

Table 3.4. Various Nanoparticles used in Cardiovascular applications.

Formulation	Nanoparticle/Drug	Significant Outcomes	Field of Application	Ref.
Carbon Nanotubes	MWCNTs/dipyridamole	enhanced dissolution	Drug delivery	101
liposome	Sirolimus	inhibit vascular restenosis		102
Niosome	Carvedilol	1.7–2.3-fold increased plasma concentrations, enhanced bioavailability, and therapeutic effect		103
Solid lipid nanoparticle	Resveratrol	enhanced oral bioavailability and controlled release		104
Liposome				104
Polymeric particle	vascular endothelial growth factor (VEGF)	tissue remodeling in an acute myocardial ischemic model		105,106
	PLGA-Heparin	Anticoagulant		107
	ligand-binding polymeric micelles	aids in visualizing and treating atherosclerotic lesions		108

(Table 4) cont.....

Formulation	Nanoparticle/Drug	Significant Outcomes	Field of Application	Ref.
Graphene and its derivatives	Boron-doped silicon nanowires	Multiple CVDs	Biosensor	109
	Cu nanoparticles/laser-induced graphene	The detection limit was between 0.001 and 6 mM for glucose		110
	Gold-graphene oxide	Electrochemical immunosensor for label-free detection of cardiac marker troponin I and myoglobin		111
	GCE/CeO2–Au nanofibers/GO	A wide detection range of 0.01–1000 µmol/l for amlodipine drug		112
Carbon Nanotubes	Au/ZnO/MWCNTs	The detection range of cholesterol was between 0.1 and 100 µM		113
	SWCNT/Collagen hydrogel	enhanced mechanical strength and electrical conductivity	Tissue engineering	114
	3D printable SWCNTs ink/bacterial nanocellulose cardiac patch	Similar conductivity and elasticity		115
Graphene and its derivatives	rGO/Gelatin methacryloyl (GelMA) hybrid hydrogel	Better mechanical, electrical properties, cellular attachment, and maturation		116
	rGO–reinforced gellan gum hydrogel	Mechanical properties are similar to the native myocardium with no cellular toxicity.		117
	Graphene oxide foam chip	Improved cell attachment, spreading, organization, and beating function		118
	Heparin loaded polycaprolactone/chitosan/ polypyrrole /functionalized graphene cardiac patch	Improved mechanical and electrical properties with biocompatibility		119

SWCNTs: Single-walled Carbon Nanotubes: MWCNTs: Multi-walled Carbon Nanotubes; rGO: reduced graphene oxide; GO: graphene oxide; Au: gold; ZnO: Zinc oxide; GCE: glassy carbon electrode; GelMA: methacrylated gelatin.

Infectious Diseases

Infectious diseases sometimes referred to as contagious diseases are caused by pathogens like bacteria, viruses, and fungi. Infectious diseases can be spread among people from an infected person to a healthy person. The use of antimicrobial drugs for treating infectious diseases is the major therapeutic approach, but with time these pathogens can develop resistance. Pathogens can develop resistance through numerous mechanisms. DNA alterations, development of multidrug efflux pumps, modification in membrane permeability, increase in the intracellular lifecycle are some of them. In such cases, the normal therapeutic doses are ineffective so, the dose administered and frequency of dosing should be increased. Chronic administration can enhance the chances of systematic adverse effects and toxicity. The use of nanoformulations can overcome such limitations and can be promising in treating infectious diseases [120]. Nanoparticles effective against some resistant strains are given in Table **3.5**.

Table 3.5. Drug-Nanoparticles effective against resistant strains.

Pathogen	Resistant to	Nanoparticle	Conjugated Drug	Ref.
C. albicans	Fluconazole	AgNP	Fluconazole	121
E. coli	Ampicillin	AuNP and AgNP	Ampicillin	122, 2
HIV-infected cells with drug efflux pumps	Multiple drug resistance	Polymeric micelles	Nelfinavir and saquinavir	123
		Silica NP	Penicillin	124
		Chitosan NP	Streptomycin	125
P. aeruginosa	Ampicillin	AgNP	Ampicillin	126
S. aureus	β-lactam, penicillin, and cephalosporins	Liposome	β-Lactam, and penicillin	127
		PLA NP	Penicillin	128
		AuNP and AgNP	Ampicillin	122, 2
***S. aureus* strains**	Vancomycin	AuNP	Vancomycin	122
Enterococcus species	Vancomycin	Liposome	Vancomycin	129
		AuNP		130
P. aeruginosa	Polycationic antibiotics	Liposome	Polymyxin B	131
Plasmodium species	Chloroquine	Liposome	Chloroquine	132
E. coli	Tetracycline	ZnO-PEI NP	Tetracycline	133
P. aeruginosa	Multidrug resistant	Chitosan AuNP	Ciprofloxacin	134

Nano formulations for infectious diseases include both polymers-based, Non-polymer based and Lipid-based NPs. Amphotericin B containing anti-fungal liposome (Ambiosome®) reduces amphotericin-associated toxicity [135]. This formulation can also be used in highly immunocompromised HIV patients. Similarly, another drug ciprofloxacin, a broad-spectrum antibiotic is marketed as Lipoquin™. It is a sustained liposomal preparation reducing systematic side effects. Furthermore, nanoparticles are also used as medical devices such as Silverline® and Acticoat™ [136 - 138]. A brief list of therapeutic nanoparticles for the treatment and prevention of infectious diseases is listed in Table **3.6**.

Table 3.6. Therapeutic nanoparticles for treatment and prevention of infectious diseases.

Pathogen	Disease Caused	Nanoparticle	Conjugated Drug	Ref.
C. Albicans	Candidiasis, UTI	Metallic nanoparticle (AgNP)	Fluconazole	121
		Solid Lipid Nanoparticles (SLNs)	Terpinene-4-ol	139
E. Coli	Pneumonia, UTI, meningitis, liver abscess, Gastroenteritis, Post-surgical wound infection	Metallic nanoparticle (AuNP and AgNP)	Ampicillin	140
		Metallic nanoparticle (ZnO-PEI)	Tetracycline	141
		PLGA NPs	Nafcillin and levofloxacin	142
		polymeric nanoparticles	Ciprofloxacin and levofloxacin	143
HIV	AIDS	Solid Lipid Nanoparticles (SLNs)	Saquinavir	144
P. Aeruginosa	Cystic fibrosis, folliculitis, acute external otitis	Metallic nanoparticle (AgNP)	Polymyxin B	145
		Metallic nanoparticle (AgNP)	Ampicillin	146
		Solid Lipid Nanoparticles (SLNs)	Ciprofloxacin	147
Plasmodium sp.	Malaria	Liposome	Chloroquine	132
S. Aureus	Impetigo, cellulitis, abscess, pneumonia, various skin infections	Liposome	β-Lactam	127
		Chitosan NP	Vancomycin	148
		Metallic nanoparticle (AuNP)		2
		Polymeric nanoparticle (PLA NP)	Penicillin	128
		Silica nanoparticle		124
		Liposome		127
		Chitosan NP	Streptomycin	125
		Metallic nanoparticle (AuNP and AgNP)	Ampicillin	122

AgNP: Silver Nanoparticles; AuNP: Gold Nanoparticles; PLA NP: polylactic acid nanoparticles; PLGA NPs: Poly (lactic-co-glycolic acid) Nanoparticles.

Cancer

Cancer is the general term used for a large group of diseases affecting any part of the body. It may arise due to the transformation of healthy cells into tumor cells in several stages. These stages can vary from a pre-cancerous lesion to a malignant tumor. This arises due to the interaction between an individual genetic factor and a carcinogen [149]. Carcinogens are usually agents that may agitate or initiate cancer in a patient. These carcinogens are usually divided into three types depending upon their source. Physical carcinogens include ionizing radiation and ultraviolet light. Asbestos, arsenic, and smoke from tobacco come under chemical carcinogens whereas infections caused by certain bacteria, fungi, and viruses are termed as biological carcinogens [150].

Cancer is the major cause of death globally with 10 million deaths in 2020 alone. Breast, lung, colon, and rectum cancer were among the top three cancers in 2020 in terms of new cases registered. While, most deaths were caused due to lung, colorectal, and liver cancer. The major therapeutic approach for cancer treatment is chemotherapy. Lack of aqueous solubility, tumor specificity, and the existence of dose-dependent toxicity and multidrug resistance is the major concern for chemotherapeutic agents [151].

The use of the nanoparticulate system for the treatment of cancers can overcome these limitations. Optimization of the therapeutic dose, and delivery of the drug in a controlled manner at the desired target site can be achieved by nanocarriers. Among all the nanoparticles used, the majority of them are focused on treating cancer. A plethora of nanoparticles is used that target the tumor cells by either passive or active targeting. Defective lymphatic drainage and leaky vasculature are some of the characteristic features of tumor cells that distinguish them from normal cells. NPs owing to their small size can exhibit enhanced permeability and retention (EPR) effect [152]. They can easily penetrate and accumulate more in tumor cells offering passive targeting. While functionalization of the nanoparticle surface with receptor-specific ligands can lead to active targeting.

Doxil®, a PEGylated liposome preparation of the drug doxorubicin was the first therapeutic nanoparticle approved by USFDA for the treatment of cancer [153]. The use of polymer polyethylene glycol (PEG) resulted in higher circulation time. Similarly, nanoliposome formulation of irinotecan is used for pancreatic and colorectal cancer. There are several other lipid-based formulations present in the market. For instance, Vyxeos® an intravenous liposome prepared using Distearoyl-phosphatidylcholine, Distearoylphosphatidylglycerol, and Cholesterol was approved by USFDA in the year 2017. It comprises daunorubicin and cytarabine in a 1:5 molar ratio recommended for acute myeloid leukemia. Table **3.7** summarizes several other nanoparticles used in cancer therapy.

Table 3.7. Nanoparticles in Cancer therapy.

Formulation Type	Product	Drug	Drug Class	Main Indication(s)	Adverse Reactions	Ref.
Lipid-based (Non-liposomal)	Onpattro®	Transthyretin targeted siRNA	-	Transthyretin-mediated amyloidosis	Upper respiratory tract infections	154

(Table 7) cont.....

Formulation Type	Product	Drug	Drug Class	Main Indication(s)	Adverse Reactions	Ref.
Liposomes	Marqibo®	Vincristine sulfate	-	Acute lymphoid leukemia	Constipation, Pyrexia, febrile neutropenia, peripheral neuropathy	155
	Doxil®	Doxorubicin	Anthracycline topoisomerase inhibitor	Ovarian cancer, AIDS-related Kaposi's Sarcoma	Anorexia, Stomatitis, neutropenia, Thrombocytopenia	156
	Mepact®	Mifamurtide	Immunomodulator, Anti-tumour	Non-metastasizing osteosarcoma	Muscle spasms, hypersensitivity reactions	157
	Onivyde®	Irinotecan	Topoisomerase inhibitor	Pancreatic cancer, Colorectal cancer	Fatigue, decreased appetite, stomatitis, pyrexia	158
	DepoCyte®	Cytarabine	nucleoside metabolic inhibitor	Neoplastic meningitis	Arachnoiditis, abnormal gait, convulsions, pyrexia	159
	DaunoXome®	Daunorubicin citrate	Anthracycline topoisomerase inhibitor	Acute myeloid leukemia	febrile neutropenia, mucositis, dyspnea, edema	159
	Vyxeos®	Daunorubicin Cytarabine	Anthracycline topoisomerase inhibitor, nucleoside metabolic inhibitor	Acute myeloid leukemia	febrile neutropenia, mucositis, dyspnea, edema	160
	Myocet®	Doxorubicin	Anthracycline topoisomerase inhibitor	Metastatic breast cancer	Fatigue, stomatitis, neutropenia, hand and foot syndrome	159
Pegylated liposome	LipoDox®	Doxorubicin	Anthracycline topoisomerase inhibitor	Acquired immune deficiency syndrome (AIDS)-related Kaposi's sarcoma	hand and foot syndrome, rash, neutropenia, thrombocytopenia, and anemia	159

(Table 7) cont.....

Formulation Type	Product	Drug	Drug Class	Main Indication(s)	Adverse Reactions	Ref.
Protein-drug conjugates	Kadcyla®	Trastuzumab	HER2-targeted antibody and microtubule inhibitor	HER2+ breast cancer	musculoskeletal pain, thrombocytopenia, headache, increased transaminases, and constipation	161
	Abraxane®	Paclitaxel	Microtubule inhibitor	Non-small lung cancer, Pancreatic cancer	neutropenia, thrombocytopenia, alopecia, peripheral neuropathy	162
	Ontak®	Denileukin diftitox	CD-25 cytotoxin	Cutaneous T-cell lymphoma	pyrexia, nausea, fatigue, rigors, peripheral edema, cough, dyspnea, and pruritus	156
	Oncaspar®	L-asparaginase enzyme	asparagine specific enzyme	Acute lymphocytic leukemia	thrombosis, coagulopathy, elevated transaminases, hyperbilirubinemia, hyperglycemia	156
Micelles	Genexol-TM ®	Paclitaxel	Microtubule inhibitor	Breast cancer and non-small cell lung cancer (NSCLC)	neutropenia, thrombocytopenia, alopecia, peripheral neuropathy	156
Metallic nanoparticles	NanoTherm ®	-	-	Glioblastoma, prostate, pancreatic cancer	-	163

Adverse reactions were obtained online from **http://labels.fda.gov**

Pulmonary diseases

Cystic fibrosis, asthma, pulmonary tuberculosis, chronic obstructive pulmonary disease (COPD), idiopathic pulmonary fibrosis (IPF), and cancers affecting the lungs are categorized into pulmonary diseases [164]. Most of these diseases can only be managed and cannot be cured completely. The currently employed pharmacotherapy utilizing a variety of peptides, drugs, and even genetic material like siRNA, shRNA, and miRNA is proven to be insufficient. The use of nanoscale carriers has proven to be effective in improving pharmacokinetic parameters and decreasing side effects owing to its unique physical properties.

Nanoparticles used in pulmonary diseases can be broadly classified into two main groups. Nanoparticles for cancerous pulmonary diseases and those for non-cancerous pulmonary disease. The early focus was more concentrated on cancerous pulmonary diseases but recent advancement in technologies has shifted the focus to other diseases like asthma, cystic fibrosis, and COPD [165]. Inhalation formulations of solid lipid nanoparticles and liposomes are used for chronic lung diseases as they are stable during aerosolization. Lipid-based particles like cholesterol and phosphatidylcholine are biocompatible and can easily be fabricated making them the obvious choice for formulations. Polymer-based NPs comprise a different set of polymers each having a unique property. For example, Polyethylene glycol (PEG) owing to its bioinert nature is used for surface functionalization [166]. PEGylated NPs can evade opsonization by immune cells. Similarly, poly ethylene imine (PEI), a cationic polymer can easily bind to nucleotides and is effective in gene delivery. Dendrimers due to their size and surface morphology can carry a large therapeutic payload and PEG-coated dendrimers have shown better pulmonary absorption after inhalation [167]. Furthermore, in experimental animal models tested for asthma and pulmonary fibrosis, SLN of curcumin was proven to be effective [168]. The results of Poly (lactic-co-glycolic acid) (PLGA) conjugated with Pirfenidone were also promising. Table **3.8** provides some insights on nanoformulations in the treatment of pulmonary diseases.

CHALLENGES IN NANOPARTICULATE DRUG DELIVERY SYSTEMS

The use of NPs as drug carriers gives promising results for the treatment of several diseases including cancer. Apart from their use as a nanocarrier, they are also used as diagnostic and biosensing agents. Unfortunately, the use of these nano-sized particles comes up with some limitations, which include nanoparticulate toxicity, immune system evasion, and elution of unnecessary immune responses [159, 178].

Table 3.8. Nanoparticles in pulmonary therapy.

Formulation Type	Composition	Drug	Indication(s)	Ref.
Polymeric nanoparticles	Poly (gamma-benzyl L-glutamate)-blo-k-hyaluronan (*PBLG-b-HYA*)	Gefitinib	Lung Cancer	169
	Poly (lactic-co-glycolic acid) (PLGA)	Celecoxib		170
	Polymeric micelles	Budesonide	Asthma	171
Dendrimers	Poly (amidoamine)	Doxorubicin	Non-Small Cell Lung Cancer	172
	Polylysine			173
Nanostructured lipid carriers	Precirol, Stearic acid, and Beeswax	Sildenafil	Pulmonary arterial hypertension	174
	Squalene and Procirol	Lumacaftor Ivacaftor	Cystic fibrosis	175

(Table 8) cont.....

Formulation Type	Composition	Drug	Indication(s)	Ref.
Liposome	Dimyristoyl phosphatidylcholine Cholesterol	Ciprofloxacin	Respiratory tract infections	176
	Egg phosphatidylcholine and Cholesterol	Procaterol	Asthma and COPD	177

The major challenge is their different *in vitro* and *in vivo* behavior, which needs to be scientifically investigated in more animal models. They mainly differ in aspects related to bioavailability, diffusion, and cellular interactions. Size can also play a vital role in its *in vivo* behavior. The smaller the size of NPs, the greater the chance of their cellular and systemic toxicity. Poor biodistribution is exhibited by some dendrimers and QDs, which may be a result of particle aggregation due to small size. Nano formulations designed to treat cancer may have concerns with the heterogeneous nature of tumors. Tumors may differ in their molecular patterns and gene expression profiles. These may limit the penetration and effectiveness of tumor-targeted NPs to a great extent [179].

Mass production of NPs may also arise questions on the upscaling procedures employed. Even, the characterization of NPs may be time-consuming and batch-to-batch variations may further hamper the production. Moreover, problems may be formulation specific. Dendrimers have limited administration routes and may exhibit particle aggregation inside the biological system. Polymers in some polymeric NPs may swell/burst on initial contact with the biological system, eluting the entire drug at once. Initial burst protection may be required in such cases. QDs irrespective of their numerous advantages exhibit cellular toxicity which cannot be neglected. Studies have also shown high toxicity in hepatocyte culture due to leakage of metal ions from QDs. Insufficient persistent emission of active pharmaceutical ingredient (API) may be seen in polymeric micelles and engineered NPs like nanocrystals [159]. Furthermore, lack of administration routes, cytotoxicity due to surfactants used, and rapid uptake by the reticuloendothelial system (RES) is the major concern in lipid-based nanoformulations.

CONCLUSION

Over the years, nanoparticulate therapeutic systems are extensively studied and are of prime importance owing to their targeted delivery. Most NPs are designed and developed for treating only one disease, but research is underway for treating more diseases. NPs made of lipids or polymer is most commonly used. The structural similarity of lipids with cell membranes helps them in reaching sites otherwise inaccessible. Polymeric NPs are also widely used but most of them require surface functionalization unlike those made of lipids. Even with limitations like cytotoxicity, biocompatibility, and difficult scaling procedure, NPs are promising in disease therapy.

The prime focus has been shifted to nanoparticle delivery systems owing to their increased bioavailability, reduced toxicity, and improved targeting. Still, clearance, metabolism, and toxicity need to be further studied and elaborated. Even though there are many studies of nanoformulations containing drugs, only a few address formulations containing genes, enzymes, and RNA/DNA. Moreover, there are many challenges on the way to the market. Ethical, financial, and regulatory being the major ones. Most clinical trials of NPs are on diseased patients or patients with no clinical benefits from conventional drugs. While the cost/benefit ratio of nanoformulations prevents them from entering clinical trials. The major concern for progressive trials is their benefit/harm ratio. Regulations laid by regulatory bodies such as FDA and EMA are not constant and undergo periodical changes that affect nanoformulations. Even designated test procedures, assays of active ingredients, and determinants in the pharmacopeia are limited to drugs and conventional dosage forms and do not address nanoformulations.

Most of the nanoformulations are still prepared using conventional methods which need further improvement and optimization. Lack of characterization/ evaluation methods and limited reports on its safety studies also hinders its chances for approval. If concerns regarding upscaling procedures, and characterization are addressed then, nanoformulations will the choice of future for effective delivery of medicines safely and effectively.

CONSENT FOR PUBLICATION

Not applicable.

CONFLICT OF INTEREST

The authors declare no conflict of interest, financial or otherwise.

ACKNOWLEDGEMENT

Declared none.

REFERENCES

[1] Thassu D, Pathak Y, Deleers M. Nanoparticulate drug-delivery systems: An overview.CRC Press 2007.
[http://dx.doi.org/10.1201/9781420008449]

[2] Yetisgin AA, Cetinel S, Zuvin M, Kosar A, Kutlu O. Therapeutic nanoparticles and their targeted delivery applications. Molecules 2020; 25(9): 2193.
[http://dx.doi.org/10.3390/molecules25092193] [PMID: 32397080]

[3] Torchilin V. Introduction. Nanocarriers for drug delivery: Needs and requirements.Nanoparticulates as drug carriers. World Scientific 2006; pp. 1-8.
[http://dx.doi.org/10.1142/p432]

[4] Reinholz J, Landfester K, Mailänder V. The challenges of oral drug delivery *via* nanocarriers. Drug Deliv 2018; 25(1): 1694-705.
[http://dx.doi.org/10.1080/10717544.2018.1501119] [PMID: 30394120]

[5] Palmer B, DeLouise L. Nanoparticle-enabled transdermal drug delivery systems for enhanced dose control and tissue targeting. Molecules 2016; 21(12): 1719.
[http://dx.doi.org/10.3390/molecules21121719] [PMID: 27983701]

[6] Chenthamara D, Subramaniam S, Ramakrishnan SG, *et al.* Therapeutic efficacy of nanoparticles and routes of administration. Biomater Res 2019; 23(1): 20.
[http://dx.doi.org/10.1186/s40824-019-0166-x] [PMID: 31832232]

[7] Mansour H, Haemosu , Wu X. Nanomedicine in pulmonary delivery. Int J Nanomedicine 2009; 4: 299-319.
[http://dx.doi.org/10.2147/IJN.S4937] [PMID: 20054434]

[8] Ghezzi M, Pescina S, Padula C, *et al.* Polymeric micelles in drug delivery: An insight of the techniques for their characterization and assessment in biorelevant conditions. J Control Release 2021; 332: 312-36.
[http://dx.doi.org/10.1016/j.jconrel.2021.02.031] [PMID: 33652113]

[9] Ghosh B, Biswas S. Polymeric micelles in cancer therapy: State of the art. J Control Release 2021; 332: 127-47.
[http://dx.doi.org/10.1016/j.jconrel.2021.02.016] [PMID: 33609621]

[10] Ringsdorf H, Ed. Structure and properties of pharmacologically active polymers.Journal of Polymer Science: Polymer Symposia. Wiley Online Library 1975.

[11] Canal F, Sanchis J, Vicent MJ. Polymer–drug conjugates as nano-sized medicines. Curr Opin Biotechnol 2011; 22(6): 894-900.
[http://dx.doi.org/10.1016/j.copbio.2011.06.003] [PMID: 21724381]

[12] Marasini N, Haque S, Kaminskas LM. Polymer-drug conjugates as inhalable drug delivery systems: A review. Curr Opin Colloid Interface Sci 2017; 31: 18-29.
[http://dx.doi.org/10.1016/j.cocis.2017.06.003]

[13] Thakor P, Bhavana V, Sharma R, Srivastava S, Singh SB, Mehra NK. Polymer–drug conjugates: Recent advances and future perspectives. Drug Discov Today 2020; 25(9): 1718-26.
[http://dx.doi.org/10.1016/j.drudis.2020.06.028] [PMID: 32629170]

[14] Tahara Y, Akiyoshi K. Current advances in self-assembled nanogel delivery systems for immunotherapy. Adv Drug Deliv Rev 2015; 95: 65-76.
[http://dx.doi.org/10.1016/j.addr.2015.10.004] [PMID: 26482187]

[15] Akiyoshi K, Deguchi S, Moriguchi N, Yamaguchi S, Sunamoto J. Self-aggregates of hydrophobized polysaccharides in water. Formation and characteristics of nanoparticles. Macromolecules 1993; 26(12): 3062-8.
[http://dx.doi.org/10.1021/ma00064a011]

[16] Neamtu I, Rusu AG, Diaconu A, Nita LE, Chiriac AP. Basic concepts and recent advances in nanogels as carriers for medical applications. Drug Deliv 2017; 24(1): 539-57.
[http://dx.doi.org/10.1080/10717544.2016.1276232] [PMID: 28181831]

[17] Hsu HJ, Bugno J, Lee S, Hong S. Dendrimer-based nanocarriers: A versatile platform for drug delivery. Wiley Interdiscip Rev Nanomed Nanobiotechnol 2017; 9(1): e1409.
[http://dx.doi.org/10.1002/wnan.1409] [PMID: 27126551]

[18] Palmerston Mendes L, Pan J, Torchilin V. Dendrimers as nanocarriers for nucleic acid and drug

delivery in cancer therapy. Molecules 2017; 22(9): 1401.
[http://dx.doi.org/10.3390/molecules22091401] [PMID: 28832535]

[19] Crucho CIC, Barros MT. Polymeric nanoparticles: A study on the preparation variables and characterization methods. Mater Sci Eng C 2017; 80: 771-84.
[http://dx.doi.org/10.1016/j.msec.2017.06.004] [PMID: 28866227]

[20] Letchford K, Liggins R, Wasan KM, Burt H. *in vitro* human plasma distribution of nanoparticulate paclitaxel is dependent on the physicochemical properties of poly(ethylene glycol)-bloc--poly(caprolactone) nanoparticles. Eur J Pharm Biopharm 2009; 71(2): 196-206.
[http://dx.doi.org/10.1016/j.ejpb.2008.08.003] [PMID: 18762253]

[21] Peng Z, Han X, Li S, *et al.* Carbon dots: Biomacromolecule interaction, bioimaging and nanomedicine. Coord Chem Rev 2017; 343: 256-77.
[http://dx.doi.org/10.1016/j.ccr.2017.06.001]

[22] Mishra V, Patil A, Thakur S, Kesharwani P. Carbon dots: Emerging theranostic nanoarchitectures. Drug Discov Today 2018; 23(6): 1219-32.
[http://dx.doi.org/10.1016/j.drudis.2018.01.006] [PMID: 29366761]

[23] Liu J, Li R, Yang B. Carbon dots: A new type of carbon-based nanomaterial with wide applications. ACS Cent Sci 2020; 6(12): 2179-95.
[http://dx.doi.org/10.1021/acscentsci.0c01306] [PMID: 33376780]

[24] Iijima S. Helical microtubules of graphitic carbon. Nature 1991; 354(6348): 56-8.

[25] Wong BS, Yoong SL, Jagusiak A, *et al.* Carbon nanotubes for delivery of small molecule drugs. Adv Drug Deliv Rev 2013; 65(15): 1964-2015.
[http://dx.doi.org/10.1016/j.addr.2013.08.005] [PMID: 23954402]

[26] Ravi Kiran AVVV, Kusuma Kumari G, Krishnamurthy PT. Carbon nanotubes in drug delivery: Focus on anticancer therapies. J Drug Deliv Sci Technol 2020; 59: 101892.
[http://dx.doi.org/10.1016/j.jddst.2020.101892]

[27] Al-Qattan MN, Deb PK, Tekade RK. Molecular dynamics simulation strategies for designing carbon-nanotube-based targeted drug delivery. Drug Discov Today 2018; 23(2): 235-50.
[http://dx.doi.org/10.1016/j.drudis.2017.10.002] [PMID: 29031623]

[28] Vashist SK, Zheng D, Pastorin G, Al-Rubeaan K, Luong JHT, Sheu FS. Delivery of drugs and biomolecules using carbon nanotubes. Carbon 2011; 49(13): 4077-97.
[http://dx.doi.org/10.1016/j.carbon.2011.05.049]

[29] Kim H, Beack S, Han S, *et al.* Multifunctional photonic nanomaterials for diagnostic, therapeutic, and theranostic applications. Adv Mater 2018; 30(10): 1701460.
[http://dx.doi.org/10.1002/adma.201701460] [PMID: 29363198]

[30] Iga AM, Robertson JH, Winslet MC, Seifalian AM. Clinical potential of quantum dots. Journal of Biomedicine and Biotechnology 2007; 2007
[http://dx.doi.org/10.1155/2007/76087]

[31] Matea C, Mocan T, Tabaran F, *et al.* Quantum dots in imaging, drug delivery and sensor applications. Int J Nanomedicine 2017; 12: 5421-31.
[http://dx.doi.org/10.2147/IJN.S138624] [PMID: 28814860]

[32] Bailey RE, Smith AM, Nie S. Quantum dots in biology and medicine. Physica E 2004; 25(1): 1-12.
[http://dx.doi.org/10.1016/j.physe.2004.07.013]

[33] Chen F, Hableel G, Zhao ER, Jokerst JV. Multifunctional nanomedicine with silica: Role of silica in nanoparticles for theranostic, imaging, and drug monitoring. J Colloid Interface Sci 2018; 521: 261-79.
[http://dx.doi.org/10.1016/j.jcis.2018.02.053] [PMID: 29510868]

[34] Bagheri E, Ansari L, Abnous K, *et al.* Silica based hybrid materials for drug delivery and bioimaging. J Control Release 2018; 277: 57-76.

[http://dx.doi.org/10.1016/j.jconrel.2018.03.014] [PMID: 29550399]

[35] Mura S, Nicolas J, Couvreur P. Stimuli-responsive nanocarriers for drug delivery. Nat Mater 2013; 12(11): 991-1003.
[http://dx.doi.org/10.1038/nmat3776] [PMID: 24150417]

[36] Torres Sangiao E, Holban AM, Gestal MC. Applications of nanodiamonds in the detection and therapy of infectious diseases. Materials (Basel) 2019; 12(10): 1639.
[http://dx.doi.org/10.3390/ma12101639] [PMID: 31137476]

[37] Man HB, Ho D. Nanodiamonds as platforms for biology and medicine. SLAS Technol 2013; 18(1): 12-8.
[http://dx.doi.org/10.1177/2211068212456198] [PMID: 22933615]

[38] Ho D, Wang CHK, Chow EKH. Nanodiamonds: The intersection of nanotechnology, drug development, and personalized medicine. Sci Adv 2015; 1(7): e1500439.
[http://dx.doi.org/10.1126/sciadv.1500439] [PMID: 26601235]

[39] Singh P, Pandit S, Mokkapati VRSS, Garg A, Ravikumar V, Mijakovic I. Gold nanoparticles in diagnostics and therapeutics for human cancer. Int J Mol Sci 2018; 19(7): 1979.
[http://dx.doi.org/10.3390/ijms19071979] [PMID: 29986450]

[40] Singh S, Vidyarthi AS, Nigam VK, Dev A. Extracellular facile biosynthesis, characterization and stability of gold nanoparticles by *Bacillus licheniformis*. Artif Cells Nanomed Biotechnol 2014; 42(1): 6-12.
[http://dx.doi.org/10.3109/21691401.2012.759122] [PMID: 23438180]

[41] Cuenca AG, Jiang H, Hochwald SN, Delano M, Cance WG, Grobmyer SR. Emerging implications of nanotechnology on cancer diagnostics and therapeutics. Cancer 2006; 107(3): 459-66.
[http://dx.doi.org/10.1002/cncr.22035] [PMID: 16795065]

[42] Masse F, Ouellette M, Lamoureux G, Boisselier E. Gold nanoparticles in ophthalmology. Med Res Rev 2019; 39(1): 302-27.
[http://dx.doi.org/10.1002/med.21509] [PMID: 29766541]

[43] Buse J, El-Aneed A. Properties, engineering and applications of lipid-based nanoparticle drug-delivery systems: Current research and advances. Nanomedicine (Lond) 2010; 5(8): 1237-60.
[http://dx.doi.org/10.2217/nnm.10.107] [PMID: 21039200]

[44] Daraee H, Etemadi A, Kouhi M, Alimirzalu S, Akbarzadeh A. Application of liposomes in medicine and drug delivery. Artif Cells Nanomed Biotechnol 2016; 44(1): 381-91.
[http://dx.doi.org/10.3109/21691401.2014.953633] [PMID: 25222036]

[45] Gabizon A, Catane R, Uziely B, *et al.* Prolonged circulation time and enhanced accumulation in malignant exudates of doxorubicin encapsulated in polyethylene-glycol coated liposomes. Cancer Res 1994; 54(4): 987-92.
[PMID: 8313389]

[46] Rahmati S, Shojaei F, Shojaeian A, Rezakhani L, Dehkordi MB. An overview of current knowledge in biological functions and potential theragnostic applications of exosomes. Chem Phys Lipids 2020; 226: 104836.
[http://dx.doi.org/10.1016/j.chemphyslip.2019.104836] [PMID: 31678051]

[47] Batrakova EV, Kim MS. Using exosomes, naturally-equipped nanocarriers, for drug delivery. J Control Release 2015; 219: 396-405.
[http://dx.doi.org/10.1016/j.jconrel.2015.07.030] [PMID: 26241750]

[48] Familtseva A, Jeremic N, Tyagi SC. Exosomes: Cell-created drug delivery systems. Mol Cell Biochem 2019; 459(1-2): 1-6.
[http://dx.doi.org/10.1007/s11010-019-03545-4] [PMID: 31073888]

[49] Wu P, Zhang B, Shi H, Qian H, Xu W. MSC-exosome: A novel cell-free therapy for cutaneous regeneration. Cytotherapy 2018; 20(3): 291-301.

[http://dx.doi.org/10.1016/j.jcyt.2017.11.002] [PMID: 29434006]

[50] de Jesus MB, Zuhorn IS. Solid lipid nanoparticles as nucleic acid delivery system: Properties and molecular mechanisms. J Control Release 2015; 201: 1-13.
[http://dx.doi.org/10.1016/j.jconrel.2015.01.010] [PMID: 25578828]

[51] Doktorovova S, Souto EB, Silva AM. Nanotoxicology applied to solid lipid nanoparticles and nanostructured lipid carriers – A systematic review of *in vitro* data. Eur J Pharm Biopharm 2014; 87(1): 1-18.
[http://dx.doi.org/10.1016/j.ejpb.2014.02.005] [PMID: 24530885]

[52] Ezzati Nazhad Dolatabadi J, Valizadeh H, Hamishehkar H. Solid lipid nanoparticles as efficient drug and gene delivery systems: Recent breakthroughs. Adv Pharm Bull 2015; 5(2): 151-9.
[http://dx.doi.org/10.15171/apb.2015.022] [PMID: 26236652]

[53] Rostami E, Kashanian S, Azandaryani AH, Faramarzi H, Dolatabadi JEN, Omidfar K. Drug targeting using solid lipid nanoparticles. Chem Phys Lipids 2014; 181: 56-61.
[http://dx.doi.org/10.1016/j.chemphyslip.2014.03.006] [PMID: 24717692]

[54] Shen H, Shi S, Zhang Z, Gong T, Sun X. Coating solid lipid nanoparticles with hyaluronic acid enhances antitumor activity against melanoma stem-like cells. Theranostics 2015; 5(7): 755-71.
[http://dx.doi.org/10.7150/thno.10804] [PMID: 25897340]

[55] Weber S, Zimmer A, Pardeike J. Solid Lipid Nanoparticles (SLN) and Nanostructured Lipid Carriers (NLC) for pulmonary application: A review of the state of the art. Eur J Pharm Biopharm 2014; 86(1): 7-22.
[http://dx.doi.org/10.1016/j.ejpb.2013.08.013] [PMID: 24007657]

[56] Luo Y, Teng Z, Li Y, Wang Q. Solid lipid nanoparticles for oral drug delivery: Chitosan coating improves stability, controlled delivery, mucoadhesion and cellular uptake. Carbohydr Polym 2015; 122: 221-9.
[http://dx.doi.org/10.1016/j.carbpol.2014.12.084] [PMID: 25817662]

[57] Junyaprasert VB, Morakul B. Nanocrystals for enhancement of oral bioavailability of poorly water-soluble drugs. Asian journal of pharmaceutical sciences 2015; 10(1): 13-23.
[http://dx.doi.org/10.1016/j.ajps.2014.08.005]

[58] Macedo LdO, Barbosa EJ, Löbenberg R, Bou-Chacra NA. Anti-inflammatory drug nanocrystals: State of art and regulatory perspective. Eur J Pharm Sci 2020; 105654.

[59] Davis ME, Chen Z, Shin DM. Nanoparticle therapeutics: An emerging treatment modality for cancer. Nanoscience and technology: A collection of reviews from nature journals 2010; 239-50.

[60] Rheumatoid Arthritis: Causes, Symptoms, Treatments and More: Arthritis Foundation 2021. Availble from: https://www.arthritis.org/diseases/rheumatoid-arthritis

[61] Chai L-x, Fan X-x, Zuo Y-h, Zhang B, Nie G-h, Xie N, *et al.* Low-dimensional nanomaterials enabled autoimmune disease treatments: Recent advances, strategies, and future challenges. Coord Chem Rev 2020; 213697.

[62] Gharagozloo M, Majewski S, Foldvari M. Therapeutic applications of nanomedicine in autoimmune diseases: From immunosuppression to tolerance induction. Nanomedicine 2015; 11(4): 1003-18.
[http://dx.doi.org/10.1016/j.nano.2014.12.003] [PMID: 25596076]

[63] Foong WC, Green KL. Retention and distribution of liposome-entrapped [3H]methotrexate injected into normal or arthritic rabbit joints. J Pharm Pharmacol 2011; 40(7): 464-8.
[http://dx.doi.org/10.1111/j.2042-7158.1988.tb05278.x] [PMID: 2904984]

[64] Choi JS, Lee DH, Ahn JB, *et al.* Therapeutic effects of celecoxib polymeric systems in rat models of inflammation and adjuvant-induced rheumatoid arthritis. Mater Sci Eng C 2020; 114: 111042.
[http://dx.doi.org/10.1016/j.msec.2020.111042] [PMID: 32993980]

[65] Salah S, Mahmoud AA, Kamel AO. Etodolac transdermal cubosomes for the treatment of rheumatoid

arthritis: *Ex vivo* permeation and *in vivo* pharmacokinetic studies. Drug Deliv 2017; 24(1): 846-56. [http://dx.doi.org/10.1080/10717544.2017.1326539] [PMID: 28535740]

[66] Wang Q, Qin X, Fang J, Sun X. Nanomedicines for the treatment of rheumatoid arthritis: State of art and potential therapeutic strategies. Acta Pharm Sin B 2021; 11(5): 1158-74. [http://dx.doi.org/10.1016/j.apsb.2021.03.013] [PMID: 34094826]

[67] Ahmed M, Khanna D, Furst DE. Meloxicam in rheumatoid arthritis. Expert Opin Drug Metab Toxicol 2005; 1(4): 739-51. [http://dx.doi.org/10.1517/17425255.1.4.739] [PMID: 16863437]

[68] Krug H, Broadwell LK, Berry M, DeLapp R, Palmer RH, Mahowald M. Tolerability and efficacy of nabumetone and naproxen in the treatment of rheumatoid arthritis. Clin Ther 2000; 22(1): 40-52. [http://dx.doi.org/10.1016/S0149-2918(00)87976-X] [PMID: 10688389]

[69] Williams GW, Kivitz AJ, Brown MT, Verburg KM. A comparison of valdecoxib and naproxen in the treatment of rheumatoid arthritis symptoms. Clin Ther 2006; 28(2): 204-21. [http://dx.doi.org/10.1016/j.clinthera.2006.01.016] [PMID: 16678642]

[70] de Castro S, Camarasa MJ. Polypharmacology in HIV inhibition: Can a drug with simultaneous action against two relevant targets be an alternative to combination therapy? Eur J Med Chem 2018; 150: 206-27. [http://dx.doi.org/10.1016/j.ejmech.2018.03.007] [PMID: 29529501]

[71] Herskovitz J, Gendelman HE. HIV and the macrophage: From cell reservoirs to drug delivery to viral eradication. J Neuroimmune Pharmacol 2019; 14(1): 52-67. [http://dx.doi.org/10.1007/s11481-018-9785-6] [PMID: 29572681]

[72] Dutta T, Garg M, Jain NK. Targeting of efavirenz loaded tuftsin conjugated poly(propyleneimine) dendrimers to HIV infected macrophages *in vitro*. Eur J Pharm Sci 2008; 34(2-3): 181-9. [http://dx.doi.org/10.1016/j.ejps.2008.04.002] [PMID: 18501568]

[73] Dembri A, Montisci MJ, Gantier JC, Chacun H, Ponchel G. Targeting of 3′-azido 3′-deoxythymidine (AZT)-loaded poly(isohexylcyanoacrylate) nanospheres to the gastrointestinal mucosa and associated lymphoid tissues. Pharm Res 2001; 18(4): 467-73. [http://dx.doi.org/10.1023/A:1011050209986] [PMID: 11451033]

[74] Löbenberg R, Maas J, Kreuter J. Improved body distribution of 14C-labelled AZT bound to nanoparticles in rats determined by radioluminography. J Drug Target 1998; 5(3): 171-9. [http://dx.doi.org/10.3109/10611869808995872] [PMID: 9606007]

[75] Chiappetta DA, Facorro G, Rubin de Celis E, Sosnik A. Synergistic encapsulation of the anti-HIV agent efavirenz within mixed poloxamine/poloxamer polymeric micelles. Nanomedicine 2011; 7(5): 624-37. [http://dx.doi.org/10.1016/j.nano.2011.01.017] [PMID: 21371572]

[76] Dutta T, Agashe HB, Garg M, Balasubramanium P, Kabra M, Jain NK. Poly (propyleneimine) dendrimer based nanocontainers for targeting of efavirenz to human monocytes/macrophages *in vitro*. J Drug Target 2007; 15(1): 89-98. [http://dx.doi.org/10.1080/10611860600965914] [PMID: 17365278]

[77] Pham K, Li D, Guo S, Penzak S, Dong X. Development and *in vivo* evaluation of child-friendly lopinavir/ritonavir pediatric granules utilizing novel *in situ* self-assembly nanoparticles. J Control Release 2016; 226: 88-97. [http://dx.doi.org/10.1016/j.jconrel.2016.02.001] [PMID: 26849919]

[78] Liptrott NJ, Giardiello M, McDonald TO, Rannard SP, Owen A. Assessment of interactions of efavirenz solid drug nanoparticles with human immunological and haematological systems. J Nanobiotechnology 2018; 16(1): 22. [http://dx.doi.org/10.1186/s12951-018-0349-y] [PMID: 29544545]

[79] Shah LK, Amiji MM. Intracellular delivery of saquinavir in biodegradable polymeric nanoparticles for

HIV/AIDS. Pharm Res 2006; 23(11): 2638-45.
[http://dx.doi.org/10.1007/s11095-006-9101-7] [PMID: 16969696]

[80] Garg M, Asthana A, Agashe HB, Agrawal GP, Jain NK. Stavudine-loaded mannosylated liposomes: In-vitro anti-HIV-I activity, tissue distribution and pharmacokinetics. J Pharm Pharmacol 2010; 58(5): 605-16.
[http://dx.doi.org/10.1211/jpp.58.5.0005] [PMID: 16640829]

[81] Komano Y, Yagi N, Onoue I, Kaneko K, Miyasaka N, Nanki T. Arthritic joint-targeting small interfering RNA-encapsulated liposome: Implication for treatment strategy for rheumatoid arthritis. J Pharmacol Exp Ther 2012; 340(1): 109-13.
[http://dx.doi.org/10.1124/jpet.111.185884] [PMID: 21994423]

[82] Moallem E, Koren E, Ulmansky R, *et al.* A liposomal steroid nano-drug for treating systemic lupus erythematosus. Lupus 2016; 25(11): 1209-16.
[http://dx.doi.org/10.1177/0961203316636468] [PMID: 26957351]

[83] Makadia HK, Siegel SJ. Poly lactic-co-glycolic acid (PLGA) as biodegradable controlled drug delivery carrier. Polymers (Basel) 2011; 3(3): 1377-97.
[http://dx.doi.org/10.3390/polym3031377] [PMID: 22577513]

[84] Calabresi PA, Kieseier BC, Arnold DL, *et al.* Pegylated interferon β-1a for relapsing-remitting multiple sclerosis (ADVANCE): A randomised, phase 3, double-blind study. Lancet Neurol 2014; 13(7): 657-65.
[http://dx.doi.org/10.1016/S1474-4422(14)70068-7] [PMID: 24794721]

[85] Deeks ED. Certolizumab pegol. Drugs 2013; 73(1): 75-97.
[http://dx.doi.org/10.1007/s40265-013-0009-3] [PMID: 23338540]

[86] Yuan B, Zhao L, Fu F, *et al.* A novel nanoparticle containing MOG peptide with BTLA induces T cell tolerance and prevents multiple sclerosis. Mol Immunol 2014; 57(2): 93-9.
[http://dx.doi.org/10.1016/j.molimm.2013.08.006] [PMID: 24084097]

[87] Leonavičienė L, Kirdaitė G, Bradūnaitė R, *et al.* Effect of gold nanoparticles in the treatment of established collagen arthritis in rats. Medicina (Kaunas) 2012; 48(2): 16.
[http://dx.doi.org/10.3390/medicina48020016] [PMID: 22491387]

[88] Tsai CY, Shiau AL, Chen SY, *et al.* Amelioration of collagen-induced arthritis in rats by nanogold. Arthritis Rheum 2007; 56(2): 544-54.
[http://dx.doi.org/10.1002/art.22401] [PMID: 17265489]

[89] Brown CL, Bushell G, Whitehouse MW, *et al.* Nanogoldpharmaceutics. Gold Bull 2007; 40(3): 245-50.
[http://dx.doi.org/10.1007/BF03215588]

[90] Yeste A, Nadeau M, Burns EJ, Weiner HL, Quintana FJ. Nanoparticle-mediated codelivery of myelin antigen and a tolerogenic small molecule suppresses experimental autoimmune encephalomyelitis. Proc Natl Acad Sci USA 2012; 109(28): 11270-5.
[http://dx.doi.org/10.1073/pnas.1120611109] [PMID: 22745170]

[91] Aghaie T, Jazayeri MH, Avan A, Anissian A, Salari AA. Gold nanoparticles and polyethylene glycol alleviate clinical symptoms and alter cytokine secretion in a mouse model of experimental autoimmune encephalomyelitis. IUBMB Life 2019; 71(9): 1313-21.
[http://dx.doi.org/10.1002/iub.2045] [PMID: 30957389]

[92] Zhang N, Zhang S, Xu C, Fu L, Liu T, Zhao Y. Decoy oligodeoxynucleotides, polysaccharides, and targeted peptide-functionalized gold nanorods for the combined treatment of rheumatoid Arthritis. Advanced healthcare materials 2019; 8(20): e1970074.

[93] Badea I, Verrall R, Baca-Estrada M, Tikoo S, Rosenberg A, Kumar P, *et al. in vivo* cutaneous interferon-γ gene delivery using novel dicationic (gemini) surfactant–plasmid complexes. The Journal of Gene Medicine: A cross-disciplinary journal for research on the science of gene transfer and its

clinical applications 2005; 7(9): 1200-14.

[94] Metselaar JM, Wauben MHM, Wagenaar-Hilbers JPA, Boerman OC, Storm G. Complete remission of experimental arthritis by joint targeting of glucocorticoids with long-circulating liposomes. Arthritis Rheum 2003; 48(7): 2059-66.
[http://dx.doi.org/10.1002/art.11140] [PMID: 12847701]

[95] Zhang H, Yamazaki T, Zhi C, Hanagata N. Identification of a boron nitride nanosphere-binding peptide for the intracellular delivery of CpG oligodeoxynucleotides. Nanoscale 2012; 4(20): 6343-50.
[http://dx.doi.org/10.1039/c2nr31189e] [PMID: 22941279]

[96] Tan KX, Pan S, Jeevanandam J, Danquah MK. Cardiovascular therapies utilizing targeted delivery of nanomedicines and aptamers. Int J Pharm 2019; 558: 413-25.
[http://dx.doi.org/10.1016/j.ijpharm.2019.01.023] [PMID: 30660748]

[97] Pala R, Anju VT, Dyavaiah M, Busi S, Nauli SM. Nanoparticle-mediated drug delivery for the treatment of cardiovascular diseases. Int J Nanomedicine 2020; 15: 3741-69.
[http://dx.doi.org/10.2147/IJN.S250872] [PMID: 32547026]

[98] Jiang W, Rutherford D, Vuong T, Liu H. Nanomaterials for treating cardiovascular diseases: A review. Bioact Mater 2017; 2(4): 185-98.
[http://dx.doi.org/10.1016/j.bioactmat.2017.11.002] [PMID: 29744429]

[99] Gioffredi E, Boffito M, Calzone S, *et al.* Pluronic F127 hydrogel characterization and biofabrication in cellularized constructs for tissue engineering applications. Procedia CIRP 2016; 49: 125-32.
[http://dx.doi.org/10.1016/j.procir.2015.11.001]

[100] Alagarsamy KN, Mathan S, Yan W, *et al.* Carbon nanomaterials for cardiovascular theranostics: Promises and challenges. Bioact Mater 2021; 6(8): 2261-80.
[http://dx.doi.org/10.1016/j.bioactmat.2020.12.030] [PMID: 33553814]

[101] Zhu W, Huang H, Dong Y, Han C, Sui X, Jian B. Multi-walled carbon nanotube-based systems for improving the controlled release of insoluble drug dipyridamole. Exp Ther Med 2019; 17(6): 4610-6.
[http://dx.doi.org/10.3892/etm.2019.7510] [PMID: 31105789]

[102] Haeri A, Sadeghian S, Rabbani S, *et al.* Effective attenuation of vascular restenosis following local delivery of chitosan decorated sirolimus liposomes. Carbohydr Polym 2017; 157: 1461-9.
[http://dx.doi.org/10.1016/j.carbpol.2016.11.021] [PMID: 27987857]

[103] Arzani G, Haeri A, Daeihamed M, Bakhtiari-Kaboutaraki H, Dadashzadeh S. Niosomal carriers enhance oral bioavailability of carvedilol: Effects of bile salt-enriched vesicles and carrier surface charge. Int J Nanomedicine 2015; 10: 4797-813.
[PMID: 26251598]

[104] Neves AR, Lúcio M, Martins S, Lima JLC, Reis S. Novel resveratrol nanodelivery systems based on lipid nanoparticles to enhance its oral bioavailability. Int J Nanomedicine 2013; 8: 177-87.
[PMID: 23326193]

[105] Formiga FR, Pelacho B, Garbayo E, *et al.* Sustained release of VEGF through PLGA microparticles improves vasculogenesis and tissue remodeling in an acute myocardial ischemia–reperfusion model. J Control Release 2010; 147(1): 30-7.
[http://dx.doi.org/10.1016/j.jconrel.2010.07.097] [PMID: 20643169]

[106] Simón-Yarza T, Formiga FR, Tamayo E, Pelacho B, Prosper F, Blanco-Prieto MJ. PEGylated-PLGA microparticles containing VEGF for long term drug delivery. Int J Pharm 2013; 440(1): 13-8.
[http://dx.doi.org/10.1016/j.ijpharm.2012.07.006] [PMID: 22814223]

[107] Lee PC, Zan BS, Chen LT, Chung TW. Multifunctional PLGA-based nanoparticles as a controlled release drug delivery system for antioxidant and anticoagulant therapy. Int J Nanomedicine 2019; 14: 1533-49.
[http://dx.doi.org/10.2147/IJN.S174962] [PMID: 30880963]

[108] Wang Y, Xu X, Zhao X, Yin Z. Functionalized polymeric hybrid micelles as an efficient

nanotheranostic agent for thrombus imaging and thrombolysis. Acta Biomater 2021; 122: 278-90. [http://dx.doi.org/10.1016/j.actbio.2020.10.015] [PMID: 33359293]

[109] Niu JJ, Wang JN, Chen YX. Boron-doped silicon nano-wires. Mater Sci Eng B 2007; 139(1): 95-8. [http://dx.doi.org/10.1016/j.mseb.2007.01.038]

[110] Zhang Y, Li N, Xiang Y, *et al.* A flexible non-enzymatic glucose sensor based on copper nanoparticles anchored on laser-induced graphene. Carbon 2020; 156: 506-13. [http://dx.doi.org/10.1016/j.carbon.2019.10.006]

[111] Liu G, Qi M, Zhang Y, Cao C, Goldys EM. Nanocomposites of gold nanoparticles and graphene oxide towards an stable label-free electrochemical immunosensor for detection of cardiac marker troponin-I. Anal Chim Acta 2016; 909: 1-8. [http://dx.doi.org/10.1016/j.aca.2015.12.023] [PMID: 26851079]

[112] Arvand M, Samie HA. Electrospun CeO2–Au nanofibers/graphene oxide 3D nanonetwork structure for the electrocatalytic detection of amlodipine. Ionics 2018; 24(6): 1813-26. [http://dx.doi.org/10.1007/s11581-017-2321-5]

[113] Ghanei Agh Kaariz D, Darabi E, Elahi SM. Fabrication of Au/ZnO/MWCNTs electrode and its characterization for electrochemical cholesterol biosensor. Journal of Theoretical and Applied Physics 2020; 14(4): 339-48. [http://dx.doi.org/10.1007/s40094-020-00390-5]

[114] Sun H, Zhou J, Huang Z, *et al.* Carbon nanotube-incorporated collagen hydrogels improve cell alignment and the performance of cardiac constructs. Int J Nanomedicine 2017; 12: 3109-20. [http://dx.doi.org/10.2147/IJN.S128030] [PMID: 28450785]

[115] Pedrotty DM, Kuzmenko V, Karabulut E, *et al.* Three-dimensional printed biopatches with conductive ink facilitate cardiac conduction when applied to disrupted myocardium. Circ Arrhythm Electrophysiol 2019; 12(3): e006920. [http://dx.doi.org/10.1161/CIRCEP.118.006920] [PMID: 30845835]

[116] Shin SR, Zihlmann C, Akbari M, *et al.* Reduced graphene oxide-gelMA hybrid hydrogels as scaffolds for cardiac tissue engineering. Small 2016; 12(27): 3677-89. [http://dx.doi.org/10.1002/smll.201600178] [PMID: 27254107]

[117] Zargar SM, Mehdikhani M, Rafienia M. Reduced graphene oxide–reinforced gellan gum thermoresponsive hydrogels as a myocardial tissue engineering scaffold. J Bioact Compat Polym 2019; 34(4-5): 331-45. [http://dx.doi.org/10.1177/0883911519876080]

[118] Wang Y, Dong Y, Chen P, *et al.* Reduced graphene oxide foam templated by nickel foam for organ-on-a-chip engineering of cardiac constructs. Mater Sci Eng C 2020; 117: 111344. [http://dx.doi.org/10.1016/j.msec.2020.111344] [PMID: 32919691]

[119] Talebi A, Labbaf S, Karimzadeh F, Masaeli E, Nasr Esfahani MH. Electroconductive graphene-containing polymeric patch: A promising platform for future cardiac repair. ACS Biomater Sci Eng 2020; 6(7): 4214-24. [http://dx.doi.org/10.1021/acsbiomaterials.0c00266] [PMID: 33463338]

[120] Zazo H, Colino CI, Lanao JM. Current applications of nanoparticles in infectious diseases. J Control Release 2016; 224: 86-102. [http://dx.doi.org/10.1016/j.jconrel.2016.01.008] [PMID: 26772877]

[121] Longhi C, Santos JP, Morey AT, *et al.* Combination of fluconazole with silver nanoparticles produced by *Fusarium oxysporum* improves antifungal effect against planktonic cells and biofilm of drug-resistant *Candida albicans*. Med Mycol 2016; 54(4): 428-32. [http://dx.doi.org/10.1093/mmy/myv036] [PMID: 26092103]

[122] Zhao Y, Jiang X. Multiple strategies to activate gold nanoparticles as antibiotics. Nanoscale 2013; 5(18): 8340-50.

[http://dx.doi.org/10.1039/c3nr01990j] [PMID: 23893008]

[123] Shaik N, Pan G, Elmquist WF. Interactions of pluronic block copolymers on P-gp efflux activity: Experience with HIV-1 protease inhibitors. J Pharm Sci 2008; 97(12): 5421-33. [http://dx.doi.org/10.1002/jps.21372] [PMID: 18393290]

[124] Wang L, Chen YP, Miller KP, *et al.* Functionalised nanoparticles complexed with antibiotic efficiently kill MRSA and other bacteria. Chem Commun (Camb) 2014; 50(81): 12030-3. [http://dx.doi.org/10.1039/C4CC04936E] [PMID: 25136934]

[125] Hussein-Al-Ali SH, El Zowalaty ME, Hussein MZ, Ismail M, Webster TJ. Synthesis, characterization, controlled release, and antibacterial studies of a novel streptomycin chitosan magnetic nanoantibiotic. Int J Nanomedicine 2014; 9: 549-57. [PMID: 24549109]

[126] Khatoon N, Alam H, Khan A, Raza K, Sardar M. Ampicillin silver nanoformulations against multidrug resistant bacteria. Sci Rep 2019; 9(1): 6848. [http://dx.doi.org/10.1038/s41598-019-43309-0] [PMID: 31048721]

[127] Abeylath SC, Turos E, Dickey S, Lim DV. Glyconanobiotics: Novel carbohydrated nanoparticle antibiotics for MRSA and Bacillus anthracis. Bioorg Med Chem 2008; 16(5): 2412-8. [http://dx.doi.org/10.1016/j.bmc.2007.11.052] [PMID: 18063370]

[128] Turos E, Reddy GSK, Greenhalgh K, *et al.* Penicillin-bound polyacrylate nanoparticles: Restoring the activity of β-lactam antibiotics against MRSA. Bioorg Med Chem Lett 2007; 17(12): 3468-72. [http://dx.doi.org/10.1016/j.bmcl.2007.03.077] [PMID: 17420125]

[129] Shimizu N, Otsuka K, Sawada H, Maejima T, Shirotake S. Bacteriolysis by vancomycin-conjugated acryl nanoparticles and morphological component analysis. Drug Dev Ind Pharm 2014; 40(6): 813-8. [http://dx.doi.org/10.3109/03639045.2013.788012] [PMID: 23594303]

[130] Gu H, Ho PL, Tong E, Wang L, Xu B. Presenting vancomycin on nanoparticles to enhance antimicrobial activities. Nano Lett 2003; 3(9): 1261-3. [http://dx.doi.org/10.1021/nl034396z]

[131] Alipour M, Halwani M, Omri A, Suntres ZE. Antimicrobial effectiveness of liposomal polymyxin B against resistant Gram-negative bacterial strains. Int J Pharm 2008; 355(1-2): 293-8. [http://dx.doi.org/10.1016/j.ijpharm.2007.11.035] [PMID: 18164881]

[132] Aditya NP, Vathsala PG, Vieira V, Murthy RSR, Souto EB. Advances in nanomedicines for malaria treatment. Adv Colloid Interface Sci 2013; 201-202: 1-17. [http://dx.doi.org/10.1016/j.cis.2013.10.014] [PMID: 24192063]

[133] Chakraborti S, Mandal AK, Sarwar S, Singh P, Chakraborty R, Chakrabarti P. Bactericidal effect of polyethyleneimine capped ZnO nanoparticles on multiple antibiotic resistant bacteria harboring genes of high-pathogenicity island. Colloids Surf B Biointerfaces 2014; 121: 44-53. [http://dx.doi.org/10.1016/j.colsurfb.2014.03.044] [PMID: 24937133]

[134] Baelo A, Levato R, Julián E, *et al.* Disassembling bacterial extracellular matrix with DNase-coated nanoparticles to enhance antibiotic delivery in biofilm infections. J Control Release 2015; 209: 150-8. [http://dx.doi.org/10.1016/j.jconrel.2015.04.028] [PMID: 25913364]

[135] Walsh TJ, Finberg RW, Arndt C, *et al.* Liposomal amphotericin B for empirical therapy in patients with persistent fever and neutropenia. N Engl J Med 1999; 340(10): 764-71. [http://dx.doi.org/10.1056/NEJM199903113401004] [PMID: 10072411]

[136] Weissig V, Pettinger T, Murdock N. Nanopharmaceuticals (part 1): Products on the market. Int J Nanomedicine 2014; 9: 4357-73. [http://dx.doi.org/10.2147/IJN.S46900] [PMID: 25258527]

[137] Bozzuto G, Molinari A. Liposomes as nanomedical devices. Int J Nanomedicine 2015; 10: 975-99. [http://dx.doi.org/10.2147/IJN.S68861] [PMID: 25678787]

[138] Beal SG, Ciurca J, Smith G, *et al.* Evaluation of the nanosphere verigene gram-positive blood culture assay with the VersaTREK blood culture system and assessment of possible impact on selected patients. J Clin Microbiol 2013; 51(12): 3988-92.
[http://dx.doi.org/10.1128/JCM.01889-13] [PMID: 24048531]

[139] Sun L, Zhang C, Li P. Characterization, antibiofilm, and mechanism of action of novel PEG-stabilized lipid nanoparticles loaded with terpinen-4-ol. J Agric Food Chem 2012; 60(24): 6150-6.
[http://dx.doi.org/10.1021/jf3010405] [PMID: 22640226]

[140] Brown AN, Smith K, Samuels TA, Lu J, Obare SO, Scott ME. Nanoparticles functionalized with ampicillin destroy multiple-antibiotic-resistant isolates of Pseudomonas aeruginosa and Enterobacter aerogenes and methicillin-resistant Staphylococcus aureus. Appl Environ Microbiol 2012; 78(8): 2768-74.
[http://dx.doi.org/10.1128/AEM.06513-11] [PMID: 22286985]

[141] Djafari J, Marinho C, Santos T, *et al.* New synthesis of gold- and silver-based nano-tetracycline composites. ChemistryOpen 2016; 5(3): 206-12.
[http://dx.doi.org/10.1002/open.201600016] [PMID: 27957408]

[142] Bastari K, Arshath M, Ng ZHM, *et al.* A controlled release of antibiotics from calcium phosphate-coated poly(lactic-co-glycolic acid) particles and their *in vitro* efficacy against Staphylococcus aureus biofilm. J Mater Sci Mater Med 2014; 25(3): 747-57.
[http://dx.doi.org/10.1007/s10856-013-5125-9] [PMID: 24370968]

[143] Cheow WS, Chang MW, Hadinoto K. Antibacterial efficacy of inhalable antibiotic-encapsulated biodegradable polymeric nanoparticles against E. coli biofilm cells. J Biomed Nanotechnol 2010; 6(4): 391-403.
[http://dx.doi.org/10.1166/jbn.2010.1116] [PMID: 21323113]

[144] Dodiya SS, Chavhan SS, Sawant KK, Korde AG. Solid lipid nanoparticles and nanosuspension formulation of Saquinavir: Preparation, characterization, pharmacokinetics and biodistribution studies. J Microencapsul 2011; 28(6): 515-27.
[http://dx.doi.org/10.3109/02652048.2011.590612] [PMID: 21728760]

[145] Salman M, Rizwana R, Khan H, *et al.* Synergistic effect of silver nanoparticles and polymyxin B against biofilm produced by *Pseudomonas aeruginosa* isolates of pus samples *in vitro*. Artif Cells Nanomed Biotechnol 2019; 47(1): 2465-72.
[http://dx.doi.org/10.1080/21691401.2019.1626864] [PMID: 31187657]

[146] Salomoni R, Léo P, Montemor A, Rinaldi B, Rodrigues M. Antibacterial effect of silver nanoparticles in *Pseudomonas aeruginosa.* Nanotechnol Sci Appl 2017; 10: 115-21.
[http://dx.doi.org/10.2147/NSA.S133415] [PMID: 28721025]

[147] Shazly GA. Ciprofloxacin controlled-solid lipid nanoparticles: Characterization, *in vitro* release, and antibacterial activity assessment. BioMed research international 2017; 2017

[148] Chakraborty SP, Sahu SK, Pramanik P, Roy S. *in vitro* antimicrobial activity of nanoconjugated vancomycin against drug resistant Staphylococcus aureus. Int J Pharm 2012; 436(1-2): 659-76.
[http://dx.doi.org/10.1016/j.ijpharm.2012.07.033] [PMID: 22841851]

[149] Chidambaram M, Manavalan R, Kathiresan K. Nanotherapeutics to overcome conventional cancer chemotherapy limitations. J Pharm Pharm Sci 2011; 14(1): 67-77.
[http://dx.doi.org/10.18433/J30C7D] [PMID: 21501554]

[150] Cancer: World Health Organization 2021. Available from:https://www.who.int/news-room/fac--sheets/detail/cancer

[151] Cancer Today: World Health Organization: International Agency for Research on Cancer 2021. Availble from: https://gco.iarc.fr/today/home

[152] Maeda H, Bharate GY, Daruwalla J. Polymeric drugs for efficient tumor-targeted drug delivery based on EPR-effect. Eur J Pharm Biopharm 2009; 71(3): 409-19.

[http://dx.doi.org/10.1016/j.ejpb.2008.11.010] [PMID: 19070661]

[153] Barenholz YC. Doxil® — The first FDA-approved nano-drug: Lessons learned. J Control Release 2012; 160(2): 117-34.
[http://dx.doi.org/10.1016/j.jconrel.2012.03.020] [PMID: 22484195]

[154] Akinc A, Maier MA, Manoharan M, *et al.* The Onpattro story and the clinical translation of nanomedicines containing nucleic acid-based drugs. Nat Nanotechnol 2019; 14(12): 1084-7.
[http://dx.doi.org/10.1038/s41565-019-0591-y] [PMID: 31802031]

[155] Silverman JA, Deitcher SR. Marqibo® (vincristine sulfate liposome injection) improves the pharmacokinetics and pharmacodynamics of vincristine. Cancer Chemother Pharmacol 2013; 71(3): 555-64.
[http://dx.doi.org/10.1007/s00280-012-2042-4] [PMID: 23212117]

[156] Gadekar V, Borade Y, Kannaujia S, Rajpoot K, Anup N, Tambe V, *et al.* Nanomedicines accessible in the market for clinical interventions. J Control Release 2020.
[PMID: 33370576]

[157] Venkatakrishnan K, Liu Y, Noe D, *et al.* Pharmacokinetics and pharmacodynamics of liposomal mifamurtide in adult volunteers with mild or moderate renal impairment. Br J Clin Pharmacol 2014; 77(6): 986-97.
[http://dx.doi.org/10.1111/bcp.12260] [PMID: 24134181]

[158] Zhang H. Onivyde for the therapy of multiple solid tumors. OncoTargets Ther 2016; 9: 3001-7.
[http://dx.doi.org/10.2147/OTT.S105587] [PMID: 27284250]

[159] Farjadian F, Ghasemi A, Gohari O, Roointan A, Karimi M, Hamblin MR. Nanopharmaceuticals and nanomedicines currently on the market: Challenges and opportunities. Nanomedicine (Lond) 2019; 14(1): 93-126.
[http://dx.doi.org/10.2217/nnm-2018-0120] [PMID: 30451076]

[160] Anselmo AC, Mitragotri S. Nanoparticles in the clinic: An update. Bioeng Transl Med 2019; 4(3): e10143.
[http://dx.doi.org/10.1002/btm2.10143] [PMID: 31572799]

[161] Kim MT, Chen Y, Marhoul J, Jacobson F. Statistical modeling of the drug load distribution on trastuzumab emtansine (Kadcyla), a lysine-linked antibody drug conjugate. Bioconjug Chem 2014; 25(7): 1223-32.
[http://dx.doi.org/10.1021/bc5000109] [PMID: 24873191]

[162] Miele E, Spinelli GP, Miele E, Tomao F, Tomao S. Albumin-bound formulation of paclitaxel (Abraxane ABI-007) in the treatment of breast cancer. Int J Nanomedicine 2009; 4: 99-105.
[PMID: 19516888]

[163] El-Boubbou K. Magnetic iron oxide nanoparticles as drug carriers: Clinical relevance. Nanomedicine (Lond) 2018; 13(8): 953-71.
[http://dx.doi.org/10.2217/nnm-2017-0336] [PMID: 29376469]

[164] Sugawara E, Nikaido H. Properties of AdeABC and AdeIJK efflux systems of Acinetobacter baumannii compared with those of the AcrAB-TolC system of Escherichia coli. Antimicrob Agents Chemother 2014; 58(12): 7250-7.
[http://dx.doi.org/10.1128/AAC.03728-14] [PMID: 25246403]

[165] Liu Q, Guan J, Qin L, Zhang X, Mao S. Physicochemical properties affecting the fate of nanoparticles in pulmonary drug delivery. Drug Discov Today 2020; 25(1): 150-9.
[http://dx.doi.org/10.1016/j.drudis.2019.09.023] [PMID: 31600580]

[166] Omlor AJ, Nguyen J, Bals R, Dinh QT. Nanotechnology in respiratory medicine. Respir Res 2015; 16(1): 64.
[http://dx.doi.org/10.1186/s12931-015-0223-5] [PMID: 26021823]

[167] Lim YH, Tiemann KM, Hunstad DA, Elsabahy M, Wooley KL. Polymeric nanoparticles in

development for treatment of pulmonary infectious diseases. Wiley Interdiscip Rev Nanomed Nanobiotechnol 2016; 8(6): 842-71.
[http://dx.doi.org/10.1002/wnan.1401] [PMID: 27016134]

[168] Jin X, Song L, Ma CC, Zhang YC, Yu S. Retracted: Pulmonary route of administration is instrumental in developing therapeutic interventions against respiratory diseases. Saudi Pharm J 2020; 28(12): 1655-65.
[http://dx.doi.org/10.1016/j.jsps.2020.10.012] [PMID: 33424258]

[169] Jeannot V, Gauche C, Mazzaferro S, *et al.* Anti-tumor efficacy of hyaluronan-based nanoparticles for the co-delivery of drugs in lung cancer. J Control Release 2018; 275: 117-28.
[http://dx.doi.org/10.1016/j.jconrel.2018.02.024] [PMID: 29474960]

[170] Said-Elbahr R, Nasr M, Alhnan MA, Taha I, Sammour O. Nebulizable colloidal nanoparticles co-encapsulating a COX-2 inhibitor and a herbal compound for treatment of lung cancer. Eur J Pharm Biopharm 2016; 103: 1-12.
[http://dx.doi.org/10.1016/j.ejpb.2016.03.025] [PMID: 27020529]

[171] Pellosi DS, d'Angelo I, Maiolino S, *et al. in vitro*/*in vivo* investigation on the potential of Pluronic® mixed micelles for pulmonary drug delivery. Eur J Pharm Biopharm 2018; 130: 30-8.
[http://dx.doi.org/10.1016/j.ejpb.2018.06.006] [PMID: 29890256]

[172] Zhong Q, Bielski ER, Rodrigues LS, Brown MR, Reineke JJ, da Rocha SRP. Conjugation to poly (amidoamine) dendrimers and pulmonary delivery reduce cardiac accumulation and enhance antitumor activity of doxorubicin in lung metastasis. Mol Pharm 2016; 13(7): 2363-75.
[http://dx.doi.org/10.1021/acs.molpharmaceut.6b00126] [PMID: 27253493]

[173] Kaminskas LM, McLeod VM, Ryan GM, *et al.* Pulmonary administration of a doxorubicin-conjugated dendrimer enhances drug exposure to lung metastases and improves cancer therapy. J Control Release 2014; 183: 18-26.
[http://dx.doi.org/10.1016/j.jconrel.2014.03.012] [PMID: 24637466]

[174] Nafee N, Makled S, Boraie N. Nanostructured lipid carriers *versus* solid lipid nanoparticles for the potential treatment of pulmonary hypertension *via* nebulization. Eur J Pharm Sci 2018; 125: 151-62.
[http://dx.doi.org/10.1016/j.ejps.2018.10.003] [PMID: 30292750]

[175] Garbuzenko OB, Kbah N, Kuzmov A, Pogrebnyak N, Pozharov V, Minko T. Inhalation treatment of cystic fibrosis with lumacaftor and ivacaftor co-delivered by nanostructured lipid carriers. J Control Release 2019; 296: 225-31.
[http://dx.doi.org/10.1016/j.jconrel.2019.01.025] [PMID: 30677435]

[176] Liu C, Shi J, Dai Q, Yin X, Zhang X, Zheng A. *In-vitro* and *in-vivo* evaluation of ciprofloxacin liposomes for pulmonary administration. Drug Dev Ind Pharm 2015; 41(2): 272-8.
[http://dx.doi.org/10.3109/03639045.2013.858740] [PMID: 24252110]

[177] Tahara K, Tomida H, Ito Y, *et al.* Pulmonary liposomal formulations encapsulated procaterol hydrochloride by a remote loading method achieve sustained release and extended pharmacological effects. Int J Pharm 2016; 505(1-2): 139-46.
[http://dx.doi.org/10.1016/j.ijpharm.2016.03.031] [PMID: 27012982]

[178] Jana P, Shyam M, Singh S, Jayaprakash V, Dev A. Biodegradable polymers in drug delivery and oral vaccination. Eur Polym J 2020; 110155.

[179] Choi YH, Han HK. Nanomedicines: Current status and future perspectives in aspect of drug delivery and pharmacokinetics. J Pharm Investig 2018; 48(1): 43-60.
[http://dx.doi.org/10.1007/s40005-017-0370-4] [PMID: 30546919]

CHAPTER 4

Nanocarriers For Drug Targeting

Bina Gidwani[1], Varsha Sahu[2], Priya Namdeo[2], Sakshi Tiwari[2], Atul Tripathi[4], Ravindra Kumar Pandey[1], Shiv Shankar Shukla[1], Veenu Joshi[3], Vishal Jain[2], Suresh Thareja[5] and **Amber Vyas[2,*]**

[1] *Columbia Institute of Pharmacy, Raipur (C.G), India*

[2] *University Institute of Pharmacy, Pt. Ravishankar Shukla University, Raipur (C.G), India*

[3] *Center of Basic Science, Pt. Ravishankar Shukla University, Raipur (C.G), India*

[4] *People's Institute of Pharmacy & Research Centre, Bhopal, (M.P.), India*

[5] *Department of Pharmaceutical Sciences and Natural Products Central University of Punjab, Bathinda, 151001, Punjab, India*

Abstract: Drug targeting specific cells/tissues of the body without their becoming a part of the systemic circulation is a prominent area of research in drug delivery, with the main emphasis on improvement in formulation and development. Drug-targeting can improve the viability, lower/minimize the adverse/side effects, and can become cost-effective. Certain limitations like short circulating half-life, bioavailability issues, rapid metabolism and degradation, poor tissue distribution and penetration in the blood-brain barrier, intestinal absorption barriers, *etc*., are associated with the delivery of various therapeutic agents. Nanocarriers have arisen in the field of drug targeting with valuable delivery of drugs to site-specific/desired areas which is a significant therapeutic advantage since it keeps drugs from being conveyed to some unacceptable spots. Nanocarriers prevent the obstacles in clinical utilization of the therapeutic agents as they decrease the serious and critical side/adverse effects by targeted drug delivery and provide slow and sustained drug release. Nanocarriers bring new trust to drug targeting by upgrading the efficacy, defeating resistance, and minimizing toxicity. This chapter mainly focuses on the role and benefits of nanocarriers in drug-targeting and nanocarriers as prominent systems for targeting and delivering drugs to achieve maximum effects with improved therapeutic response.

Keywords: Bioavailability, Blood-brain barrier, Drug delivery, Drug efficacy, Drug resistance, Drug targeting, Half-life, Intestinal barrier, Metabolic degradation, Nanocarriers, Site of action, Site-specific targets, Sustained release, Targeted drug delivery, Tissue distribution.

* **Corresponding author Amber Vyas**: University Institute of Pharmacy, Pt. Ravishankar Shukla University, Raipur, Chhattisgarh, India; Tel: 9926807999; E-mail: **ambervyas@gmail.com**

Akhlesh K. Jain & Keerti Mishra (Eds.)

INTRODUCTION

In the world of medicine, there is continuous development in drug delivery, which involves the delivery of drugs to their particular site in a specific amount. Recent advances in pharmaceutical science are to discover a new therapeutic molecule ranging from micro molecules to macromolecules such as proteins and peptides. But the actual aim of drug delivery is to achieve disease-free conditions in the person's body; minimizing the physicochemical hurdles, and reducing the overdose to biological targets are necessary [1, 2]. Disease like cardiovascular, cancer, viral disease, inflammatory, microbial disease, and neurological diseases can be treated through conventional available drug delivery system, but there is some limitation like the short half-life of the drug, low efficacy, side effects, some biological barriers, low penetration, and low bioavailability, *etc.*, which limit their use [3]. To overcome this problem and enhance their *in-vivo* drug action, prepare such type of formulation that facilitates the improved pharmacokinetic and biodistribution of the drug, thereby enhancing the drug's safety and efficacy. The targeted delivery system is a newer system of drug delivery [4, 5]. In 1906, Paul Ehrlich suggested the targeted delivery through a magic bullet. The therapeutic efficiency is improved by reducing the non-specific drug distribution and minimizing the side effect. Drug targeting a particular site improves the therapeutic profile in the body. Delivering the drug at a specific site at the right time and the right place to maximize the therapeutic effect is the main aim of targeted delivery [6].

A targeted system is a type of specific delivery system, where the drug is precisely targeted or delivered to the specific or desired site. These results show minimum drug accumulation in non-targeted tissue [7]. It delivers a particular amount of drug for a longer period at the target site, which improves its efficacy and reduces the side effect [2, 8]. The pharmacokinetics and pharmacodynamics of the drugs are improved through targeted delivery. The major factor for drug delivery depends on the biological characteristic of the targeted area. The targeted delivery is achieved by:

1. Drugs directly apply to the site of action, such as topical application of drugs in skin disease.

2. Used external stimuli for targeted action of drugs such as ultrasound.

3. Modification of physicochemical properties of drugs.

4. Using nanocarriers for delivery of drug to a particular site such as liposomes, solid lipid nanoparticles, nanoemulsion, polymeric nanoparticles, *etc* [2].

Targeted drug delivery can be achieved by some direct invasive techniques such as direct injection, gene gun, catheter, *etc.* But these techniques are a bit expensive, not patient compliance, and not applicable to many conditions. Therefore, targeted drug delivery also involves chemical and physical modification of drugs [7, 9]. Changes in the physicochemical property of drugs make them suitable for targeted delivery. *E.g.*, prodrugs can be led to improvement in the kinetics of drugs. In prodrugs, the drug is chemically modified by attaching some moiety and makes them pharmacological inactive and *in vivo* metabolically active after reaching their target site. Some of the small molecule and lipophilic nature of drugs are suitable for brain drug delivery through the crossing of the blood-brain barrier [8, 10]. Another method for targeted drug delivery is to incorporate the drug into nanocarriers. This involves the use of drug carriers such as liposomes, polymeric nanoparticles, solid lipid nanoparticles, nanogels, *etc.* These nanocarriers are effective for the delivery of drugs, genes, and proteins. The great advantage of this is the pharmacokinetic property of nanocarriers [2, 11]. This drug is added to nanocarriers, and the biodistribution of the drug depends on the pharmacokinetic property of nanocarriers in which targeting is controlled by further modification.

Some of the basic properties of drugs that are used for the preparation of targeted drug delivery [10]:

1. If a drug has a short half-life.

2. If a drug has low stability.

3. If a drug has poor absorption.

4. If a drug has a narrow therapeutic index.

5. If a drug has low specificity.

In the field of nanotechnology, various nanostructures have been involved that benefit conventional available systems for the delivery of medicine, such as nanoparticles, nanofibers, and nanocomposites which are used in the treatment of various diseases. This nanostructured molecule works as a carrier that carries various drugs, genes, proteins, enzymes, *etc.*, and is delivered to a particular targeted site or tissue [12, 13]. These nanocarriers provide a longer half-life, minimize drug degradation, overcome first-pass metabolism, provide sustained or targeted drug release, reduce the side effect and improve the pharmacological response of the drug [9]. All these properties provide better treatment of diseases. The targeted drug delivery system is designed to overcome the drawback and limitations associated with conventional drug delivery systems.

Nanocarriers are nanoparticles in the form of colloids, which work as a carrier to carry therapeutic agents or other substances to the target site. The size of nanocarriers ranges from 1-100nm in diameter. Nanocarriers have biocompatible, chemically inert, have long blood circulation, have a large surface area, and different shape; therefore, it is used in drug delivery [14, 15]. It enhanced the pharmacokinetics and biodistribution of drugs such as:

1. Nanocarriers enhance drug stability by protecting through environmental factors

2. It enhances the solubility of drugs

3. It provides sustained and targeted drug delivery

4. It reduces the toxicity of drugs by targeting a particular site

Nanocarriers have optimized physicochemical and biological properties of drugs which are easily taken up by the cells as compared to large molecules. The method of conjugating the drug to nanocarriers is essential for targeted delivery. A drug may be adsorbed or covalently attached or encapsulate into nanocarriers. If the drug is covalently attached to nanocarriers, it enables control of the release of the drug [8, 16]. Cell-specific targeting through nano-sized carriers can be achieved by active or passive targeting mechanisms. This targeting involves recognizing low molecular weight ligands for cell surface receptors. g. folate receptor, peptide, *etc* [17]. Active targeting is achieved by manipulation of physical or external stimuli, such as temperature, magnetism, and pH. Passive targeting is obtained by enhancing the vascular permeability and retention (EPR) and releasing the therapeutic agent [18]. Some of the nanocarriers provide controlled release by altering the physiological environment, such as pH, temperature, and osmotic pressure. Nanocarriers used in the biomedical field for drug delivery and diagnosis must be biocompatible and non-toxic. Some of the side effects of nanocarriers are related to their size, shape, route of administration, their surface property, and their residence time in blood circulations. *E.g.*, some reports show that a smaller size has a large surface area and is highly reactive, but in generalized form, a size ranging from 10-to 100nm is the optimum size for drug delivery [19, 20]. Smaller nanocarriers undergo renal clearance or extravasation while larger sizes are removed from blood circulation *via* macrophages of the reticuloendothelial system. The key parameters to observe for designing nanocarriers include the size, shape, surface chemistry or functionalization, and other parameters. Nanocarriers are available in various forms, which provide a wide range of possibilities for targeted delivery of drugs, and because of this, recent research is ongoing to explore their potential. The ideal characteristics for nanocarriers are:

1. It should be biodegradable.

2. It should be stable.

3. It should be non-immunogenic.

4. It should be easy and cost-effective to fabricate.

5. It should provide the desired release of the therapeutic agent at the target-specific site [21].

Importance of Targeted Drug Delivery [5 - 18]

1. It facilitates delivering of drug molecules to a particular site or specific cell.

2. It protects the drug and gene from degradation through environmental factors such as pH, enzyme, *etc.*

3. It gives reduced side effects of the drug by targeting a particular site or minimal concentration in non-specific cell

4. It can easily deliver small and effective amounts of drugs.

5. The targeted system overcomes the first-pass metabolism of the drug.

Advantages of Nanocarriers in Drug Targeting

1. These nano-sized carriers are prepared using natural or synthetic polymers, providing better stability and surface modification.

2. Nanocarriers can be easily tailored to achieve controlled and targeted drug release.

3. Nanocarriers enhance the EPR effect (enhanced permeability and retention) on the target site.

4. Nanocarriers also provide a synergistic effect in drug delivery.

5. Nanocarriers improve bioavailability and solubility.

6. Nanocarriers protect the drug from degradation caused by the enzymes present in the body and environment.

MECHANISM OF DRUG TARGETING [1, 18]

Various types of drug targeting mechanisms (Fig. **4.1**) have been discussed below:

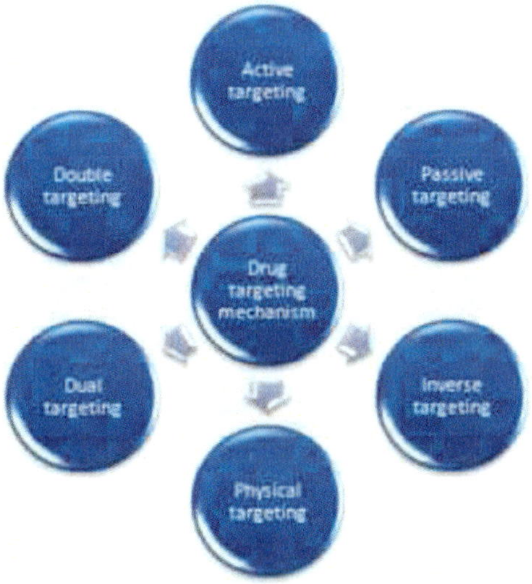

Fig. (4.1). Mechanism of Drug Targeting.

Active Targeting

In the active drug targeting mechanism, the ligand attached to the drug delivery system targets the receptor present on the cell or tissue, causing intracellular localization of the drug. The targeting ligand is either antibodies or proteins [2]. The surface modification and functionalization of drug carriers help them target the specific receptor, cell markers, tissue, or organ. Active targeting has 3 types which includes:

First-order Targeting/ Organ Targeting

It particularly targets an organ like the lymphatic cavity, cerebral ventricle, pleural cavity, eye, joints, *etc.*

Second-order Targeting/Cell Targeting

These types of targeting refers to delivering the drug or targeting a particular cell such as kupffer cell, tumor cell, *etc.*

Third-order Targeting/ Intracellular Targeting

These types of targeting deliver the drug to specific intracellular target sites, such as ligand-based target receptors, through the endocytosis process.

Inactive targeting, the addition of a small targeting ligand on the nanocarrier is actively bound with specific receptors and retained in a particular site and easily actively taken up by the disease cell or tissue. The targeting ligand has the affinity for the particular receptors, which are overexpressed in diseased cells and absent in normal cells. Such as, in tumor cells, overexpressed receptors are present on their surface. The targeting ligand involves hormones, lipoproteins, some peptides, glycoproteins, and some low molecular weight vitamins [22]. The nanocarriers can target multiple receptors because it has high surface volume. It can reduce the MDR (multidrug resistance). Some of the receptors are overexpressed in cancer cells, such as epidermal growth factor, folate receptor present in lungs, and/or ovarian cancer. In summary form, active targeting has more effective targeting because it does not involve with EPR (enhanced permeation and retention) effect. It is reported that the folate receptor is used for active targeting of anticancer drugs.

Passive Targeting

Passive targeting occurs naturally in the human body. *E.g.*, Neurotransmitters and hormones tend to target their receptor and show pharmacological responses. This system is used for drug targeting. The passive targeting system targets the systemic circulation through the body's natural response to the Physico-chemical properties of the drug and/or carrier system. In diseased conditions, there are pathological changes in the body, which are used as passive targeting for drug or drug carriers [2]. *E.g.*, in an inflammatory condition such as inflammatory rheumatoid arthritis and tumor tissue, leaky vasculature of blood vessels is present, which are used as passive targeting for drug or drug carriers. Some of the drug carriers can be taken up by the Reticuloendothelial system (RES), which makes them suitable for the passive targeting system. Surface modification in nanocarriers provides long blood circulation and avoids the RES, which is useful for the accumulation of the drug in a particular target site [1, 18]. Some of the internal stimuli also help in passive targeting, such as low pH in the tumor cell.

The enhanced Permeability and Retention effect is the basic route for passive targeting. In cancer cells, there are some physiological conditions such as leaky vasculature, lymphatic drainage, increased dimension of endothelial cells, *etc.* therefore, nanocarriers can extravasate through this physiological condition of an inflamed region or tumor cells. Targeting these conditions provides entry of nanocarriers through interstitial space in a particular area and enhanced accumulation of nanocarrier drug conjugate at the diseased site; this is called the enhanced permeability and retention effect. This effect provides the target-specific accumulation of the drug and reduces the undesirable side effects. The accumulation of nanocarriers depends on the size of surface charges. It is reported that the hydrophilic surface of nanocarriers of size less than 200nm shows an EPR effect due to their high blood circulation. It is reported that the micelles conjugated with salinomycin provide passive targeting in breast cancer and stem cell cancer.

Inverse Targeting

Inverse targeting is used to bypass or avoid the uptake of drug delivery through the RES system; these are achieved by suppressing the uptake function of RES and suppressing the defense mechanism [1, 18]. These are widely used to target the non- RES organ. *E.g.*, Inverse targeting is used for targeting methotrexate to peritoneal tumors.

Physical Targeting

Physical targeting is done by changes in external changes in the drug delivery system, which allows to target them at a specific site. Physical changes involve alterations in temperature, pH and electric field. These are frequently utilized for cancer treatment by gene targeting therapy [18]. *E.g.*, it is reported that physical targeting is used in gene therapy.

Dual Targeting

Dual targeting method involves drug carrier and drug, in which drugs, as well as nanocarrier both, have the therapeutic effect which causes a synergistic effect on the overall drug delivery system. *E.g.*, Anti-viral drugs loaded with the carrier, which also has antiviral properties, this system increases the therapeutic effect [1, 18]. It is also reported that delivery of paclitaxel and curcumin for brain tumors is done by dual targeting.

Double Targeting

It is a targeting method that involves the temporal and spatial delivery of the drug. In spatial delivery targeting, the drug to a particular target site in the cell, tissue, or organ and temporal delivery involves controlling the drug release rate at the target site [1, 18]. *E.g.*, Anti-cancer drug conjugate with dendrimer targeting to tumor site through Double targeting mechanism.

TYPES OF NANOCARRIERS FOR TARGETING

Targeting of drugs can be achieved through many nano-sized carrier systems. The selection of nanocarrier is based on targeting cells, tissue, or organ. In this, the nanocarriers are categorized according to the materials used for their preparation (Fig. **4.2**) [10, 17, 20, 23]. They are:

Lipid-based Nanocarriers

These types of nanocarriers are prepared from lipids or oils such as lecithin, cholesterol, oils, *etc.* Nanocarriers included in the lipid base are liposomes, nanoparticles (SLNs and NLCs), exosomes, and nanoemulsion [23].

Polymer-based Nanocarriers

This type of nanocarriers are usually from a synthetic polymer such as polyethylene glycol, polyesters, polydioxanones, *etc.*, and natural polymers such as chitosan, gelatin, *etc* [20]. This type of nanocarriers involves polymeric nanoparticles, drug conjugate, nanogel polymeric micelles, and dendrimers.

Non-Polymers-based Nanocarriers

These types of nanocarriers are prepared from inorganic/non-polymeric materials such as silica nanoparticles, gold nanoparticles, carbon nanotubes, quantum dots, metallic nanoparticles, *etc* [10].

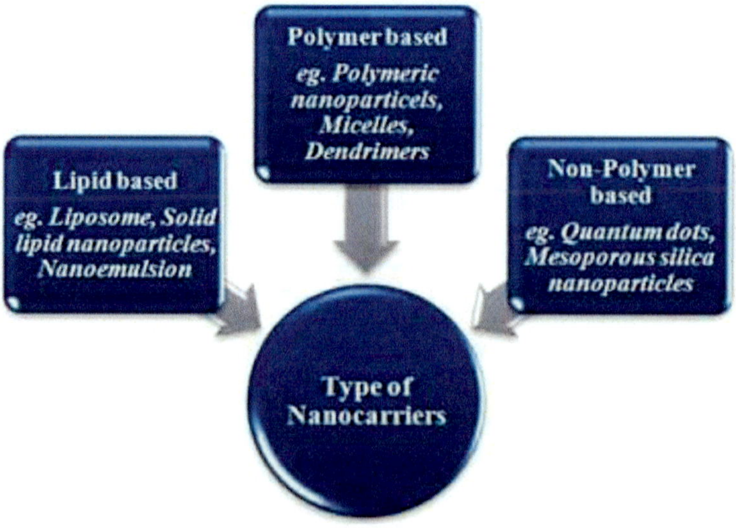

Fig. (4.2). Nanocarriers for drug targeting.

Liposome

It is the first nanocarriers that are investigated for targeting. They are colloidal nano-sized carriers composed of phospholipids and cholesterol or surfactant. It is a bilayer vesicle enclosed in an aqueous core and forms spherical vesicles. It can be delivered by both hydrophilic as well as a lipophilic drugs [17, 24, 25].

Liposomes have the property of increasing water solubility and improving the pharmacokinetic properties of drugs. Drug release from liposomes depends on various parameters *viz.* pH, osmotic gradients, composition, and the cellular environment [26]. The liposomal system also provides longer residence time in the cell which increases the duration of action. Liposomes will interact with cell through adsorption, endocytosis, fusion, and lipid transfer. Liposomes are classified according to their structure and size [27 - 29].

Liposomes are available in various sizes and formed from lipid incorporated in an aqueous environment. Due to hydrophobic force, the amphiphilic molecules aggregates and form liposome through sonication and homogenizations [30, 31]. Various methods are available for the preparation of liposomes and drug loadings, such as active drug loading, in which the drug is entrapped after vesicle formation and passive loading, in which the drug is encapsulated during vesicle formation in Table **4.1**.

Table 4.1. Types of Liposomes.

S.No.	Type of liposome	Size in nm
1.	Unilamellar	All size ranges
2.	Small unilamellar	20–100 nm
3.	Medium unilamellar	>100 nm
4.	Large unilamellar	>100 nm
5.	Oligolamellar	0.1–1 mm
6.	Multilamellar	>0.5 mm
7.	Multivesicular	>1 mm

There are some common methods available that are used for the preparation of liposomes [31 - 33].

a. ***Thin-film method***: It is the most common method. Thin films of lipid in the rotary evaporate formed with the help of lipid dissolved in the organic solvent. Then after complete drying, the film is hydrated with an aqueous/buffer solution [32]. The lipophilic drug which is encapsulated in the liposome, is added with lipid before film formation, and the hydrophilic drug should be added with an aqueous solvent or buffer solution. The advantage of this techniqúc is high reproducibility, and the disadvantage is low encapsulation efficiency.
b. ***Proliposome technique***: This is quite a simple method as compared to the thin-film technique. It has high encapsulation efficiency. In this technique, the

lipid is dissolved in water and alcohol (ethanol) at 60 °C and forms a smooth paste, then, after the lipid is cooled, and through stirring, water or buffer is added dropwise. This method is widely used for the preparation of large quantities of liposomes [32]. For encapsulation of lipophilic drugs, the drug is added in ethanol, and for hydrophilic drugs, the drug is added in water or buffer solution.

c. ***Ethanol injection method***: As the name justifies, the injection of lipid solution prepared in ethanol is added into the aqueous phase while stirring then the solvent is removed. This technique is used for the preparation of SUV liposomes in the size range of 30-170nm. It has some drawbacks, such as low encapsulation efficiency for hydrophilic drugs, and the solubility of lipid in ethanol is limited [31, 33].In this method, the size of the liposome depends on two factors, *viz.,* the lipid concentration and the injection speed.
d. ***Ether Injection technique***: This method is almost similar to the above-mentioned ethanol injection method; in place of ethanol, ether is used as an organic solvent, and this solvent is not miscible with water. The liposome formation technique is the same as the ethanol injection technique in which lipid is injected into the water while stirring. Some exception is that the ether is not soluble in water, so both the phases organic and aqueous phase has to be at different temperature during the injection process [31, 32]. The rate of injection should be slow as compared to ethanol injection, and sometimes, it is also used under vacuumed conditions. This technique provides LUV with high encapsulation efficiency.
e. ***Emulsification technique***: This method involves using water and organic solvents to dissolve the lipid. In this technique, the organic solvent is not removed, and this solution forms the emulsion. A monolayer of lipid is formed around water droplets then the organic solvent is evaporated and produces liposomes. This technique provides high drug encapsulation.

Some of the drugs that have liposome preparation include some neurotransmitters, antibiotics, and anti-inflammatory and anti-cancer drugs. Some of the properties of Liposomes is an accumulation of liposomes in cells, *e.g.*, Liver macrophages, which are other than the target site and show undesirable effect depending on therapeutic agents such as cellular necrosis [29, 34] Recently, multifunctional liposome have been used that contain specific protein, antigen, and ligands which act on particular target site. These multifunctional liposomes are widely used for targeted drug delivery systems. It is reported that cationic liposome is used as a gene delivery carrier [35].

Solid Lipid Nanoparticles (SLNs)

These are nanocarrier systems containing a solid lipid matrix. SLNs are stable as compared to liposomes, micelles, and nanoemulsions. They can be easily synthesized without organic solvent. It is composed of lipid which is solid at room temperature and surfactant [4, 36]. It is prepared by dispersed melting lipid in an aqueous surfactant through micro-emulsification or high-pressure homogenization technique. This carrier system is absorbed through dermal, parenteral, ocular, pulmonary, and rectal routes. SLNs are made up of solid lipids like triglycerides, complex glycerides, and waxes which are stabilized by various types of surfactants such as sodium cholate, sodium glycolate, soya lecithin, *etc* [17, 37]. SLN has good physical stability, protects the drug from degradation, has a large surface area, improves bioavailability, has high drug loading capacity, encapsulates both hydrophilic/lipophilic drugs, and provides desired drug release [10, 37]. SLNs are easily cross the blood-brain barrier or taken up by brain cells, bypass the liver, escape from the reticuloendothelial system (RES) and show the least toxicity due to the biodegradable nature of lipid [26, 38]. Some of the drawbacks of SLN are low drug loading capacity, drug expulsion, and high-water content. The methods for the preparation of SLNs are discussed below [36, 39]:

a. ***High-pressure Homogenization Technique (HPH)***: This is the most preferred method for the preparation of SLN and nanoemulsion at a large scale. It is based on the particle size reduction concept under different pressure conditions. In this technique, high pressure is applied to liquids which generate high shear stress and reduce the particle size up to nano ranges. This process is continued till the desired uniform particle size is not obtained. This technique provides an easy, less time-consuming, and scale-up facility. In the HPH technique, there are two approaches; one is Hot HPH, in which the lipid phase is heated 5-10 °C more than the melting point of solid lipid and mixed with a drug to form a homogenous mixture and then dispersed in a surfactant-containing aqueous phase at the same temperature; this pre-emulsion is homogenized at the same temperature. The desired formulation was obtained after 3-5 cycles at 500-1500 bars. Finally obtained emulsion was cooled down at room temperature to solidify SLN. This technique is not useful for heat-sensitive hydrophilic drugs [36]. Another is the Cold HPH technique, in which drug added melt lipid phase is cool down through liquid nitrogen to solidify and then ground with the help of a mortar pestle to form microparticles, and this is dispersed in the surfactant-containing cool aqueous phase to form pre-emulsion. Then this emulsion is homogenized at room temperature in HPH.
b. ***Microemulsion Technique***: In this technique, microemulsion dilutes in a cold aqueous phase which forms SLN or lipid nanoparticles by precipitation. A drug is dissolved in melted lipids particular temperature and surfactant-containing aqueous phase heated at the same temperature. Then hot aqueous phase is then added to melted lipid through stirring at the same temperature to

form a microemulsion [36]. The oil in water microemulsion is then dispersed in cold water through gentle mixing and crystallized to form SLN. This technique is simple, reproducible, and for large scale-up. Excess water from SLN can be removed through lyophilization or ultra-filtration.

c. ***Solvent Emulsification***- *evaporation technique:* In this method, a lipid is dissolved in a water-immiscible organic solvent such as acetone, cyclohexane, *etc.* In this technique, the drug is added to a lipid-containing organic solvent. While continuing stirring oily organic phase is added to the aqueous surfactant-containing phase [39]. The stirring is continued till the organic solvent is completely vaporized and obtained nanoemulsion is cooled to solidify the SLNs. This technique is highly suitable for heat-sensitive drugs. Its only disadvantage is that it requires toxic organic solvent.
d. ***Ultrasonication Method***: In this technique, both the drug and lipid are dissolved in organic solvent and heated. Surfactant or emulsifier containing aqueous phase is also heated at the same temperature. After partial vaporization of the organic solvent aqueous phase is added to the organic phase with stirring at high speed. Then formed emulsion is sonicated for a particular time and cooled in an ice bath to solidify SLNs [36, 39]. It is a simple and cost-effective method.
e. ***Double Emulsion Technique***: This technique is based on the solvent emulsification evaporation technique. It is used for the preparation of hydrophilic drug-loaded SLNs. In this technique, hydrophilic drugs and stabilizers are dissolved in the aqueous phase and emulsified with melted lipid in the water-immiscible organic phase. These primary emulsions are dispersed in a hydrophilic emulsifier containing an aqueous phase to form water in oil in water emulsion. After solvent evaporation due to precipitation SLNs or NLCs is prepared [39]. This stabilizer is used for the prevention of drug partitioning to the external phase during solvent evaporation.

Polymeric Nanoparticles (PNPs)

Polymeric Nanoparticles (PNPs) are colloidal nanocarriers prepared from synthetic polymers such as polyacrylate, polyacrylamide, poly e-caprolactone, *etc.*, and natural polymers such as albumin, chitosan, gelatin, *etc.* PNPs are classified based on *in vivo* behavior, such as biodegradable (*e.g.*, poly-L-lactide, poly-glycolide) and non-biodegradable (*e.g.*, Polyurethane) [38]. To reduce intermolecular interaction or immunological interactions, PNPs are coated with a nonionic surfactant. The drug can be added to PNPs after polymerization reaction or can be encapsulated during polymerization steps [40, 41]. It can work as a reservoir in which the drug is dissolved or dispersed in the core or matrix of polymeric material, which can conjugate or adsorb the drug. In the body, polymeric nanoparticles produce monomers that can be easily degraded by metabolic pathways. Drugs can be released from PNPs through desorption, diffusion, and nanoparticle erosion [42]. It was reported in a study that nanoparticles that contained biodegradable thermoresponsive chitosan-g-po-y-biopolymer delivered 5-fluorouracil to the cancer cell. Nanocarriers which are composed of biodegradable material, get metabolized through hydrolysis and form biodegradable monomers such as lactic acid and glycolic acid, which shows minimum toxicity and are applicable for biomedical use. Drugs which are encapsulated in biodegradable polymer nanocarriers are stable in blood, non-thrombogenic and non-toxic [23, 43]. Drugs such as doxorubicin are entrapped in polymeric nanoparticles are the potential to target the cancer cell. Polymeric nanoparticles it has the potential to produce multifunctional polymeric nanoparticles, which can incorporate multiple drugs at the same time [44, 45]. These are also synthesized for targeted delivery through stimuli such as low pH, redox, *etc.* Methods used for the preparation of polymeric nanoparticles (PNPs) are discussed below [23, 41, 46]:

a. ***Solvent Evaporation***: This is the technique used for the preparation of PNPs from a preformulated polymer. The organic phase is prepared by dissolving the drug in an organic solvent such as ethyl acetate. This organic phase is emulsified with a surfactant-containing aqueous phase through ultra-sonication or high-speedhomogenization [23]. The organic solvent is evaporated, and the solidified NPs can be collected.
b. ***Emulsification Technique/solvent Diffusion***: O/Wtype emulsion is prepared using water as aqueous phase and partial water-miscible solvent as organic phase [41]. The drug and polymer are dissolved in a water-miscible organic solvent such as ethyl acetate, benzyl alcohol, *etc.*, and are incorporated into a large amount of surfactant-containing aqueous phase to form a dispersed phase into a continuous phase which results in the formation of colloidal particles.
c. ***Emulsification/Reverse salting-out technique***: This technique is based on the separation of organic solvent from the aqueous phase through the salting-out effect and produces PNPs. In this technique, the o/w emulsion is formed with the help of water-miscible polymer-solvent and gel, stabilizer, or salting-out agent-containing aqueous phase through continuous stirring. And then diluted with an appropriate volume of deionized water. The remaining solvent or salting-out agents should be removed through cross-flow filtration [23, 46]. Magnesium chloride, calcium chloride, and magnesium acetate are a few salting-out agents used for PNPs preparation.
d. ***Nanoprecipitation***: In this method, two miscible solvents are used. First is the internal phase, which consists of a polymer containing organic solvents such as acetone or acetonitrile. It is miscible in water therefore, it can be easily evaporated with water. The second phase is the surfactant-containing aqueous

phase. The first polymer containing the organic phase is added to the aqueous phase with continuous stirring. When solvent diffuses out from droplets, it forms a precipitate in the form of PNPs [23, 41].

Dendrimer

These are unique types of nanocarriers with well define dendritic structure and size. This structure is similar to some biological molecules such as amylopectin, glycogen, and proteoglycan. In dendrimer, it contains several structures: a core, dendrons, and a surface-active group. The core is a single molecule or atom in which dendrons are attached [42]. Dendrons are also called dendrimer arms; these are monomers of the molecule which attached to the core and formed a different layer with successive generations. Dendrimer also contains some surface-active groups responsible for the biocompatibility and physicochemical properties of nanocarrier. In dendrimer number of surface-active groups on the surface is called polyvalence [4, 47]. The selection of core material, type of monomer, and surface-active agents decide the applicability of dendrimer in the biomedical field. The toxicity of dendrimer depends on the core material and is also affected by the dendrimer surface. *E.g.*, Changes in the surface of the hydroxyl group from the amine group reduce the toxicity level. Dendrimer contains several functional groups on the surface, which enables it to interact with no. of receptors and increase its activity [48, 49]. The addition of a drug to dendrimer depends on the drug's properties. The drug can be chemically attached to dendrimer or physically adsorbed on the surface of dendrimer, or encapsulated in the internal structure of dendrimer. The encapsulation method is used for drugs that are highly toxic or poorly soluble. Chemical attachment of drug controls the amount of drug in dendrimer [50]. In some cases, both methods provide targeted delivery by attaching targeting agents such as folic acid or epidermal growth factor. The dendrimer surface provides a platform for attaching the specific ligand for targeting delivery such as folic acid, antibodies, *etc.* Poly amido amide (PAMAM) is a type of dendrimer which are widely used in biological applications [51]. This dendrimer grows up to G 1-10 generations, and their size up to 1.1-12.4nm. It is reported that cisplatin is conjugate with PAMAM dendrimer, which shows slow drug release, low toxicity, and increased drug accumulation in the tumor cell.

The synthesis of the dendrimer is concerned with polymer and molecular chemistry. Dendrimers are related to molecular chemistry through their controlled synthesis and polymer chemistry for their particular structure [47]. The structures are synthesized through a repetitive sequence of reactive groups and form first generation, second generation, and so on. Dendrimers are prepared from divergent and convergent methods.

a. ***Divergent Method***: The synthesis of dendrimer starts from the core to the arms in a stepwise manner. Polyamidoamines (PAMAMs) dendrimer is the first synthesized dendrimer. The divergent synthesis starts from a multifunctional core such as ethylenediamine, and then two arms are added to the nitrogen of EDA after that, in the second step, EDA is again reacted, and four arms are added [47]. These steps are repeated multiple times and form different generations. This technique gives a higher yield value with low purity.
b. ***Convergent Method***: In the convergent method synthesis of a dendrimer starts from the exterior part of molecules that configure the outermost arm of the final dendrimer. This is an easy technique to purify the formulation. This method does not provide a high-generation dendrimer [47, 52, 53].

Nanoemulsion

It is a type of liquid-based formulation used for systemic or local targeted delivery systems. These are non-equilibrium emulsions with size ranges from 20-200nm. Nanoemulsions are transparent and stable systems [54]. There is the energy required for the preparation of nanoemulsion. It can be prepared through phase inversion and self-emulsifying techniques. Its droplet remains stable in stress conditions. Nanoemulsion has various properties, including high drug loading capacity, protection of drug load from the biological environment, increased bioavailability, provide sustained release, which makes them suitable for targeted delivery and biomedical application [55]. There are 3 types of nanoemulsion - oil in water (o/w), water in oil (w/o), and bicontinuous nanoemulsion. In oil in water (o/w), nanoemulsion oil droplets are dispersed in the aqueous continuous phase, whereas in water in oil (w/o), nanoemulsion water droplets are dispersed in the oil continuous phase. In bicontinuous nanoemulsion, amounts of water and oil are similar. In preparation of nanoemulsion, other than oil and water, surfactant or cosurfactant are also used, which cause the interaction of oil and water phase. The structure of formulations is affected by the ratio of oil and water [56]. The oil in water (o/w) nanoemulsion has lipophilic, which can be helpful in the accumulation of nanocarrier in lipid reach portions such as skin; therefore, it is used in the local targeting system. It has a very small size which can help in achieving the target by EPR (enhanced permeation and retention) effect. The nanoemulsion surface can be modified by conjugating with specific ligands which target their specific receptor overexpressed in disease conditions. In nanoemulsion formation, additives and emulsifiersused [57]. Various methods are involved in the preparation of nanoemulsion. These two methods are used: the high energy emulsification technique involves high energy stirring, ultrasonic emulsification, high-pressure homogenization, *etc.*, and the low energy emulsification technique involves emulsion inversion and spontaneous emulsification. Some of the methods are available for nanoemulsion preparation [57 - 59].

a. ***Ultrasonic emulsification technique***: This technique is worked based on the high-energy emulsification technique. This method provides energy through a sonicator probe and provides mechanical vibration and cavitation. The Ultrasonication method is very effective for reducing droplet size. It is mostly used for laboratory purposes.
b. ***High-pressure homogenization***: This technique also works based on the high-energy emulsification technique. In this technique, a high-pressure homogenizer is used to produce the desired size of nanoemulsion. In this technique, various forces are involved, such as hydraulic shear, turbulence, and cavitation, to produce nanosize ranges of nanoemulsion. In the HPH technique, resultant products are re-entered till the desired size of nanoemulsion is not prepared [57, 58].
c. ***Microfluidization method***: It is a mixing technology through a microfluidizer device. This technique used high energy, which forces the formulation to flow through the microchannel present in the device to reduce the particle size in nano ranges. In this technique, firstly, two solutions, aqueous or oily solution, are mixed and processed in a homogenizer to form a coarse emulsion; after that, this pre-emulsion is placed in a microfluidizer repeatedly to further size reduction and obtain a stable nanoemulsion. The emulsion is then filtered through nitrogen to remove large particles [57, 59].
d. ***Phase Inversion temperature (PIT) technique***: In nanoemulsions, because of their small size, their sedimentation or creaming is the main reason for their breakdown. Phase inversion temperature technique used for temperature-dependent solubility of nonionic surfactants to modify their affinity for water or oil. In this technique, the oily phase is mixed with the surfactant-containing aqueous phase at room temperature and forms o/w microemulsion. In this emulsion, surfactants form a monolayer. When the emulsion is heated gradually, the surfactant change into lipophilic and is completely solubilized in the oily phase and undergo phase inversion and make w/o emulsion [57, 58]. This method is not suitable for thermolabile drug substances.
e. ***Solvent displacement technique***: This technique is used for the spontaneous formation of nanoemulsion. In this technique, the oily phase is dissolved in water-miscible organic solvents such as ethanol, acetone, *etc.* Then this organic phase is poured into the surfactant-containing aqueous phase with continued stirring to form spontaneous nanoemulsion [46, 57, 59]. This method is simple, reliable, and used at room temperature. This technique is widely used for the preparation of nanoemulsion parenteral formulation.

Quantum Dots

These are a type of fluorescent semiconductor inorganic nano-sized particles from 2-10nm. Quantum dots are composed of core material and capped with shell materials. It consists of heavy metals such as Cd, Pb, Hg, In, Zn, and Se. These atoms are involved in group II-VI or II-V elements in the periodic table. Cadmium selenide (CdSe) and cadmium telluride (CdTe) are two common examples of quantum dots [10]. The size of the quantum dots depends on their light emissions range, such as UV and IR regions. QDs which are smaller in size (~2nm) emit blue fluorescence and larger QDs (~5nm) show red to orange fluorescence [60, 61]. Quantum dots have unique optical properties, high photostability, high fluorescence and good chemical property, making them suitable for biomedical applications in drug delivery, biosensor, labeling, bioimaging, and diagnosis. It shows the various advantages over traditional organic dyes [62]. Quantum dots transmit the light near-infrared region, which is suitable for imaging tissue *in-vivo* and *in-vitro*. It provides various surface functionalization, which makes them suitable for biological applications through the attachment of various drugs, proteins, and targeting ligands and provide targeting delivery of drugs. It also provides water solubility and high photostability [61, 63]. The quantum dots are also used in tagging nanocarriers, or self serves as nanocarriers for targeting a specific cell, tissue, or organ. The major drawback of quantum dots is their toxicity. Some QDs, such as CdSe, CdTe, *etc.*, release cadmium after metabolism and generate oxidative free radicals that accumulate in liver or kidney cells and cause toxicity. The toxicity is also caused by the amount of QDs, their shell or capping material, and surface chemistry [64]. The toxicity of QDs leads to cell death or hepatotoxicity. It is reported that Peptide conjugates with the peptide used for *in-vivo* tumor vasculature targeting. Research shows that QDs are conjugated with streptavidin and IgG to target HER2 on live breast cancer cells [63, 64].

The synthesis of various techniques is used according to desired size and property [62, 64].

a. ***High-temperature synthesis***: This technique is used for the preparation of monodisperse QDs at high temperatures. In this method, dimethyl cadmium is used as starting material at high temperatures. This technique is a toxic, expensive method. Therefore, various alternate precursors are used for this technique to reduce their toxicity.
b. ***Microwave-assisted method***: Microwave-assisted method worked on either pulse wave mode or continuous mode. The fast heating accelerates the decomposition of substance and provides uniform crystal nucleation, which results in the formation of QDs [64]. The size and shape of QDs depend on the intensity of microwavc radiation, the concentration of substrates, polymer concentration, and temperature. The microwave-assisted technique provides uniform heat transfer and nucleation [63]. This technique is used for the

preparation of CdS, CdSe, carbon quantum dots, *etc.*

c. ***Sol-gel Method***: This is a very simple, quick, and cheap technique for the preparation of QDs. The precursor materials are used in the form of solution and grow at low temperatures to form a gel [63, 64]. This can be optimized through thermal annealing. This process can yield QDs sizes ranging from 4-20nm. This process is widely used for the preparation of Au, Cu, and Zn containing QDs.

These are some common methods for the preparation of QDs because of the high toxicity of Cd compounds. At present, carbon-QDs, graphene QDs, and ZnO QDs are widely used for biological applications. In Fig. (**4.3**), some common C-QDs preparation methods are shown [64].

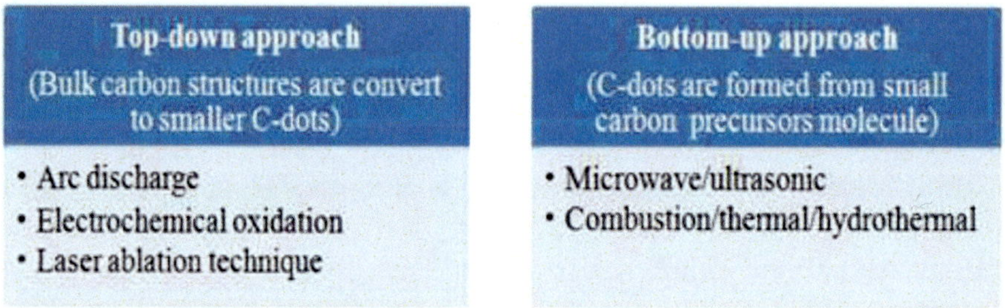

Fig. (4.3). Methods of preparation of Quantum dots.

Mesoporous Silica Nanoparticles

It is a type of nanoparticle suitable for drug targeting because of its various physicochemical properties, good stability, smaller size, large surface area, and biocompatibility. It possesses a smaller size which provides efficient and targeted delivery of drugs at a controlled rate [42]. The large surface area of silica nanoparticles allows different functionalization for targeting the therapeutic agents to their particular target site [10]. It has a porous honeycomb structure that provides encapsulation of therapeutic agents, which protects from environmental degradation or immune system as well as reduced the side effect. It can encapsulate hydrophilic as well as lipophilic drug, which can be binded with suitable ligands for targeted drug delivery [26]. It has a high drug loading capacity, is biocompatible, has a large pore volume or surface area, and is thermodynamic stable. It possesses active or passive targeting in the cancer cell. It is widely applicable in targeted delivery, diagnosis, bio-sensing, and cosmetics.

The synthesis process of microporous silica nanoparticles was firstly discovered by Stober therefore, this technique is called Stober synthesis. The MSNs synthesis is done under acidic, basic, or neutral conditions. For the synthesis of MSNs, some conditions are considered, such as pH of the reaction mixture, source of silica, temperature, the concentration of surfactant, *etc.* Altering the condition leads to changes in the size and shape of MSNs. Other than this technique, some other approaches are also used for the preparation of MSNs [35, 65, 66].

a. ***Sol-gel technique***: This process is widely used to synthesize inorganic materials, where hydrolysis and condensation of alkoxide monomer occur to form a colloidal solution. This solution act as a precursor material to form a gel-like structure of polymer [35]. This process involves the use of some acidic or basic catalyst. The alkoxide groups get hydrolyzed based on the molar ratio of Si/H_2O and reaction conditions. Then multiple condensations of solution lead to the formation of gel and form MSNs.
b. ***Evaporation-induced self-assembly technique***: In this technique, the desired amount of precursor formulation was prepared with the help of surfactant in ethanol/water. This solution is injected into the aerosol generator and forms monodisperse droplets [65, 66]. During the drying process, the alcohol evaporated, formed micelles, and turned into solid particles.

Polymeric Micelles

This is the new type of nanocarrier. Micelles are the colloidal aggregate that is prepared through the mixing of detergent and water. Polymeric micelles are amphiphilic in which a non-polar or hydrophobic region is present in the center, and a polar head or hydrophilic region is present in contact with the external solvent. The micelles are best suited for hydrophobic therapeutic agents, poorly soluble drugs, genes, and imaging agents. Critical micelle concentration (CMC) is the key parameter during the preparation of micelles. Below critical micellar concentration, micelles were not formed [40, 42, 67]. Polymeric micelles are self-assembled structures. It is made up of two-layer first is the inner core layer which encapsulates the hydrophobic drug or works as a drug reservoir. The second is the outer shell which works as a protective layer and provides protection to the drug from the external environment and also helps to attain long circulation in the blood. They are prepared from different types of blocked copolymers such as PEGylated polylactic acid (PEG-PLA), PEGylated polyaspartic acid, PEGylated polyglutamic acid, and PEGylated poly(lactic-*co*-glycolic acid), *etc.* in which one copolymer is soluble in the solvent while other is insoluble in water. It provides high drug loading and stability in the biological environment [68]. Low molecular weight drug is conjugated with polymeric micelles, which give changes in pharmacokinetic properties of drugs at the cellular level; this provides passive targeting of tumor cells via EPR effect. It is reported that polymeric micelles are used as a drug carrier for amphotericin B to target the particular site and reduce drug toxicity. Polymeric micelles coated with sugar or peptide moieties are used to target the specific receptor in the cell. It is also reported that drug-polymer conjugate contains galactosamine, which directs the HPMA- tetrapeptidyl-doxorubicingalactosamine to target the asialoglycoprotein receptor in hepatocytes for treatment of liver cancer. In hair follicle-related diseases, polymeric micelles are highly used to target the pilosebaceous gland, such as adapalene encapsulated within polymeric micelle and increase its target efficacy [69]. It is also reported that the target delivery of nucleic acid to a cancer cell is achieved through pH-responsive micelle nanocarrier with conjugation of the fluorescent-labeled aptamer. Polymeric micelles are widely used as nanocarriers in the treatment of cancer. Most anticancer drugs have limited aqueous solubility; polymeric micelles allow the hydrophobic drug to be entrapped within and increase their water solubility [26, 70]. The smaller size of the polymeric nanocarriers provides prolonged blood circulation and accumulates in the tumor site by the EPR effect. Other than passive targeting polymeric micelles also allows active targeting of cancer cell by surface modifications. The methods for the preparation of polymeric micelles are mentioned under [67, 70]:

a. ***Direct dissolution technique***: In this method, drug and block copolymer are mixed with an aqueous solvent through heating. As the temperature increase, dehydration of core-forming molecules occurs and forms polymeric micelles [67]. This technique is commonly used for hydrophobic copolymers such as poloxamer.
b. ***Solvent evaporation method***: In this technique, in place or aqueous solvent, organic solvents are used for mixing drug and copolymer. Both are dissolvent in the same organic solvent, which is immiscible with an aqueous phase [67]. Then the organic solvent can be removed through evaporation, and the thin film of drug and copolymer is formed, and water is added additionally to the film to produce polymeric micelles.
c. ***Dialysis technique***: In this technique, drug and block copolymer were mixed with organic solvent and passed through the dialysis membrane or bags, which are placed in a water-containing beaker. Organic solution and water is moved in and out [70]. This method is used for drugs which are poor solubility.

Some of the nanocarrier systems used in the targeting system are mentioned in Table **4.2**.

STRATEGIES FOR DRUG LOADING IN NANOCARRIERS OR THEIR RELEASE

For targeting delivery, nanocarriers play an important role to target the particular cell, tissue, or organ. The loading of drugs into nanocarriers and their release depends on their surface chemistry or functional group present on their surface [9, 71]. There are 3 strategies for drug loading within nanocarriers:

- 1^St Strategy: Conjugation of drug with nanocarriers through covalent bonding
- 2nd strategy: Electrostatic interaction of drug with nanocarriers
- 3rd Strategy: Encapsulation of drug within nanocarriers.

Table 4.2. Nanocarrier system used in targeting system.

S. No.	Type of Nanocarrier	Size (in nm)	Definition	Advantage	Disadvantage
1	Liposome	50–100	It is the type of spherical vesicle with a phospholipid bilayer. They are microscopic vesicular structures in which aqueous volume is enclosed by a lipid bilayer.	bilayer vesicle, Biocompatible, biodegradable, less toxicity, entrapping the hydrophilic or lipophilic drug	Leakage of a drug, rapid uptake by RES, poor stability, and phospholipid cause oxidation or hydrolysis
2	Dendrimer	1–10	It originated from the Greek dendron, meaning "tree" Dendrimer are highly branched 3D structures, consisting of three components: core, branches, and end groups.	It is the colloidal carrier, has Thermodynamic stability, acts as a solubility enhancer, the controllable size, functional groups on the surface, and uniform size distribution biodegradable	Low drug loading capacity, burst release, cellular toxicity, and high cost for synthesis.
3	Polymer micelles	10–100	It is a block of polymers, typically having a core-shell structure. The core contains the drugs, while the shell interacts with the solvent making the nanoparticles stable in the liquid	Useful for poorly water-soluble drugs, reduced side effects, stability, maximum	Used only for lipophilic drugs, stability, prone to deformation, depends on the CMC
4	Quantum dots	2–10	It is an inorganic type of semiconductor nanoparticles that are composed of heavy metals; it contains core or capping materials.	Electronic properties, luminescence, and narrow emission spectra provide surface functionalization, continuous absorption spectra, high light stability, and large surface area.	High cellular toxicity, shows photo-blinking effects, accumulation of QDs in RES

(Table 2) cont.....

S. No.	Type of Nanocarrier	Size (in nm)	Definition	Advantage	Disadvantage
5	Nanoemulsion	10-200	An emulsion is generally described as a heterogonous system composed of two immiscible liquids: one dispersed uniformly as fine droplets throughout the other. An emulsion is generally described as a heterogonous system composed of two immiscible liquids: one dispersed uniformly as fine droplets throughout the other. An emulsion is generally described as a heterogonous system composed of two immiscible liquids: one dispersed uniformly as fine droplets throughout the other. It is defined as a colloidal dispersion of 2 immiscible liquids which is thermodynamic unstable.	Stable, improved water solubility, biocompatible, biodegradable,	A high amount of surfactant needed
6	Solid lipid nanoparticles	50–100	It is the 1st generation of lipid-based nanocarriers that are prepared from solid lipid at room temperature and emulsifiers.	Colloidal carrier, better stability, ease of upgradeability, biodegradable	drug expulsion, Low drug loading capacity, burst release
7	Polymeric nanoparticles	10–100	Polymeric nanoparticles are a type of nanoparticles that are made up of synthetic or biodegradable polymer, in which drugs are entrapped or surface-adsorbed onto the polymeric core.	Effective cell membrane permeation, stability in the bloodstream, biodegradable	Difficult to scale up, physical handling is difficult, and low drug loading capacity.
8	Mesoporous Silica Nanoparticles	1–100	It is a special type of nanoparticles made up of inorganic material silica. It is small, rigid, and non-biodegradable.	good biocompatibility, high loading capacity, stable, controllable pore, high drug payload, versatility for drugs	Difficult in preparation, it causes cell lysis through the silanol group which is present in silica.

1st Strategy: It involves conjugation of drug with nanocarriers by covalent binding at high concentration through the presence of the suitable surface functional group. The drug is covalently attached to nanocarriers due to the presence of the various functional group. This covalent conjugation can be broken through enzymatic cleavage or chemical cleavage of the hydrolytic bond. This conjugation release or diffuse the drug at the specific target site and provide controlled drug release [9, 71]. This covalent conjugated stable nanocarriers system is suitable for targeted drug delivery systems.

2nd Strategy: The second strategy is the electrostatic interaction of drugs and nanocarriers. Some of the nanocarriers have surface functional groups, such as amine or carboxyl, which increase drug solubility. These functional groups enable to the making of the electrostatic bond between drugs and nanocarrier [71]. Certain drugs, such as ciprofloxacin, ibuprofen, indomethacin, *etc.* incorporated with nanocarriers through electrostatic interaction.

3rdStrategy: This strategy involves in encapsulation of drugs within nanocarriers. In some nanocarriers, such as polymeric nanoparticles, liposomes, dendrimers, *etc.*, there is some hollow space in which the drug is encapsulated. The hydrophobic core of the hollow cavity enables to encapsulation of the drug with hydrophobic bond interaction or hydrogen bonding. Sometimes, this drug encapsulation is also done by physical interaction [9]. Example: In liposomes, encapsulation occurs through active or passive loading. From the conjugation of drug-nanocarrier, the drug is released through pH neutralization by hydrolysis or thiolysis, *etc.*

Marketed Formulations, Patents, And Recent Developments

Marketed nanocarriers formulations, including formulations in clinical trials, are mentioned in Table **4.3**, while patents and recent developments in nanocarriers for drug targeting are mentioned in Table **4.4**.

Table 4.3. Marketed nanocarriers formulations, including formulations in clinical trials.

Nanocarrier	Product name	Detail	Disease is used	Market Status
Liposomes	Doxil (USA)	PEGylated doxorubicin HCl liposomes with EGFR targeting ligand	Kaposi's sarcoma, breast cancer, ovarian cancer	Available commercially
	Daunoxome	Daunorubicin citrate	advanced HIV-associated Kaposi's sarcoma	Available commercially
	MBP-426	Oxaliplatin with Her2 ligand	Gastroesophageal adenocarcinoma	Phase 1

Liposomes	ThermoDox®	Lyso-thermosensitive Liposomal Doxorubicin	Liver Tumor	Phase 1
	DepoCyte	liposome-encapsulated cytarabine	Acute Lymphoblastic Leukemia	Phase 2/ Phase 3
	Marqibo®	vincristine sulfate liposomes	Acute Lymphoblastic Leukemia (ALL)	Phase 2
	C225-ILS-DOX	Anti-EGFR-immunoliposomes loaded with doxorubicin	Glioblastoma	Phase 1
Polymeric micelles	Genexol PM	Polymeric Micelle Formulation of Paclitaxel	breast cancer, pancreatic cancer, and non-small cell lung cancer.	Available commercially
Polymeric nanoparticles	Cetuximab nanoparticles	Polymeric Nanoparticles Loaded with Cetuximab and Decorated with Somatostatin Analogue for Targeting of Colon Cancer	Colon Cancer or Colorectal Cancer	Phase 1

Table 4.4. Patents and recent developments in nanocarriers for drug targeting

Type of nanocarriers	Patent title	Patent number	Year	Ref.
Polymeric nanoparticles	Nanoparticles for cytoplasmic drug delivery to cancer cells	WO2007001356A3	2005	[72]
	Intravenous nanoparticles for targeting drug delivery and sustained drug release	US20060233883A1	2004	[73]
Polymeric nanoparticles	Targeted nanoparticle conjugates	US20140044791A1	2012	[74]
	Nanoparticles for drug delivery	US20070190160A1	2004	[75]
	Therapeutic composition with enhanced vessel targeting	US9456983B1	2006	[76]
	Bone targeting of biodegradable drug-containing nanoparticles	EP1620079A1	2004	[77]

(Table 4) cont.....

Type of nanocarriers	Patent title	Patent number	Year	Ref.
Liposome	Drug delivery system with two-step targeting	US6562316B1	1997	[78]
	Responsive liposomes for ultrasonic drug delivery	US20060002994A1	2005	[79]
	Drug delivery nanocarriers targeted by landscape phage	US8137693B2	2006	[80]
	Immunoliposome composition for targeting a HER2 cell receptor	US2006069542A1	2006	[80]
	Reversible masking of liposomal complexes for targeted delivery	US7037520B2	2003	[81]
	Composition and preparation method of targeting liposome-cyclic dinucleotide and application of targeting liposome-cyclic dinucleotide to anti-tumor	CN106667914A	2017	[82]
-	Tumor-targeted liposomal drug delivery system	WO2014046630A1	2012	[83]
	Lipid composition used for construction of liposomal genetic drug carrier targeted with antibodies, and use thereof	WO2015160271A1	2014	[84]
	Utilize liposome of natural sugar antibody target tumor immunotherapy and preparation method thereof	CN106146824A	2016	[85]
	A kind of Paclitaxel liposome preparation with tumor-targeting function and its preparation method and application	CN107019673A	2017	[86]
Nanoemulsion	Albendazolenanoemulsion and preparation method thereof	CN102973505A	2012	[87]
	A kind of tilmicosinnano-emulsion antibacterial drug and preparation method thereof	CN10142432A	2008	[88]
Dendrimer	Dendrimers targeting nanoparticles and preparation and application thereof	CN101327328B	2008	[89]
	Tree-like polymer nanometer drug delivery carrier targeting doxorubicin and its preparation method	CN103127525A	2013	[90]
	Dendrimers for use in targeted delivery	WO2003033027A2	2001	[91]
Polymeric micelle	Preparation method of block polymer micelle administration system with targeting effect	CN101507705A	2009	[92]
	Brain-targeted amphotericin B (AmB) polymer micelle administration system	CN102614105A	2011	[93]
Mesoporous silica nanoparticles	Folic acid-functionalized drug-loaded mesoporous silica and preparation method thereof	CN102805869B	2011	[94]
	High-yield mesoporous silica nano-particle and folic acid targeting modification method thereof	CN105905912A	2016	[95]

(Table 4) cont.....

Type of nanocarriers	Patent title	Patent number	Year	Ref.
Solid lipid nanoparticles	A suspension containing andrographolide solid lipid nanoparticles as well as preparation method and application of suspension	CN102716080B	2012	[96]
	Docetaxel solid lipid nanoparticles and preparation method thereof	CN102579341A	2011	[97]
Quantum dots	Preparation method of targeted grapheme nano-drug carrier	WO2014026435A1	2012	[98]
	Drugs for treating tumors and preparation method thereof	CN105288623A	2015	[99]
	Fluorescence carbon quantum dot with targeted recognition function on cancer cells, and preparation method and application thereof	CN103980894A	2014	[100]

CONCLUSION

Targeted delivery is an upcoming concept for a drug molecule to be delivered at a particular/desired/specific site or cell in the human body. The target delivery system provides dose reduction, and therefore, it reduces the side effect of the drug. This approach effectively treats various life-threatening diseases like cancer, neurological disorder, anti-inflammatory disorder. For drug targeting, various nanocarriers are used, such as liposomes, solid lipid nanoparticles, dendrimers, quantum dots, nanoemulsions, polymeric nanoparticles or micelles, *etc.* There is continuous progress in the drug targeting field to overcome the conventional drug delivery system. Nanocarriers can overcome the hurdles related to drug delivery or target a variety of cells. Nanocarriers have the capacity for the drug to pass the various biological barriers and target a particular cell. Nanocarriers have enormous potential for targeted delivery systems and clinical applications. Other than smaller size nanocarriers have various physicochemical properties, such as colloidal properties, controlled release, stability, biodegradation, protection of therapeutic agents, and improved pharmacokinetic and pharmacodynamic property of drugs. Nanocarriers are prepared at a scalable level at a low cost. Therefore, nanocarriers have a special ability for targeted drug delivery and overcome various drawbacks from conventional delivery systems.

CONSENT FOR PUBLICATION

Not applicable.

CONFLICT OF INTEREST

The authors declare no conflict of interest, financial or otherwise.

ACKNOWLEDGEMENTS

The authors acknowledge the Department of Science and Technology, New Delhi, India (DST/INSPIRE Fellowship/2019/IF190329 and DST/NM/NT/2018/20) for providing financial assistance for the successful completion of this work.

REFERENCES

[1] Kumar A, Nautiyal U, Kaur C, Goel V, Piarchand N. Targeted drug delivery system : Current and novel approach. Int J Pharm Med Res J 2017; 5: 448-54.

[2] Torchilin V. Multifunctional nanocarriers. Adv Drug Deliv Rev 2006; 58(14): 1532-55. [http://dx.doi.org/10.1016/j.addr.2006.09.009] [PMID: 17092599]

[3] Hameed GS, Sabar MH. Nano-carriers as a selective treatment for cancer. Al Mustansiriyah J Pharm Sci 2020; Vol. 20.

[4] Öztürk-Atar K, Eroğlu H, Çalış S. Novel advances in targeted drug delivery. J Drug Target 2018; 26(8): 633-42. [http://dx.doi.org/10.1080/1061186X.2017.1401076] [PMID: 29096554]

[5] Carbone C, Cupri S, Leonardi A, Puglisi G, Pignatello R. Lipid-based nanocarriers for drug delivery and targeting: A patent survey of methods of production and characterization. Pharm Pat Anal 2013; 2(5): 665-77. [http://dx.doi.org/10.4155/ppa.13.43] [PMID: 24237173]

[6] Garnett MC. Targeted drug conjugates: Principles and progress. Adv Drug Deliv Rev 2001; 53(2): 171-216. [http://dx.doi.org/10.1016/S0169-409X(01)00227-7] [PMID: 11731026]

[7] Pushpalatha R, Selvamuthukumar S, Kilimozhi D. Nanocarrier mediated combination drug delivery for chemotherapy – A review. J Drug Deliv Sci Technol 2017; 39: 362-71. [http://dx.doi.org/10.1016/j.jddst.2017.04.019]

[8] A review on targeted drug delivery. Am J PharmTech Res 2018; 8: 1-11. [http://dx.doi.org/10.46624/ajptr.2018.v8.i4.001]

[9] Solaro R, Chiellini F, Battisti A. Targeted delivery of protein drugs by nanocarriers. Materials (Basel) 2010; 3(3): 1928-80. [http://dx.doi.org/10.3390/ma3031928]

[10] Cui W, Li J, Decher G. Self-assembled smart nanocarriers for targeted drug delivery. Adv Mater 2016; 28(6): 1302-11.https://doi.org/https://doi.org/10.1002/adma.201502479 [http://dx.doi.org/10.1002/adma.201502479] [PMID: 26436442]

[11] Mura S, Nicolas J, Couvreur P. Stimuli-responsive nanocarriers for drug delivery. Nat Mater 2013; 12(11): 991-1003. [http://dx.doi.org/10.1038/nmat3776] [PMID: 24150417]

[12] Kumar Khanna V. Targeted delivery of nanomedicines. ISRN Pharmacol 2012; 2012: 1-9. [http://dx.doi.org/10.5402/2012/571394] [PMID: 22577576]

[13] Yu X, Trase I, Ren M, Duval K, Guo X, Chen Z. Design of nanoparticle-based carriers for targeted drug delivery. J Nanomater 2016; 2016: 1-15. [http://dx.doi.org/10.1155/2016/1087250]

[14] Din F, Aman W, Ullah I, *et al.* Effective use of nanocarriers as drug delivery systems for the treatment of selected tumors. Int J Nanomedicine 2017; 12: 7291-309. [http://dx.doi.org/10.2147/IJN.S146315] [PMID: 29042776]

[15] Kumari P, Ghosh B, Biswas S. Nanocarriers for cancer-targeted drug delivery. J Drug Target 2016;

24(3): 179-91.
[http://dx.doi.org/10.3109/1061186X.2015.1051049] [PMID: 26061298]

[16] Wilczewska AZ, Niemirowicz K, Markiewicz KH, Car H. Nanoparticles as drug delivery systems. Pharmacol Rep 2012; 64(5): 1020-37.
[http://dx.doi.org/10.1016/S1734-1140(12)70901-5] [PMID: 23238461]

[17] Daima HK, Navya PN, Ranjan S, Dasgupta N, Lichtfouse E. Nanoscience in Medicine. Springer Nature 2020; Vol. 1.

[18] Jabr-Milane L, van Vlerken L, Devalapally H, *et al.* Multi-functional nanocarriers for targeted delivery of drugs and genes. J Control Release 2008; 130(2): 121-8.
[http://dx.doi.org/10.1016/j.jconrel.2008.04.016] [PMID: 18538887]

[19] Singh AP, Biswas A, Shukla A, Maiti P. Targeted therapy in chronic diseases using nanomaterial-based drug delivery vehicles. Signal Transduct Target Ther 2019; 4(1): 33.
[http://dx.doi.org/10.1038/s41392-019-0068-3] [PMID: 31637012]

[20] Begines B, Ortiz T, Pérez-Aranda M, *et al.* Polymeric nanoparticles for drug delivery: Recent developments and future prospects. Nanomaterials (Basel) 2020; 10(7): 1403.
[http://dx.doi.org/10.3390/nano10071403] [PMID: 32707641]

[21] Xia W, Tao Z, Zhu B, *et al.* Targeted delivery of drugs and genes using polymer nanocarriers for cancer therapy. Int J Mol Sci 2021; 22(17): 9118.
[http://dx.doi.org/10.3390/ijms22179118] [PMID: 34502028]

[22] Salahpour Anarjan F. Active targeting drug delivery nanocarriers: Ligands. Nano-Structures & Nano-Objects 2019; 19: 100370.
[http://dx.doi.org/10.1016/j.nanoso.2019.100370]

[23] Khan I, Saeed K, Khan I. Nanoparticles: Properties, applications and toxicities. Arab J Chem 2019; 12(7): 908-31.https://doi.org/https://doi.org/10.1016/j.arabjc.2017.05.011
[http://dx.doi.org/10.1016/j.arabjc.2017.05.011]

[24] Bulbake U, Doppalapudi S, Kommineni N, Khan W. Liposomal formulations in clinical use: An updated review. Pharmaceutics 2017; 9(4): 12.
[http://dx.doi.org/10.3390/pharmaceutics9020012] [PMID: 28346375]

[25] Sharma G, Anabousi S, Ehrhardt C, Ravi Kumar MNV. Liposomes as targeted drug delivery systems in the treatment of breast cancer. J Drug Target 2006; 14(5): 301-10.
[http://dx.doi.org/10.1080/10611860600809112] [PMID: 16882550]

[26] Mudshinge SR, Deore AB, Patil S, Bhalgat CM. Nanoparticles: Emerging carriers for drug delivery. Saudi Pharm J 2011; 19(3): 129-41.
[http://dx.doi.org/10.1016/j.jsps.2011.04.001] [PMID: 23960751]

[27] Bardania H, Tarvirdipour S, Dorkoosh F. Liposome-targeted delivery for highly potent drugs. Artif Cells Nanomed Biotechnol 2017; 45(8): 1478-89.
[http://dx.doi.org/10.1080/21691401.2017.1290647] [PMID: 28278584]

[28] Fan Y, Zhang Q. Development of liposomal formulations: From concept to clinical investigations. Asian J Pharm Sci 2013; 8: 81-7.https://doi.org/https://doi.org/10.1016/j.ajps.2013.07.010

[29] Šturm L, Poklar Ulrih N. Basic methods for preparation of liposomes and studying their interactions with different compounds, with the emphasis on polyphenols. Int J Mol Sci 2021; 22(12): 6547.
[http://dx.doi.org/10.3390/ijms22126547] [PMID: 34207189]

[30] Akbarzadeh A, Rezaei-Sadabady R, Davaran S, *et al.* Liposome: Classification, preparation, and applications. Nanoscale Res Lett 2013; 8(1): 102.
[http://dx.doi.org/10.1186/1556-276X-8-102] [PMID: 23432972]

[31] Allen TM, Cullis PR. Liposomal drug delivery systems: From concept to clinical applications. Adv Drug Deliv Rev 2013; 65(1): 36-48.

[http://dx.doi.org/10.1016/j.addr.2012.09.037] [PMID: 23036225]

[32] Nekkanti V, Kalepu S. Recent advances in liposomal drug delivery: A review. Pharm Nanotechnol 2015; 3(1): 35-55.https://doi.org/http://dx.doi.org/10.2174/2211738503666150709173905 [http://dx.doi.org/10.2174/2211738503666150709173905]

[33] Beltrán-Gracia E, López-Camacho A, Higuera-Ciapara I, Velázquez-Fernández JB, Vallejo-Cardona AA. Nanomedicine review: Clinical developments in liposomal applications. Cancer Nanotechnol 2019; 10(1): 11. [http://dx.doi.org/10.1186/s12645-019-0055-y]

[34] Chenthamara D, Subramaniam S, Ramakrishnan SG, *et al.* Therapeutic efficacy of nanoparticles and routes of administration. Biomater Res 2019; 23(1): 20. [http://dx.doi.org/10.1186/s40824-019-0166-x] [PMID: 31832232]

[35] Narayan R, Nayak U, Raichur A, Garg S. Mesoporous silica nanoparticles: A comprehensive review on synthesis and recent advances. Pharmaceutics 2018; 10(3): 118. [http://dx.doi.org/10.3390/pharmaceutics10030118] [PMID: 30082647]

[36] Haley B, Frenkel E. Nanoparticles for drug delivery in cancer treatment. Urol Oncol 2008; 26(1): 57-64. [http://dx.doi.org/10.1016/j.urolonc.2007.03.015] [PMID: 18190833]

[37] Duong VA, Nguyen TTL, Maeng HJ. Preparation of solid lipid nanoparticles and nanostructured lipid carriers for drug delivery and the effects of preparation parameters of solvent injection method. Molecules 2020; 25(20): 4781. [http://dx.doi.org/10.3390/molecules25204781] [PMID: 33081021]

[38] El-Say KM, El-Sawy HS. Polymeric nanoparticles: Promising platform for drug delivery. Int J Pharm 2017; 528(1-2): 675-91. [http://dx.doi.org/10.1016/j.ijpharm.2017.06.052] [PMID: 28629982]

[39] Mohammadi-Samani S, Ghasemiyeh P. Solid lipid nanoparticles and nanostructured lipid carriers as novel drug delivery systems: Applications, advantages and disadvantages. Res Pharm Sci 2018; 13(4): 288-303. [http://dx.doi.org/10.4103/1735-5362.235156] [PMID: 30065762]

[40] Prabahar K, Alanazi Z, Qushawy M. Targeted drug delivery system: Advantages, carriers, and strategies. Indian Journal of Pharmaceutical Education and Research 2021; 55(2): 346-53. [http://dx.doi.org/10.5530/ijper.55.2.72]

[41] Zielińska A, Carreiró F, Oliveira AM, *et al.* Polymeric nanoparticles: Production, characterization, toxicology and ecotoxicology. Molecules 2020; 25(16): 3731. [http://dx.doi.org/10.3390/molecules25163731] [PMID: 32824172]

[42] Singh R, Lillard JW Jr. Nanoparticle-based targeted drug delivery. Exp Mol Pathol 2009; 86(3): 215-23. [http://dx.doi.org/10.1016/j.yexmp.2008.12.004] [PMID: 19186176]

[43] Mary Ealias A. M P S. A review on the classification, characterization, synthesis of nanoparticles and their application. IOP Conf Ser Mater Sci Eng. 263: 32019. [http://dx.doi.org/10.1088/1757-899X/263/3/032019]

[44] Selvakumaran S, Muhamad I, Md Lazim NA. Designing Polymeric Nanoparticles for Targeted Drug Delivery System 2014; 287-313.

[45] Kumar A. A comprehensive review on polymeric micelles: A promising drug delivery carrier. J Anal Pharm Res 2021; 10(3): 102-7. [http://dx.doi.org/10.15406/japlr.2021.10.00372]

[46] Abasian P, Shakibi S, Maniati MS, Nouri Khorasani S, Khalili S. Targeted delivery, drug release strategies, and toxicity study of polymeric drug nanocarriers. Polym Adv Technol 2021; 32(3): 931-44.https://doi.org/https://doi.org/10.1002/pat.5168

[http://dx.doi.org/10.1002/pat.5168]

[47] Abbasi E, Aval SF, Akbarzadeh A, *et al.* Dendrimers: Synthesis, applications, and properties. Nanoscale Res Lett 2014; 9(1): 247. [http://dx.doi.org/10.1186/1556-276X-9-247] [PMID: 24994950]

[48] Patra JK, Das G, Fraceto LF, *et al.* Nano based drug delivery systems: Recent developments and future prospects. J Nanobiotechnology 2018; 16(1): 71. [http://dx.doi.org/10.1186/s12951-018-0392-8] [PMID: 30231877]

[49] Mittal P, Saharan A, Verma R, *et al.* Dendrimers: A new race of pharmaceutical nanocarriers. BioMed Res Int 2021; 2021: 1-11. [http://dx.doi.org/10.1155/2021/8844030] [PMID: 33644232]

[50] Pandita D, Poonia N, Kumar S, Lather V, Madaan K. Dendrimers in drug delivery and targeting: Drug-dendrimer interactions and toxicity issues. J Pharm Bioallied Sci 2014; 6(3): 139-50. [http://dx.doi.org/10.4103/0975-7406.130965] [PMID: 25035633]

[51] Alavi M, Karimi N, Safaei M. Application of various types of liposomes in drug delivery systems. Adv Pharm Bull 2017; 7(1): 3-9. [http://dx.doi.org/10.15171/apb.2017.002] [PMID: 28507932]

[52] Chauhan A, Patil C, Jain P, Kulhari H. 14 - Dendrimer-based marketed formulations and miscellaneous applications in cosmetics, veterinary, and agriculture.Chauhan A, Kulhari HBT-PA of D. Elsevier 2020; pp. 325-34.https://doi.org/https://doi.org/10.1016/B978-0-12-814527-2.00014-7

[53] Chis AA, Dobrea C, Morgovan C, *et al.* Applications and limitations of dendrimers in biomedicine. Molecules 2020; 25(17): 3982. [http://dx.doi.org/10.3390/molecules25173982] [PMID: 32882920]

[54] Jaiswal M, Dudhe R, Sharma PK. Nanoemulsion: An advanced mode of drug delivery system. 3 Biotech 2015; 5: 123-7. [http://dx.doi.org/10.1007/s13205-014-0214-0]

[55] Mahato R. Nanoemulsion as targeted drug delivery system for cancer therapeutics. J Pharm Sci Pharmacol 2017; 3(2): 83-97. [http://dx.doi.org/10.1166/jpsp.2017.1082]

[56] Bharti C, Gulati N, Nagaich U, Pal AK. Mesoporous silica nanoparticles in target drug delivery system: A review. Int J Pharm Investig 2015; 5(3): 124-33. [http://dx.doi.org/10.4103/2230-973X.160844] [PMID: 26258053]

[57] Abasian P, Ghanavati S, Rahebi S, Nouri Khorasani S, Khalili S. Polymeric nanocarriers in targeted drug delivery systems: A review. Polym Adv Technol 2020; 31(12): 2939-54. https://doi.org/https://doi.org/10.1002/pat.5031 [http://dx.doi.org/10.1002/pat.5031]

[58] Lovelyn C, Attama AA. Current state of nanoemulsions in drug delivery. J Biomater Nanobiotechnol 2011; 2(5): 626-39. [http://dx.doi.org/10.4236/jbnb.2011.225075]

[59] Kumar M, Bishnoi RS, Shukla AK, Jain CP. Techniques for formulation of nanoemulsion drug delivery system: A review. Prev Nutr Food Sci 2019; 24(3): 225-34. [http://dx.doi.org/10.3746/pnf.2019.24.3.225] [PMID: 31608247]

[60] Matea C, Mocan T, Tabaran F, *et al.* Quantum dots in imaging, drug delivery and sensor applications. Int J Nanomedicine 2017; 12: 5421-31. [http://dx.doi.org/10.2147/IJN.S138624] [PMID: 28814860]

[61] Zhao MX, Zhu BJ. The research and applications of quantum dots as nano-carriers for targeted drug delivery and cancer therapy. Nanoscale Res Lett 2016; 11(1): 207. [http://dx.doi.org/10.1186/s11671-016-1394-9] [PMID: 27090658]

[62] Jha S, Mathur P, Ramteke S, Jain NK. Pharmaceutical potential of quantum dots. Artif Cells Nanomed Biotechnol 2018; 46(sup1): 57-65. [http://dx.doi.org/10.1080/21691401.2017.1411932] [PMID: 29216759]

[63] Obonyo O, Fisher E, Edwards M, Douroumis D. Quantum dots synthesis and biological applications as imaging and drug delivery systems. Crit Rev Biotechnol 2010; 30(4): 283-301. [http://dx.doi.org/10.3109/07388551.2010.487184] [PMID: 20528252]

[64] Ezzati Nazhad Dolatabadi J, Valizadeh H, Hamishehkar H. Solid lipid nanoparticles as efficient drug and gene delivery systems: Recent breakthroughs. Adv Pharm Bull 2015; 5(2): 151-9. [http://dx.doi.org/10.15171/apb.2015.022] [PMID: 26236652]

[65] Amiji M, Tiwari S. Nanoemulsion Formulations for Tumor-Targeted Delivery 2006; 723-39. [http://dx.doi.org/10.1201/9781420006636.sec7]

[66] Sharma N, Mishra S, Sharma S, Deshpande R, Sharma R. Preparation and optimization of nanoemulsions for targeting drug delivery. Int J Drug Dev Res 2013; 5: 37-48.

[67] Ahmad Z, Shah A, Siddiq M, Kraatz HB. Polymeric micelles as drug delivery vehicles. RSC Advances 2014; 4(33): 17028-38. [http://dx.doi.org/10.1039/C3RA47370H]

[68] Kulthe SS, Choudhari YM, Inamdar NN, Mourya V. Polymeric micelles: Authoritative aspects for drug delivery. Des Monomers Polym 2012; 15(5): 465-521. [http://dx.doi.org/10.1080/1385772X.2012.688328]

[69] Qiu L, Zheng C, Jin Y, Zhu K. Polymeric micelles as nanocarriers for drug delivery. Expert Opin Ther Pat 2007; 17(7): 819-30. [http://dx.doi.org/10.1517/13543776.17.7.819]

[70] Valizadeh A, Mikaeili H, Samiei M, *et al.* Quantum dots: Synthesis, bioapplications, and toxicity. Nanoscale Res Lett 2012; 7(1): 480. [http://dx.doi.org/10.1186/1556-276X-7-480] [PMID: 22929008]

[71] Wang N, Cheng X, Li N, Wang H, Chen H. Nanocarriers and their loading strategies. Adv Healthc Mater 2019; 8(6): 1801002.https://doi.org/https://doi.org/10.1002/adhm.201801002 [http://dx.doi.org/10.1002/adhm.201801002] [PMID: 30450761]

[72] Marciej Radosz, Youqing Shen TH. Nanoparticles for cytoplasmic drug delivery to cancer cells WO2007001356A2, 2005.

[73] Tsutomu Ishihara YM. Intravenous nanoparticles for targeting drug delivery and sustained drug release US20060233883A1, 2004.

[74] Basilion James BC. Targeted nanoparticle conjugates US20140044791A1, 2012.

[75] Turos Edward J-YS. Nanoparticles for drug-delivery US20070190160A1, 2004.

[76] Faiyaz Ahmed Hossainy Syed, Niklas Ludwig Florian, Stephen DP. Therapeutic composition with enhanced vessel targeting US9456983B1, 2006.

[77] Garlich Joseph R, Durden Donald L, Brannon-Peppas L, Smith Tim C. Bone targeting of biodegradable drug-containing nanoparticles EP1620079A1, 2004.

[78] Edwards Katarina, JörgenCarlsson SS. Drug delivery system with two-step targeting US6562316B1, 1997.

[79] James Thomas, Hung-Yin Lin, Natalia Rapoport. Responsive liposomes for ultrasonic drug delivery US20060002994A1, 2005.

[80] PV A. Drug delivery nanocarriers targeted by landscape phage US8137693B2, 2006.

[81] Smyth TN. Reversible masking of liposomal complexes for targeted delivery US7037520B2, 2003.

[82] Tan Yingxuan, Xiang Daofeng, Lu Xing TX. Composition and preparation method of targeting

liposome-cyclic dinucleotide and application of targeting liposome-cyclic dinucleotide to anti-tumor CN106667914A, 2017.

[83] Banerjee Sreeparna, Tezcaner Asli Erdog Aysen. Tumor targeted liposomal drug delivery system WO2014046630A1, 2012.

[84] Monika Toporkiewicz, Justyna Meissner, Kuliczkowski Kazimierz, Aleksander Sikorski. Lipid composition used for construction of liposomal genetic drug carrier targeted with antibodies, and use thereof WO2015160271A1, 2014.

[85] Wen Yi, Rao Xiongjian. Utilize liposome of natural sugar antibody target tumor immunotherapy and preparation method thereof CN106146824A, 2016.

[86] Cai Lulu, Yan Junfeng, Daiwen Zeng, BaiJiaojiao YC. A kind of Paclitaxel liposome preparation with tumor-targeting function and its preparation method and application CN107019673A, 2017.

[87] Shuai Hu, Nan Fan, Li Kunpeng. Albendazole nanoemulsion and preparation method thereof CN102973505A, 2012.

[88] OuyangWuqing LX. A kind of tilmicosinnano-emulsion antibacterial drug and preparation method thereof CN101422432A, 2008.

[89] Shufang Luo, Weilu Zhang, Shunying Liu, Na Li. Dendrimers targeting nanoparticle and preparation and application thereof CN101327328B, 2008.

[90] Ye Yang, Chunyan Gu, Xiaoquan Sun, Meiling Lu, Wan Li WX. Tree-like polymer nanometer drug delivery carrier targeting doxorubicin and its preparation method CN103127525A, 2013.

[91] Uchegbu Ijeoma Florence, Munro Avril, GerhartSchatzlein Andreas, Alexander Irvine Gray BZ. Dendrimers for use in targeted delivery WO2003033027A2, 2001.

[92] Hua Song, Cui Daxiang, He Rong G. Preparation method of block polymer micelle administration system with targeting effect CN101507705A, 2009.

[93] Jiang Chen, Shao Kun, KeWeilun RH. Brain targeted amphotericin B (AmB) polymer micelle administration system CN102614105A, 2011.

[94] Fang Chenjie, Guo Rui TZ. Folic acid-functionalized drug-loaded mesoporous silica and preparation method thereof CN102805869B, 2011.

[95] Jin Chang, Bin Zheng, Wang Hanjie, Chen Hongbin, Pan Huizhuo, Chen Deguang. High-yield mesoporous silica nano-particle and folic acid targeting modification method thereof CN105905912A, 2016.

[96] Yu Zhang, Guang Han, Gangjun Du, Shengjie Zhang, Wenwen Jiao, Su Hua. Suspension containing andrographolide solid lipid nanoparticles as well as preparation method and application of suspension CN102716080B, 2012.

[97] Wang Dongkai, Xiang Li, Xiao Xue. Docetaxel solid lipid nanoparticle and preparation method thereof CN102579341A, 2011.

[98] Lin Quangui, Huang Xiaojie, Yong Liu, *et al.* Preparation method of targeted graphene nano-drug carrier WO2014026435A1, 2012.

[99] RenTianbin , Zhiyong Wu, Yan Li, Haiqing Dong, Yongyong Li. Drug for treating tumors and preparation method thereof CN105288623A, 2015.

[100] Quan Lin, Xue Yang, Yang Xudong, *et al.* Fluorescence carbon quantum dot with targeted recognition function on cancer cells, and preparation method and application thereof CN103980894A, 2014.

CHAPTER 5

Nanomaterials as Diagnostic Tools and Drug Carriers

Ashish K. Parashar[1], **Preeti Patel**[2], **Monika Kaurav**[3], **Krishna Yadav**[4], **Dilpreet Singh**[2], **G.D. Gupta**[2] and **Balak Das Kurmi**[2,*]

[1] *Chameli Devi Institute of Pharmacy, Indore-452020, (M.P.), India*

[2] *ISF College of Pharmacy, Moga-142001, Punjab, India*

[3] *KIET School of Pharmacy, Ghaziabad-201206, (U.P.), India*

[4] *Raipur Institute of Pharmaceutical Education and Research (RIPER), Sarona, Raipur-492010, (C.G.), India*

Abstract: Nanotechnology is a multidisciplinary field of study that bridges chemistry, engineering, biology, and medicine. The utilization of the nanotechnological approach for the development of theranostic nanocarrier system is capable of being loaded as drug therapy/delivery and diagnostic vehicles/means. A very recent term, theranostic nanomedicine, has gained much attention as a favorable model for various types of progressive disease. Theranostic nanocarriers' strategy utilizes the diagnostic excellence mediated treatment of such illnesses that required individual therapy, such as in cancer. These can impart an essential role in improving public health regarding high-stress lifestyle-related challenges in diabetes, asthma, cancer, hypertension, and many infectious diseases, as the diagnosis of these circumstances and the treatment strategy, are also possible with biomedical applications of these nanomaterials. It includes benefits from both worlds: highly powerful nanocarriers to drug delivery and diagnosis spawned the concept, enabling the emergence of personalized medicine. This chapter discusses the state of various nanocarriers' art in the form of NPs and nanodevices applications in medical diagnosis and disease treatments. It presents key insights and current advancements into the intriguing biomedical applications of NPs, including bioimaging of biological surroundings and their significance as a critical early detection tool for various diseases. It also describes their types and limitations concerning conventional means. The topic has attracted significant attention and interest as diagnostic and treating nanocarriers' can target various illnesses faced by the healthcare providers suggested by several researchers over the past decade. Additionally, with recent advances in nanoscience and nanoscale materials, the creation of different diagnostic or therapeutic devices is also discussed briefly. Along with nanocarrier systems' therapeutic and diagnostic aims, physicochemical advantages even considerable potential to be studied concerning health system, which is useful for protecting active drug molecules from degradation, targeted and site-specific drug deli-

* **Corresponding author Balak Das Kurmi:** ISF College of Pharmacy, Moga-142001,(Punjab), India; Tel: +919754275553; E-mail: bdkurmi@gmail.com

Akhlesh K. Jain & Keerti Mishra (Eds.)

veries are also discussed. Despite the numerous technological, scientific, regulatory, and legal hurdles that nanomedicine faces, researchers are driven to develop new medications and nanomedicine devices. As a result, the development of nanoparticle-based drug delivery and diagnostic devices could help improve patient comfort and convenience while also lowering treatment costs.

Keywords: Bio-imaging, Cancer, Carbon nanotube, Cardiovascular diseases, Central nervous system diseases, Dendrimer, Drug targeting, Drug delivery, Diagnosis, Liposome, Metallic nanomaterials, MRI imaging, Nanocarriers, Nano-engineering, Nanomedicine, Nanoprobes, Photodynamic therapy, Polymeric micelle, Polymer conjugates, Pharmaceutical technology, Quantum dots, Theranostic.

INTRODUCTION

Diagnostics, nanomedicine, and pharmaceutical technology advancements have accelerated the drug discovery and development process, resulting in various innovative, compelling, and therapeutic candidates with a specific target for theranostic uses. Additionally, recent developments in pharmaceutical technology and nanotechnology have enabled theranostics to be used as realistic programmable moieties capable of performing sophisticated operations in order to correctly detect each patient's sickness status [1]. In 2002, Funkhouser invented the term "theranostics," which he defines as the product that combines two modalities, that is therapy and diagnostic imaging, along with a single set" to overcome unwanted biodistribution and therapeutic efficacy differences [2].

Using theranostic nanomedicine incorporates theranostic NPs with multiple capabilities, including stimuli-responsive systems, sustained or controlled release dosage form, increased endocytosis mediated transport efficiency, and multimodality diagnosis and therapy, to treat lethal cancers and other serious illnesses. Thus, theranostic nanomedicine has the potential to revolutionize cancer treatment and other serious diseases. Pharmacokinetics, pharmacodynamics, and biodistribution of each therapy may be optimized by using theranostic nanomedicine to deliver medicines at the right time, place, and quantity [1].

Theranostic nanomedicine allows for systemic circulation, circumvents host defence systems, and distributes medicines and diagnostic materials directly to the place of need, allowing for cellular and molecular diagnosis and therapy. When used in conjunction with theranostic nanomedicine, precise spatial and temporal regulation of therapeutic molecule development can achieve drug release based on the specific patient's sickness state, increasing therapeutic benefits while decreasing adverse effects.

Nanomedicine combines therapeutic and diagnostic agents into a single theranostic scaffold that may subsequently be attached with biological ligands to transport the agents to their targeted targets. The theranostic efficacy of NPs will steadily improve using "smart and distinctive" biomaterials in combination with NPs. Numerous biological factors, including temperature, pH, enzyme activity, or the presence of a particular targeting moiety, might result in the production of theranostic NPs that enable system-specific drug delivery while limiting damage to healthy tissues [1 - 3].

CONCEPT OF NANOTHERANOSTICS

Nanotheranostics is distinguished by three key characteristics: nanoscale size, diagnostic and therapeutic properties. By integrating several functionalities within a single particle, nanotheranostics have been shown to improve the solubilization and release profile of the medicaments, as well as the accumulation of contrast and medicinal chemicals at the site of action. Fig. **(5.1)** demonstrates the easy and simple concept of theranostics [1].

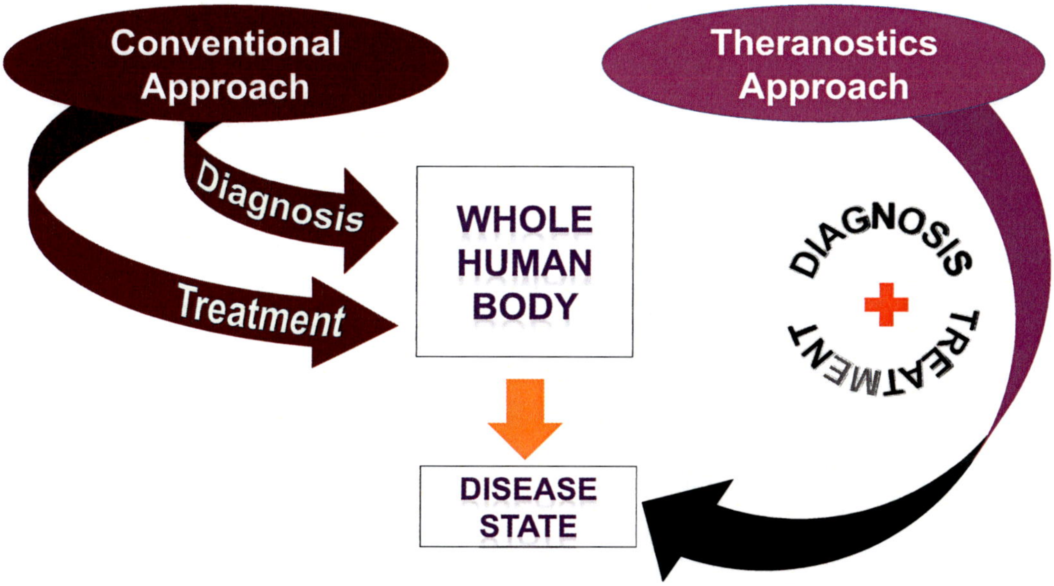

Fig. (5.1). Nanotheranostics concept.

Nanomedicine is currently generating innovative and promising uses in diagnosing and non-invasive treatment of many diseases. Although still important, developing innovative devices with superior imaging properties, which can aid in the early identification of diseases, is still a top priority. Nanotherapeutics, in addition to this, are essential components in the treatment of severe diseases. Although the approach was originally developed to treat cancer, it has since been expanded to include inflammatory diseases, autoimmune disorders, cardiovascular diseases, and neurological issues [4, 5].Nanotheranostics can be used to improve the efficacy of magnetic resonance imaging (MRI), positron emission tomography (PET), fluorescence imaging, and photoacoustic tomography [6].

There have been several approaches investigated for the production of nanotheranostics. These include polymeric, metal and inorganic NPs and conjugates, carbon nanotubes, solid lipid NPs, micelles, liposomes and dendrimers are just a few examples. Theranostic nanomedicine nanocarriers are intended to deliver diagnostic and therapeutic substances in a prolonged, controlled, and targeted way, as a result, theranostic benefits are boosted while adverse effects are minimised. Additionally, the incorporation of reporter system in sensor based theranostic devices to detect diseases allows *in vivo* evaluation for the treatment efficacy after implantation. Through the use ofnanotheranostics, it is possible to distribute siRNA in conjunction with other drugs, release drugs in response to stimuli, provide drugs orally, transfer drugs through the blood-brain barrier, and circumvent the intracellular autophagy [1]. Fig. **(5.2)** demonstrates how nanosystems may be used to personalize treatment for each patient, therefore boosting their odds of survival.

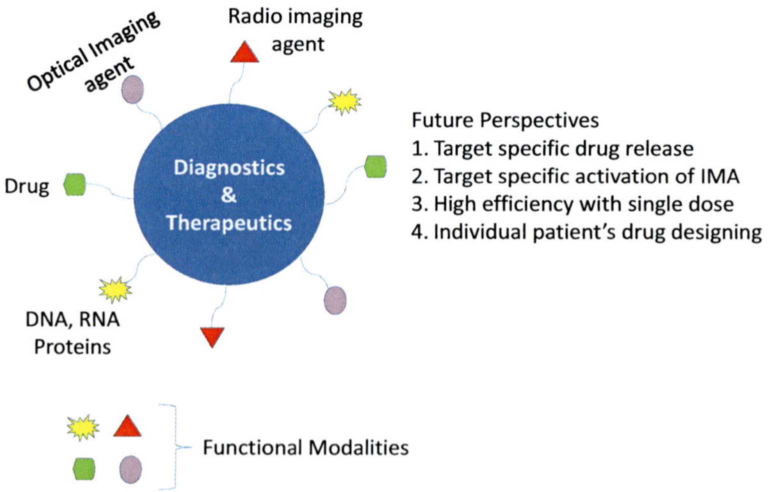

Fig. (5.2). Advancements in nanotheranostics are represented schematically.

NANOMATERIALS AS NANOTHERANOSTICS

Theranostic methods have demonstrated significant potential in terms of drug distribution monitoring. Physicochemical characteristics of a theranostic agent must allow for simple biological investigation while being stable under physiological circumstances throughout delivery [7, 8]. Furthermore, the theranostic drug must pass through biological barriers on its way to the target tissue or organ without causing severe harm [8]. It is necessary to have a therapeutic agent, a carrier for the therapeutic payload, targeting ligands, and signal emitters that are covalently or non-covalently attached to the delivery platform to function as a theranostic agent. Nanotheranosticmedicines have the potential to outperform other theranostics because it combines advanced capabilities in a single platform, including sustained/controlled release, targeted delivery, synergetic performance (*e.g.*, combination therapy, siRNA co-delivery), stimulus-responsive drug release (*i.e.,* smart delivery), increased transport efficiency *via* endocytosis, and multimodality diagnosis [9, 10].

Typically, nanotheranostics are developed using sophisticated synthetic procedures that enable numerous functionalities to a single delivery platform. As a result, nanotheranostics is frequently targeted *via* particle passive accumulation in diseased tissue *via* the increased permeability and retention effect (EPR), which is generally achieved by biological coatings (*e.g.*, albumin, peptides) or surface modification with polyethylene glycol (PEG).

Nanotheranostics is perhaps the most promising of the several techniques employed to date to design a theranostic approach properly. The method manipulates NPs by using their numerous unique features, including their large surface area, optical and magnetic capabilities, low melting point, and mechanical strength [10 - 13]. To improve the transport and treatment of biological and conventional therapies (drugs, ligands, and antibodies), nanotheranostic agents such as gold, silver, and magnetic nanoparticles (NPs), as well as nanoshells and nanocages, can be used [11]. NP-based medicines can be used as theranostic agents for a range of diseases. Theranostic NPs against plaque angiogenesis in macrophage-rich atherosclerotic lesions has been shown to irradiate inflammatory macrophages by their photodynamic action, as established in several studies [12]. It has been demonstrated that theranostic siRNA nanoprobes can protect adoptively transferred pancreatic islet transplants from immunological rejection [13], allowing for the suppression of a critical non-invasive monitoring of the graft's survival and the major histocompatibility complex domains *via* magnetic resonance imaging.

In recent years, there has been a surge in interest in using nanomaterials that offer various physical imaging modalities and therapeutic possibilities. In general, theranostic nanomaterials are composed of the following chemical components: moiety for selective cellular binding, therapeutics, diagnostics, and a polymer matrix for colloidal stability for the nanomaterials. The properties of nanomaterials, both individually and in combination, are essential in defining their path through biological systems and their biological function and immunological fate in the body. The surface decoration of NPs with carbohydrates, proteins, polyethylene glycol and zwitterion moieties prevents their intake by cells *via* phagocytosis, resulting in longer circulation time in blood as well as theranostics efficacy of the nanomaterials [14, 15].

TYPES OF NANOTHERANOSTIC SYSTEMS

Following are the different types of nanocarriers used as nanotheranostics for drug delivery and diagnosis and presented in Fig. **(5.3)** and Table **(5.1)**.

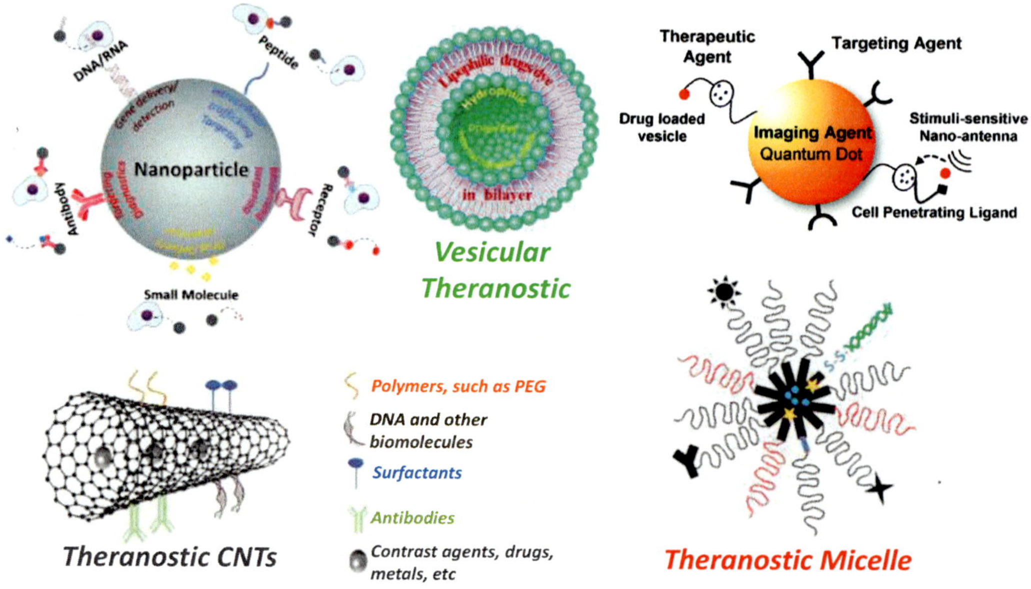

Fig. (5.3). Different types of nanotheranostic systems.

Table 5.1. Types and applications of nanotheranostic systems.

Particle Type	Examples	Size	Properties	Applications
Polymeric and Lipid NPs	PLGA, Chitosan, SLNs	5-100 nm	Biodegradable	Drug targeting and controlled release
Metalic NPs	Gold, Siver, Iron	5-100 nm	Biocompatible	Hyperthermia therapy, Drug delivery and targeting

(Table 1) cont.....

Particle Type	Examples	Size	Properties	Applications
Quantum dots	CdSe, CdTe, Ag2S	5-100 nm	Broad excitation, no photobleaching, tunable emission	Optical imaging and drug delivery
Lipid	Liposomes, micelles	50-500 nm	Carry hydrophilic and hydrophobic drugs, Biocompatible	Drug delivery and targeting
Silica	Mesoporous particles	500 nm	Biocompatible	Drug delivery and contrast agent
Magnetic	Iron oxide, Cobalt based	10 nm	Superparamagnetic	Hyperthermia therapy and MRI agent
Carbon based	CNTs, GO	3-30 nm	Biocompatible	Drug delivery

Theranostic Quantum Dots

Colloidal quantum dots (QDs) are nanometer-sized quantum mechanical crystals with semiconductor colloidal characteristics. The electrical properties of QDs display both semiconductivity and discrete molecule features [15]. QDs are particularly well-suited for multicolor fluorescent applications due to their remarkable optical features, which include small, symmetrical, and size based emission spectra as well as broad excitation spectra. The smallest QDs (2 nm) exhibit blue fluorescence (380-440 nm), whereas the largest (5 nm) emit red fluorescence (605-630 nm). QDs have several advantages over conventional organic dye molecules. Due to their inorganic nature, they are more durable and stable light emitters than organic dye molecules and are less prone to photobleaching. They are suitable for long-term cell monitoring due to their photostability [16]. Several surface modifications of QDs were carried out [17]. As new uses for QDs in therapeutic delivery, the possibility of multifunctional QDs functioning as theranostic agents becomes more feasible. The non-specific internalization and toxicity of QDs have hindered their use in the biomedical area.

Metallic Nanomaterials for Theranostics

Metallic NPs are used in various medical applications, including diagnostics, drug administration, gene transfer, and non-invasive treatment techniques like hyperthermia and PTT. Additionally, they can be utilized in cancer theranostics when appropriately functionalized with ligands or polymers.

Superparamagnetic Iron Oxide NPs(SPIONs)

In the biological sciences, SPIONs are frequently utilized for numerous purposes, including magnetic separation, medication administration through temperature, cancer treatment, and MRI contrast agents [18]. Because of their remarkable superparamagnetic characteristics, SPIONs with iron oxide cores can be utilized for magnetically controlled medication or gene delivery [19]. Biopolymers like dextran or carboxyl dextran are used to coat SPIONs, making them more stable and more biocompatible. To ensure long-term immune evasion and *in vivo* survival, SPIONs must hide their foreignness and avoid being recognized by the immune system.

Heat is produced when a high-frequency AMF activates magnetic hyperthermic SPIONs. Cancerous cells can be destroyed with only a little amount of localized heat. The key challenge will be to fine-tune the magnetic field properties of the NPs to generate enough heat for therapeutic use.

SPIONs have been utilized to manufacture pharmaceuticals and biotherapeutics, including nucleic acids, proteins, and cells, for long-term circulation and targeted delivery in various incurable illnesses [20]. By selectively targeting the medicine with a targeting ligand, SPIONs can be utilized to replace invasive methods of delivering medication to the brain [21]. SPIONs are a suitable drug carrier, and they have also been studied for gene delivery [22]. SPIONs' surfaces can be modified with cationic lipids or polymers to enhance the attachment of negatively charged nucleic acids (siRNA/miRNA and plasmids).

Combining SPIONs with a PDT/PTT agent simplifies pictorial data regarding the target site (MRI), successful drug delivery, and NIR hyperthermia. Urries *et al.* studied magnetic resonance imaging (MRI), positron emission tomography (PTT), and drug delivery using hybrid double-shell NPs made of gold (Au) and SPIONs [23].

They may cluster in the mononuclear phagocyte system due to SPION's pharmacokinetic characteristics, making them appropriate for MRI scans of primary and secondary lymphoid organs (bone marrow, liver, spleen and lymph nodes). Kupffer cells in normal liver tissue absorb SPIONs of size 10-100. SPION *in vivo* applications relies on the circulation to deliver NPs to specific organs and tissues. Perfluorocarbon NPs can be utilized to administer thrombolytic drugs such as staphylokinase streptokinase and recombinant tissue plasminogen activator and deliver ultrasonically contrast agents like ultrasound-echogenic liposomes and iron oxide NPs. The use of nanotheranostics in diagnosing and treating cardiovascular diseases (CVDs) is possible [24].

Gold NPs as Nanotheranostic Carrier

A gold (Au) nanostructure is a broad word that encompasses various types of gold NPs (AuNPs). Due to its diversity and complexity, it has garnered growing interest as a platform for biological applications. It has been proven that gold NPs have the ability to be employed as theranostic agents. They have the advantages of being simple to synthesize, bioconjugate, and modify the surface of gold NPs, increasing biocompatibility and decreasing cytotoxicity. Compared to MNPs, gold NPs have comparable multimodal imaging capabilities and application flexibility, allowing for a larger range of therapeutic and diagnostic uses in cancer therapy [25]. By properly controlling the intensity of light and the volume of injected nanomaterials, the possible adverse effects of utilizing Au nanostructures for cancer treatment may be minimized, making it a highly selective material for cancer treatment.

Gold NPs are utilized to deliver siRNA safely, accurately, and effectively in cancer-based gene therapy, attracting thiol and amine groups to the gold surface. As a result, nucleic acids that have been thiolated can be linked through an Au–thiol bond. By immobilizing single-stranded antisense siRNA and assembling *via* complementary hybridization with AuNPs containing the opposing single-stranded sense siRNA, gold NPs have been demonstrated to crosslink multimerized siRNA [26].

Proper metal surface functionalization enables the use of gold NPs as a drug carrier since it inhibits the drug from interacting directly with the gold. By conjugating paclitaxel (PTX) with polyvalent DNA and coating it with a gold surface containing thiol linkages, Zhang *et al.* identified a way for enhancing the solubility and potency of the hydrophobic medication. The fluorophore-labeled DNA linker allowed medication dispersion throughout cells to be visualized [27].

Apart from their high biocompatibility and basic chemical surface properties, Au nanostructures can function as photothermal transducers. Gold NPs absorb NIR light, which increases light-to-heat conversion in PTT and may also be designed to absorb light at a longer wavelength, such as the near-infrared region. Hollow gold NPs have recently been demonstrated to be capable of being loaded with medicines such as DOX and thermal ablation along with increased radiosensitization of the tumour was achieved by utilizing near-infrared light to release the medication [28].

Carbon-Based Nanomaterials for Theranostics

Carbon nanomaterials (CNMs) have demonstrated efficacy as carriers of genes, drugs, and diagnostic tools. In drug delivery, hydrophobic medications are loaded into CNMs *via* the π–π interaction [29]. However, despite their high surface area, which allows for increased drug loading, CNMs have some drawbacks, including toxicity, renal passage problems, and poor solubility. These disadvantages can be mitigated by surface decoration with carbon structures containing oxygen [30].

Graphene Oxide as Nanotheranostics

Graphene Oxide GO has a two-dimensional single-layered sp^2orbitals hybrid structure with adequate hydrophilic groups on surface to create stable colloids in water. However, GO clumps due to salts in physiological buffers, resulting in a charge screening effect [29]. Graphene oxide (GO) and its reduced form (rGO) can absorb near-infrared, visible, ultraviolet light and fluoresce at specific wavelengths. The processes underlying the fluorescence, on the other hand, remain unclear. Shang *et al.* discovered that three distinct functional groups on GO, C–O, C=Oand O–C–OH, were involved in GO fluorescent property [31].

Since GO absorbs more NIR light, it is a highly effective photothermal agent. PEGylated rGO had a 6 times more NIR absorbance over ultrasmall GO, and irradiation with an 808 nm laser resulted in a temperature increase to 55°C and a concentration increase in 8 minutes [32]. Numerous studies have shown that GO may be loaded with DOX and coupled with other ligands like folic acid or chlorotoxin [33] for targeted cancer treatment and PTT. Graphene and its derivatives, as one of the most intriguing and versatile materials, offer a relatively basic yet highly integrated and multipurpose nanotheranostic platform for biological applications. To better understand the compound's action, biodegradability, and toxicological profiles in a complex biological environment, additional systemic research is needed.

Polymer-Based Theranostics Nanomaterials

Polymers, both synthetic and natural, have been utilized to carry medicines, genes, and imaging agents in theranostic applications.Synthetic polymers surpass natural polymers by a wide margin when it comes to the long-term release of medicinal substances. Biodegradable polymers have been utilized in conjunction with different nanoplatforms, including GO, SPIONs, and gold NPs since they enhance solubility and biocompatibility while simultaneously serving as a site for biomolecule conjugation [34]. Typical designs include dendrimers, liposomes, polymeric NPs (NPs),conjugated polymers, micelles, and carbon nanotubes. They may be formed from viral capsids. They have various applications when they are employed as colloids to transport medicines or DNA, coat materials, or serve as templates in various industrial processes.

Theranostic Liposomes

Liposomes are round unilamellar or multilamellar phospholipid- and cholesterol-rich lipid bilayer vesicular structure comprised of phospholipids and cholesterol similar to live cells. This bilayer shape allows for the cohabitation of both hydrophilic as well as lipophilic and drug or genetic materials, resulting in biocompatible, non-toxic, and biodegradable multifunctional NPs with a wide range of functions and applications. They can passively collect in tumors through increased permeability and retention or actively accumulate in tumors by selectively targeting cancer cells. Due to this flexible and changing feature, liposomes can encapsulate functional molecules in their core, insert them into the bilayer, or adhere them to the bilayer membrane surface. As a result, their application in multifunctional platforms such as treatment and imaging has been proposed. They shield amphiphilic, hydrophobic, and hydrophilic therapeutic drugs from a range of obstacles that might otherwise result in their dilution and degradation.

PEG is coated on the surface of liposomes to form stealth liposomes that are not identified by the reticuloendothelial system for extended periods of blood circulation due to liposome instability, drug leakage, and delayed-release kinetics in the tumour [35]. while utilizing stealth liposomes nanosize structure still show slow drug transport, to this problem various approaches have been employedincluding:

1. Polymers with high pH sensitivity for polymeric liposomes.

2. Probes that are sensitive to enzymes linked to cancer.

3. Internalization and release of medications can be improved by tagging with hyaluronic acid (HA) which shows higher expression on cancer cells.

Liposomes were grafted with natural polymers like chitosan and HA to improve their stability and biocompatibility. HA was also used as a backbone for the formulations to target cancer cells with liposomes and polymeric micelles. PEG–HA–liposome was proven to have equal tumour accumulation to PEG–liposome in solid tumours, despite its higher cellular internalization [36]. As previously mentioned, the hydrophobic diethylenetriaminepentaacetic acid (C18) employed by Smith *et al.* was conjugated with chitosan to increase the concentration of gadolinium at the target site for MRI contrast. Chitosan was easier to attach to the liposome because of the hydrophobic chain [37].

L–QD hybrid vesicles have been used theranostically in the past. Using the pH gradient loading technique, Tian *et al.* examined the release of doxorubicin (DOX) from DOX-loaded L–QD hybrid vesicles and assessed and monitored the release of DOX using dynamic light scattering (DLS) [38]. Muthu *et al.* created theranostic liposomes containing folic acid-conjugated quantum dots and docetaxel for targeted co-delivery [9]. Liposomes have been used to examine the effects of cancer therapy by integrating both drugs and imaging agents. Kostarelos and colleagues co-encapsulated the color indocyanine green (ICG) and the anticancer medication doxorubicin in an HSPC-supported liposome and functionalized it with a humanized MUC-1 antibody [39]. This theranostic liposome was investigated in a mouse model of breast cancer and revealed the capacity to combine tumor-specific targeted treatment with optoacoustic tomography diagnostics. Apomorphine and QDs were encapsulated in multifunctional liposomes for brain targeting and imaging, and the findings revealed that these liposomes may accumulate considerably in the brain.

Theranostic Carbon Nanotube (CNT)

CNTs display a diverse range of electrical and optical properties due to their cylindrical carbon structure and have been investigated for usage in biological applications. Because of their mechanical strength and optical properties, carbon nanotubes have been used as tissue scaffolds, drug delivery systems, and imaging. CNTs, like GO, exhibit a near-infrared optical transition, making them ideal for NIR fluorescence microscopy and optical coherence tomography.

To be employed in theranostic applications, carbon nanotubes must have the following properties:

1. The drugs or genes transport ability.

2. The PTT properties.

3. The sensitivity to Raman scattering.

Due to the high sensitivity of CNTs to Raman scattering as a result of their broad symmetric carbon bonds, selective PTT in tumor cells may be done using CNTs with unique Raman spectrum fingerprints [40]. Carbon nanotubes can be used in theranostic applications when coupled with silver and gold NPs or SPIONs [41]. MRI and SPECT contrast agents tagged with technetium-99m were recently developed using SPIONs-coated multiwalled carbon nanotubes (SWCNTs). SMWCNTs were functionalized with bisphosphonate (dipicolylamine-alendronate) and subsequently coated with SPIONs to enable radiolabeling. SWCNTs can be used as a theranostics agent because their high NIR absorption capacity permits photothermal therapy, far more selective and less aggressive than traditional chemo- or radiation. The high specificity is mostly due to SWCNTs' bioactivity and cellular absorption, which may render them hazardous. Individual (or bundled) SWCNT suspensions or micron-sized SWCNT agglomerates are utilized in biomedical diagnostics and treatment [42].

Polymeric Micelle NPs as Nanotheranostic

Micelles are formed when surfactants and lipids self-assemble supramolecular [43]. Micelles are produced when amphiphilic molecules in water become hydrophobic, resulting in colloidal aggregation of these molecules. Micelles are spherical particles produced in an aqueous solution by amphipathic lipid molecules. Polymeric micelles are made up of a polymer backbone and a hydrophobic unit; the hydrophobic core can include hydrophobic medications, dye molecules, or SPIONs, enabling for imaging and drug/gene delivery at the same time. It's a great transporter for hydrophobic and water-insoluble medications or colours. Polymeric micelles have the extended circulation kinetics and increased solubility needed for medicine accumulation at tumour target sites.

Although amphiphilic di-block copolymers (for example, polystyrene and poly(ethylene glycol)) and triblock copolymers (for example, poloxamers) are the most frequently used polymers for micelle development, graft (for example, G-chitosan) and ionic copolymers (for example, poly(ethylene glycol)-poly(-capro-lactone)-g-polyethyleneimine) copolymers Typically, the hydrophilic segment is composed of PEG (polyethylene glycol), but other polymers such as poly (acryl-oylmorpholine), poly(vinyl pyrrolidone), or poly(trimethylene carbonate) are also used; the hydrophobic segment is typically composed of poly(propylene oxide), glycolic and lactic acid polymers, or polyesters such as poly(-caprolactone)and copolymers [44].

Micelles can be formed during or after the manufacturing process, depending on the manufacturing technique and the physicochemical characteristics of the medication. Dialysis, emulsion evaporation with solvent (or co-solvent) evaporation, and solution casting followed by film hydration are some of the other ways of preparation. The approach taken is determined by the polymer and drug properties, and specific publications [45] provide extensive information on this topic. Because the micelles' features, such as polarity and degree of hydration, vary depending on the carrier, the drug can be stored in a variety of locations, including close to the surface or deep into the carrier. The inner core is frequently used to load and store hydrophobic medications.

However, the polymeric micelle-based drug delivery method is inefficient for systemic drug administration due to its low stability and rapid drug release. Self-assembled polymeric micelles produced from amphiphilic block copolymers are a form of nanovehicle for delivering therapeutic genes and anticancer drugs. Xiong*et al.* devised a polymeric micelle delivery method for DOX and siRNA administration into cells. In MDA-MB-435/LCC6MDR1-resistant tumor animal models, the polymeric micelle proved effective in preserving and delivering siRNA to target areas, as well as achieving pH-sensitive DOX release [46].

Theranostic Dendrimers

Dendrimers are large, hyperbranched polymers with a central core that radiates radially. They are monodisperse macromolecules in the form of stars with nanometer-scale dimensions. Dendrimers are made up of three parts:

- A central core
- An interior dendritic structure (the branches)
- An exterior surface with functional surface groups [47]

Dendrimers can include drugs, imaging agents, and targeting ligands into a single molecule due to their multifunctionality. The interior space may be used to hold molecules *via* electrostatic interactions. At the same time, the outer surface can be conjugated to and complexed with molecules, implying that dendrimers are excellent nanoplatforms for theranostics. Dendrimers have been utilized in the biomedical industry for *in vitro* diagnostics, as contrast agents in combination with other molecules in magnetic resonance imaging, as drug delivery systems, and as vectors for gene transfer in regenerative medicine [48]. It is common to combine drug- or gene-loaded dendrimers with FIs for *in vitro* fluorescence imaging. Research into theranostic dendrimers has increased for diagnostic applications, including MRI, CT, PET, and SPECT, are relevant *in vivo*.

Dendrimers' multifunctional properties make them excellent for use with imaging agents, medications, and targeting ligands in biomedical applications. To create theranostic dendrimers for fluorescence imaging, a fluorescent dye is added to the drug- and gene-loaded dendrimer NP. Dendrimers are having gadolinium (III) chelates display enhanced relaxivities in MRI, and dendrimers containing Gd (III) chelates are advantageous for theranostic applications. Dendrimers encapsulated in Au NP can be used in theranostic applications requiring CT imaging.

SPIO NPs coated with dendrimers are an excellent choice for theranostic applications. These complexes are especially advantageous due to their adaptability, biocompatibility, and low toxicity. SPIO's surface functionalization with dendrimers improves its stability and targeting capabilities and its ability to encapsulate medicines or other particular conjugate ligands. These integrated structures have various therapeutic applications, including the induction of magnetic hyperthermia utilizing AMF, controlled medication delivery *via* pH and temperature, and gene therapy *via* gene delivery.

Taratula *et al.* [49] introduced a new dendrimer-based theranostic platform for delivery of tumor-targeted phthalocyanine (Pc). Dendrimers have considerable promise as an effective NIR theranostic agent, as demonstrated by his work. The technique involves adding a hydrophobic linker to the Pc molecule, which dramatically improves the hydrophobic drug's physical encapsulation into a 4.0G polypropylene imine (4.0G PPI) dendrimer. The Pc- 4.0G PPI complexes' surfaces were further tailored with PEG and the LHRH peptide to enhance tumor-targeted distribution and biocompatibility, respectively. The phthalocyanine derivative produced and encapsulated in the dendrimer-based nanocarrier exhibits distinctive near-infrared absorption (700 nm) and fluorescence emission (710 and 815 nm), which are required for successful photodynamic therapy and fluorescence imaging. The intrinsic fluorescent properties of encapsulated phthalocyanine allowed for assessing the nanocarrier's subcellular localization *in vitro* and organ distribution *in vivo*. For up to 24 hours, the proposed formulation exhibited significant cytotoxicity and photodynamic therapy. *In vitro* and *in vivo* imaging investigations demonstrated that the LHRH-targeted theranostic dendrimer could efficiently internalize and accumulate tumor cells.

Polymer Conjugates

Due to their potential to perform both therapy and diagnosis or imaging tasks in a single system, polymer conjugates combined with an imaging agent and therapeutic medicines are theranostic agents. Polymer conjugates are covalently linked polymer chains attached to a drug or protein in hydrophilic hybrid molecules. Chemically, polymer conjugates are macromolecules that include pharmacological or biologically active molecules linked together by an intervening macromolecule.The spacer molecule may have a breaking point that allows the drug to be released at the target location. The majority of polymer conjugate applications are in the therapeutic and nanomedical fields [50]. Polymer conjugates have been shown to improve the pharmacokinetic characteristics of medicines, increase their resistance to degradation, provide high loading capacity and prolonged release patterns, and minimize premature drug release. It is feasible to transport both hydrophobic and hydrophilic medicines using the polymer conjugate method, which is often problematic with drug-loaded NPs produced by physical encapsulation and relying on hydrophobic contact as the primary mode of action.

Numerous polymers are being investigated for their potential as nanotheranostics *via* the creation of polymer-drug conjugates. The polymer chain's free functional groups enable them to be linked with various therapeutic, imaging, and targeting moieties, making them a potential material for nanotheranostic applications. PDCs are formulated using both synthetic and natural polymers. Poly N-(2-hydroxy-propyl)-methacrylamide (poly-HPMA), polyphosphazene, polyphosphoesters

(PPEs), polylactic acid (PLA), poly(lactic-co-glycolic acid) (PLGA), polyethylene glycol (PEG),and polyglycerol are all synthetic polymers used to create PDCs. Natural polymers such as polyglutamic acid, albumin, gelatin, alginate, chitosan, hyaluronic acid, and hydroxyethyl starch have been investigated for use in the production of PDCs. While natural polymers are the most plentiful and biodegradable, batch-to-batch differences (reproducibility) and microbial contamination (purity) frequently occur within this class of polymers, posing a source-related transmission risk.

THERAPEUTIC APPLICATIONS OF NANOTHERANOSTICS

Applications of Nanotheranostics in Therapy

Photodynamic Therapy

Photodynamic treatment (PDT) has been utilized to treat a wide variety of malignant and noncancerous illnesses for decades. A photosensitizing substance absorbs light at a particular wavelength in PDT. It degrades molecular oxygen ($3O_2$) in cells' cytoplasm to singlet oxygen ($1O_2$), causing cell death *via* apoptosis or necrosis [2, 51].

After the incident light is absorbed, the electrons in the photosensitizer transition from the ground state to the excited state. Rather than decaying to the ground state, the electrons undertake intersystem crossing, transferring energy to additional photosensitizer molecules or potentially damaging intermediates such as h. It causes apoptosis or necrosis in cells in either case by destroying organelles such as mitochondria or the nucleus (DNA), leading to the selective removal of sick cells [52].

A photosensitizing agent, also known as a photosensitizer, is a chemical compound that absorbs light to impact chemical processes occurring within cells. It has been shown in preclinical studies to have potentially beneficial qualities for PDT [53]. PDT photosensitizers such as morphine, chlorins, and phthalocyanine derivatives have been extensively used in clinical and experimental cancer therapy [54].

PDT has been used to treat malignancies such as head, brain, and neck cancer in clinical settings. Still, it is also used to treat ophthalmic diseases,dermatological problems, urological diseases, and cardiovascular conditions. The primary drawback of PDT is that photosensitizers in the patient's circulation for an extended period cause them to be light-sensitive [55]. As a result, patients must be kept in the darkroom following treatment to avoid further phototoxicity. On the other hand, by targeting diseased cells, PDT employing a nanotheranostics platform can be rendered safe and effective.

Photothermal Therapy

Following near-infrared irradiation (NIR), photothermal therapy (PTT) agents absorb light/energy from cancer cells and electrons transition from the ground state to the excited state at the subatomic level. Then, when the particle returns to its ground state *via* nonradiative decay pathways, kinetic energy is released, resulting in heat energy generation in the tumor's immediate surroundings. The produced heat energy ruptures the cell membrane, causing protein and other biological components to breakdown (Fig. **5.4**). The increased thermal output in the tumor region relative to normal tissues is due to the tumor tissue's insufficient circulatory system, leading to inefficient heat dissipation. Consequently, the produced an amount of heat which does not cause any harm to normal tissue and is used only to ablate tumor tissue thermally. When exposed to light, both organic and inorganic nanoparticles become excitable, according to PTT. Noble metals like gold and silver, as well as carbon-based nanomaterials like graphene oxide (GO) or carbon nanotube (CNT), have been used in cancer photothermal ablation.This method has been chiefly used to treat cancer, but it has also been used to treat other disorders such as Alzheimer's disease [56].Apart from drug delivery, PTT may be achieved by fine-tuning and implementing specific functionalization methods in GO and CNT [57].

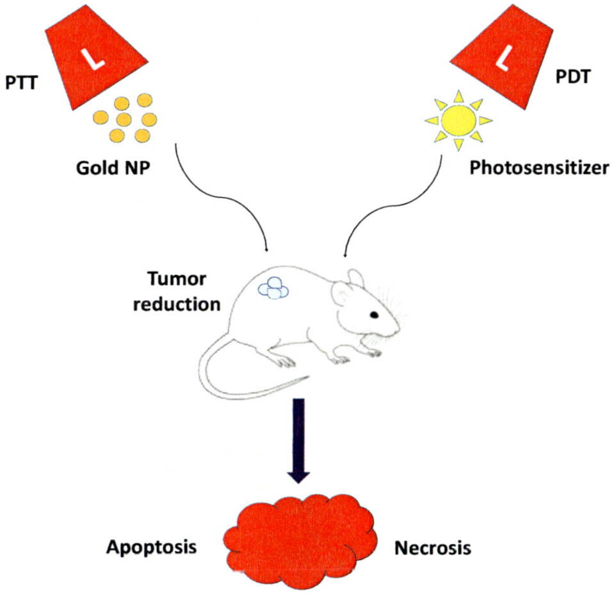

Fig. (5.4). Application of PTT and PDT in cancer treatment.

Hyperthermia Treatment

Laser thermotherapy employs a laser to target the tumor location and creates heat energy, killing cancer cells. The term "hyperthermia" is frequently used to refer to this form of therapy. While high temperatures (40-45°C) destroy cancer cells, healthy cells are preserved by merely heating tumor tissues. When cancer cells are exposed to hyperthermia, the following processes occur:

(1) proteins begin to denature,

(2) apoptotic agents cause apoptosis,

(3) DNA repair processes are slowed, and

(4) heat shock protein production is slowed [30].

Apart from these basic activities, the tumor microenvironment increases the sensitivity of the cells to heat.Special consideration must be given to the neurological system when employing this method, as nerve cells are highly heated sensitive and can sustain irreversible damage. As a result, exposure duration and temperature must be maintained constant while concentrating on the target region [58].

The unique features of the materials change according to the source type; for example, when a magnetic field is applied, magnetic NPs (MNP) with increased magnetic characteristics create heat [59], whereas gold NPs with a high absorption coefficient generate heat when a laser is applied [60]. (photothermal). The most often used method for performing this non-invasive procedure without causing damage to healthy tissues is MNP-based hyperthermia. An alternating magnetic field (AMF) causes the MNPs to vibrate, which releases heat energy when measured as the specific absorption rate (SAR) [60]. MR T2 relaxivity of MNPs makes them potential candidates for SAR and MRI-guided thermal cancer ablation [61].

Applications of Nanotheranostics for Imaging

Optical Imaging

Molecular identification and imaging using optical imaging have become a powerful non-invasive, sensitive, and real-time method. Unionization makes optical imaging more affordable, simpler, and safer. PET, SPECT, and MRI are all imaging modalities used in conjunction with optical imaging. Image-guided surgery (IGS) and tumor diagnostic methods that employ bioluminescence and fluorescence imaging are most commonly used *in vivo*. For tiny malignancies such as polyps in the stomach or breast cancer tumors, IGS is the most commonly utilized therapy [61]. This avoids the loss of healthy tissue or cancer metastases, and further treatment regimens can be established as needed.

By integrating optical imaging techniques with cancer-specific imaging agents, a barrier prevents cancer recurrence due to tumor margins. To achieve cancer cell selectivity, the imaging dye can be combined with biomolecules such as antibodies, cell-penetrating peptides, cyclic RGD, or medicinal drugs. Metal NPs can also be utilized for theranostics, which uses fluorescence imaging to provide anticancer treatment. Silver NPs with increased metal fluorescence are beneficial for cell imaging [62].

MRI Imaging

Solid tumours and brain tumours are frequently diagnosed with magnetic resonance imaging (MRI). It is usually regarded as the most efficient and non-invasive imaging approach due to its superior spatial resolution and sensitivity. MRI develops a detailed map of the body's anatomical structure, diagnoses lesions, and provides information on how the body functions. In the presence of a regulated magnetic field, RF radiation is employed in MRI to give high-quality cross-sectional images of the body in any plane. All hydrogen atoms align along the outside region when a magnetic field is introduced, and they become excited when radio frequency is applied. Excited atoms generate energy, which is detected by the MRI equipment's wire coils, and MR mapping is performed by a computer.

Magnetic resonance imaging contrast agents are divided into two types: paramagnetic agents with a permanent magnetic moment, such as gadolinium (Gd^{3+}) or manganese (Mn^{2+}), and superparamagnetic agents, such as iron oxide cores or Fe/Mn composite metal cores embedded in a polymer matrix, which have a larger magnetic moment than paramagnetic agents [63]. MRI has a good spatial resolution (0.2–1 mm), however it has a low sensitivity (10–3–10–5 mol/L). As a result, MRI is frequently used in conjunction with other imaging modalities to increase image quality and reveal tissue architecture and function [64].

Ultrasound Imaging

Ultrasonic imaging is well-established, non-invasive, flexible, and often used in people as a diagnostic tool. Ultrasonic imaging does not require contrast agents, and the vascular information gained by color or power Doppler imaging is usually adequate to make an accurate diagnosis. Ultrasound imaging, on the other hand, is required to scan inflammatory areas or thromboses. The discovery of microbubbles (MBs) prompted interest in contrast ultrasonic imaging for theranostics [64]. For targeted imaging within the body, these MBs can be conjugated to a specific antibody, peptide, or ligand. They can also deliver medications and genes to specific cells, including cancer cells.

The use of drug-loaded MBs targeting vascular endothelial growth factor to treat brain glioma tumours in rats was proven by Fan *et al.*, with drug release aided by an ultrasound-guided burst of MBs across the blood-brain barrier (BBB). Drug molecules entered the tumor site and enhanced tumor death during the brief opening [65].

A single nanoparticle with dual scattering/reflection capabilities has been shown to improve ultrasonic imaging in recent study. Zhang *et al.* developed a rattle-type mesoporous silica nanostructure with two contributing surfaces that disperses and reflects incoming ultrasound twice inside the nanoparticle [66].

Nanotheranostics in Cancer Treatment

Theranostic nanomedicine seeks to enhance cancer diagnosis and treatment efficacy and the systemic toxicity associated with these therapies [9]. As a result, therapeutic medications must reach and target specific regions. Indeed, improved theranostic nanomedicines with a targeting moiety can recognize, bind to, and be internalized *via* specialized mechanisms such as receptor-mediated endocytosis [67].

Another significant benefit of theranostic nanomedicine in cancer treatment is its ability to assess treatment outcomes in specific patients in real-time to plan further therapy or determine whether to repeat a therapeutic session. Researchers think that combining magnetic NPs with MRI imaging can assist in advancing the notion of personalized nanomedical theranostic cancer treatment for a specific patient [67]. Due to the widespread availability of MRI scanners in hospitals, this appears to be the most effective method for monitoring the effects of cancer nanomedicine therapy.

In comparison to solid tumors, research on nanotheranostic uses in the treatment of liquid malignancies is still in its early stages. The majority of techniques taken thus far have been aimed towards diagnosing and treating blood malignancies such as lymphoma and leukemia. It's remarkable to notice that, even though blood malignancies have a distinct physicochemical profile than solid tumors, the same types of nanomaterials are utilized. The employment of metal NPs demonstrates this to ablate solid and liquid tumors thermally. The nanomaterial is attached to the tumor's surface in solid tumors, allowing for efficient and non-invasive ablation.

Nonetheless, the target element is always in circulation in liquid tumours and could cause tissue ablation. When polymeric and lipid NPs are used as drug delivery vehicles in solid and liquid tumours, they have a similar effect. The criteria for blood-brain barrier penetration, stability, and renal clearance are still unknown. This issue must be addressed, and more study into nanotheranostics for *in vivo* applications in circulating malignancies is needed.

Because of its high drug loading capacity and low toxicity, SPIONs have emerged as an interesting theranostic NPs platform for the translational development of new image-guided cancer treatment agents. Human ovarian cancer cell lines were treated with gold-coated SPIONs and cisplatin to test the efficacy of medication delivery [68]. Due to tumor target specific and intratumoral accumulation of theranostic NPs without the use of invasive techniques is critical for image-guided cancer phototherapy, as it enables the therapy to be given precisely and at the ideal moment (Fig. **5.5**).

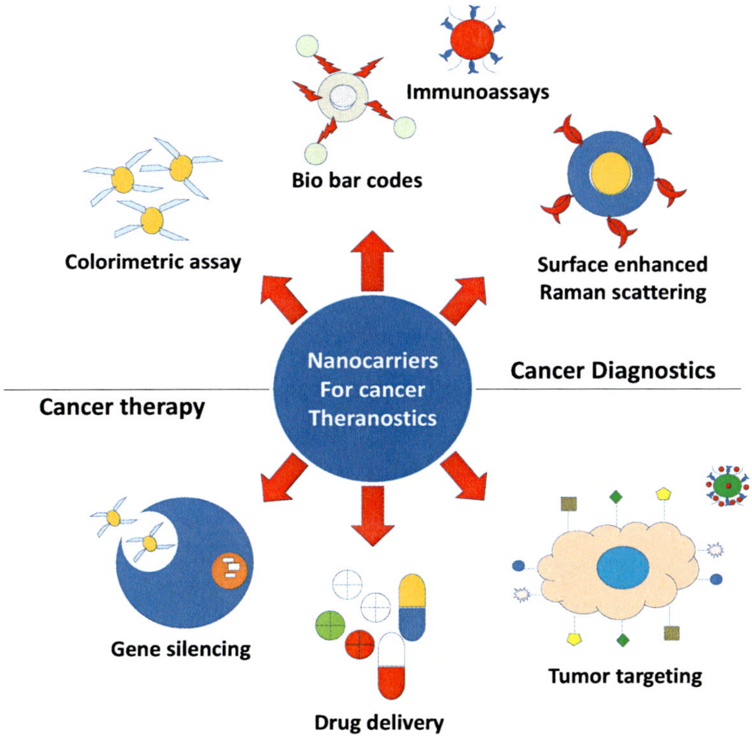

Fig. (5.5). Functional architecture of nanomaterials and theranostic modalities.

Nanotheranostics for Photothermal and Photodynamic Cancer Therapy

Nanotechnology-based photothermal therapy (PTT) has emerged as a promising and less invasive cancer treatment method in recent years. It can deliver precise photo energy to the tumor site, boosting treatment efficacy while causing little harm to healthy tissues. Noble metal-based nanostructures such as gold nanospheres, gold nanorods, gold nanoshells, gold nanocages, and copper-based semiconductor NPs are the most effective nanomaterials for NIR laser-induced PTT [69]. However, their potentially transformative therapeutic uses have been largely limited because of the PTT mentioned above drugs' inherent toxicity and unknown long-term toxicity.

Engineered Mammalian Cell-Based Theranostic Agents for Cancer Therapy

In recent years, it's been possible to create new theranostic chemicals in mammalian cells. Engineered T cells have been used in cancer theranostics studies in the past [70]. It was discovered that T cells taken from a cancer patient could tell the difference between benign and malignant cells because they were genetically engineered to produce cancer-specific receptors. After that, the T cells were reintroduced into the patient's body to target just the cancer cells. Scientists believe that engineered mammalian cells have a better chance of successfully detecting and administering medicines than tiny molecules and NPs.

When exposed to a sufficient dose of medication or blue light, engineered mammalian cells can also release a therapeutic protein to treat metabolic diseases like diabetes. Therapeutic proteins can be accurately and dynamically regulated in response to external stimuli using next-generation theranostic agents, cells modified to do just that. To trigger specially engineered cells to secrete additional therapeutic proteins targeted against associated diseases such as obesity and hyperglycemia, the concentration of a drug targeting one aspect of a disease state [71], like hypertension, could be used. This would allow simultaneous treatment of multiple pathologies and circumvent the limitations of a one-drug one-disease approach. It is possible to employ reprogrammed mammalian cells in diagnostic and therapeutic procedures.

Theranostic Nanomedicine in Cardiovascular Diseases (CVD)

Numerous preclinical findings have been made on nanotheranostic devices in cardiovascular disease research and clinical translation. These discoveries might be used in future non-invasive real-time cardiovascular study methods. MRI and near-infrared fluorescence are commonly utilized in cardiovascular disease studies to detect atherosclerotic plaque without causing any harm. One of the most active research areas involves searching for effective treatments for atherosclerosis and its side effects. Few details about the dose, pharmacokinetics, long-term impact and toxin profile of most NPs are now being utilized in research. Nanotheranostics, such as IOPs, were among the first used to treat atherosclerosis when they were initially developed. This non-invasive imaging technique based on NPs evaluated drug therapy in patients with atherosclerosis. CVDs can be treated using targeted theranostic microbubbles, another type of theranostics [72]. Platelets may be observed using *in vivo* ultrasound molecular imaging because they are covalently linked to them. To avoid thrombus and blood clots, they may benefit from clot-specific enrichment of fibrinolytic activity. When it comes to creating and testing new therapeutic methods for cardiovascular disease, Nanotheranostics may help. NPs' biocompatibility (such as blood half-life) and immunogenicity should be assessed more thoroughly in future studies, as should the development of precision medicine administration and early detection of atherosclerotic plaque [72].

Nanotheranostics for the imaging of pulmonary diseases

Respiratory disorders encompass a broad range of ailments affecting the upper and lower respiratory systems. Nanomedicine has demonstrated efficacy in treating a variety of chronic obstructive lung illnesses, including asthma [73], as well as hereditary diseases such as cystic fibrosis. Additionally, nanoplatforms can be used to diagnose and cure pulmonary TB and lung cancer. The lung is easily targeted, mainly *via* inhaled aerosols, due to the ease these nanosystems may be transported to the airways. Imaging nanoplatforms for the diagnosis of pulmonary illnesses are few. Numerous methods, however, have been created. For instance, Aillon *et al.* demonstrated that iodine-doped nanoclusters may potentially be used as a contrast agent for lung imaging [74]. PET and MRI are the most often used imaging modalities for NPs in lung imaging. The nano delivery methods employed to treat pulmonary illnesses are many [75]. Despite this, the combination of imaging and therapeutic nanosystems is very restricted. For the treatment of asthma, Lanza *et al.* developed lipase-labile phospholipid prodrugs of fumagillin or docetaxel. We investigated the anti-angiogenic efficacy of v3-targeted micelles in asthma using MR simultaneous dual 19F/1H neovascular molecular imaging. They were coupled with a biocompatible antibody to evaluate the *in vivo* impact of superparamagnetic iron oxide NPs following pulmonary injection. The proposed method enables precise targeting and imaging of a specific macrophage subpopulation in a mouse model of chronic obstructive lung disease caused by lipopolysaccharide [76].

Theranostics for Treatment of Diseases of the Central Nervous System

Neurodegenerative diseases are various disorders that result in the gradual degeneration of specific neural systems and, eventually, cognitive skills. Alzheimer's disease (AD), Parkinson's disease (PD), amyotrophic lateral sclerosis (ALS), and Huntington's disease are the prototypes of degenerative diseases. AD is the most frequent neurodegenerative disease, and hence the majority of nanotheranostic methods for brain diseases are aimed against it. Significant progress has been achieved in administering therapeutic or diagnostic contrast probes over the blood-brain barrier into the nervous system, as in the case of glioblastoma, while preserving the ability to target specific brain or spinal cord subregions [77].

In this context, nanotechnology-based techniques and nanotheranostics hold tremendous promise for improving the applied effect of central nervous system imaging, studying critically sick states, and advancing neurosurgical treatment. Bioimaging is without a doubt the most advantageous use. Magnetic resonance imaging is the most critical technique for diagnosing brain disorders (MRI). PET imaging is not far off from being used to monitor the course of different nervous system diseases and the pathogenesis of Alzheimer's disease. It has already aided in disease knowledge. This has been proposed using radiolabeled amyloid ligands [78, 79]. Nanomedicine and nanotheranostics have the potential to aid in the study of the pathophysiology and genesis of neurodegenerative disorders [80].

Theranostics for Treatment of Autoimmune Diseases

Our immune system defends us against sickness and infection. However, if a person has an autoimmune disorder, the body's defensive mechanism will target particular host cells, tissues, and organs. Autoimmune disorders can manifest in various ways and have a significant impact on the patient's well-being. Environmental, viral, and genetic variables may all have a role in developing or exacerbating autoimmune disorders. Rheumatoid arthritis (RA) is a chronic inflammatory illness that causes significant cartilage, bone loss, and widespread synovial joint inflammation. Currently, there is no cure for rheumatoid arthritis. Metallic NPs have been effectively applied to the treatment of rheumatoid arthritis due to their small size and magnetic characteristics, which enable them to operate as multifunctional drug delivery and theranostic platform. Nanomaterials are primarily used to target the scavenger receptor on activated macrophages. NPs enable extended bloodstream circulation and passive buildup of medicines in inflamed synovial tissues, resulting in controlled drug release at targeted action locations. Cu is a necessary component of the human body, playing a role in osteogenesis and chondrogenesis. Cu-based NPs are superior PTT agents and photosensitizers for PDT. Cu-based NPs have been recommended as a therapy for rheumatoid arthritis due to their high biocompatibility and ease of production. Concerns about safety (biodistribution in nontargeted organs, propensity for inflammation, biodegradability, biocompatibility, and clearance) are the primary impediment to the clinical use of the majority of rheumatoid arthritis nanomedicine.

CONCLUSION

Theranostic nanomedicine attempts to optimize each treatment's pharmacokinetics, pharmacodynamics, and biodistribution to ensure that medicines are delivered to the correct location, at the appropriate time, and in the right amount. Nanomaterials can be synthesized in response to changes in the biological environment, such as temperature, pH, enzyme activity, or the presence of a particular targeting moiety, enabling system-specific medication release while minimizing damage to healthy tissues. Theranostics can penetrate the bloodstream, circumvent host defenses, and transport medicines and diagnostic agents to the target location, enabling cellular and molecular diagnosis and therapy.

Pharmaceutical and diagnostic companies have concentrated their efforts on creating a single drug capable of treating life-threatening illnesses such as cancer. Although theranostics is predominantly used to treat cancer, it is also used to treat other chronic diseases such as cardiovascular, autoimmune, and neurological disorders such as Alzheimer's disease. Nanotheranostics can forecast treatment responses by integrating information about the general location of the target site with non-invasive imaging insights into the medication and carrier material distribution at the target site. Each nanomaterial's strengths and weaknesses, notably its possible side effects/toxicities, should be thoroughly studied before creating them with substantial effectiveness and clinical benefits.

FUTURE PROSPECTS

Theranostics is a rapidly developing area where diagnostic and mainly targeted therapies are integrated to provide a more individualized therapeutic approach to each patient. In nuclear medicine clinical practice, theranostics will be frequently applied by labeling the same molecule with two distinct radionuclides and comparing the results. The theranostics process is based on the magnitude of alterations in functioning and structure in the development. Simultaneously, the genetic changes in various diseases lead to the development of different targets that will be exploited for imaging, and treatment is expressed or increased in abundance. In recent years, this theranostic notion has gained more prominence in personalized medicine, particularly in oncology, where advanced malignancies can be treated efficiently and with minimal side effects using targeted therapies.

CONSENT FOR PUBLICATION

Not applicable.

CONFLICT OF INTEREST

The authors declare no conflict of interest, financial or otherwise.

ACKNOWLEDGEMENTS

The authors would like to acknowledge all of their associated institutions to compile this work for providing the necessary resources.

REFERENCES

[1] Enrico C. Nanotheranostics and theranostic nanomedicine for diseases and cancer treatment.Elsevier BV 2018.
[http://dx.doi.org/10.1016/B978-0-12-813669-0.00002-6]

[2] Kalash RS, Lakshmanan VK, Cho C-S, Park I-K. Theranostics. Biomaterials Nanoarchitectonics. Elsevier 2016; pp. 197-215.
[http://dx.doi.org/10.1016/B978-0-323-37127-8.00012-1]

[3] Caldorera-Moore ME, Liechty WB, Peppas NA. Responsive theranostic systems: Integration of diagnostic imaging agents and responsive controlled release drug delivery carriers. Acc Chem Res 2011; 44(10): 1061-70.
[http://dx.doi.org/10.1021/ar2001777] [PMID: 21932809]

[4] Patel SK, Janjic JM. Macrophage targeted theranostics as personalized nanomedicine strategies for inflammatory diseases. Theranostics 2015; 5(2): 150-72.
[http://dx.doi.org/10.7150/thno.9476] [PMID: 25553105]

[5] Chakravarthy M, AlShamaileh H, Huang H, *et al.* Development of DNA aptamers targeting low-molecular-weight amyloid-β peptide aggregates *in vitro*. Chem Commun (Camb) 2018; 54(36): 4593-6.
[http://dx.doi.org/10.1039/C8CC02256A] [PMID: 29670956]

[6] Ma Z, Wan H, Wang W, *et al.* A theranostic agent for cancer therapy and imaging in the second near-infrared window. Nano Res 2019; 12(2): 273-9.
[http://dx.doi.org/10.1007/s12274-018-2210-x] [PMID: 31832124]

[7] Roy Chowdhury M, Schumann C, Bhakta-Guha D, Guha G. Cancer nanotheranostics: Strategies, promises and impediments. Biomed Pharmacother 2016; 84: 291-304.
[http://dx.doi.org/10.1016/j.biopha.2016.09.035] [PMID: 27665475]

[8] Sahoo AK, Banerjee S, Ghosh SS, Chattopadhyay A. Simultaneous RGB emitting Au nanoclusters in chitosan nanoparticles for anticancer gene theranostics. ACS Appl Mater Interfaces 2014; 6(1): 712-24.
[http://dx.doi.org/10.1021/am4051266] [PMID: 24281656]

[9] Muthu MS, Leong DT, Mei L, Feng SS. Nanotheranostics - application and further development of nanomedicine strategies for advanced theranostics. Theranostics 2014; 4(6): 660-77.
[http://dx.doi.org/10.7150/thno.8698] [PMID: 24723986]

[10] Horikoshi S, Serpone N, Eds. Microwaves in nanoparticle synthesis: Fundamentals and applications.Weinheim, Germany: Wiley-VCH Verlag 2013.
[http://dx.doi.org/10.1002/9783527648122]

[11] Mody V, Siwale R, Singh A, Mody H. Introduction to metallic nanoparticles. J Pharm Bioallied Sci 2010; 2(4): 282-9.
[http://dx.doi.org/10.4103/0975-7406.72127] [PMID: 21180459]

[12] Kim H, Kim Y, Kim IH, Kim K, Choi Y. ROS-responsive activatable photosensitizing agent for

imaging and photodynamic therapy of activated macrophages. Theranostics 2014; 4(1): 1-11. [http://dx.doi.org/10.7150/thno.7101] [PMID: 24396511]

[13] Wang P, Yigit MV, Ran C, *et al.* A theranostic small interfering RNA nanoprobe protects pancreatic islet grafts from adoptively transferred immune rejection. Diabetes 2012; 61(12): 3247-54. [http://dx.doi.org/10.2337/db12-0441] [PMID: 22923469]

[14] Wong XY, Sena-Torralba A, Álvarez-Diduk R, Muthoosamy K, Merkoçi A. Nanomaterials for nanotheranostics: Tuning their properties according to disease needs. ACS Nano 2020; 14(3): 2585-627. [http://dx.doi.org/10.1021/acsnano.9b08133] [PMID: 32031781]

[15] Murray CB, Kagan CR, Bawendi MG. Synthesis and characterization of monodisperse nanocrystals and close-packed nanocrystal assemblies. Annu Rev Mater Sci 2000; 30(1): 545-610. [http://dx.doi.org/10.1146/annurev.matsci.30.1.545]

[16] Michalet X, Pinaud F, Lacoste TD, *et al.* Properties of fluorescent semiconductor nanocrystals and their application to biological labeling. Single Mol 2001; 2(4): 261-76. [http://dx.doi.org/10.1002/1438-5171(200112)2:4<261::AID-SIMO261>3.0.CO;2-P]

[17] Wu X, Liu H, Liu J, *et al.* Erratum: Corrigendum: Immunofluorescent labeling of cancer marker Her2 and other cellular targets with semiconductor quantum dots. Nat Biotechnol 2003; 21(4): 452-2. [http://dx.doi.org/10.1038/nbt0403-452b]

[18] Zhang E, Kircher MF, Koch M, Eliasson L, Goldberg SN, Renström E. Dynamic magnetic fields remote-control apoptosis *via* nanoparticle rotation. ACS Nano 2014; 8(4): 3192-201. [http://dx.doi.org/10.1021/nn406302j] [PMID: 24597847]

[19] Mahmoudi M, Sant S, Wang B, Laurent S, Sen T. Superparamagnetic iron oxide nanoparticles (SPIONs): Development, surface modification and applications in chemotherapy. Adv Drug Deliv Rev 2011; 63(1-2): 24-46. [http://dx.doi.org/10.1016/j.addr.2010.05.006] [PMID: 20685224]

[20] Veiseh O, Gunn JW, Zhang M. Design and fabrication of magnetic nanoparticles for targeted drug delivery and imaging. Adv Drug Deliv Rev 2010; 62(3): 284-304. [http://dx.doi.org/10.1016/j.addr.2009.11.002] [PMID: 19909778]

[21] Stephen ZR, Kievit FM, Veiseh O, *et al.* Redox-responsive magnetic nanoparticle for targeted convection-enhanced delivery of O6-benzylguanine to brain tumors. ACS Nano 2014; 8(10): 10383-95. [http://dx.doi.org/10.1021/nn503735w] [PMID: 25247850]

[22] Mok H, Zhang M. Superparamagnetic iron oxide nanoparticle-based delivery systems for biotherapeutics. Expert Opin Drug Deliv 2013; 10(1): 73-87. [http://dx.doi.org/10.1517/17425247.2013.747507] [PMID: 23199200]

[23] Liu W, Lo YL, Hsu C, *et al.* CS-PEI/Beclin-siRNA downregulate multidrug resistance proteins and increase paclitaxel therapeutic efficacy against NSCLC. Mol Ther Nucleic Acids 2019; 17: 477-90. [http://dx.doi.org/10.1016/j.omtn.2019.06.017] [PMID: 31336235]

[24] McCarthy JR. Multifunctional agents for concurrent imaging and therapy in cardiovascular disease. Adv Drug Deliv Rev 2010; 62(11): 1023-30. [http://dx.doi.org/10.1016/j.addr.2010.07.004] [PMID: 20654664]

[25] Draz MS, Fang BA, Zhang P, *et al.* Nanoparticle-mediated systemic delivery of siRNA for treatment of cancers and viral infections. Theranostics 2014; 4(9): 872-92. [http://dx.doi.org/10.7150/thno.9404] [PMID: 25057313]

[26] Hong CA, Nam YS. Functional nanostructures for effective delivery of small interfering RNA therapeutics. Theranostics 2014; 4(12): 1211-32. [http://dx.doi.org/10.7150/thno.8491] [PMID: 25285170]

[27] Zhang XQ, Xu X, Lam R, Giljohann D, Ho D, Mirkin CA. Strategy for increasing drug solubility and

efficacy through covalent attachment to polyvalent DNA-nanoparticle conjugates. ACS Nano 2011; 5(9): 6962-70.
[http://dx.doi.org/10.1021/nn201446c] [PMID: 21812457]

[28] Park J, Park J, Ju EJ, *et al.* Multifunctional hollow gold nanoparticles designed for triple combination therapy and CT imaging. J Control Release 2015; 207: 77-85.
[http://dx.doi.org/10.1016/j.jconrel.2015.04.007] [PMID: 25863273]

[29] Liu J, Cui L, Losic D. Graphene and graphene oxide as new nanocarriers for drug delivery applications. Acta Biomater 2013; 9(12): 9243-57.
[http://dx.doi.org/10.1016/j.actbio.2013.08.016] [PMID: 23958782]

[30] Lim EK, Kim T, Paik S, Haam S, Huh YM, Lee K. Nanomaterials for theranostics: Recent advances and future challenges. Chem Rev 2015; 115(1): 327-94.
[http://dx.doi.org/10.1021/cr300213b] [PMID: 25423180]

[31] Shang J, Ma L, Li J, Ai W, Yu T, Gurzadyan GG. The origin of fluorescence from graphene oxide. Sci Rep 2012; 2(1): 792.
[http://dx.doi.org/10.1038/srep00792] [PMID: 23145316]

[32] Loh KP, Bao Q, Eda G, Chhowalla M. Graphene oxide as a chemically tunable platform for optical applications. Nat Chem 2010; 2(12): 1015-24.
[http://dx.doi.org/10.1038/nchem.907] [PMID: 21107364]

[33] Wang H, Gu W, Xiao N, Ye L, Xu Q. Chlorotoxin-conjugated graphene oxide for targeted delivery of an anticancer drug. Int J Nanomedicine 2014; 9: 1433-42.
[PMID: 24672236]

[34] Krasia-Christoforou T, Georgiou TK. Polymeric theranostics: Using polymer-based systems for simultaneous imaging and therapy. J Mater Chem B Mater Biol Med 2013; 1(24): 3002-25.
[http://dx.doi.org/10.1039/c3tb20191k] [PMID: 32261003]

[35] Molineux G. Pegylation: Engineering improved pharmaceuticals for enhanced therapy. Cancer Treat Rev 2002; 28 (Suppl. A): 13-6.
[http://dx.doi.org/10.1016/S0305-7372(02)80004-4] [PMID: 12173407]

[36] Qhattal HSS, Hye T, Alali A, Liu X. Hyaluronan polymer length, grafting density, and surface poly(ethylene glycol) coating influence *in vivo* circulation and tumor targeting of hyaluronan-grafted liposomes. ACS Nano 2014; 8(6): 5423-40.
[http://dx.doi.org/10.1021/nn405839n] [PMID: 24806526]

[37] Smith CE, Shkumatov A, Withers SG, *et al.* A polymeric fastener can easily functionalize liposome surfaces with gadolinium for enhanced magnetic resonance imaging. ACS Nano 2013; 7(11): 9599-610.
[http://dx.doi.org/10.1021/nn4026228] [PMID: 24083377]

[38] Tian G, Sun X, Bai J, *et al.* Doxorubicin-loaded dual-functional hyaluronic acid nanoparticles: Preparation, characterization and antitumor efficacy *in vitro* and *in vivo*. Mol Med Rep 2019; 19(1): 133-42.
[PMID: 30483793]

[39] Al-Jamal WT, Kostarelos K. Liposomes: From a clinically established drug delivery system to a nanoparticle platform for theranostic nanomedicine. Acc Chem Res 2011; 44(10): 1094-104.
[http://dx.doi.org/10.1021/ar200105p] [PMID: 21812415]

[40] Bhirde AA, Liu G, Jin A, *et al.* Combining portable Raman probes with nanotubes for theranostic applications. Theranostics 2011; 1: 310-21.
[http://dx.doi.org/10.7150/thno/v01p0310] [PMID: 21769298]

[41] Modugno G, Ménard-Moyon C, Prato M, Bianco A. Carbon nanomaterials combined with metal NPs for theranostic applications: Carbon nanomaterials for theranostic applications. Br J Pharmacol 2015; 172(4): 975-91.

[http://dx.doi.org/10.1111/bph.12984] [PMID: 25323135]

[42] Wang JTW, Cabana L, Bourgognon M, *et al.* Magnetically decorated multiwalled carbon nanotubes as dual MRI and SPECT contrast agents. Adv Funct Mater 2014; 24(13): 1880-94. [http://dx.doi.org/10.1002/adfm.201302892] [PMID: 26097444]

[43] Kurmi BD, Kayat J, Gajbhiye V, Tekade RK, Jain NK. Micro- and nanocarrier-mediated lung targeting. Expert Opin Drug Deliv 2010; 7(7): 781-94. [http://dx.doi.org/10.1517/17425247.2010.492212] [PMID: 20560777]

[44] Tekchandani P, Kurmi BD, Paliwal R, Paliwal SR. Galactosylated TPGS micelles for docetaxel targeting to hepatic carcinoma: Development, characterization, and biodistribution study. AAPS PharmSciTech 2020; 21(5): 174. [http://dx.doi.org/10.1208/s12249-020-01690-4] [PMID: 32548786]

[45] Makhmalzadeh BS, Molavi O, Vakili MR, *et al.* Functionalized caprolactone-polyethylene glycol based thermo-responsive hydrogels of silibinin for the treatment of malignant melanoma. J Pharm Pharm Sci 2018; 21(1): 143-59. [http://dx.doi.org/10.18433/jpps29726] [PMID: 29789104]

[46] Xiong XB, Lavasanifar A. Traceable multifunctional micellar nanocarriers for cancer-targeted co-delivery of MDR-1 siRNA and doxorubicin. ACS Nano 2011; 5(6): 5202-13. [http://dx.doi.org/10.1021/nn2013707] [PMID: 21627074]

[47] Kurmi BD, Gajbhiye V, Kayat J, Jain NK. Lactoferrin-conjugated dendritic nanoconstructs for lung targeting of methotrexate. J Pharm Sci 2011; 100(6): 2311-20. [http://dx.doi.org/10.1002/jps.22469] [PMID: 21491447]

[48] Oliveira JM, Salgado AJ, Sousa N, Mano JF, Reis RL. Dendrimers and derivatives as a potential therapeutic tool in regenerative medicine strategies—A review. Prog Polym Sci 2010; 35(9): 1163-94. [http://dx.doi.org/10.1016/j.progpolymsci.2010.04.006]

[49] Taratula O, Schumann C, Duong T, Taylor KL, Taratula O. Dendrimer-encapsulated naphthalocyanine as a single agent-based theranostic nanoplatform for near-infrared fluorescence imaging and combinatorial anticancer phototherapy. Nanoscale 2015; 7(9): 3888-902. [http://dx.doi.org/10.1039/C4NR06050D] [PMID: 25422147]

[50] Kurmi BD, Paliwal R, Paliwal SR. Dual cancer targeting using estrogen functionalized chitosan nanoparticles loaded with doxorubicin-estrone conjugate: A quality by design approach. Int J Biol Macromol 2020; 164: 2881-94. [http://dx.doi.org/10.1016/j.ijbiomac.2020.08.172] [PMID: 32853621]

[51] Kim C, Kim SY, Lim YT, Lee TS. Synthesis of conjugated polymer nanoparticles with core-shell structure for cell imaging and photodynamic cancer therapy. Macromol Res 2017; 25(6): 572-7. [http://dx.doi.org/10.1007/s13233-017-5104-y]

[52] Calzavara-Pinton PG, Venturini M, Sala R. Photodynamic therapy: Update 2006 Part 1: Photochemistry and photobiology. J Eur Acad Dermatol Venereol 2007; 21(3): 293-302. [http://dx.doi.org/10.1111/j.1468-3083.2006.01902.x] [PMID: 17309449]

[53] Berg K, Selbo PK, Weyergang A, *et al.* Porphyrin-related photosensitizers for cancer imaging and therapeutic applications. J Microsc 2005; 218(2): 133-47. [http://dx.doi.org/10.1111/j.1365-2818.2005.01471.x] [PMID: 15857375]

[54] Allison RR, Downie GH, Cuenca R, Hu XH, Childs CJH, Sibata CH. Photosensitizers in clinical PDT. Photodiagn Photodyn Ther 2004; 1(1): 27-42. [http://dx.doi.org/10.1016/S1572-1000(04)00007-9] [PMID: 25048062]

[55] Kurmi BD, Patel P, Paliwal R, Paliwal SR. Molecular approaches for targeted drug delivery towards cancer: A concise review with respect to nanotechnology. J Drug Deliv Sci Technol 2020; 57: 101682. [http://dx.doi.org/10.1016/j.jddst.2020.101682]

[56] Li M, Yang X, Ren J, Qu K, Qu X. Using graphene oxide high near-infrared absorbance for

photothermal treatment of Alzheimer's disease. Adv Mater 2012; 24(13): 1722-8. [http://dx.doi.org/10.1002/adma.201104864] [PMID: 22407491]

[57] Robinson JT, Tabakman SM, Liang Y, *et al.* Ultrasmall reduced graphene oxide with high near-infrared absorbance for photothermal therapy. J Am Chem Soc 2011; 133(17): 6825-31. [http://dx.doi.org/10.1021/ja2010175] [PMID: 21476500]

[58] Sharma M, Easha P, Tapasvi G, Reetika R. Nanomaterials in biomedical diagnosis. Nanomaterials in Diagnostic Tools and Devices. Elsevier 2020; pp. 57-83. [http://dx.doi.org/10.1016/B978-0-12-817923-9.00002-X]

[59] Bañobre-López M, Teijeiro A, Rivas J. Magnetic nanoparticle-based hyperthermia for cancer treatment. Rep Pract Oncol Radiother 2013; 18(6): 397-400. [http://dx.doi.org/10.1016/j.rpor.2013.09.011] [PMID: 24416585]

[60] Shah RR, Davis TP, Glover AL, Nikles DE, Brazel CS. Impact of magnetic field parameters and iron oxide nanoparticle properties on heat generation for use in magnetic hyperthermia. J Magn Magn Mater 2015; 387: 96-106. [http://dx.doi.org/10.1016/j.jmmm.2015.03.085] [PMID: 25960599]

[61] Kumar CSSR, Mohammad F. Magnetic nanomaterials for hyperthermia-based therapy and controlled drug delivery. Adv Drug Deliv Rev 2011; 63(9): 789-808. [http://dx.doi.org/10.1016/j.addr.2011.03.008] [PMID: 21447363]

[62] Gao M, Yu F, Chen H, Chen L. Near-infrared fluorescent probe for imaging mitochondrial hydrogen polysulfides in living cells and *in vivo*. Anal Chem 2015; 87(7): 3631-8. [http://dx.doi.org/10.1021/ac5044237] [PMID: 25751615]

[63] Amiri S, Shokrollahi H. The role of cobalt ferrite magnetic nanoparticles in medical science. Mater Sci Eng C 2013; 33(1): 1-8. [http://dx.doi.org/10.1016/j.msec.2012.09.003] [PMID: 25428034]

[64] Bennett KM, Jo J, Cabral H, Bakalova R, Aoki I. MR imaging techniques for nano-pathophysiology and theranostics. Adv Drug Deliv Rev 2014; 74: 75-94. [http://dx.doi.org/10.1016/j.addr.2014.04.007] [PMID: 24787226]

[65] Lu X, Liu Q, Wang L, Jiang W, Zhang W, Song X. Multifunctional triple-porous Fe_3O_4@SiO_2 superparamagnetic microspheres for potential hyperthermia and controlled drug release. RSC Advances 2017; 7(51): 32049-57. [http://dx.doi.org/10.1039/C7RA00899F]

[66] Zhang K, Chen H, Guo X, *et al.* Double-scattering/reflection in a single nanoparticle for intensified ultrasound imaging. Sci Rep 2015; 5(1): 8766. [http://dx.doi.org/10.1038/srep08766] [PMID: 25739832]

[67] Catalano E. Magnetic nanomaterial-based anticancer therapy. Advanced Magnetic and Optical Materials. Hoboken, NJ, USA: John Wiley & Sons, Inc. 2016; pp. 141-63.

[68] Wagstaff AJ, Brown SD, Holden MR, *et al.* Cisplatin drug delivery using gold-coated iron oxide nanoparticles for enhanced tumour targeting with external magnetic fields. Inorg Chim Acta 2012; 393: 328-33. [http://dx.doi.org/10.1016/j.ica.2012.05.012]

[69] Zhou M, Zhang R, Huang M, *et al.* A chelator-free multifunctional [64Cu]CuS nanoparticle platform for simultaneous micro-PET/CT imaging and photothermal ablation therapy. J Am Chem Soc 2010; 132(43): 15351-8. [http://dx.doi.org/10.1021/ja106855m] [PMID: 20942456]

[70] Barrett DM, Singh N, Porter DL, Grupp SA, June CH. Chimeric antigen receptor therapy for cancer. Annu Rev Med 2014; 65(1): 333-47. [http://dx.doi.org/10.1146/annurev-med-060512-150254] [PMID: 24274181]

[71] Ye H, Charpin-El Hamri G, Zwicky K, Christen M, Folcher M, Fussenegger M. Pharmaceutically

controlled designer circuit for the treatment of the metabolic syndrome. Proc Natl Acad Sci USA 2013; 110(1): 141-6.
[http://dx.doi.org/10.1073/pnas.1216801110] [PMID: 23248313]

[72] Wang X, Gkanatsas Y, Palasubramaniam J, *et al.* Thrombus-targeted theranostic microbubbles: A new technology towards concurrent rapid ultrasound diagnosis and bleeding-free fibrinolytic treatment of thrombosis. Theranostics 2016; 6(5): 726-38.
[http://dx.doi.org/10.7150/thno.14514] [PMID: 27022419]

[73] Durham AL, Caramori G, Chung KF, Adcock IM. Targeted anti-inflammatory therapeutics in asthma and chronic obstructive lung disease. Transl Res 2016; 167(1): 192-203.
[http://dx.doi.org/10.1016/j.trsl.2015.08.004] [PMID: 26334389]

[74] Aillon KL, El-Gendy N, Dennis C, Norenberg JP, McDonald J, Berkland C. Iodinated NanoClusters as an inhaled computed tomography contrast agent for lung visualization. Mol Pharm 2010; 7(4): 1274-82.
[http://dx.doi.org/10.1021/mp1000718] [PMID: 20575527]

[75] Ding B, Siddiqui S, DePietro M, Petersson G, Martin UJ. Inhaler usability of a pressurized metered dose inhaler and a soft mist inhaler in patients with COPD: A simulated-use study. Chron Respir Dis 2019; 16
[http://dx.doi.org/10.1177/1479972318787914] [PMID: 30016880]

[76] Lanza GM, Jenkins J, Schmieder AH, *et al.* Anti-angiogenic nanotherapy inhibits airway remodeling and hyper-responsiveness of dust mite triggered asthma in the brown norway rat. Theranostics 2017; 7(2): 377-89.
[http://dx.doi.org/10.7150/thno.16627] [PMID: 28042341]

[77] Alam MI, Beg S, Samad A, *et al.* Strategy for effective brain drug delivery. Eur J Pharm Sci 2010; 40(5): 385-403.
[http://dx.doi.org/10.1016/j.ejps.2010.05.003] [PMID: 20497904]

[78] Jack CR Jr, Knopman DS, Jagust WJ, *et al.* Tracking pathophysiological processes in Alzheimer's disease: An updated hypothetical model of dynamic biomarkers. Lancet Neurol 2013; 12(2): 207-16.
[http://dx.doi.org/10.1016/S1474-4422(12)70291-0] [PMID: 23332364]

[79] Ni R, Gillberg PG, Bergfors A, Marutle A, Nordberg A. Amyloid tracers detect multiple binding sites in Alzheimer's disease brain tissue. Brain 2013; 136(7): 2217-27.
[http://dx.doi.org/10.1093/brain/awt142] [PMID: 23757761]

[80] Smith BR, Gambhir SS. Nanomaterials for *in vivo* imaging. Chem Rev 2017; 117(3): 901-86.
[http://dx.doi.org/10.1021/acs.chemrev.6b00073] [PMID: 28045253]

CHAPTER 6

Targeting Potential of Nanocarriers for Efficient Treatment of *H. Pylori* Infection

Sunil K. Jain[1,*], **Kuldeep Rajpoot**[1], **K. Kesavan**[1], **Awesh Yadav**[2], **Umesh Gupta**[3] and **Prem N. Gupta**[4]

[1] *Department of Pharmacy, Guru Ghasidas Vishwavidyalaya (A Central University), Bilaspur (C.G.) 495 009, India*

[2] *Department of Pharmaceutics, National Institute of Pharmaceutical Education and Research, Raebareli, India*

[3] *Department of Pharmacy, Central University of Rajasthan, Ajmer, Rajasthan 305801, India*

[4] *CSIR-Indian Institute of Integrative Medicine, Canal Road, Jammu-180001, India*

Abstract: *Helicobacter pylori* (*H. pylori*), a prevalent human-specific pathogen, plays a key role in the development of peptic ulcer disease, gastric carcinoma, and gastric mucosa associated lymphoid tissue lymphoma. Once infected, those bacteria reside below the gastric mucosa adherent to the gastric epithelium, and entry of drugs to this target site is very difficult. The bacteria can also acquire resistance to commonly used antimicrobial drugs. Thus, an effective antimicrobial concentration cannot be achieved in the gastric mucous layer or on the epithelial cell surfaces where *H. pylori* exist and caused inefficient treatment. Such challenges have encouraged researchers into developing some therapies based on nanotechnology.

Keywords: Antibiotics, Gastro-retentive delivery system, *H. pylori*, Nanoparticles, pH responsive nanoparticles, Herbal approach, Liposomes, Lectins, Nanogels, Nanoparticulate vaccine, Mucoadhesion, Nanocarriers, Nanolipobeads, Polymeric nano-micelles, Receptor mediated targeting.

INTRODUCTION

The incidence of Helicobacter pylori (*H. pylori*) is found to be between 85 to 95% in developing countries such as India, Malaysia, *etc* and 30 to 50% in developed countries such as the USA, Australia, UK, *etc*. The epidemiology of *H. pylori* infection has been changed with improved sanitation and methods of eradication.

* **Corresponding author Sunil K. Jain**: Institute of Pharmaceutical Sciences, Guru Ghasidas Vishwavidyalaya (A Central University), Bilaspur (C.G.) 495 009, India; Tel: +91 94254 52174; E-mail: suniljain25in@yahoo.com

On the other hand, the occurrence of *H. pylori* is still plentiful all around the world [1, 2]. The incidences of *H. pylori* remain at the maximum in developing countries, and it is very much directly related to socioeconomic conditions and levels of sanitation. It was observed that after the year 2000, the prevalence of *H. pylori* was found to become lower than before in European countries. However, in Asia, the status/condition remains the same [3, 4]. The highest reported occurrence was reported in Africa (70.1%) and the lowest occurrence was reported in Switzerland (18.9%). Pakistan and India have shown the highest *H. pylori* prevalence 81% and 63.5%, respectively.

H. pylori is classified as a Class I carcinogen by the World Health Organization (WHO) and considered as an infectious disease. It is associated with dyspepsia, gastritis, peptic ulcer disease, gastric carcinoma, and mucous associated lymphoid tissue (MALT) lymphoma [5, 6]. It is a gram-negative spiral, 3.5 mm long, 0.6 mm thick, with 4-7 sheathed flagella at one end, which colonizes on the surface of the epithelium (beneath the mucus layer) of the gastric antrum [7, 8]. It is usually adhered to the inner lining of the gastric region and developed suitable surroundings to cultivate [9]. During *H. pylori* infection, urease hydrolyses the urea that is present in gastric epithelium into the ammonia and carbamate, which ultimately augmented the pH of the gastric region [10, 11].

All research communities and healthcare professionals are continuously involved to develop controlled release formulations of antimicrobial agents with the combination of certain newer drug molecules. Both unit dosage forms and multiunit dosage forms were developed and it was found that nanocarriers are getting more success in the effective treatment of *H. pylori* infection [12]. Gastro retentive drug delivery systems (GRDDS) have the immense potential and ability to effectively answer the problem of high bacterial load.

NANO APPROACHES

Nanocarriers are getting much attention from formulation scientists/researchers due to their effective surface area, uptake ability and penetration power. Several researchers have found the possibility of immunologically mediated prevention of *H. pylori* infection using an oral vaccine. Various nanocarriers *i.e.* nanoparticles, nanocapsules, nanolipobeads, nanosize liposomes with the various novel concepts with a target to treat *H. pylori* infection effectively were developed in past by researchers. There were various approaches utilized for the effective treatment of *H. pylori* (Fig. **6.1**).

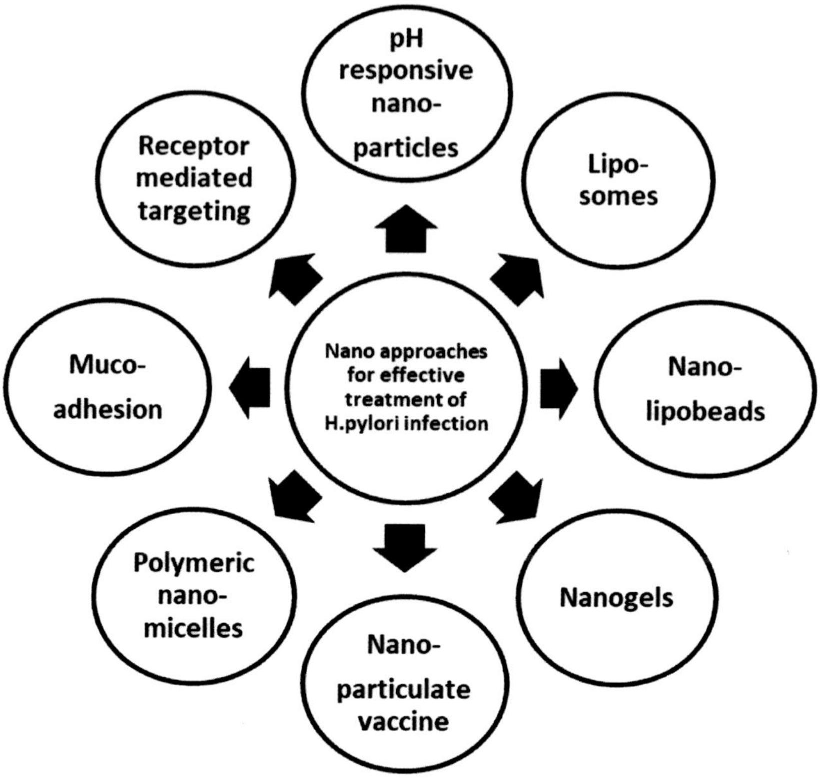

Fig. (6.1). Schematic showing various nano approaches for effective treatment of *H. pylori*.

Mucoadhesion Approach

Mucoadhesion has played a very important role in developing treatment strategies for *H. pylori* infection [13]. Different polymers have varied mucoadhesive abilities because of their inherent nature and properties. Fig. **6.2** is showing the mechanism of mucoadhesion of polymers. Nowadays, a variety of polymers such as methylcellulose, sodium carboxymethylcellulose, hydroxyethylcellulose, sodium alginate, karya gum, guar gum, retene, tragacanth and poly(ethylene glycol) (PEG) have been found to exhibit mucoadhesive properties and are widely used (Table **6.1**).

Since most of the existing drug delivery systems have failed on account of either improper mucoadhesion or muco-penetration. Now research is focused on the use of mucoadhesive nanocarriers that are based on the fact that these mucoadhesive nanoparticulate delivery systems show longer retention in the gastric region and deliver the antibiotic locally in the gastric mucosa for a longer period of time [14, 15].

Table 6.1. Classification of Mucoadhesive polymers.

Based on Specificity	**Specific bio-adhesive polymers They have the ability to adhere to specific chemical structures within the biological molecules**	**Lectins, Fimbrin**
	Non-specific bio-adhesive polymers They have the ability to bind with both the cell surface and the mucosal layer	Polyacrylic acid, Cyanoacrylates
According to their source	Natural and semisynthetic	Chitosan, Agarose, Gelatin, Pectin, CMC, HPMC
	Synthetic	Carbopol, PVA, PVP, Methacrylic acid, poly carbophil

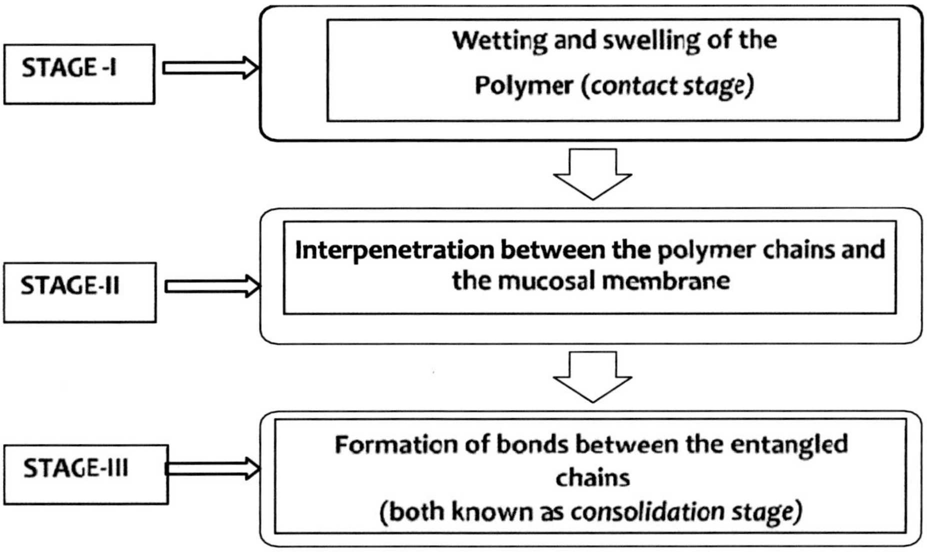

Fig. (6.2). Mechanism of mucoadhesion.

It is reported that mucoadhesive gliadin nanoparticles containing amoxicillin (AGNP) were found to be a suitable delivery system for effective treatment of *H. pylori* [16]. Formulations showed a stronger mucoadhesive propensity and specificity of GNP toward the stomach. It was also observed that Amoxicillin and AGNP both showed anti-*H. pylori* effects in infected Mongolian gerbils. AGNP eradicated *H. pylori* from the GI tract more effectively than amoxicillin because of the prolonged GI time attributed to mucoadhesion. Ramteke and Jain prepared and evaluated the oral mucoadhesive sustained release nanoparticles of clarithromycin and omeprazole [17]. *In vitro* antibacterial activity of these mucoadhesive nanoparticles was performed on an isolated culture of *H. pylori*.

The study showed a better eradication effect of formulations containing both drugs as compared to formulations containing single drug and plain drugs. Arora *et al.* developed mucoadhesive chitosan-alginate polyelectrolyte complex (CS-ALG PEC) nanoparticles of amoxicillin for complete eradication of *H. pylori* [18]. The optimized FITC labeled formulations had shown excellent muco-penetration and localization as observed with increased fluorescence in gastric mucosa continuously over 6 h. The pharmaceutical suspension containing Carbopol®-loaded amoxicillin nanospheres was developed as a newer delivery system for eradication of *H. pylori* [19]. The nanospheres had shown prolonged release of drug for more than 12 h. Similarly, amoxicillin-loaded gelatin nanoparticles also showed sustained release of the drug for more than 12 h [20].

Pan-In *et al.* reported the development of ethyl cellulose (EC) nanoparticles containing clarithromycin. Formulations had shown enhanced anti-adhesion activity when tested with *H. pylori* and Hep-2 cells, but also gave significant enhancement of *H. pylori* clearance in the gastric region of C57BL/6 mice infected with the bacteria [21]. Mucoadhesive pectin sulfate (PECS) nanoparticles of amoxicillin were prepared [22]. The mixed lipids such as the combination of rhamnolipid and phospholipids as the outer layer of nanoparticles and PECS as the inner core produces a system capable of significantly disrupting *H. pylori* biofilm by eliminating the extracellular polymeric substances (EPS) as well as inhibiting the adherence and colonization of bacteria.

Bacterial adhesion also plays a very important function in supporting effective antimicrobial delivery and also providing an original bioinspired targeting approach *via* specific EPS-mediated adsorption. Ping *et al.* reported such type of bioinspired approach to utilize bacteria-targeting and membrane-disruptive nanoparticles for the efficient antibiotic therapy of *H. pylori* infection [23]. Antibacterial nanoparticles were developed using montmorillonite (eMMT) and cationic linear polyethyleneimine (lPEI) *via* electrostatic interactions. eMMT serves as a bioinspired adhesive agent and membrane-disruptive lPEI function is to effectively lyse the bacterial outer membrane to let topical transmembrane delivery of antibiotic agents such as metronidazole into the intracellular cytoplasm.

Protein/polysaccharide core-shell-corona (PP-CSC) nanocarrier based delivery systems (NDS) were prepared by using bovine serum albumin (BSA) and chitosan (CS) [24]. CS polymer caused to control the release, provide mucoadhesion, and also stability of ε-PL loaded C(B)NDS in simulated gastric fluid due to their innate antimicrobial and mucoadhesive properties. BSA proteins progress the penetration power into bacterial biofilms for better eradication of *H. pylori*. The chitosan (CS) is harmless, biocompatible, biodegradable, and hydrophilic polymer. CS is derived from chitin, having the capability to set up electrostatic interactions with the mucin sialic acid residues [25 - 27]. Recently, Mucoadhesive nanostructured polyelectrolyte complexes (nano PECs) using chitosan (CS) and hypromellose phthalate (HP) of metronidazole were formulated [28]. Zafar *et al.* developed amoxicillin loaded nanoformulation using polycarbophil (PCP), thiolated polycarbophil (PCP-Cys), and papain modified thiolated polycarbophil (PCP-Cys-PAP) that allows it to reach the bacterium, hiding in deeper mucus layers and lengthen its availability at infection site [29].

pH Responsive Nanoparticles

These pH responsive nanoparticles are playing a very important role in the effective treatment strategy of *H. pylori* infection. Many researchers are continuously working in this field. During *H. pylori* infection, it was observed that the pH of gastric region is changed drastically and the management of pH can be an effective strategy against this infection. The pH-responsive nanoparticles were prepared by the addition of heparin solution to a chitosan solution with continuous magnetic stirring at room temperature [30]. The developed nanoparticles were found to be stable at pH 1.2-2.5, allowing them to protect an incorporated drug from destructive gastric acids. Further, it was attempted to incorporate Chitosan/poly-gamma-glutamic acid nanoparticles into pH-sensitive hydrogels that were developed as an effective carrier for delivery of amoxicillin [31]. These pH-sensitive hydrogels protect nanoparticles from being destructed by gastric acid and make possible amoxicillin contact specifically with intercellular spaces where *H. pylori* infection resides.

Thamphiwatana *et al.* reported a pH-responsive gold nanoparticle-stabilized liposome system of doxycycline. The developed formulation has a great potential to stay in the gastric region for a longer period of time and also dynamic ability to fight against bacteria residing in the mucus layer of the gastric region [32].

H. pylori can specifically express the urea transport protein on its membrane to transport urea into the cytoplasm for urease to produce ammonia, which protects the bacterium in the acid milieu of the stomach. Researchers utilized that concept and developed formulations. Covalently modified ureido-conjugated chitosan derivatives UCCs-1 and UCCs-2 and TPP were used to develop multifunctional nanoparticles of amoxicillin [33, 34]. These formulations displayed constructive pH-sensitive properties, which could delay the release of amoxicillin at gastric acids and allow the drug to deliver and target *H. pylori* efficiently.

Receptor Mediated Targeting

The receptor mediated targeting is getting much attention nowadays due to its better success ratio as compared to other approaches. The key points are (1) this approach increases the selectivity and effectiveness of drugs at the targeted site and to also reduce the toxicological aspects on other body organs (2) this approach offer protection and improves the pharmacokinetics of various drugs, and (3) it helps to triumph over the systemic toxicity and adverse effects mainly due to non-selective nature of most therapeutic agents. *H. pylori* identifies particular carbohydrate receptors, such as the fucose receptor, and produces the vacuolating cytotoxin, which induces inflammatory responses and modulates the cell-cell junction integrity of the gastric epithelium.

A very important ligand such as Concanavalin-A (Con-A) is found to be valuable mucoadhesive carrier. This ligand shown better specificity to bind mono-, oligo- and poly-saccharides with terminal non-reducing R-D-mannopyranosyl, R-D-glucopyranosyl or D-fructofuranosyl residues makes it appropriate candidate to execute the bioadhesive objectives in formulations [35, 36]. (Fig. **6.3**) Umamaheswari *et al.* developed fucose-specific and mannose-specific lectin-conjugated gliadin particles that have the ability to attach effectively at the carbohydrate receptors present at the location of *H. pylori* and provide an effective means of treatment [37].

Acetohydroxamic acid loaded Phosphatidyl ethanolamine (PE) liposomes anchored polyvinyl alcohol (PVA) xerogel beads (lipobeads) were developed as a receptor-mediated drug delivery system for use in blocking adhesion of *H. pylori* and thereby preventing the shriek of persistent stomach infections [38]. It was found that the surface of *H. pylori* contains lectins or adhesins, which may influence its adherence to the membrane of surface mucous cells [39]. Furthermore, the surface-associated antigens such as mannose and fucose are also present which may be utilized for targeting purpose [40, 41].

Ramteke *et al.* employed the triple therapy using amoxicillin, clarithromycin and omeprazole and developed gliadin nanoformulations. Triple therapy is found to be very useful due to its synergic and additive effects and also prevent the development of antibiotic resistance [42]. The lectin-conjugated formulations had shown superior *in vivo* clearance efficacy as compared to the non-conjugated formulations and plain drugs. UlexEuropaeus Agglutinin I (UEA I) and Con-A conjugated gliadin nanoparticles of acetohydroxamic acid (AHA) were developed. These lectin-conjugated gliadin nanoparticles have shown great potential as a targeted drug delivery for effective treatment of *H. pylori*. Ramteke *et al.* also reported another excellent strategy to combat *H. pylori* infection. They have developed targeted nanoparticles of chitosan-glutamic acid conjugates containing triple therapy for *H. pylori* to improve its therapeutic effect and reduce its dose-related side effect [43].

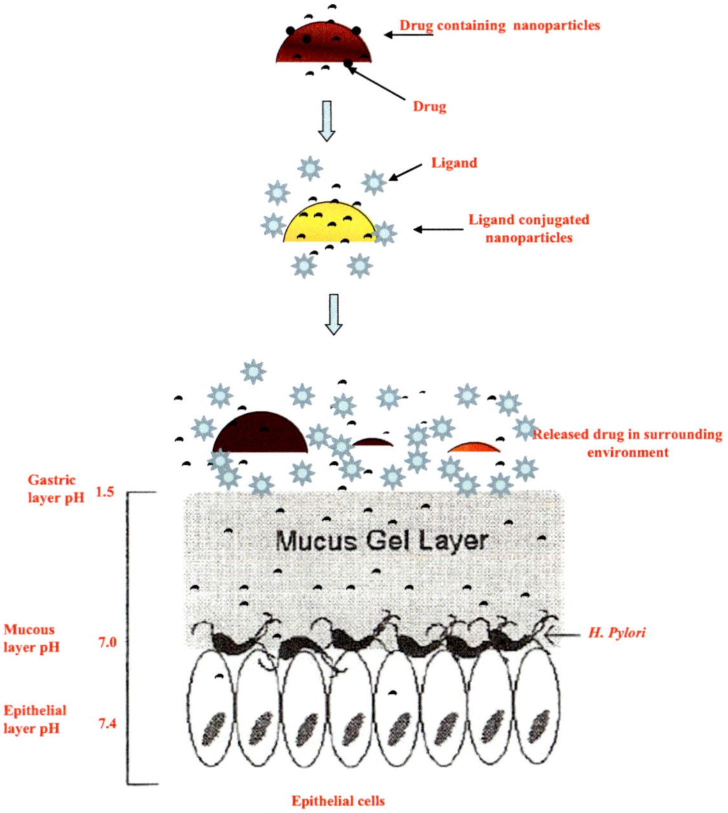

Fig. (6.3). Schematic showing working principle of ligand conjugated nanoparticles for treatment of *H. pylori.*

Lin *et al*. reported a novel combined fucose-conjugated chitosan and genipin-cross-linking approach to target region of microorganism on the gastric epithelium by developing nanoparticles of amoxicillin [44]. It was observed that the nanoparticles effectively control drug release at stomach acids and further released in an *H. pylori* survival situation to inhibit *H. pylori* growth and reduce disruption of the cell-cell junction protein in areas of *H. pylori* infection. Our research group developed Con-A conjugated gastro-retentive poly (lactic-co-glycolic acid) (PLGA) nanoparticles of acetohydroxamic acid (AHA) and clarithromycin (CLR) and evaluated under *in vitro* conditions [45]. A chemical process was adopted for the conjugation of PLGA with Con-A (Fig. **6.4**).

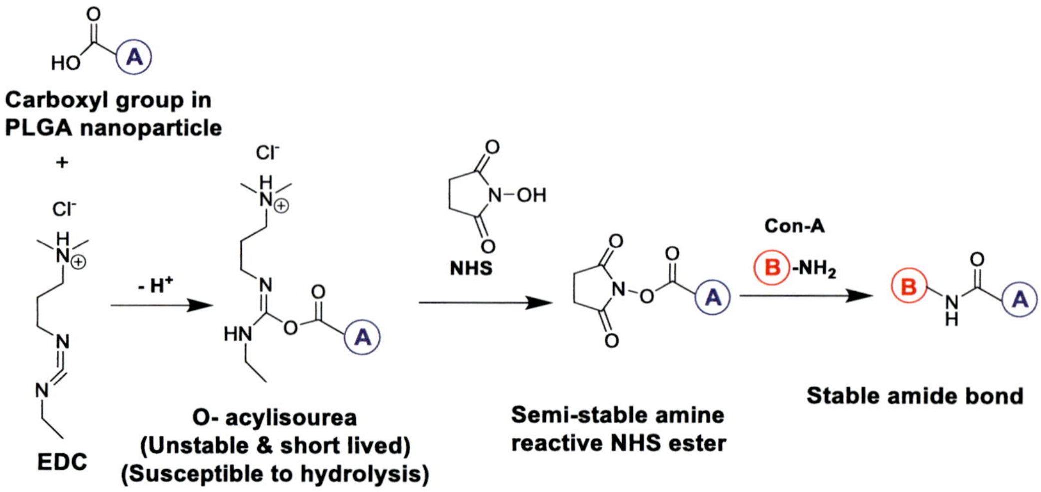

Fig. (6.4). Schematic diagram of chemical reaction for lectin conjugation with PLGA nanoparticles. [Adopted from: AAPS PharmSciTech, Jain *et al.*, 2016].

The conjugation process was straightforward two-step cross-linking procedure. The particle size of non-conjugated formulations was found to be between 400 nm to 600 nm whereas conjugated formulations ranged between 550-700 nm. The TEM analysis showed that both conjugated and non-conjugated formulations were almost observed spherical in shape and confirms their size range within the nano-limits (Fig. **6.5**).

Over a period of 8h, PLGA nanoparticles of AHA *i.e.*, AF7 and PLGA nanoparticles of AHA *i.e.* CF7 showed cumulative % drug release upto the extent of 37.69±0.10% and 30.80±0.43%, respectively whereas Con-A conjugated PLGA nanoparticles of AHA *i.e.* LAF7 and Con-A conjugated PLGA nanoparticles of AHA *i.e.* LCF7 showed a cumulative % drug release of 34.90±0.17% and 29.09±0.25%, respectively (Fig. **6.6**). L(CF7-AF7) exhibited potent inhibitory properties with zone of inhibition (ZOI) values 28.3 and 26.4 mm at 1000 and 500 µg/ml, respectively. LCF7 exhibited potent inhibitory properties alone with ZOI values 24.0 and 21.6 mm at 1000 and 500 µg/ml, respectively. LAF7 have least inhibitory properties with ZOI values 12.4 mm and 16.3 mm at 500 and 1000 µg/ml, respectively.

The fluorescence microscopy confirmed the interaction between Con-A conjugated nanoparticles and gastric mucosa. The outcome of the study suggested that the bioadhesive property of Con-A conjugated nanoparticles on rat gastric mucosa may be due to the true lectin-specific binding.

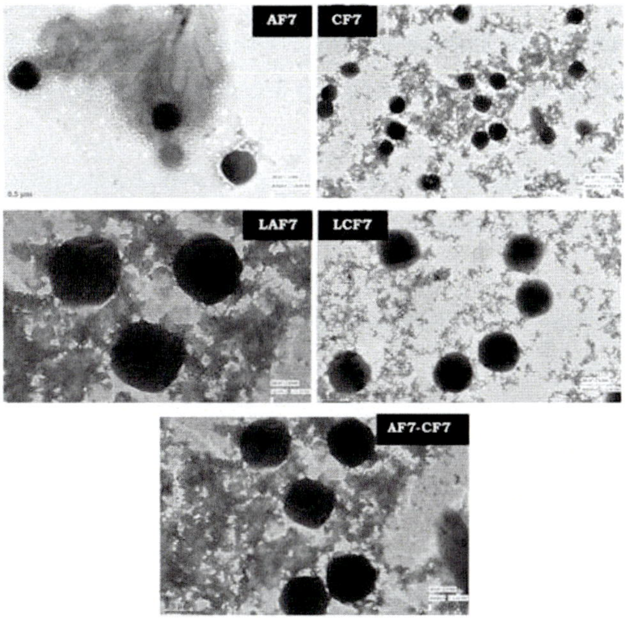

Fig. (6.5). TEM images of drug loaded nanoparticles (AF7 and CF7), lectin conjugated nanoparticles (LAF7 and LCF7) and combination batch (AF7-CF7). [Adopted from: AAPS PharmSciTech, Jain *et al.*, 2016].

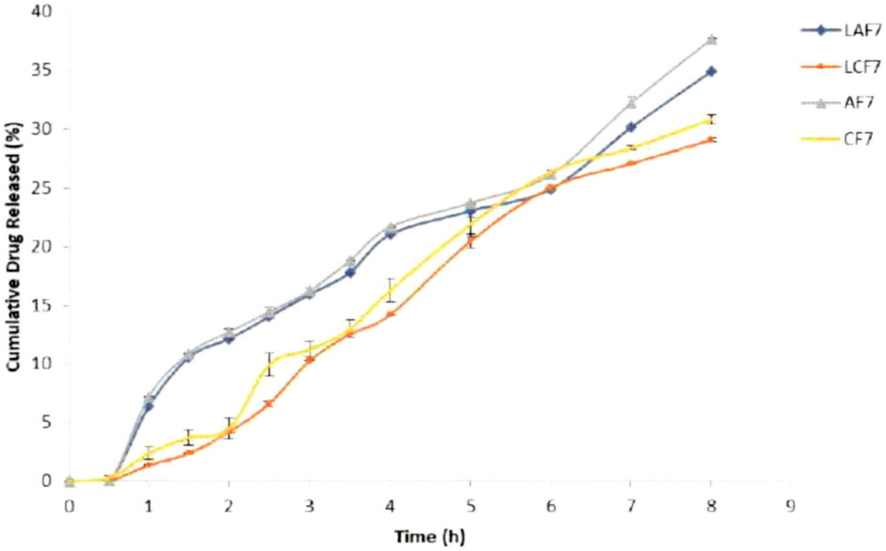

Fig. (6.6). Comparative cumulative % drug release profile of AF7, LAF7, CF7 and LCF7. CF7 = Formulation containing CLR as a drug; AF7 = Formulation containing AHA as a drug; LCF7 = Lectin conjugated formulation containing CLR as a drug; LAF7 = Lectin conjugated formulation containing AHA as a drug. Values are mean ± s.d. (n=3). [Adopted from: AAPS PharmSciTech, Jain *et al.*, 2016]

Liposomes

Liposomes are nano sized vesicular drug delivery systems, which have shown great potential for efficient treatment of *H. pylori* [46]. Bardonnet *et al.* [2008] reported formulation of targeted liposome loaded with certain antimicrobial agents such as ampicillin and metronidazole [47]. It was found that the inclusion of fucosyled glycolipids in the vesicle membrane leads to the formation of liposomes that are able to interact with the bacteria either in their spiral or in their coccoid forms. Jain *et al.* designed a gastro-retentive drug delivery system of amoxicillin and metronidazole, purposely suited for the abolition of *H. pylori* infection due to its mucoadhesiveness in the presence of polyelectrolyte polymers [48].

The developed formulations hold the advantages of both vesicular and particulate carriers, and it was prepared by the alternative coating of polyanion [poly (acrylic acid), PAA] and polycation [poly (allylamine hydrochloride), PAH] using liposomes as the core. These polyelectrolytes based multilayered formulations (nanocapsules) gave prolonged drug release in simulated gastric fluid, which is well suited for drug delivery against *H. pylori* infection in the stomach. The phosphatidylethanolamine (PE) lipid anchored double liposomes (DL) was used to incorporate two drugs such as amoxicillin trihydrate and ranitidine bismuth citrate in a single system [49]. The developed system had shown great potential against *H. pylori.* A newer concept was utilized by Thamphiwatana *et al.*, by adsorbing small charged nanoparticles onto liposome surfaces to stabilize them against fusion and payload leakage. They engineered a liposome formulation with a lipid composition sensitive to bacterium-secreted phospholipase A2 (PLA_2) and adsorbed chitosan-modified gold nanoparticles (AuChi) onto the liposome surface [50].

Jung *et al.* formulated a novel liposomal LipoLLA formulation, which showed potent bactericidal activity against several clinical isolated antibiotic-resistant strains of *H. pylori* including both the spiral and coccoid form [51]. Pectin-coated liposomes with encapsulated amoxicillin were developed [52]. This liposomal formulation aggravates direct interaction and subsequent binding of the particles to surface structures of *H. pylori*, and interaction with mucus from porcine stomach and mucus secreted by HT29-MTX cells.

Nanolipobeads, Polymeric Nano-micelles And Nanogels

Nanolipobeads, nano-micelles and nanogels offer great potential for designing anti-*H. pylori* treatment strategies. Nanolipobeads of polyvinyl alcohol loaded with amoxicillin were prepared and evaluated for targeting *H. pylori* infection

[53]. Polymeric micelles are nanosized molecules of core-shell structure that are formed by the self-association of amphiphilic block copolymers when they are added to an aqueous solvent. Polymeric micelles are among the most promising delivery systems in nanomedicine. Cong *et al.*, developed polymeric nano-micelle system of clarithromycin [54]. Initially, carboxymethyl chitosan (CMCS) was hydrophobically tailored with stearic acid (SA), and the obtained CMCS-g-SA co-polymers were additionally conjugated with urea to obtain U-CMCS-g-SA co-polymers. The prepared nano-micelle had shown an excellent retention time (almost 24 h) in the stomach and the shown effective results for effective targeting of *H. pylori*.

The nanogels are the nanosized particles formed by either physically or chemically crosslinked polymer networks that are swell in a good solvent. Genipin-crosslinked low molecular weight fucoidan/chitosan-N-arginine nanogels (FCSA) were prepared for targeted delivery of amoxicillin to the site of *H. pylori* infected AGS gastric epithelial cells [55]. The negatively charged nanogels (n-FCSA) had shown adhesion with the *H. pylori* bacteria and also displayed pH-responsive drug release properties.

Herbal Approach

Many herbal constituents are reported with anti-*H. pylori* activity. These herbal constituents were incorporated into nanocarriers and had shown very good results. The plant alkaloid berberine is identified to considerably reduce the proliferation of *H. pylori*. Chang *et al.* developed a berberine loaded novel nanoparticle with a heparin shell [56]. Results had shown that the designed formulation effectively controlled the release of berberine, which interacted specifically with the intercellular space at the site of *H. pylori* infection. In addition, the nanoparticles considerably increased the oppressive effect of berberine on *H. pylori* growth at the same time efficiently reducing cytotoxic effects in *H. pylori*-infected cells. Lin *et al.* prepared Fucose-chitosan/heparin nanoparticle-encapsulated berberine. It was demonstrated that these nanoparticles control the drug release as well as enhance the suppressive effect of berberine on *H. pylori* growth [57].

Nanoparticulate Vaccine

Due to very high incidences of diseases caused by *H. pylori*, predominantly in the developing countries, and the faster appearance of antibiotic resistance among clinical isolates, there is a strong need for the development of an effective vaccine against *H. pylori*. Svennerholm and Lundgren described the identification of diverse kinds of immune responses that may be related to protection against symptoms based on comparisons of *H. pylori*-infected patients with duodenal ulcers or gastric cancer and asymptomatic carriers [58]. There is still a need for strong clarification about the main protective immune mechanisms against *H. pylori* as well as to recognize a mixture of strong protective antigens, or recombinant bacterial strains that express such antigens that could be administered by a regimen that gives rise to effectual immune responses in human beings (Table **6.2**).

A lot of scientists have studied the prospect of immunologically-mediated prevention of *H. pylori* infection using an oral vaccine. The multiple oral immunization with *H. pylori*-PLG nanoparticles induced major *H. pylori*-specific mucosal IgA responses as well as serum IgG responses [59]. Milani *et al.* elucidated newer candidate vaccines and prophylactic or therapeutic immunization strategies for use against *H. pylori.* They also illustrated recognition of different types of immune responses that may be related to protection against *H. pylori* infection [60].

Table 6.2. Vaccine Candidates of *H. pylori.*

Type	Vaccine Candidate
Live	1. Recombinant strains expressing protective antigens 2. Attenuated *H. pylori* strain expressing protective antigens
Killed (administered with effective mucosal adjuvant)	1. Mixture of killed *H. pylori* bacteria with or without toxin/enzyme antigens 2. Mixture of purified (recombinant) *H. pylori* antigens

CONCLUSION

Till now advancements in the field of nanotechnology based effective formulations have been made since the first isolation of *H. pylori.* The sequencing of two strains of *H. pylori* has not only provided a wealth of data for understanding the pathogenesis of disease and microbial evolution but also highlighted potential therapeutic targets. Further, the invention of some novel strategies based on some newer antimicrobial agents and novel concepts will also help in modulating the immune system for effective treatment of infections.

CONSENT FOR PUBLICATION

Not applicable.

CONFLICT OF INTEREST

The authors declare no conflict of interest, financial or otherwise.

ACKNOWLEDGEMENT

Declared none.

REFERENCES

[1] Eusebi LH, Zagari RM, Bazzoli F. Epidemiology of Helicobacter pylori infection. Helicobacter 2014; 19 (Suppl. 1): 1-5.
[http://dx.doi.org/10.1111/hel.12165] [PMID: 25167938]

[2] Park JS, Jun JS, Seo JH, Youn HS, Rhee KH. Changing prevalence of Helicobacter pylori infection in children and adolescents. Clinical and Experimental Pediatrics 2021; 64(1): 21-5.
[http://dx.doi.org/10.3345/cep.2019.01543] [PMID: 32668822]

[3] Hooi JKY, Lai WY, Ng WK, *et al.* Global prevalence of Helicobacter pylori infection: Systematic review and meta-analysis. Gastroenterology 2017; 153(2): 420-9.
[http://dx.doi.org/10.1053/j.gastro.2017.04.022] [PMID: 28456631]

[4] Khoder G, Muhammad J, Mahmoud I, Soliman S, Burucoa C. Prevalence of *Helicobacter pylori* and its associated factors among healthy asymptomatic residents in the United Arab Emirates. Pathogens 2019; 8(2): 44.
[http://dx.doi.org/10.3390/pathogens8020044] [PMID: 30939800]

[5] Liu G, Xie J, Lu ZR, *et al.* Fifth Chinese national consensus report on the management of *Helicobacter pylori* infection. Zhonghua Nei Ke Za Zhi 2017; 56(7): 532-45.
[PMID: 28693066]

[6] Verma A, Dubey J, Hegde RR, Rastogi V, Pandit JK. *Helicobacter pylori* : Past, current and future treatment strategies with gastroretentive drug delivery systems. J Drug Target 2016; 24(10): 897-915.
[http://dx.doi.org/10.3109/1061186X.2016.1171326] [PMID: 27027827]

[7] Tanih NF, Ndip LM, Clarke AM, Ndip RN. An overview of pathogenesis and epidemiology of Helicobacter pylori infection. Afr J Microbiol Res 2010; 4(6): 426-36.

[8] Marshall B, Warren JR. Unidentified curved bacilli in the stomach of patients with gastritis and peptic ulceration. Lancet 1984; 323(8390): 1311-5.
[http://dx.doi.org/10.1016/S0140-6736(84)91816-6] [PMID: 6145023]

[9] Prasanthi C, Prasanthi N, Manikiran S, Rao NR. Focus on current trends in the treatment of *Helicobacter pylori* infection: An update. Int J Pharm Sci Rev Res 2011; 9(1): 42-51.

[10] Burne RA, Chen YYM. Bacterial ureases in infectious diseases. Microbes Infect 2000; 2(5): 533-42.
[http://dx.doi.org/10.1016/S1286-4579(00)00312-9] [PMID: 10865198]

[11] Rektorschek M, Weeks D, Sachs G, Melchers K. Influence of pH on metabolism and urease activity of Helicobacter pylori. Gastroenterology 1998; 115(3): 628-41.
[http://dx.doi.org/10.1016/S0016-5085(98)70142-8] [PMID: 9721160]

[12] O'Mahony R, Vaira D, Holton J, Basset C. Helicobacter pylori: Current status and future prospects. Sci Prog 2004; 87(4): 269-96.
[http://dx.doi.org/10.3184/003685004783238481] [PMID: 16028836]

[13] Smart J. The basics and underlying mechanisms of mucoadhesion. Adv Drug Deliv Rev 2005; 57(11): 1556-68.
[http://dx.doi.org/10.1016/j.addr.2005.07.001] [PMID: 16198441]

[14] Carvalho FC, Bruschi ML, Evangelista RC, Gremião MPD. Mucoadhesive drug delivery systems. Braz J Pharm Sci 2010; 46(1): 1-17.
[http://dx.doi.org/10.1590/S1984-82502010000100002]

[15] Nagahara N, Akiyama Y, Nakao M, Tada M, Kitano M, Ogawa Y. Mucoadhesive microspheres containing amoxicillin for clearance of Helicobacter pylori. Antimicrob Agents Chemother 1998;

42(10): 2492-4.
[http://dx.doi.org/10.1128/AAC.42.10.2492] [PMID: 9756746]

[16] Umamaheshwari RB, Jain NK. Receptor-mediated targeting of lipobeads bearing acetohydroxamic acid for eradication of Helicobacter pylori. J Control Release 2004; 99(1): 27-40.
[http://dx.doi.org/10.1016/j.jconrel.2004.06.006] [PMID: 15342178]

[17] Ramteke S, Jain NK. Clarithromycin- and omeprazole-containing gliadin nanoparticles for the treatment of *Helicobacter pylori.* J Drug Target 2008; 16(1): 65-72.
[http://dx.doi.org/10.1080/10611860701733278] [PMID: 18172822]

[18] Arora S, Gupta S, Narang RK, Budhiraja RD. Amoxicillin loaded chitosan-alginate polyelectrolyte complex nanoparticles as mucopenetrating delivery system for *h. Pylori.* Sci Pharm 2011; 79(3): 673-94.
[http://dx.doi.org/10.3797/scipharm.1011-05] [PMID: 21886911]

[19] Harsha S. Dual drug delivery system for targeting H. pylori in the stomach: Preparation and *in vitro* characterization of amoxicillin-loaded Carbopol® nanospheres. Int J Nanomedicine 2012; 7: 4787-96.
[http://dx.doi.org/10.2147/IJN.S34312] [PMID: 22969298]

[20] Harsha S. Pharmaceutical suspension containing both immediate/sustained-release amoxicillin-loaded gelatin nanoparticles: Preparation and *in vitro* characterization. Drug Des Devel Ther 2013; 7: 1027-33.
[http://dx.doi.org/10.2147/DDDT.S39956] [PMID: 24101859]

[21] Pan-In P, Banlunara W, Chaichanawongsaroj N, Wanichwecharungruang S. Ethyl cellulose nanoparticles: Clarithomycin encapsulation and eradication of *H. pylori.* Carbohydr Polym 2014; 109: 22-7.
[http://dx.doi.org/10.1016/j.carbpol.2014.03.025] [PMID: 24815396]

[22] Cai J, Huang H, Song W, *et al.* Preparation and evaluation of lipid polymer nanoparticles for eradicating *H. pylori* biofilm and impairing antibacterial resistance *in vitro.* Int J Pharm 2015; 495(2): 728-37.
[http://dx.doi.org/10.1016/j.ijpharm.2015.09.055] [PMID: 26417849]

[23] Ping Y, Hu X, Yao Q, *et al.* Engineering bioinspired bacteria-adhesive clay nanoparticles with a membrane-disruptive property for the treatment of Helicobacter pylori infection. Nanoscale 2016; 8(36): 16486-98.
[http://dx.doi.org/10.1039/C6NR05551F] [PMID: 27605059]

[24] Niaz T, Ihsan A, Abbasi R, Shabbir S, Noor T, Imran M. Chitosan-albumin based core shell-corona nano-antimicrobials to eradicate resistant gastric pathogen. Int J Biol Macromol 2019; 138: 1006-18.
[http://dx.doi.org/10.1016/j.ijbiomac.2019.07.165] [PMID: 31356942]

[25] Gatti THH, Eloy JO, Ferreira LMB, *et al.* Insulin-loaded polymeric mucoadhesive nanoparticles: Development, characterization and cytotoxicity evaluation. Braz J Pharm Sci 2018; 54(1)
[http://dx.doi.org/10.1590/s2175-97902018000117314]

[26] Calixto GMF, de Annunzio SR, Victorelli FD, *et al.* Chitosan-based drug delivery systems for optimization of photodynamic therapy: A review. AAPS PharmSciTech 2019; 20(7): 253.
[http://dx.doi.org/10.1208/s12249-019-1407-y] [PMID: 31309346]

[27] Fonseca-Santos B, Chorilli M. An overview of carboxymethyl derivatives of chitosan: Their use as biomaterials and drug delivery systems. Mater Sci Eng C 2017; 77: 1349-62.
[http://dx.doi.org/10.1016/j.msec.2017.03.198] [PMID: 28532012]

[28] Chaves de Souza MP, de Mattos NH, Pedreiro LN, *et al.* Design of mucoadhesive nanostructured polyelectrolyte complexes based on chitosan and hypromellose phthalate for metronidazole delivery intended to the treatment of *Helicobacter pylori* infections. Pharmaceutics 2020; 12(12): 1211.
[http://dx.doi.org/10.3390/pharmaceutics12121211] [PMID: 33327588]

[29] Zafar H, Kiani MH, Raza F, *et al.* Design of enzyme decorated mucopermeating nanocarriers for

eradication of *H. pylori* infection. J Nanopart Res 2020; 22(1): 4.
[http://dx.doi.org/10.1007/s11051-019-4719-7]

[30] Lin YH, Chang CH, Wu YS, Hsu YM, Chiou SF, Chen YJ. Development of pH-responsive chitosan/heparin nanoparticles for stomach-specific anti-Helicobacter pylori therapy. Biomaterials 2009; 30(19): 3332-42.
[http://dx.doi.org/10.1016/j.biomaterials.2009.02.036] [PMID: 19299008]

[31] Chang CH, Lin YH, Yeh CL, *et al.* Nanoparticles incorporated in pH-sensitive hydrogels as amoxicillin delivery for eradication of Helicobacter pylori. Biomacromolecules 2010; 11(1): 133-42.
[http://dx.doi.org/10.1021/bm900985h] [PMID: 19924885]

[32] Thamphiwatana S, Fu V, Zhu J, Lu D, Gao W, Zhang L. Nanoparticle-stabilized liposomes for pH-responsive gastric drug delivery. Langmuir 2013; 29(39): 12228-33.
[http://dx.doi.org/10.1021/la402695c] [PMID: 23987129]

[33] Jing ZW, Jia YY, Wan N, *et al.* Design and evaluation of novel pH-sensitive ureido-conjugated chitosan/TPP nanoparticles targeted to Helicobacter pylori. Biomaterials 2016; 84: 276-85.
[http://dx.doi.org/10.1016/j.biomaterials.2016.01.045] [PMID: 26851392]

[34] Arif M, Dong QJ, Raja MA, Zeenat S, Chi Z, Liu CG. Development of novel pH-sensitive thiolated chitosan/PMLA nanoparticles for amoxicillin delivery to treat Helicobacter pylori. Mater Sci Eng C 2018; 83: 17-24.
[http://dx.doi.org/10.1016/j.msec.2017.08.038] [PMID: 29208276]

[35] Borrebaeck C, Mattiasson B. A study of structurally related binding properties of concanavalin A using differential scanning calorimetry. Eur J Biochem 1980; 107(1): 67-71.
[http://dx.doi.org/10.1111/j.1432-1033.1980.tb04625.x] [PMID: 7398639]

[36] Jain SK, Gupta M, Sahoo AK, Pandey AN, Jain AK. Lectin conjugated gastro-retentive microspheres of amoxicillin for effective treatment of Helicobacter pylori. Curr Sci 2014; 106(2): 267-76.

[37] Umamaheshwari RB, Jain NK. Receptor mediated targeting of lectin conjugated gliadin nanoparticles in the treatment of Helicobacter pylori. J Drug Target 2003; 11(7): 415-24.
[http://dx.doi.org/10.1080/10611860310001647771] [PMID: 15203930]

[38] Umamaheshwari RB, Ramteke S, Jain NK. Anti-Helicobacter pylori effect of mucoadhesive nanoparticles bearing amoxicillin in experimental gerbils model. AAPS PharmSciTech 2004; 5(2): 60-8.
[http://dx.doi.org/10.1208/pt050232] [PMID: 15760090]

[39] Khin MM, Hua JS, Ng HC, Wadstrom T, Bow H. Agglutination of Helicobacter pylori coccoids by lectins. World J Gastroenterol 2000; 6(2): 202-9.
[PMID: 11819557]

[40] Borlace GN, Butler RN, Brooks DA. Monocyte and macrophage killing of helicobacter pylori: Relationship to bacterial virulence factors. Helicobacter 2008; 13(5): 380-7.
[http://dx.doi.org/10.1111/j.1523-5378.2008.00625.x] [PMID: 19250513]

[41] Fedwick JP, Lapointe TK, Meddings JB, Sherman PM, Buret AG. Helicobacter pylori activates myosin light-chain kinase to disrupt claudin-4 and claudin-5 and increase epithelial permeability. Infect Immun 2005; 73(12): 7844-52.
[http://dx.doi.org/10.1128/IAI.73.12.7844-7852.2005] [PMID: 16299274]

[42] Ramteke S, Ganesh N, Bhattacharya S, Jain NK. Triple therapy-based targeted nanoparticles for the treatment of *Helicobacter pylori*. J Drug Target 2008; 16(9): 694-705.
[http://dx.doi.org/10.1080/10611860802295839] [PMID: 18982518]

[43] Ramteke S, Ganesh N, Bhattacharya S, Jain NK. Amoxicillin, clarithromycin, and omeprazole based targeted nanoparticles for the treatment of *H. pylori*. J Drug Target 2009; 17(3): 225-34.
[http://dx.doi.org/10.1080/10611860902718649] [PMID: 19241256]

[44] Lin YH, Tsai SC, Lai CH, Lee CH, He ZS, Tseng GC. Genipin-cross-linked fucose–chitosan/heparin

nanoparticles for the eradication of Helicobacter pylori. Biomaterials 2013; 34(18): 4466-79.
[http://dx.doi.org/10.1016/j.biomaterials.2013.02.028] [PMID: 23499480]

[45] Jain SK, Haider T, Kumar A, Jain A. Lectin-conjugated clarithromycin and acetohydroxamic acid-loaded PLGA nanoparticles: A novel approach for effective treatment of *H. pylori.* AAPS PharmSciTech 2016; 17(5): 1131-40.
[http://dx.doi.org/10.1208/s12249-015-0443-5] [PMID: 26566630]

[46] Bardonnet PL, Faivre V, Boullanger P, Ollivon M, Falson F. Glycosylated liposomes against Helicobacter pylori: Behavior in acidic conditions. Biochem Biophys Res Commun 2009; 383(1): 48-53.
[http://dx.doi.org/10.1016/j.bbrc.2009.03.117] [PMID: 19324015]

[47] Bardonnet P, Faivre V, Boullanger P, Piffaretti J, Falson F. Pre-formulation of liposomes against Helicobacter pylori: Characterization and interaction with the bacteria. Eur J Pharm Biopharm 2008; 69(3): 908-22.
[http://dx.doi.org/10.1016/j.ejpb.2008.01.018] [PMID: 18362065]

[48] Jain P, Jain S, Prasad KN, Jain SK, Vyas SP. Polyelectrolyte coated multilayered liposomes (nanocapsules) for the treatment of Helicobacter pylori infection. Mol Pharm 2009; 6(2): 593-603.
[http://dx.doi.org/10.1021/mp8002539] [PMID: 19718807]

[49] Singh DY, Prasad NK. Double liposomes mediated dual drug targeting for treatment of Helicobacter pylori infections. Pharmazie 2011; 66(5): 368-73.
[PMID: 21699071]

[50] Thamphiwatana S, Gao W, Pornpattananangkul D, *et al.* Phospholipase A2-responsive antibiotic delivery *via* nanoparticle-stabilized liposomes for the treatment of bacterial infection. J Mater Chem B Mater Biol Med 2014; 2(46): 8201-7.
[http://dx.doi.org/10.1039/C4TB01110D] [PMID: 25544886]

[51] Jung SW, Thamphiwatana S, Zhang L, Obonyo M. Mechanism of antibacterial activity of liposomal linolenic acid against Helicobacter pylori. PLoS One 2015; 10(3): e0116519.
[http://dx.doi.org/10.1371/journal.pone.0116519] [PMID: 25793403]

[52] Gottesmann M, Goycoolea FM, Steinbacher T, Menogni T, Hensel A. Smart drug delivery against Helicobacter pylori: Pectin-coated, mucoadhesive liposomes with antiadhesive activity and antibiotic cargo. Appl Microbiol Biotechnol 2020; 104(13): 5943-57.
[http://dx.doi.org/10.1007/s00253-020-10647-3] [PMID: 32399588]

[53] Jain AK, Jain SK. Development and characterization of nanolipobeads-based dual drug delivery system for *H. Pylori* targeting. J Drug Target 2013; 21(6): 593-603.
[http://dx.doi.org/10.3109/1061186X.2013.784978] [PMID: 23597027]

[54] Cong Y, Geng J, Wang H, *et al.* Ureido-modified carboxymethyl chitosan-graft-stearic acid polymeric nano-micelles as a targeted delivering carrier of clarithromycin for Helicobacter pylori: Preparation and *in vitro* evaluation. Int J Biol Macromol 2019; 129: 686-92.
[http://dx.doi.org/10.1016/j.ijbiomac.2019.01.227] [PMID: 30772413]

[55] Lin YH, Lu KY, Tseng CL, Wu JY, Chen CH, Mi FL. Development of genipin-crosslinked fucoidan/chitosan- *N* -arginine nanogels for preventing *Helicobacter* infection. Nanomedicine (Lond) 2017; 12(12): 1491-510.
[http://dx.doi.org/10.2217/nnm-2017-0055] [PMID: 28524785]

[56] Chang CH, Huang WY, Lai CH, *et al.* Development of novel nanoparticles shelled with heparin for berberine delivery to treat Helicobacter pylori. Acta Biomater 2011; 7(2): 593-603.
[http://dx.doi.org/10.1016/j.actbio.2010.08.028] [PMID: 20813208]

[57] Lin YH, Lin JH, Chou SC, *et al.* Berberine-loaded targeted nanoparticles as specific *Helicobacter pylori* eradication therapy: *In vitro* and *in vivo* study. Nanomedicine (Lond) 2015; 10(1): 57-71.
[http://dx.doi.org/10.2217/nnm.14.76] [PMID: 25177920]

[58] Svennerholm AM, Lundgren A. Progress in vaccine development against *Helicobacter pylori*. FEMS Immunol Med Microbiol 2007; 50(2): 146-56. [http://dx.doi.org/10.1111/j.1574-695X.2007.00237.x] [PMID: 17442014]

[59] Kim SY, Doh HJ, Jang MH, Ha YJ, Chung SI, Park HJ. Oral immunization with Helicobacter pylori-loaded poly(D, L-lactide-co-glycolide) nanoparticles. Helicobacter 1999; 4(1): 33-9. [http://dx.doi.org/10.1046/j.1523-5378.1999.09046.x] [PMID: 10352085]

[60] Milani M, Sharifi Y, Rahmati-Yamchi M, Somi MH, Akbarzadeh A. Immunology and vaccines and nanovaccines for *Helicobacter pylori* infection. Expert Rev Vaccines 2015; 14(6): 833-40. [http://dx.doi.org/10.1586/14760584.2015.1008460] [PMID: 25645086]

CHAPTER 7

Gastro-retentive Nanocarriers in Drug Delivery

Kuldeep Rajpoot[1,*], **Sunil K. Jain**[1] and **Saroj Dangi Rajpoot**[2]

[1] *Institute of Pharmaceutical Sciences, Guru Ghasidas Vishwavidyalaya (A Central University), Bilaspur, C.G. 495009, India*

[2] *Mahatma Gandhi Homoeopathic Medical College, Rani Durgavati Vishwavidyalaya, Jabalpur, M.P. 482001, India*

Abstract: The oral route is an extremely accepted route for the administration of several drug delivery systems. This route exhibits several merits for the controlled and sustained release of different formulation types to attain enhanced therapeutic responses. Gastro-retentive nanocarriers (NCs) (GRNCs) have advantages due to their aptitude for extended retaining potential in the stomach environment and thereby elevate gastric retention and augmenting bioavailability of the drug molecules. This chapter covers various merits and demerits of gastro-retentive NCs. Further, it also discusses some gastro-retentive strategies and their applications in the therapy of various illnesses, for instance, swelling NCs, porous NCs, floating/non-floating NCs, lipid NCs, Polymeric NCs, bioadhesive NCs, and magnetic NCs, *etc*.

Keywords: Bioavailability, Controlled drug release, Drug delivery, Eudragit L100, Floating systems, Gastric cancer, Gastro-retentive carriers, Gastric retention time, Gastric emptying time, Gastrointestinal, HPMC, Ion-exchange resin, Lipids nanocarriers, Mucoadhesive nanocarriers, Magnetic nanocarriers, Polymer, Polymeric nanocarriers, Stomach, Sustained drug release, Super porous systems.

INTRODUCTION

Oral administration of formulations exhibits several merits such as flexibility in preparation, low price, ease of delivery, easy transport, as well as elevated patient compliance. Despite this, it is associated with some demerits like low bioavailability of drugs owing to the heterogeneity of the gastrointestinal (GI) environment, the poor gastric retention time (GRT) of the product, enzymatic actions, pH conditions of the GI tract (GIT), and surface area [1]. Furthermore, traditional drug delivery systems (DDS) have not shown great potential to combat the challenges levied by the GIT, for instance, imperfect drug release, less

* **Corresponding author Kuldeep Rajpoot**: Institute of Pharmaceutical Sciences, Guru Ghasidas Vishwavidyalaya (A Central University), Bilaspur (C.G.) 495 009, India; Tel: +919993965153; E-mail: **kuldeep_sagar06@rediffmail.com**

Akhlesh K. Jain & Keerti Mishra (Eds.)

efficiency of the drug, as well as the compulsion of recurrent dosing. Hence, to overcome these issues associated with traditional DDS and for enhancing the retaining aptitude of drugs in gastric conditions, it becomes essential to develop gastro-retentive nanocarriers (NCs) (GRNCs) [2].

GRNCs may offer various advantages like prolonged GRT of developed products especially in the harsh conditions of the stomach for many hours, improving therapeutic efficiency of drugs in different ways such as by elevating drug absorption and bioavailability, as well as *via* opening the door of possibilities for targeted delivery of the drug in the stomach using different NCs. Besides, GRNCs can augment sustained and controlled delivery *via* constantly releasing many drugs at the desired rate at preferred absorption sites [1, 3, 4]. GRNCs show good feasibility for drugs, which usually have poor absorption ability in the inferior part of the GIT and are not stable in the harsh condition of the stomach. Further, they are also a strong candidate for drugs that are poorly soluble in the basic pH environment, and having a short half-life. In this regard, numerous formulation approaches are being implemented and developed for attaining controlled release of the drug, for instance, porous NCs (*e.g.*, hydrogel (HG), porous silicon NCs) [5, 6], mucoadhesive NCs [7], raft-forming nanosystems [8], magnetic NCs [9], *etc.*

PHYSIOLOGICAL ASPECTS OF STOMACH

The physiology of the stomach plays a vital role in the development of NCs. Hence, for the successful development of GRNCs, deep insight into anatomy as well as the physiology of the stomach is essential. Moreover, anatomically, the stomach is classified as proximal stomach and distal stomach. The proximal part represents the fundus and body, while the distal region includes the antrum as well as pylorus (Fig. **7.1**).

In the stomach, food content is crushed, and then, it transfers slowly into the next part (*i.e.*, duodenum) [10]. On the other hand, the fundus along with the body mainly reserves the undigested food contents. In contrast, the antrum pumps the content *via* utilizing a propelling action and facilitates gastric emptying [10, 11]. Diverse phases in the mobility of food content through the stomach are called migrating myoelectric complex (MMC) (Fig. **7.2**). The gastric emptying pattern significantly fluctuates during fed and fast states [1, 10, 12]. In the fast state, particles having a smaller size over the diameter of the pyloric sphincter can effortlessly clear from the pylorus and reach into the duodenum [12]. In contrast, in the fed state, motor action plays a crucial role and can produce its motor effect after 5–10 min following ingestion of food. Further, this effect remains until the food is present in the stomach, which can interrupt gastric emptying speed.

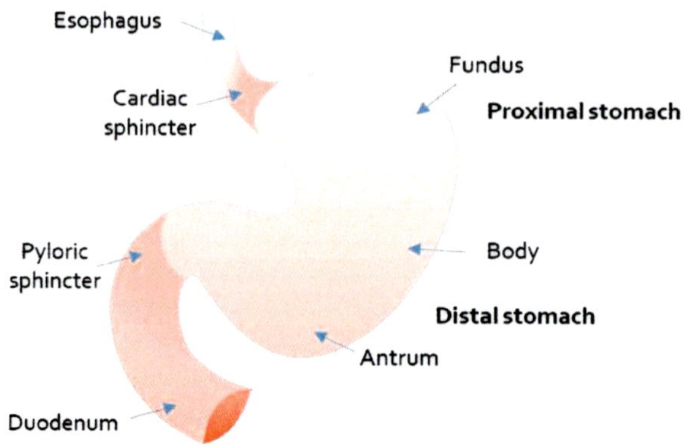

Fig. (7.1). Schematic view on the anatomy of the stomach.

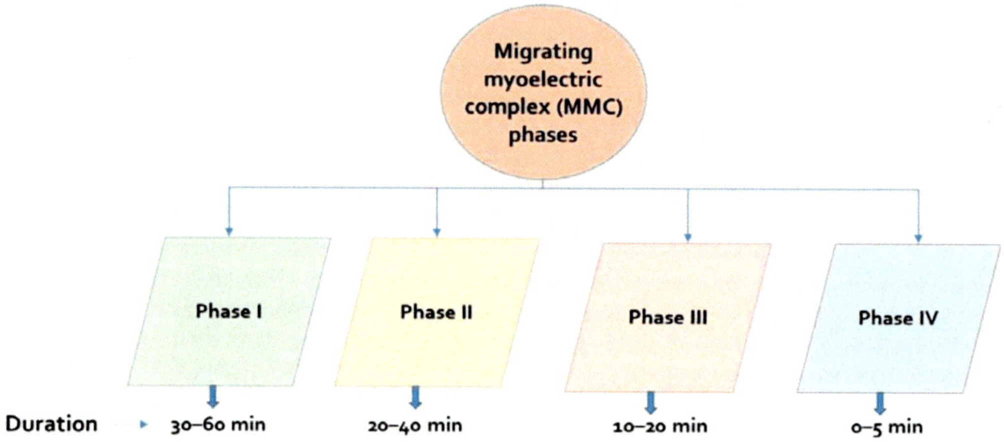

Fig. (7.2). Four phases of the MMC.

FACTORS INFLUENCING THE ACTIVITY OF GRNC$_S$ IN THE STOMACH

Various factors affect the performance of GRNCs. These factors are mainly categorized into pharmaceutical factors, physiological factors, and patient-related factors (Fig. **7.3**).

Physiological Factors

In the stomach, several extrinsic factors may affect GRTs of drugs, for example, nature and content of meal, nature, and density of calories, eating habits, exercise, position and movement of the body, and duration of sleep [1, 13 - 15]. During MMC phases (every 1.5-2 h) in a fast state, the undigested food content is swept through the stomach owing to motor activity. Therefore, if the timing of the dosing formulation overlaps with MMC, then it results in a decrease in the GRT of the formulation. In contrast, in the fed state, the MMC phases do not have a significant effect, hence GRT is extended [10]. Similarly, an enhanced caloric density substantially augments the GRT of formulation while the nature of calories slightly influences GRT [14, 16]. Besides, elevated food viscosity also leads to enhancement in the GRT of the formulation [17, 18].

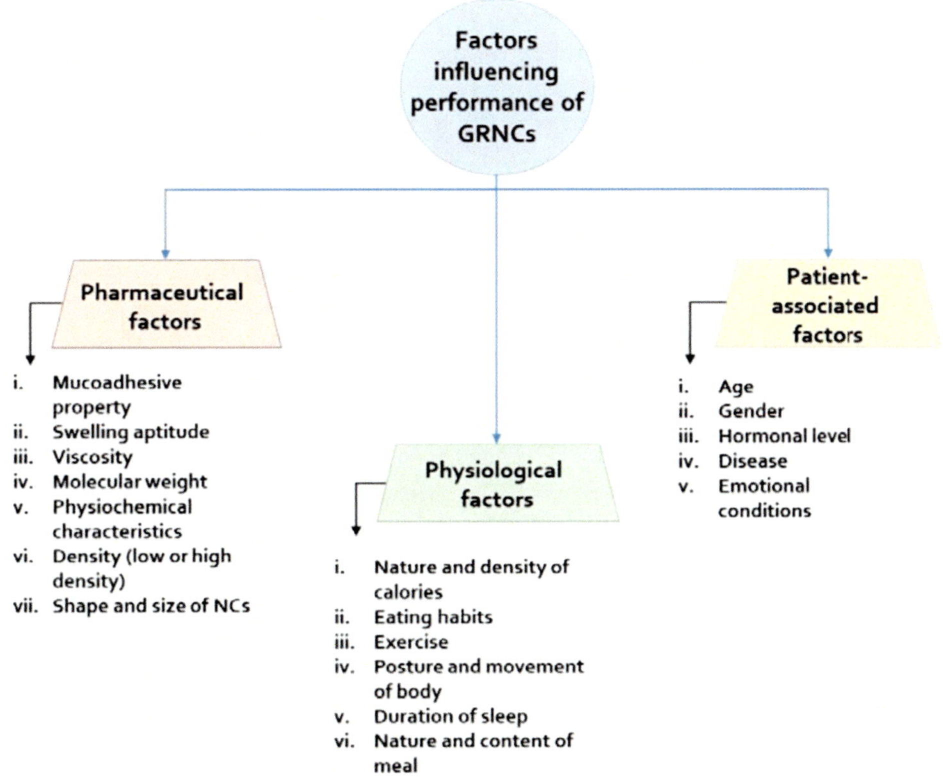

Fig. (7.3). A summary of factors affecting the performance of GRNCs.

Additionally, body posture also has a great effect on the GRT [1]. For instance, during upright posture, the floating DDS normally enhances GRT owing to the floating of formulation in the gastric fluid for an extended period. On the other hand, in the case of the non-floating system, formulations settle down in the stomach and sweep across rapidly owing to the effect of the peristaltic contraction [1], while in the supine condition, the non-floating DDS exhibit a prolonged GRT over floating DDS [19, 20].

Patient-associated Factors

Some patient-related factors can also significantly influence the efficacy of GRNCs by varying gastric emptying time, for instance, age of the patient, gender, hormonal level, disease, and emotional conditions. For example, females exhibit slower gastric emptying speed compared to males [21]. Hormone-related variations may increase GRT in females over males, for example, males produce extra gastric acid than females [22]. An emotional state like depression can decline gastric emptying rate in patients while patients suffering from anxiety may experience elevated gastric emptying rate [13]. Aged patients show augmented GRT for formulations over younger patients [23]. Moreover, the disease of the patient can substantially influence the GRT of GRNCs. For example, patients suffering from Parkinson's disease normally show long-lasting GRT, which is often associated with constipation [24]. On the other hand, diabetic patients experience decreased gastric emptying time by 30 to 50% [25].

Pharmaceutical Factors

It is vital to employ the right polymers along with other excipients to design the desired GRNC. For instance, if we are designing a mucoadhesive NC, then employed polymers should have good mucoadhesive properties. Some mucoadhesive polymers including hydroxypropyl methylcellulose (HPMC) and Carbopol can be used for designing the mucoadhesive NCs. Similarly, in the case of an expandable system, the polymers possessing high swelling aptitude can be used.

Besides, some other factors can also affect the success of NCs, which include shape and size of NCs (ring shape or tetrahedron-shape), viscosity, molecular weight, as well as physicochemical characteristics of polymers [13]. Likewise, density (low or high density) also play a crucial role, for instance, during the designing of low-density NCs, their density must be lesser than that of the gastric fluid (1.004 g/cm^3) so that they can easily float in the gastric medium [26, 27]. However, by improving the floating ability of NCs we can also enhance the GRT of the low-density formulations. Moreover, this can be significantly influenced by the food [28]. In contrast, in high-density NCs, their density must be higher than the density of gastric fluid so that they remain to sink in the extremity of the stomach so that gastric emptying may be avoided. Moreover, the GRT of the NCs can be enhanced by elevating the density (>2.500 g/cm^3) [29].

GRNCS-BASED APPROACHES FOR IMPROVING GRT OF NC$_S$

Several approaches are generally applied for extending the GRT of a drug such as designing sinking, floating, porous, swelling, ion-exchange resin, mucoadhesive, effervescent, raft forming, as well as magnetic type NCs (Fig. **7.4**). Further, GRNCs investigated for improving GRT have been listed in Table **7.1**. Some important approaches are being discussed here.

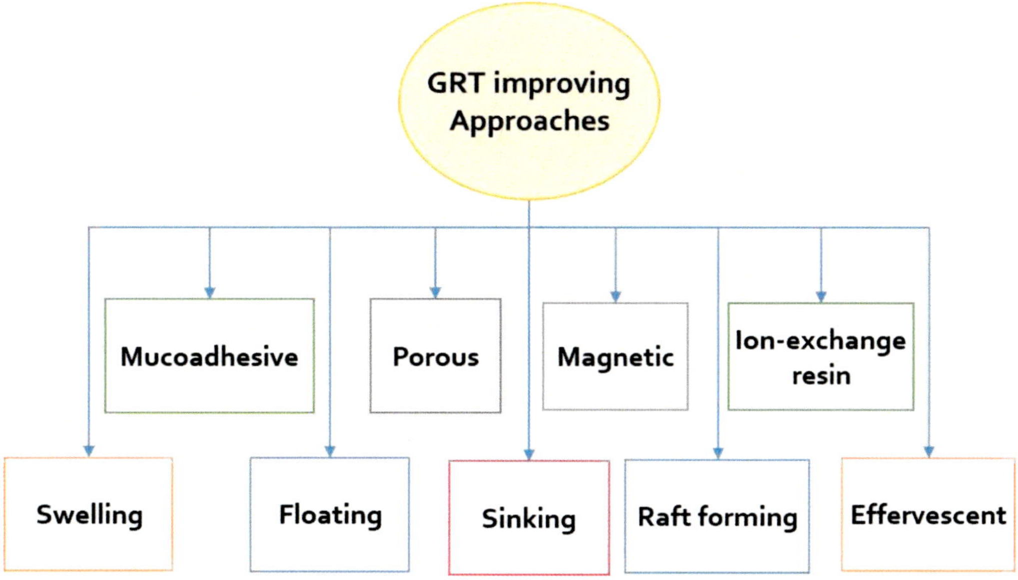

Fig. (7.4). Diagram depicting different approaches for improving GRT of NCs.

Table 7.1. List of NCs for improving GRT.

Drug	Formulation Type	Approach Used	Indications	References
Carvedilol	Nanoparticles	Mucoadhesive	Antihypertensive	[30]
Emodin	Nanomicelles	Floating mucoadhesive	Gastric cancer	[31]
-	Hydrophobin-coated porous silicon nanoparticle	Mucoadhesive	-	[32]
Rifampicin	Mussel-inspired polymeric nanoparticles	Mucoadhesive	Antibiotic	[33]
Pramipexole	Electrospun nanofiber membranes	Effervescence-based floating	Parkinson's disease	[34]
Ofloxacin	Gellan/PVA nanofibers	Mucoadhesive	Antimicrobial activity	[35]
-	Alginate microspheres	Mucoadhesive	-	[36]

Sink-approach Based NCs

In the sink approach, high-density materials (*e.g.*, zinc oxide, titanium dioxide, barium sulfate, and iron powder) are employed to develop NCs as they have a higher density compared to gastric fluid [10]. High-density substances generally exhibit less GRT as compared to light-density materials. In this regard, a study revealed that tiny pellets having a high density can refrain from peristaltic activities in the stomach owing to their stay in the antrum rugae or bends, which normally enhance their GI retention time usually from 5.8 to 25 h [19]. In another investigation, Zamani *et al.* synthesized zinc oxide and titanium dioxide NCs for controlled and targeted delivery of curcumin. The NCs revealed a pH-reliant drug release profile and exhibited maximum release of curcumin in the neutral pH over-acidic medium. Further, MTT analysis advocated significant toxicity of NCs suggesting their anticancer effects [37]. Besides, diverse titanium dioxide NCs indicated inhibition in cell proliferation and caused apoptosis of the cancer cells. For instance, brookite BSA titanium dioxide NCs hindered cell invasion. On the other hand, PEG-amorph titanium dioxide NCs elevated cell invasion, which suggests the potential of titanium dioxide NCs for cancer therapy [38]. Titanium dioxide NCs were reported after loading ibuprofen and gentamicin drugs. Both drugs loaded NCs exhibited a prolonged drug release pattern, regardless of their structure [39].

Porous NCs

Porous NCs have attracted researchers for attaining controlled release of the drug through formulations owing to their elevated mechanical power as well as elastic qualities [40]. They swell speedily owing to the uptake of water through several pores already present at the surface. However, traditional formulations (*e.g.*, HG) exhibit a slow process (spend many hours to attain equilibrium state), therefore, these formulations are easily emptied through the stomach. On the other hand, super porous HGs exhibit fast swelling (~100-folds) with sufficient mechanical power to combat the pressure generated by gastric contraction, which leads to an elevation in the GRT. Moreover, the development of these formulations uses some highly swellable polymers (*e.g.*, sodium alginate and croscarmellose sodium) [41, 42].

In a study, Sarparanta *et al.* developed a bioadhesive oral DDS. These GRNCs were usually relied on thermally-hydrocarbonized porous silicon (THCPSi). They were loaded with hydrophobin (HFBII) and functionalized using a self-assembled amphiphilic protein. Findings suggested that HFBII-THCPSi NCs were non-cytotoxic. further, they showed the mucoadhesive property in AGS cells. After oral delivery, HFBII-THCPSi NCs revealed significantly slower passage through the rat GIT over unfunctionalized THCPSi. GRNCs also exhibited prolonged GRT in the stomach owing to mucoadhesive property (~3 h) [32]. In another investigation, mesoporous silica nanoparticles (MSN) were synthesized possessing varying positive charges at the surface. However, a positive surface charge on MSN was introduced *via* employing trimethylammonium (TA) groups (MSN–TA). When these MSN–TA NCs were employed in the buffer of pH 7.4, it produced a partial negative charge owing to the deprotonation of silanol groups. Further, this results in the development of strong electrostatic repulsion, which prompted a sustained release effect of the entrapped drugs. Eventually, the author concluded that MSN–TA NCs can be effectively employed for the pH-reliant release of anionic molecules following oral administration of NCs [43].

Shrestha *et al.* prepared insulin-loaded chitosan-conjugated porous silicon NCs (CSUn NCs). Here, they used thermally responsive undecylenic acid-modified hydrocarbon, which encouraged not only mucoadhesion but also cellular interactions of NCs and improved their intestinal permeability. Findings revealed enhanced mucoadhesion as well as the permeability of CSUn NCs. Additionally, the surface of these NCs was further derivatized using either cell-penetrating peptide (CPP-CSUn NCs) or l-cysteine (CYS-CSUn NCs). Finally, CPP-CSUn and CYS-CSUn NCs exhibited 12- and 17-times more permeability of insulin through intestinal cells, respectively, in diabetic rats. Besides, CYS-CSUn NCs confirmed 2.03- and 1.86-fold higher relative bioavailability over oral insulin solution and drug-free NCs, respectively [44].

Recently, Juere *et al.* synthesized amino-functionalized MCM-48-type MSNs using a protein (succinylated beta-lactoglobulin). Afterward, they delivered resveratrol and omeprazole drugs loaded MSNs after transforming into a versatile tablet *via* the oral route. pH-gating attributes of employed protein desisted resveratrol from releasing in the simulated gastric fluid while due to efficient nanopore it fruitfully elevated the release of drug in the simulated intestinal environment [45].

Ion-exchange Resin NCs

The synthesis of ion-exchange resin NCs involves the application of a resin (water-insoluble cross-linked polymer). However, this resin can be of either type (*i.e.*, cationic or anionic). The main intention to design this kind of NCs is to attain the sustained and controlled release of drugs through the system. As we require the release of drugs in the stomach environment, therefore, the cationic resin is preferred for the synthesis of the drug-resin complex (called resinates). When these resinates expose to hydrogen ions in the stomach, the hydrogen ions are replaced with the drug ions already existing in the resinate system [46 - 49].

Moreover, the release profile of the drug from resins entirely relies on the intrinsic qualities of the resins (*e.g.*, size of the particle, kind of ionogenic moiety, and cross-linking density). On the other hand, in the case of a drug, it relies on the nature of the active agents employed, testing solution, as well as ionic conditions [46]. For instance, if an ion exchange resin is extremely cross-linked, then the loading capacity of the drug is reduced [50, 51].

Floating NCs

Floating GRNCs can enhance sustained drug release by extending the GRT of the NCs. For the synthesis of floating NCs, normally low-density materials are selected [1, 10, 52, 53]. In this kind of NCs, the bulk density of the NCs should be less as compared to the density of the gastric fluid, which generally lets NCs stay buoyant in the gastric environment for an extended time, on the same time, it allows the drug to release at the prerequisite rate through NCs [1, 10, 54]. However, these NCs can be of non-effervescent or effervescent floating types.

Effervescent floating NCs usually consist of gas-generating substances (*e.g.*, sodium bicarbonate, calcium carbonate, citric acid, and tartaric acid) along with volatile liquids. These NCs when reacting with gastric fluid, they generate carbon dioxide owing to the interaction of these effervescent components with gastric contents [13]. In this approach, hydrophilic polymers are frequently employed to regulate the drug release profile. In a study, Tort *et al.* developed electrospun nanofiber membranes. This nanofiber was aimed at a self-inflating effervescence-based system, which was developed *via* incorporating polyethylene oxide/sodium bicarbonate. Further, Eudragit RL and RS were employed to control the release kinetics of pramipexole. Outcomes from floating nanofiber pouches revealed the poorer primary release of the drug (*i.e.*, 20-57%), over non-floating nanofiber pouches (*i.e.*, 40–82%) after 2 h study. Eventually, effervescent floating nanofibers proved to be potential GRNCs for the delivery of the drug especially in the upper GIT [34].

In contrast, in the case of non-effervescent NCs, gel-forming polymers or extremely swellable cellulose derivatives are employed. The development of non-effervescent NCs usually comprises amalgamation drugs with a gel-developing polymer. Several types of non-effervescent NCs have been reported, for instance, nano micelles, GR-beads, multiwalled carbon nanotubes (MWCNTs), hollow microspheres, gastric-floating pill (GFP), single- and double-layer floating microbaloons, hydrodynamically balanced system (HBS), *etc.* Several formulation constraints, for example, the nature of the solvent, the proportion of plasticizer as well as polymer, and quantity of polymer can have great influence not only on the floating behavior but also drug release from these NCs [55].

In an investigation, Chen *et al.* synthesized novel emodin-loaded nano micelles (ENM)-incorporated gastro retentive (GR) beads (ENM-beads). Cytotoxicity (*in vitro*) study on SGC-7901 cells revealed the potential of ENM and exhibited elevated antitumor activity over emodin suspensions. Further, GRT behavior (*in vivo*) of ENM-beads indicated elevated retaining behavior (8 h) in the rabbit stomach [31]. On the other hand, HBS is a single unit formulation that usually consists of one or more gel-developing hydrophilic polymers (*e.g.*, agar, HPMC, hydroxyethylcellulose, sodium carboxymethylcellulose, carrageenan, hydroxypropyl cellulose (HPC), alginic acid, *etc.*) [10, 56]. Besides, drug-incorporated microbaloons are also being developed by employing different polymers (*e.g.*, low-methoxylated pectin, polycarbonate, calcium alginate, agar, Eudragit S, cellulose acetate, *etc.*).

Zhang *et al.* synthesized levofloxacin-loaded multiwalled carbon nanotubes (MWCNTs) and coated them with liquid crystalline molecularly imprinted polymers (LC-MIP) (MWCNT@LC-MIP). Further, they were prepared by employing 9-vinyl anthracene to produce high-density modified MWCNTs. Afterward, its polymerization was carried out at the surface of MWCNTs *via* employing an amalgamation of 4-methyl phenyl dicyclohexyl ethylene, ethylene glycol dimethacrylate, and methacrylic acid. *In vitro* release study revealed a zero-order drug release through MWCNT@LC-MIP. Moreover, *in vivo* study from gastro-floating MWCNT@LC-MIP indicated nearly 578.9% relative bioavailability of drug over 11.7% for blank MWCNT and 58.0% for MWCNT@MIP [57]. Besides, a gastric-floating pill (GFP) incorporating dihydromyricetin drug was developed for obtaining sustained drug release effect. The outcome revealed a significant increase in the drug content along with elevated floating aptitude from GFP over conventional tablets. Furthermore, it remarkably extended GRT, elevated the bioavailability of the drug, and as well increased the anti-inflammatory response of the drug (*in vivo*) [58].

Magnetic NCs

Magnetic NCs are constructed by employing the internal core of the magnet along with drugs and excipients. To achieve the targeting effect, an extracorporeal magnet is usually positioned just over the stomach to regulate the correct position of the NCs (Fig. **7.5**) [10]. However, both the magnetic field strength as well as position of the extracorporeal magnet produces a significant effect on the GRT [59] and can improve GRT in the stomach. Further, they may enhance the efficacy of the drug. For instance, Jin *et al.* synthesized polyethyleneimine-based magnetic NCs for efficient delivery of siRNAs. In this regard, the authors tested these magnetic NCs against BCL2 and BIRC5 cancer cells. Outcomes suggested the substantial potential of siRNAs-loaded NCs with significant inhibition of cancer cells [60]. In another study, Boya *et al.* synthesized iron oxide NCs by employing β-cyclodextrin or pluronic 127, or both. Results revealed that they together immensely interacted and attached with mucin. In addition, they also transferred through mucin over other single magnetic NCs [61].

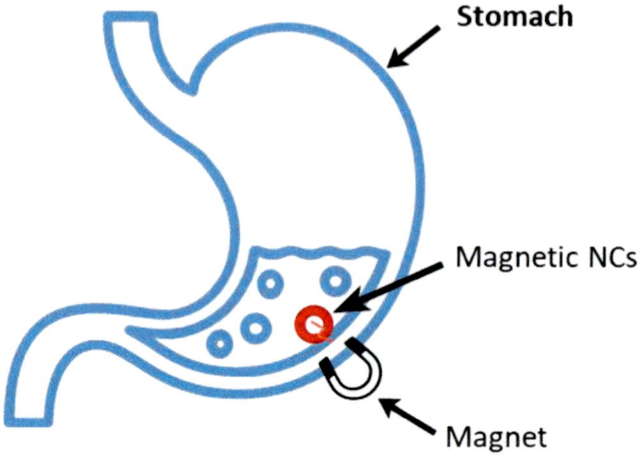

Fig. (7.5). Schematic depicting magnetic NCs for targeting effect in the stomach.

Further, ceftriaxone incorporated iron oxide magnetic NCs were also reported. Here, magnetic NCs were further modified with lactobionic acid and investigated for their potential. Thus, produced magnetic NCs exhibited promising effects for improving the oral delivery of a drug [9]. Recently, Zamani *et al.* reported magnetic NCs that were modified with gum arabic for attaining elevated oral delivery of Dunaliella salina extract. After investigation, findings revealed the high potency of these magnetic NCs for improved delivery of antioxidants [62].

Mucoadhesive NCs

In this approach, the NCs are usually developed by incorporating drugs along with a mucoadhesive (natural or synthetic) polymer. The mucoadhesion of NCs with the mucosal surface is supposed to establish by the formation of bonds amidst mucosal surface and NCs [63].

Several GI mucoadhesive NCs (*i.e.*, microbeads, microspheres, films, *etc.*) are being developed [64]. Some commonly employed mucoadhesive polymers are poly(acrylic acid), chitosan, carbopol, polyethylene glycol, sodium alginate, and HPMC [10, 41]. Mucoadhesive polymers along with drug materials normally help them in binding with the mucosal surfaces, which results in the prolongation of drug retention in the stomach. Moreover, a perfect mucoadhesive polymer should have some desired qualities like non-toxic, inert, adhering aptitude to the mucosal surface, non-irritating, and site-specificity. Further, they should adequately interact with the mucin *via* different bonding such as hydrogen, electrostatic, hydrophobic, and disulfide bonding [65].

The mucoadhesive property of polymers plays a vital role in the GRT of NCs. There are several examples of the application of mucoadhesive polymers in the development of GRNCs for augmenting the retention of drugs in gastric conditions. For instance, Sunoqrot *et al.* synthesized mussel-assisted polydopamine tailored NCs of methoxy polyethylene glycol-b-poly-ε-caprolactone). Further, they investigated the mucoadhesive property of NCs (*in vitro*) by employing mucin in the stomach environment. The interactions of mucin-NCs were confirmed using dynamic light scattering. Outcomes suggested noteworthy variation in the size distribution of NCs at different ratios of mucin and NCs (*i.e.*, 1:1, 1:2, and 1:4, w/w). Moreover, an ex vivo study on excised sheep stomachs indicated that nearly 78% of coated NCs were stayed attached with mucosa for 8 h over 33% of uncoated NCs [33]. In another investigation, a polysaccharide obtained from Bletilla striata was used for increasing the mucoadhesive property of the microspheres. For this purpose, the author's employed sodium alginate to synthesize microspheres to improve GRT. Finally, findings revealed discrete as well as the spherical attribute of microspheres. On the other hand, mucoadhesion results exhibited much longer retention of polysaccharide-containing microspheres than microspheres comprising only sodium alginate in the stomach [36].

Further, ofloxacin incorporated GR gastro retentive nanofibers of gellan/polyvinyl alcohol were developed for enhancing retention time, along with bioavailability of the drug in the stomach. The optimized nanofibers exhibited biphasic drug-release attribute along with substantial mucoadhesive property in the rat. Findings indicated the significant potential of GR nanofibers *via* oral delivery [35].

Diverse investigations have been performed by combining floating and mucoadhesive processes to augment the GRT of the NCs by forming mucoadhesive floating DDS [65 - 69]. In this regard, Liu *et al.* synthesized a psoralen-loaded hollow-bioadhesive microsphere. In this NC, they used glycerol monooleate as a mucoadhesive polymer. These NCs revealed potential mucoadhesive activity along with decent buoyancy (*in vitro* and *in vivo*).

Swelling NCs

Swelling DDS exhibits longer GRT due to enhance in volume or size. For the development of these formulations, normally three points are widely considered *viz.*, tiny size to enable easy intake *via* the oral route, swelling form to inhibit their movement in the stomach to cross the pyloric sphincter, and finally, the decrease in the size following the entire discharge of drug to ease the emptying [1, 41, 70].

However, swelling and unfolding are the two important mechanisms by which expansion of the system takes place [11, 70]. The swelling and release of the drug through formulation occur *via* the diffusion process. For this purpose, it requires the use of hydrophilic polymers (*e.g.*, HPMC, polyethylene oxide, and carbopol), which can not only absorb water in the gastric fluids but also enhance the size of the system. Similarly, in unfolding types, the polymer along with the drug remains in the folded or compressed form in the gelatin capsule. Eventually, the gelatin of the capsule gets dissolved when they expose to gastric fluid and discharge the drug [41]. However, it is important to choose an appropriate biodegradable polymer having some desired qualities like swelling properties, molecular weight, and viscosity grade to affirm sustained release characteristics of the formulation [41, 71].

Several novel polymers exhibit swelling properties when they come in contact with fluid in the GI. In this regard, Sivaneswari *et al.* synthesized novel levetiracetam-loaded unfolding GRNCs by using carbopol 934 P, HPMC, and xanthum gum. In this investigation, it was aimed to adhere to the gastric mucosa and then to release the drug for extended times [71]. Thomas *et al.* prepared rifampicin incorporated alginate NCs by employing the green technique. Swelling, as well as drug release (*in vitro*) investigations, suggested that the system obeyed not only pH-reliant swelling but also followed the pH-responsive release of the drug. Further, findings confirmed the lower release of drugs in an acid environment while higher release in the intestine. Moreover, *in vitro* cytotoxicity analysis also confirmed the non-toxic aptitude of NCs [72]. In a similar study, alginate-based nanocrystal-hybrid NCs were developed after incorporating rifampicin. The synthesized NCs also showed pH-reliant swelling as well as drug release patterns (*in vitro*). Moreover, an MTT assay was conducted for confirming the biocompatibility of the NCs, which revealed the non-toxic property of the NCs. Final results advocated elevated encapsulation efficacy as well as the sustained release of rifampicin owing to the incorporation of the cellulose nanocrystals in the NCs [73].

Stimuli-triggered layer-by-layer (LbL) microcapsules also show pH-reliant swelling properties owing to the alteration in the charge density accompanied by polyelectrolytes in terms of pH. Further, this prompts the electrostatic interactions amongst polyelectrolyte layers, which lead to changes in the permeability of these microcapsules [74]. For example, Mauser *et al.*, developed empty microcapsules using poly (methacrylic acid) and polyallylamine hydrochloride, which depicted a pH-dependent aptitude. In this investigation, microcapsules were able to reversibly swell or shrink in response to pH in a size range from 4 to 8 μm [75]. Hence, the LbL approach can be employed to adjust the size of NCs in nano-range to improve the properties of the product. For instance, stimuli-triggered multi-layered nanocapsules have been synthesized for delivery of curcumin by employing four polyelectrolytes *viz*., chitosan, poly-L-arginine, Eudragit L100, and sodium alginate. The findings revealed the potential of nanocapsules to guard the curcumin not only in the gastric condition but also encouraged the release of the drug in the lower GIT [76].

NC$_S$ FOR SUSTAINED EFFECT OF DRUG IN GIT

Lipid NCs

Lipids NCs can be employed for attaining not only sustained release of the drug but also to protect the drug from gastric harsh conditions [77, 78]. In this regard, Lopes-de-Campos *et al*. loaded amoxicillin in the lipid NCs to improve the GRT at the site of interest (*i.e*., infection in the gastric mucosa). Further, this guarded drug from the adverse environment of the stomach. The outcome indicated good stability of lipid NCs (~6 months) at 4°C. On the other hand, *in vitro* investigations advocated low cytotoxicity response against gastric cell lines including fibroblast [79]. Besides, lipid NCs loading oxaliplatin and irinotecan were developed [80, 81] and further incorporated into the alginate microbeads for protecting them from harsh conditions of the stomach. Further, these microbeads following oral delivery exhibited promising results in the treatment of colorectal cancer [82, 83].

In another investigation, Zhang *et al*. produced triptolide incorporated lipid NCs with decreased gastric irritation. The developed NCs exhibited sustained release of the drug (*in vitro*) with appreciable stability for 3 h in the simulated gastric environment [84]. Ofloxacin-containing lipid NCs also supported sustained-release effects along with the elevated antibacterial response (*in vitro*). Further, pharmacokinetic findings indicated increased bioavailability of the drug (2.27-times), as well prolonged residence time of the ofloxacin [85].

Polymeric NCs

Gastro-responsive polymeric NCs have been widely explored for their GRT effect [86 - 89]. For instance, Betala *et al*. have synthesized NCs after incorporating carvedilol *via* employing diverse hydrophilic polymers (*e.g*., HPMC K100M, chitosan, and gelatin). Moreover, chitosan-based NCs exhibited promising results when examined for various parameters like particle size (312 nm), polydispersity index (0.681), zeta potential (33.2 mV), and loading and entrapment efficiency (17.54% and 73.4%, respectively) [30].

In another study, GI-responsive polymeric NCs of HPMC phthalate was developed by employing the emulsification solvent diffusion technique. the NCs were developed for elevated efficiency of insulin through the oral route. Outcomes for drug release (*in vitro*) study indicated a constant enhancement in the release of drugs from NCs while the pH of the medium was steadily enhanced from 3.0 to 7.4. Further, enzyme resistance investigation revealed improved drug protection (>60%) under a simulated GI environment. Moreover, an oral hypoglycemic study exhibited the potential of insulin-entrapped NCs for a significant decrease in the blood sugar level in diabetic rats. Further, *ex vivo* imaging using rat tissues revealed enhanced absorption of insulin in both sites (*i.e.*, ileum and colon) [90]. Intending to enhance the oral absorption and bioavailability of drugs (*i.e.*, doxorubicin), the authors have developed PEGylated-poly-lactic-co-glycolic acid NCs. Findings indicated a significant elevation in the bioavailability (6.8-times) from drug-loaded NCs over drug solution [91].

CONCLUSIONS

GRNCs have shown immense aptitude in the delivery of drug agents, which are unstable in basic pH. GRNCs enhance the therapeutic efficiency of drugs not only by elevating their stay time in the stomach but also by increasing the solubility of drugs in the gastric environment. They can be the best carrier systems for loading poor absorption window drugs. Further, the augmented drug delivery effect of GRNCs can be attained by a thorough understanding of gastric conditions and their impacts on drug delivery systems, and the development of formulations by applying quality by design (QbD) approaches. In addition, the QbD approach can be efficiently employed to increase understanding of the influence of process variables and their impact on product functioning. Several types of GRNCs (*e.g.*, low/high-density GRNCs, magnetic GRNCs, mucoadhesive GRNCs, *etc.*) are under investigation to improve the bioavailability of drugs and enhance maximum utilization of drugs. However, they still require thorough clinical investigations to be understood.

CONSENT FOR PUBLICATION

Not applicable.

CONFLICT OF INTEREST

The authors declare no conflict of interest, financial or otherwise.

ACKNOWLEDGEMENT

Declared none.

REFERENCES

[1] Lopes CM, Bettencourt C, Rossi A, Buttini F, Barata P. Overview on gastroretentive drug delivery systems for improving drug bioavailability. Int J Pharm 2016; 510(1): 144-58. [http://dx.doi.org/10.1016/j.ijpharm.2016.05.016] [PMID: 27173823]

[2] Rajpoot K, Jain SK. The role of nanoparticles in the treatment of gastric cancer. In: Yadav AK, Gupta U, Sharma R, Eds. Nano Drug Delivery Strategies for the Treatment of Cancers. Academic Press 2021; pp. 165-89. [http://dx.doi.org/10.1016/B978-0-12-819793-6.00008-4]

[3] Jain SK, Jain AK, Rajpoot K. Expedition of Eudragit® polymers in the development of novel drug delivery systems. Curr Drug Deliv 2020; 17(6): 448-69. [http://dx.doi.org/10.2174/1567201817666200512093639] [PMID: 32394836]

[4] Rouge N, Buri P, Doelker E. Drug absorption sites in the gastrointestinal tract and dosage forms for site-specific delivery. Int J Pharm 1996; 136(1-2): 117-39. [http://dx.doi.org/10.1016/0378-5173(96)85200-8]

[5] Cisneros-Covarrubias CA, Gómez-Durán CFA, Aguirre-Bañuelos P, Hernández-Esquivel RA, Palestino G. Tramadol extended-release porous silicon microcarriers: A kinetic, physicochemical and biological evaluation. J Drug Deliv Sci Technol 2022; 69: 103132. [http://dx.doi.org/10.1016/j.jddst.2022.103132]

[6] Juthi AZ, Wang B. Super porous hydrogel: A promising gastroretentive drug delivery system. World J Pharm Pharm Sci 2017; 6(5): 129-59.

[7] Souza MPC, Sábio RM, Ribeiro TC, Santos AM, Meneguin AB, Chorilli M. Highlighting the impact of chitosan on the development of gastroretentive drug delivery systems. Int J Biol Macromol 2020; 159: 804-22. [http://dx.doi.org/10.1016/j.ijbiomac.2020.05.104]

[8] Hanif M, Shah S, Rasul A, *et al.* Enhancement of oral bioavailability of ibandronate through gastroretentive raft forming drug delivery system: *In vitro* and *in vivo* evaluation. Int J Nanomedicine 2020; 15: 4847-58. [http://dx.doi.org/10.2147/IJN.S255278] [PMID: 32764922]

[9] Kawish M, Jabri T, Elhissi A, *et al.* Galactosylated iron oxide nanoparticles for enhancing oral bioavailability of ceftriaxone. Pharm Dev Technol 2021; 26(3): 291-301. [http://dx.doi.org/10.1080/10837450.2020.1866602] [PMID: 33475034]

[10] Prajapati VD, Jani GK, Khutliwala TA, Zala BS. Raft forming system—An upcoming approach of gastroretentive drug delivery system. J Control Release 2013; 168(2): 151-65. [http://dx.doi.org/10.1016/j.jconrel.2013.02.028] [PMID: 23500062]

[11] Mandal UK, Chatterjee B, Senjoti FG. Gastro-retentive drug delivery systems and their *in vivo* success: A recent update. Asian Journal of Pharmaceutical Sciences 2016; 11(5): 575-84. [http://dx.doi.org/10.1016/j.ajps.2016.04.007]

[12] Prinderre P, Sauzet C, Fuxen C. Advances in gastro retentive drug-delivery systems. Expert Opin Drug Deliv 2011; 8(9): 1189-203. [http://dx.doi.org/10.1517/17425247.2011.592828] [PMID: 21671821]

[13] Talukder R, Fassihi R. Gastroretentive delivery systems: A mini review. Drug Dev Ind Pharm 2004; 30(10): 1019-28. [http://dx.doi.org/10.1081/DDC-200040239] [PMID: 15595568]

[14] Streubel A, Siepmann J, Bodmeier R. Drug delivery to the upper small intestine window using gastroretentive technologies. Curr Opin Pharmacol 2006; 6(5): 501-8.
[http://dx.doi.org/10.1016/j.coph.2006.04.007] [PMID: 16890020]

[15] Arora S, Ali J, Ahuja A, Khar RK, Baboota S. Floating drug delivery systems: A review. AAPS PharmSciTech 2005; 6(3): E372-90.
[http://dx.doi.org/10.1208/pt060347] [PMID: 16353995]

[16] Calbet JA, MacLean DA. Role of caloric content on gastric emptying in humans. J Physiol 1997; 498((Pt 2)): 553-9.

[17] Juvonen KR, Purhonen AK, Salmenkallio-Marttila M, *et al.* Viscosity of oat bran-enriched beverages influences gastrointestinal hormonal responses in healthy humans. J Nutr 2009; 139(3): 461-6.
[http://dx.doi.org/10.3945/jn.108.099945] [PMID: 19176745]

[18] Zhu Y, Hsu WH, Hollis JH. The impact of food viscosity on eating rate, subjective appetite, glycemic response and gastric emptying rate. PLoS One 2013; 8(6): e67482.
[http://dx.doi.org/10.1371/journal.pone.0067482] [PMID: 23818981]

[19] Garg R, Gupta GD. Progress in controlled gastroretentive delivery systems. Trop J Pharm Res 2008; 7(3): 1055-66.
[http://dx.doi.org/10.4314/tjpr.v7i3.14691]

[20] Nguyen NQ, Debreceni TL, Burgstad CM, *et al.* Effects of posture and meal volume on gastric emptying, intestinal transit, oral glucose tolerance, blood pressure and gastrointestinal symptoms after Roux-en-Y gastric bypass. Obes Surg 2015; 25(8): 1392-400.
[http://dx.doi.org/10.1007/s11695-014-1531-4] [PMID: 25502436]

[21] Wang YT, Mohammed SD, Farmer AD, *et al.* Regional gastrointestinal transit and pH studied in 215 healthy volunteers using the wireless motility capsule: Influence of age, gender, study country and testing protocol. Aliment Pharmacol Ther 2015; 42(6): 761-72.
[http://dx.doi.org/10.1111/apt.13329] [PMID: 26223837]

[22] Feldman M, Barnett C. Fasting gastric pH and its relationship to true hypochlorhydria in humans. Dig Dis Sci 1991; 36(7): 866-9.
[http://dx.doi.org/10.1007/BF01297133] [PMID: 2070698]

[23] Mojaverian P, Vlasses PH, Kellner PE, Rocci ML Jr. Effects of gender, posture, and age on gastric residence time of an indigestible solid: Pharmaceutical considerations. Pharm Res 1988; 5(10): 639-44.
[http://dx.doi.org/10.1023/A:1015922903843] [PMID: 3244616]

[24] Krygowska-Wajs A, Cheshire WP Jr, Wszolek ZK, *et al.* Evaluation of gastric emptying in familial and sporadic Parkinson disease. Parkinsonism Relat Disord 2009; 15(9): 692-6.
[http://dx.doi.org/10.1016/j.parkreldis.2009.04.003] [PMID: 19451015]

[25] Triantafyllou K, Kalantzis C, Papadopoulos AA, *et al.* Video-capsule endoscopy gastric and small bowel transit time and completeness of the examination in patients with diabetes mellitus. Dig Liver Dis 2007; 39(6): 575-80.
[http://dx.doi.org/10.1016/j.dld.2007.01.024] [PMID: 17433797]

[26] Timmermans J, Moës AJ. How well do floating dosage forms float? Int J Pharm 1990; 62(2-3): 207-16.
[http://dx.doi.org/10.1016/0378-5173(90)90234-U]

[27] Chauhan MS, Kumar A, Pathak K. Osmotically regulated floating asymmetric membrane capsule for controlled site-specific delivery of ranitidine hydrochloride: Optimization by central composite design. AAPS PharmSciTech 2012; 13(4): 1492-501.
[http://dx.doi.org/10.1208/s12249-012-9870-8] [PMID: 23104305]

[28] Ali J, Arora S, Ahuja A, *et al.* Formulation and development of hydrodynamically balanced system for metformin: *In vitro* and *in vivo* evaluation. Eur J Pharm Biopharm 2007; 67(1): 196-201.

[http://dx.doi.org/10.1016/j.ejpb.2006.12.015] [PMID: 17270409]

[29] Clarke GM, Newton JM, Short MD. Gastrointestinal transit of pellets of differing size and density. Int J Pharm 1993; 100(1-3): 81-92.
[http://dx.doi.org/10.1016/0378-5173(93)90078-T]

[30] Betala S, Mohan Varma M, Abbulu K. Formulation and evaluation of polymeric nanoparticles of an antihypetensive drug for gastroretention. J Drug Deliv Ther 2018; 8(6): 82-6.
[http://dx.doi.org/10.22270/jddt.v8i6.2018]

[31] Chen N, Niu J, Li Q, *et al.* Development and evaluation of a new gastroretentive drug delivery system: Nanomicelles-loaded floating mucoadhesive beads. J Drug Deliv Sci Technol 2019; 51: 485-92.
[http://dx.doi.org/10.1016/j.jddst.2019.03.024]

[32] Sarparanta MP, Bimbo LM, Mäkilä EM, *et al.* The mucoadhesive and gastroretentive properties of hydrophobin-coated porous silicon nanoparticle oral drug delivery systems. Biomaterials 2012; 33(11): 3353-62.
[http://dx.doi.org/10.1016/j.biomaterials.2012.01.029] [PMID: 22285465]

[33] Sunoqrot S, Hasan L, Alsadi A, Hamed R, Tarawneh O. Interactions of mussel-inspired polymeric nanoparticles with gastric mucin: Implications for gastro-retentive drug delivery. Colloids Surf B Biointerfaces 2017; 156: 1-8.
[http://dx.doi.org/10.1016/j.colsurfb.2017.05.005] [PMID: 28499200]

[34] Tort S, Han D, Steckl AJ. Self-inflating floating nanofiber membranes for controlled drug delivery. Int J Pharm 2020; 579: 119164.
[http://dx.doi.org/10.1016/j.ijpharm.2020.119164] [PMID: 32081796]

[35] Vashisth P, Raghuwanshi N, Srivastava AK, Singh H, Nagar H, Pruthi V. Ofloxacin loaded gellan/PVA nanofibers - Synthesis, characterization and evaluation of their gastroretentive/ mucoadhesive drug delivery potential. Mater Sci Eng C 2017; 71: 611-9.
[http://dx.doi.org/10.1016/j.msec.2016.10.051] [PMID: 27987752]

[36] Wu Y, Zhang W, Huang J, *et al.* Mucoadhesive improvement of alginate microspheres as potential gastroretentive delivery carrier by blending with Bletilla striata polysaccharide. Int J Biol Macromol 2020; 156: 1191-201.
[http://dx.doi.org/10.1016/j.ijbiomac.2019.11.156] [PMID: 31756485]

[37] Zamani M, Rostami M, Aghajanzadeh M, Kheiri Manjili H, Rostamizadeh K, Danafar H. Mesoporous titanium dioxide@ zinc oxide–graphene oxide nanocarriers for colon-specific drug delivery. JMatS 2017; 53(3): 1634-45.

[38] Nasr R, Hasanzadeh H, Khaleghian A, Moshtaghian A, Emadi A, Moshfegh S. Induction of apoptosis and inhibition of invasion in gastric cancer cells by titanium dioxide nanoparticles. Oman Med J 2018; 33(2): 111-7.
[http://dx.doi.org/10.5001/omj.2018.22] [PMID: 29657679]

[39] Jarosz M, Pawlik A, Szuwarzyński M, Jaskuła M, Sulka GD. Nanoporous anodic titanium dioxide layers as potential drug delivery systems: Drug release kinetics and mechanism. Colloids Surf B Biointerfaces 2016; 143: 447-54.
[http://dx.doi.org/10.1016/j.colsurfb.2016.03.073] [PMID: 27037782]

[40] Omidian H, Rocca JG, Park K. Advances in superporous hydrogels. J Control Release 2005; 102(1): 3-12.
[http://dx.doi.org/10.1016/j.jconrel.2004.09.028] [PMID: 15653129]

[41] Bardonnet PL, Faivre V, Pugh WJ, Piffaretti JC, Falson F. Gastroretentive dosage forms: Overview and special case of Helicobacter pylori. J Control Release 2006; 111(1-2): 1-18.
[http://dx.doi.org/10.1016/j.jconrel.2005.10.031] [PMID: 16403588]

[42] Bhalla S, Nagpal M. Comparison of various generations of superporous hydrogels based on chitosan-acrylamide and *in vitro* drug release. ISRN Pharm 2013; 2013: 1-8.

[http://dx.doi.org/10.1155/2013/624841] [PMID: 23984106]

[43] Lee CH, Lo LW, Mou CY, Yang CS. Synthesis and characterization of positive-charge functionalized mesoporous silica nanoparticles for oral drug delivery of an anti-inflammatory drug. Adv Funct Mater 2008; 18(20): 3283-92.
[http://dx.doi.org/10.1002/adfm.200800521]

[44] Shrestha N, Araújo F, Shahbazi MA, *et al.* Thiolation and cell-penetrating peptide surface functionalization of porous silicon nanoparticles for oral delivery of insulin. Adv Funct Mater 2016; 26(20): 3405-16.
[http://dx.doi.org/10.1002/adfm.201505252]

[45] Juère E, Caillard R, Kleitz F. Pore confinement and surface charge effects in protein-mesoporous silica nanoparticles formulation for oral drug delivery. Microporous Mesoporous Mater 2020; 306: 110482.
[http://dx.doi.org/10.1016/j.micromeso.2020.110482]

[46] Gaur PK, Mishra S, Bhardwaj S, Puri D, Kumar SS. Ion exchange resins in gastroretentive drug delivery: Characteristics, selection, formulation and applications. J Pharm Sci Pharmacol 2014; 1(4): 304-12.
[http://dx.doi.org/10.1166/jpsp.2014.1037]

[47] Jain SK, Kumar A, Kumar A, Pandey AN, Rajpoot K. Development and *in vitro* characterization of a multiparticulate delivery system for acyclovir-resinate complex. Artif Cells Nanomed Biotechnol 2016; 44(5): 1266-75.
[http://dx.doi.org/10.3109/21691401.2015.1024841] [PMID: 25813568]

[48] Jain SK, Prajapati N, Rajpoot K, Kumar A. A novel sustained release drug–resin complex-based microbeads of ciprofloxacin HCl. Artif Cells Nanomed Biotechnol 2016; 44(8): 1891-900.
[http://dx.doi.org/10.3109/21691401.2015.1111233] [PMID: 26698089]

[49] Nayak D, Rajpoot K, Jain SK. Development and evaluation of cholestyramine-amoxicillin trihydrate-loaded gastro-retentive microspheres for attaining extended therapeutic effect against H. Pylori infection. Biomed J Sci Tech Res 2020; 29(4): 22728-38.

[50] Jeong SH, Berhane NH, Haghighi K, Park K. Drug release properties of polymer coated ion-exchange resin complexes: Experimental and theoretical evaluation. J Pharm Sci 2007; 96(3): 618-32.
[http://dx.doi.org/10.1002/jps.20677] [PMID: 17080409]

[51] Jeong SH, Park K. Drug loading and release properties of ion-exchange resin complexes as a drug delivery matrix. Int J Pharm 2008; 361(1-2): 26-32.
[http://dx.doi.org/10.1016/j.ijpharm.2008.05.006] [PMID: 18565701]

[52] Choi BY, Park HJ, Hwang SJ, Park JB. Preparation of alginate beads for floating drug delivery system: Effects of CO_2 gas-forming agents. Int J Pharm 2002; 239(1-2): 81-91.
[http://dx.doi.org/10.1016/S0378-5173(02)00054-6] [PMID: 12052693]

[53] Patrey NK, Rajpoot K, Jain AK, Jain SK. Diltiazem loaded floating microspheres of Ethylcellulose and Eudragit for gastric delivery: *In vitro* evaluation. AJBR 2016; 2(2): 71-7.

[54] Rossi A, Conti C, Colombo G, *et al.* Floating modular drug delivery systems with buoyancy independent of release mechanisms to sustain amoxicillin and clarithromycin intra-gastric concentrations. Drug Dev Ind Pharm 2016; 42(2): 332-9.
[http://dx.doi.org/10.3109/03639045.2015.1054397] [PMID: 26065531]

[55] Kawashima Y, Niwa T, Takeuchi H, Hino T, Itoh Y. Hollow microspheres for use as a floating controlled drug delivery system in the stomach. J Pharm Sci 1992; 81(2): 135-40.
[http://dx.doi.org/10.1002/jps.2600810207] [PMID: 1372046]

[56] Reddy LHV, Murthy RSR. Floating dosage systems in drug delivery. Crit Rev Ther Drug Carrier Syst 2002; 19(6): 553-85.
[http://dx.doi.org/10.1615/CritRevTherDrugCarrierSyst.v19.i6.20] [PMID: 12822735]

[57] Zhang LP, Tan XX, Huang YP, Liu ZS. Floating liquid crystalline molecularly imprinted polymer

coated carbon nanotubes for levofloxacin delivery. Eur J Pharm Biopharm 2018; 127: 150-8. [http://dx.doi.org/10.1016/j.ejpb.2018.02.012] [PMID: 29438726]

[58] Liu H, Gan C, Shi H, *et al.* Gastric floating pill enhances the bioavailability and drug efficacy of dihydromyricetin *in vivo*. J Drug Deliv Sci Technol 2021; 61: 102279. [http://dx.doi.org/10.1016/j.jddst.2020.102279]

[59] Awasthi R, Kulkarni GT. Decades of research in drug targeting to the upper gastrointestinal tract using gastroretention technologies: Where do we stand? Drug Deliv 2016; 23(2): 378-94. [http://dx.doi.org/10.3109/10717544.2014.936535] [PMID: 25026414]

[60] Jin L, Wang Q, Chen J, Wang Z, Xin H, Zhang D. Efficient delivery of therapeutic siRNA by Fe_3O_4 magnetic nanoparticles into oral cancer cells. Pharmaceutics 2019; 11(11): 615. [http://dx.doi.org/10.3390/pharmaceutics11110615] [PMID: 31744202]

[61] Boya VN, Lovett R, Setua S, *et al.* Probing mucin interaction behavior of magnetic nanoparticles. J Colloid Interface Sci 2017; 488: 258-68. [http://dx.doi.org/10.1016/j.jcis.2016.10.090] [PMID: 27837716]

[62] Zamani H, Rastegari B, Varamini M. Antioxidant and anti-cancer activity of Dunaliella salina extract and oral drug delivery potential *via* nano-based formulations of gum Arabic coated magnetite nanoparticles. J Drug Deliv Sci Technol 2019; 54: 101278. [http://dx.doi.org/10.1016/j.jddst.2019.101278]

[63] Smart J. The basics and underlying mechanisms of mucoadhesion. Adv Drug Deliv Rev 2005; 57(11): 1556-68. [http://dx.doi.org/10.1016/j.addr.2005.07.001] [PMID: 16198441]

[64] Patil H, Tiwari RV, Repka MA. Recent advancements in mucoadhesive floating drug delivery systems: A mini-review. J Drug Deliv Sci Technol 2016; 31: 65-71. [http://dx.doi.org/10.1016/j.jddst.2015.12.002]

[65] Shtenberg Y, Goldfeder M, Prinz H, *et al.* Mucoadhesive alginate pastes with embedded liposomes for local oral drug delivery. Int J Biol Macromol 2018; 111: 62-9. [http://dx.doi.org/10.1016/j.ijbiomac.2017.12.137] [PMID: 29292143]

[66] Chen YC, Ho HO, Lee TY, Sheu MT. Physical characterizations and sustained release profiling of gastroretentive drug delivery systems with improved floating and swelling capabilities. Int J Pharm 2013; 441(1-2): 162-9. [http://dx.doi.org/10.1016/j.ijpharm.2012.12.002] [PMID: 23237874]

[67] Dey SK, De PK, De A, *et al.* Floating mucoadhesive alginate beads of amoxicillin trihydrate: A facile approach for H. pylori eradication. Int J Biol Macromol 2016; 89: 622-31. [http://dx.doi.org/10.1016/j.ijbiomac.2016.05.027] [PMID: 27177460]

[68] Darandale SS, Vavia PR. Design of a gastroretentive mucoadhesive dosage form of furosemide for controlled release. Acta Pharm Sin B 2012; 2(5): 509-17. [http://dx.doi.org/10.1016/j.apsb.2012.05.004]

[69] Bera H, Kandukuri SG, Nayak AK, Boddupalli S. Alginate–sterculia gum gel-coated oil-entrapped alginate beads for gastroretentive risperidone delivery. Carbohydr Polym 2015; 120: 74-84. [http://dx.doi.org/10.1016/j.carbpol.2014.12.009] [PMID: 25662690]

[70] Klausner EA, Lavy E, Friedman M, Hoffman A. Expandable gastroretentive dosage forms. J Control Release 2003; 90(2): 143-62. [http://dx.doi.org/10.1016/S0168-3659(03)00203-7] [PMID: 12810298]

[71] Sivaneswari S, Karthikeyan E, Chandana PJ. Novel expandable gastro retentive system by unfolding mechanism of levetiracetam using simple lattice design – Formulation optimization and *in vitro* evaluation. Bull Fac Pharm Cairo Univ 2017; 55(1): 63-72. [http://dx.doi.org/10.1016/j.bfopcu.2017.02.003]

[72] Thomas D, KurienThomas K, Latha MS. Preparation and evaluation of alginate nanoparticles prepared

by green method for drug delivery applications. Int J Biol Macromol 2020; 154: 888-95.
[http://dx.doi.org/10.1016/j.ijbiomac.2020.03.167] [PMID: 32209372]

[73] Thomas D, Latha MS, Thomas KK. Synthesis and *in vitro* evaluation of alginate-cellulose nanocrystal hybrid nanoparticles for the controlled oral delivery of rifampicin. J Drug Deliv Sci Technol 2018; 46: 392-9.
[http://dx.doi.org/10.1016/j.jddst.2018.06.004]

[74] Wohl BM, Engbersen JFJ. Responsive layer-by-layer materials for drug delivery. J Control Release 2012; 158(1): 2-14.
[http://dx.doi.org/10.1016/j.jconrel.2011.08.035] [PMID: 21925219]

[75] Mauser T, Déjugnat C, Möhwald H, Sukhorukov GB. Microcapsules made of weak polyelectrolytes: Templating and stimuli-responsive properties. Langmuir 2006; 22(13): 5888-93.
[http://dx.doi.org/10.1021/la060088f] [PMID: 16768525]

[76] Elbaz NM, Owen A, Rannard S, McDonald TO. Controlled synthesis of calcium carbonate nanoparticles and stimuli-responsive multi-layered nanocapsules for oral drug delivery. Int J Pharm 2020; 574: 118866.
[http://dx.doi.org/10.1016/j.ijpharm.2019.118866] [PMID: 31765776]

[77] Rajpoot K. Lipid-based nanoplatforms in cancer therapy: Recent advances and applications. Curr Cancer Drug Targets 2020; 20(4): 271-87.
[http://dx.doi.org/10.2174/1568009620666200115160805] [PMID: 31951180]

[78] Rajpoot K. Solid lipid nanoparticles: A promising nanomaterial in drug delivery. Curr Pharm Des 2019; 25(37): 3943-59.
[http://dx.doi.org/10.2174/1381612825666190903155321] [PMID: 31481000]

[79] Lopes-de-Campos D, Pinto RM, Lima SAC, *et al.* Delivering amoxicillin at the infection site - a rational design through lipid nanoparticles. Int J Nanomedicine 2019; 14: 2781-95.
[http://dx.doi.org/10.2147/IJN.S193992] [PMID: 31114195]

[80] Rajpoot K, Jain SK. Colorectal cancer-targeted delivery of oxaliplatin *via* folic acid-grafted solid lipid nanoparticles: Preparation, optimization, and *in vitro* evaluation. Artif Cells Nanomed Biotechnol 2018; 46(6): 1236-47.
[http://dx.doi.org/10.1080/21691401.2017.1366338] [PMID: 28849671]

[81] Rajpoot K, Jain SK. Irinotecan hydrochloride trihydrate loaded folic acid-tailored solid lipid nanoparticles for targeting colorectal cancer: Development, characterization, and *in vitro* cytotoxicity study using HT-29 cells. J Microencapsul 2019; 36(7): 659-76.
[http://dx.doi.org/10.1080/02652048.2019.1665723] [PMID: 31495238]

[82] Rajpoot K, Jain SK. ^{99m} Tc-labelled and pH-awakened microbeads entrapping surface-modified lipid nanoparticles for the augmented effect of oxaliplatin in the therapy of colorectal cancer. J Microencapsul 2020; 37(8): 609-23.
[http://dx.doi.org/10.1080/02652048.2020.1829141] [PMID: 32985297]

[83] Rajpoot K, Jain SK. Oral delivery of pH-responsive alginate microbeads incorporating folic acid-grafted solid lipid nanoparticles exhibits enhanced targeting effect against colorectal cancer: A dual-targeted approach. Int J Biol Macromol 2020; 151: 830-44.
[http://dx.doi.org/10.1016/j.ijbiomac.2020.02.132] [PMID: 32061847]

[84] Zhang C, Gu C, Peng F, *et al.* Preparation and optimization of triptolide-loaded solid lipid nanoparticles for oral delivery with reduced gastric irritation. Molecules 2013; 18(11): 13340-56.
[http://dx.doi.org/10.3390/molecules181113340] [PMID: 24172242]

[85] Xie S, Zhu L, Dong Z, Wang Y, Wang X, Zhou W. Preparation and evaluation of ofloxacin-loaded palmitic acid solid lipid nanoparticles. Int J Nanomedicine 2011; 6: 547-55.
[PMID: 21468357]

[86] Pandey AN, Rajpoot K, Jain SK. 5-Fluorouracil loaded orally administered wga-decorated

poly(lacticco- glycolic acid) nanoparticles for treatment of colorectal cancer: *In vivo* evaluation. Curr Nanomed 2021; 11(1): 51-60.
[http://dx.doi.org/10.2174/2468187310999201123195233]

[87] Pandey AN, Rajpoot K, Jain SK. Using 5-fluorouracil-encored PLGA nanoparticles for the treatment of colorectal cancer: The *in-vitro* characterization and cytotoxicity studies. Nanomed J 2020; 7(3): 211-24.

[88] Jain SK, Patel K, Rajpoot K, Jain A. Development of a berberine loaded multifunctional design for the treatment of Helicobacter pylori induced gastric ulcer. Drug Deliv Lett 2019; 9(1): 50-7.
[http://dx.doi.org/10.2174/2210303108666181120110756]

[89] Jain SK, Dubey V, Rajpoot K. D-mannose-decorated chitosan nanoparticles for enhanced targeting of 5-fluorouracil in the therapy of colon cancer. International Journal of Pharmaceutical Sciences and Nanotechnology 2021; 14(1): 5315-22.
[http://dx.doi.org/10.37285/ijpsn.2021.14.1.7]

[90] Fang Y, Wang Q, Lin X, *et al.* Gastrointestinal responsive polymeric nanoparticles for oral delivery of insulin: Optimized preparation, characterization, and *in vivo* evaluation. J Pharm Sci 2019; 108(9): 2994-3002.
[http://dx.doi.org/10.1016/j.xphs.2019.04.020] [PMID: 31047941]

[91] Ahmad N, Ahmad R, Alam MA, Ahmad FJ. Enhancement of oral bioavailability of doxorubicin through surface modified biodegradable polymeric nanoparticles. Chem Cent J 2018; 12(1): 65.
[http://dx.doi.org/10.1186/s13065-018-0434-1] [PMID: 29796830]

CHAPTER 8

Nanocarrier-based Targeted Delivery in Cancer

Shyam S. Pancholi[1,*], **Aseem Setia**[2], **Manu Singhai**[2] and **Atul Chaudhary**[2]

[1] *Shree S.K. Patel College of Pharmaceutical Education and Research, Ganpat University, 384012, Mahesana, Gujarat, India*

[2] *Department of Pharmaceutics, ISF College of Pharmacy, Moga, Punjab, 142001, India*

Abstract: Anticancer agents are known for their cytotoxic action against tumors, but the spread of their activity to noncancerous tissue is highly undesirable and may be toxic. The conventional methods of drug delivery pose numerous restrictions, involving side effects, lack of patient compliance, *etc.* Nanocarrier-based drug delivery alternatives offer the potential for the management of cancer, as they not only confer better delivery but also efficient targeting to the tissues with limited toxicity. Nanoparticles offer localization in tumors in the vicinity of capillaries, that accounts for improved penetration and prolonged detainment of drug in tumors. Under the tremendous potential of nanoparticles. The exploitation of multi-functional nanocarrier approaches is a burgeoning research subject, driven by increasing medical needs in the area of cancer therapy. Several nano-formulation have been approved for the treatment of cancer. This chapter is an attempt to provide an overview of the recent developments in nanoparticle formulations for cancer treatment and presents a comprehensive outlook of the clinical studies and utilization in different prevalent cancers affecting the brain, lung, breast, colon, cervix, and prostate, *etc.*

Keywords: Brain, Breast, Cancer, Cervical, Chemotherapeutic agents, Colon, Nanocarriers, Lung, Localized delivery, Prostate.

INTRODUCTION

Cancer is a disorder in which aberrant cells proliferate uncontrollably and it remains the most deadly ailment humanity is suffering from [1], accounting for one out of every six fatalities globally [2]. The latest data published in 2020 shows that 10 million people suffer from malignancies of various forms as shown in Fig. **(8.1)** the breast cancer tops the tally followed by prostate (**https://gco.iarc.fr/**). Low- and middle-income countries account for over 70% of deaths (WHO). Cancerous cell properties that make them challenging to deal with

* **Corresponding author S.S. Pancholi:** Shree S.K. Patel College of Pharmaceutical Education and Research, Ganpat University, 384012, Mahesana, Gujarat, India; Tel: 7023459497; E-mail: **sspancholi@gmail.com**

Akhlesh K. Jain & Keerti Mishra (Eds.)

include–uncontrolled, limitless replication potential, angiogenesis stimulation,and resistance to cell death with the ability to elude growth suppressors, and invasive metastasis, *etc.* This allows them to enter far-flung locations and cause cancer in areas other than the primary ones [3].

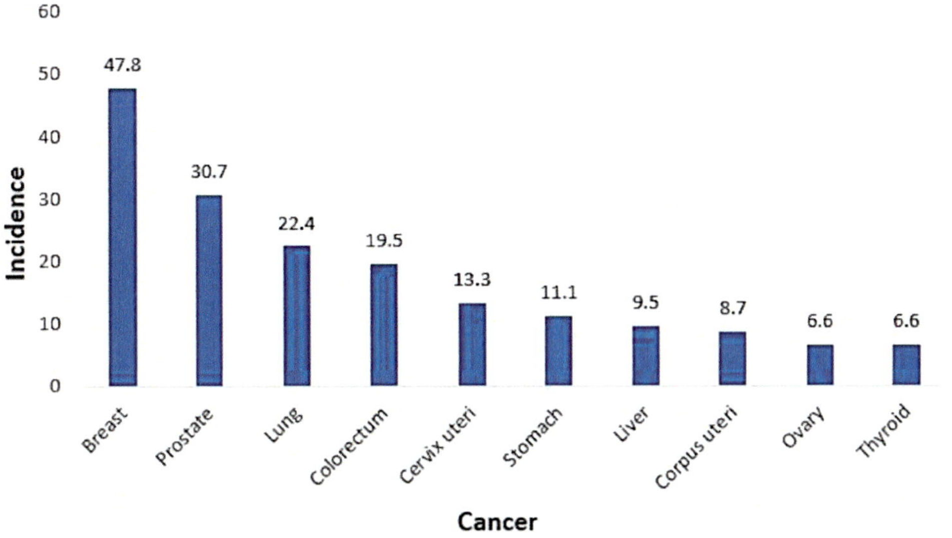

Fig. (8.1). Estimated cancer incidences in 2020. (Source: https://www.gco.iarc.fa/).

Chemotherapy remains the most effective cancer treatment approach though associated with several limitations of delivery and toxic effects. Chemotherapeutic agents are intended to eliminate the malfunctioning of cancer cells while causing no harm to healthy cells in the body [4]. Nano-pharmaceuticals have several advantages over traditional medicines, including superior targeting capabilities with high precision, as well as improved stability and sustainability in the target areas [5]. The exploitation of multi-functional nanocarrier approaches is a burgeoning research subject, driven by increasing medical needs. Several nano-formulation have been approved recently by USFDA as summarized in Table **8.1**. Nanocarriers technology has been adapted not just to deliver pharmaceuticals to target sites but also in diagnostics and drug monitoring throughout cancer treatment [6] for example image-guided drug delivery involves monitoring biodistribution, circulation, and targeting behavior of drug nanoparticles using magnetic resonance imaging (MRI) [7]. This chapter deals with available information regarding various nanocarrier systems, and their site-specific utilization for the treatment of various cancers. We have also tried to bring to the readers' knowledge various recent clinical trials on nano carrier-based formulations and their outcomes for the management of carcinoma.

Table 8.1. Anti-cancer Nanoformulations recently approved by FDA.

S. No.	Drug Product	API	Manufacturer	Indications
1.	TRODELVY	Sacituzumab Govitecan	Immunomedics Inc.	Locally advanced or metastatic triple-negative breast cancer
2.	ERBITUX	Cetuximab	ImClone LLC	EGFR-expressing colorectal cancer
3.	LORBRENA	Lorlatinib	Pfizer Inc.	Metastatic non-small-cell lung cancer
4.	LIBTAYO	Cemiplimab	Regeneron Pharmaceuticals, Inc.	Advanced non-small cell lung cancer
5.	TEPMETKO	Tepotinib	EMD Serono Inc.	Metastatic non-small-cell lung cancer
6.	TAGRISSO	Osimertinib	AstraZeneca Pharmaceuticals LP	Non-small cell lung cancer
7.	ORGOVYX	Relugolix	Myovant Sciences	Advanced prostate cancer
8.	MARGENZA	Margetuximab	MacroGenics	Metastatic HER2-positive breast cancer
9.	KEYTRUDA	Pembrolizumab	Merck & Co.	Metastatic triple-negative breast cancer
10.	GAVRETO	Pralsetinib	Blueprint Medicines Corporation	Non-small cell lung cancer
11.	KEYTRUDA	Pembrolizumab	Merck & Co.	Colorectal cancer
12.	ZEPZELCA	Lurbinectedin	Pharma Mar S.A.	Metastatic small cell lung cancer
13.	CYRAMZA	Ramucirumab	Eli Lilly and Company	Metastatic non-small-cell lung cancer
14.	OPDIVO	Nivolumab	Bristol-Myers Squibb Co.	Metastatic or recurrent non-small cell lung cancer
15.	ALUNBRIG	Brigatinib	ARIAD Pharmaceuticals Inc.	Metastatic or recurrent non-small cell lung cancer
16.	LYNPARZA	Olaparib	AstraZeneca Pharmaceuticals, LP	Gene-mutated metastatic castration-resistant prostate cancer
17.	TECENTRIQ	Atezolizumab	Genentech Inc.	Metastatic non-small-cell lung cancer
18.	RUBRACA	Rucaparib	Clovis Oncology, Inc.	Metastatic castration-resistant prostate cancer
19.	OPDIVO+ YERVOY	Nivolumab+ Ipilimumab	Bristol-Myers Squibb Co.	Metastatic non-small-cell lung cancer

(Table 1) cont.....

S. No.	Drug Product	API	Manufacturer	Indications
20.	RETEVMO	Selpercatinib	Eli Lilly and Co.	Non-small cell lung cancer

(Source: https://www.accessdata.fda.gov,https://www.fda.gov/drugs/resources).

Nanocarriers and Drug Targeted Delivery System

The physicochemical qualities of nanoparticles (NPs) have a substantial impact on their usefulness. Nanoscale formulations can be formulated using various materials such as lipids, polymers, proteins, *etc.* [8]. Unless all the administered chemotherapeutic agent reaches the tumorous cells, it can permeate other cells and cause damage. The systemically disseminated nanomaterials, however, will pass through the barriers and reach the target tumor tissue with minimal volume and activity loss [9]. The nanocarrier approach is employed by researchers to improve drug distribution, safety, solubility, and stability. The delivery of antineoplastic drugs to target tumor tissue has been achieved by the complexation of drug nanoparticles with ligands like aptamers, peptides, folic acid, *etc.* to confer site-specific targeting and a wide range of drug delivery vehicles offer options with fewer negative effects and improved pharmacokinetics [10]. The nano-size, increased surface area: volume ratio, form, charge, and composition of nanostructures make them ideal careers for anticancer agents in tumor treatment [11]. Different types of nanocarriers such as gold nanoparticles, micelles, magnetic nanoparticles, quantum dots, self-emulsifying systems, polymeric hydrogels, nanoporous silica, dendrimers, liposomes, *etc.* as depicted in Fig. **(8.2)** have been widely used for targeting drugs to different malignancies of breast, lung, brain, colon, prostate, and cervical, *etc.* Active and passive targeting approaches have been used to distribute NPs to cancerous tissue *via* blood circulation. Particles or carriers ranging in dimensions from 20 to 200 nm, can benefit from the leaky tumor vasculature resulting in better permeability and retention accounting for tissue-specific agglomeration. NPs provide optimal targeting based on size and surface qualities that influence the EPR such that the nanocarriers can swiftly infiltrate through the membranes of microcapillaries with inferior build in an angiogenic tumor [12]. The tumor tissue is known to have higher interstitial pressure in its center as compared to the periphery owing to its limited lymphatic function, thus permitting nanocarriers to enter the interstitial region and stay there for a long period, increasing their therapeutic potential in malignancies [13].

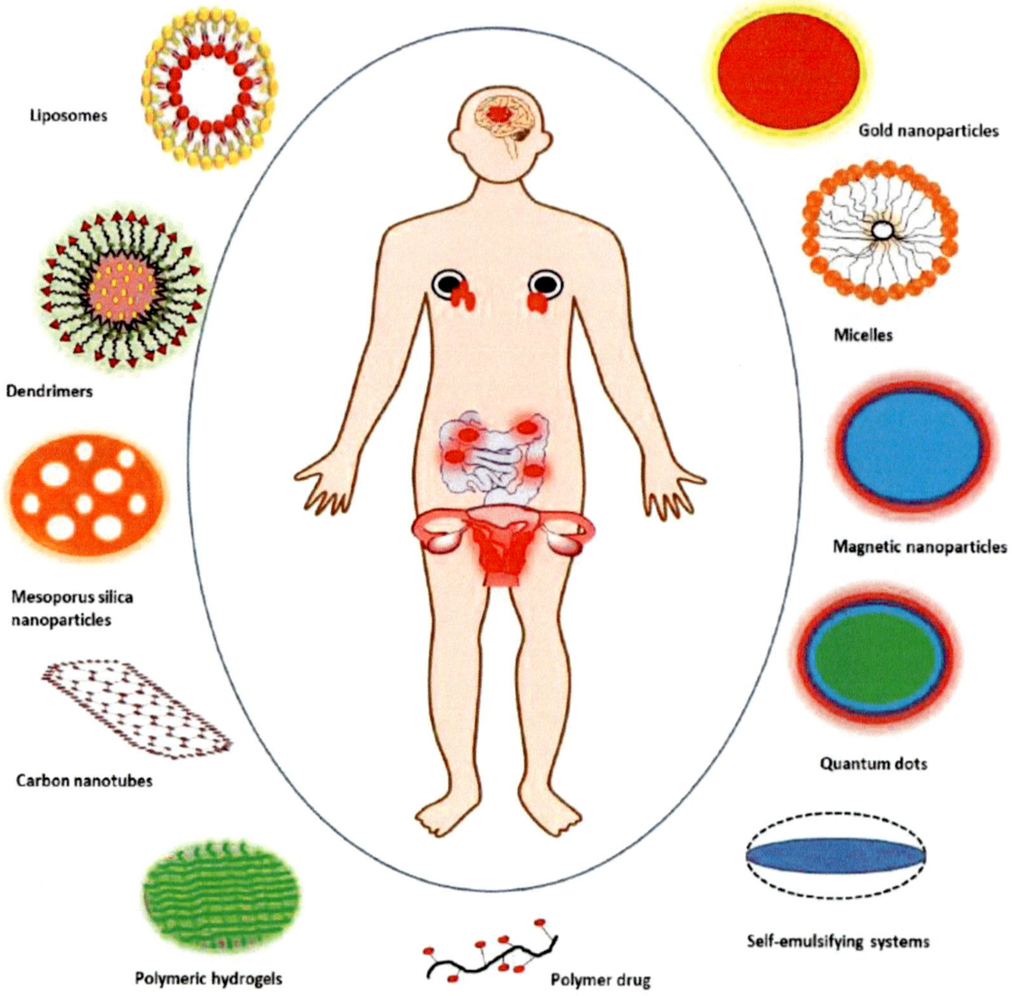

Fig. (8.2). Various types of nanocarriers for tumor targeting.

Tumor Targeting Approaches

Cancer is a serious threat to deaths worldwide affecting all age groups. The conventional therapies to manage the malignancies suffers from lots of demerits, and therefore a lot of focus has been dedicated to research aiming to develop site-specific delivery systems for different types of cancers as reflected in recent literature and reported in Table **8.2.**

Table 8.2. Drugs and their delivery systems for various types of cancer.

S. No.	Carrier and delivery system	Drug	Indication	Ref.
1.	Mannosylated liposomes	Dihydroartemisinin (DHA) Doxorubicin (Dox)	Colon cancer	[14]
2.	Folic acid conjugated liposomes	5-Fluorouracil	Colon cancer	[15]
3.	Mannosylated liposomes	Paclitaxel (PTX)	Colon cancer cells	[16]
4.	PAMAM dendrimers	siRNA	Breast cancer	[17]
5.	Conjugated Gold nanoparticle	Quercetin	Breast cancer	[18]
6.	Novel hollow gold nanoflowers	Trastuzumab	Breast cancer	[19]
7.	Gold nanoparticles & nanofibers	Enzyme glucose oxidase	Breast cancer	[20]
8.	Transferrin (Tf) nanoparticles	Temozolomide (TMZ)	Glioma stem cell-mediated therapy	[16]
9.	Polymeric nano-micelles	Geraniol	Brain cancer	[21]
10.	Nanoliposomes	Curcumin	Breast cancer	[22]
11.	Liposomes	Resveratrol and p53	Cervical Cancer	[23]
12.	Vaginal contraception delivery	Cisplatin-infused poly (Ethylene-co-vinyl acetate) (EVAc)	Cervical cancer	[24]
13.	Glutathione-responsive hydrogel	Paclitaxel	Cervical cancer	[25]
14.	Magnetic nanoparticle-incorporated nano hydrogel	Doxorubicin	Cervical cancer	[26]
15.	Mesoporous silica nanoparticles	Doxorubicin	Prostate cancer	[27]
16.	Co-delivery nanoparticles	Docetaxel and Doxorubicin	Prostate cancer	[28]

Colon/Colorectal Cancer Targeting

Colon cancer or colorectal cancer is among the most common type of human cancers [29]. Colorectal cancer is associated with many risk factors like age, race, gender, and dietary, as well as past exposure to adenomatous polyps, ovary, uterine, or breast tumors, human papillomavirus (HPV) infection, smoking and alcohol consumption habits, *etc.* [30]. A specialized drug delivery system for targeting the colon should be designed to shield the active molecule while it travels from the stomach to the colon, preventing the release of the drug or absorption in the gastrointestinal tract. The drug molecule should not get deactivated at the dissolution site or *en route* until it reaches the colon [31]. Various formulation strategies, such as pH-sensitive systems, enzyme-triggered systems, and receptor-mediated drug carriers, have been investigated to enhance the colonic dispersion of medication (Fig. **8.3**). *Kang X.J. et al.,* studied the anti-

MDR impact of dihydroartemisinin (DHA) in combination with doxorubicin (Dox), HCT8/ADR cells by encapsulating them together in mannosylated liposomes (Man-liposomes) to targeting colon delivery. Delivery of Man-liposomes resulted in an 88.59 percent tumor suppression rate in a subcutaneous tumor xenograft model, compared to 47.46 percent and 70.54 percent for free Dox and free Dox+DHA, respectively [14]. *Handali S. et al.,* created and characterized tailored liposomes carrying 5-fluorouracil (5FU) to improve the drug's efficacy and safety. For targeting ligand (folic acid) was used. The outcomes of investigation from the models were found to agree with the predicted values. DSC measurements revealed the amorphous nature of the active ingredient in the preparation, and TEM revealed that the nanoparticles were spherical. Folate-liposomal 5FU displayed stronger cytotoxic action on cancer cells in an MTT assay. In HT-29 cells, targeted liposomes caused cell death primarily through necrosis as a result of excessive ROS generation and show a reduction in tumor volume *in vivo*. The tailored liposomes of 5FU show improved therapeutic efficacy while reducing the harmful effects [15].

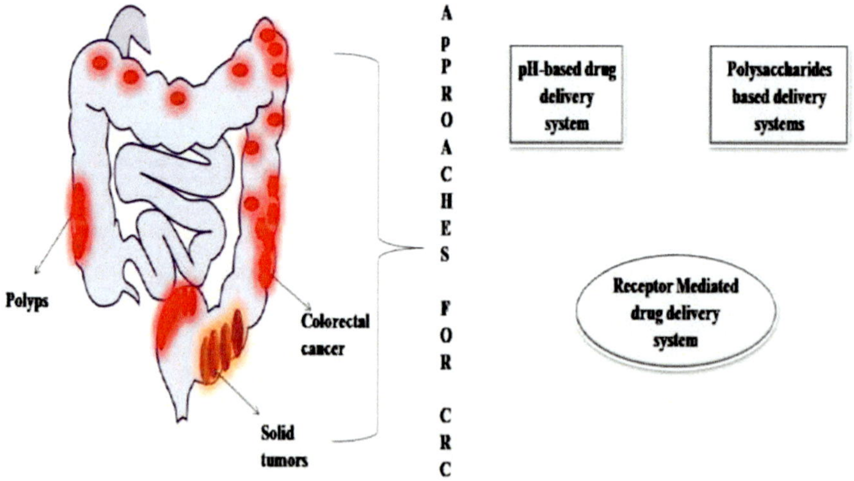

Fig. (8.3). The diagram illustrates treatment approaches for colon cancer.

pH-based Medication For Colon Targeting

The pH of the stomach lies between 1 and 2 when fasting, nevertheless rising after a meal. The small intestine pH is approximately 6.5, whereas the pH distal part of the small intestine is around 7.5. From the ileum to the colon, the pH drops dramatically. The pH of the cecum is around 6.4. In healthy people, however, pH levels in the ascending colon have been measured as low as 5.7 [32]. The pH of the transverse section lies around 6.6, while the descending colon has a pH of 7.0.

The pH fluctuations are the basis of the utilization of pH-dependent polymers. The hydrophilic or hydrophobic polymer-coated over the surface of the drug molecule and the external surface were encased with pH-sensitive polymer for colon targeting [33]. They are designed to be stable at low pH levels and then release medications at higher pH levels. Enteric coatings are widely utilized in the pharmaceutical sector and have undergone extensive testing to ensure that they are effective in targeting the colon [34]. The key differences between pH-dependent solid preparations for colonic delivery and typical enteric-coated drugs are the target location and the diversity of enteric polymers utilized. The coating method is a fundamental formulation technique for colon-specific dispersion [35]. *Liu et al.* employed a dual coating strategy comprising the inner layer with an alkaline aqueous eudragit S solution containing buffers. Whereas, for the outer layer an organic eudragit S solution was employed to accelerate medication release at a pH of more than 7 [36]. *Varum et al.* observed *in vivo* efficiency of double-coated devices in humans and found that dual-coated tablets disintegrated mostly in the lower intestine system [37].

Polysaccharides Based Delivery Systems

The natural polymers of monosaccharides are numerous, widely available, inexpensive, and available in a range of forms with different characteristics, and are gaining usage for colon targeting [38]. It includes polysaccharides obtained naturally from plants, animals, algae, and microbes [39]. Some of the novel polysaccharides, like arabinoxylans, *etc.* are newly identified polysaccharides in colon-specific delivery [38]. Persistent interaction between the mucosal surface and drug delivery vehicles may help in absorption due to the mucoadhesive properties of polysaccharides. Additional advantages of polysaccharide-based delivery methods include wide availability, lesser amount, minimal toxicity and immunogenicity, good biocompatibility, and biodegradability [40]. *Song et al.* formulated an oral therapeutic agent for the management of orthotopic colon cancer. Polyacrylic acid and chitosan were linked to Gadolinium-doped mesoporous hydroxyapatite nanoparticles (Gd-MHNPs). When administered through the oral route, they impart sustain release characteristics along with localization of therapeutic agent at the tumor site. NPs created by encapsulating 5-FU and gefitinib in Gd-MHAp demonstrated a synergistic stimulating efficacy, implying its potential use in managing orthotopic colon cancer with drug delivery systems [41].

Receptor-Mediated Drug Delivery System

Colorectal treatments are given intravenously due to their cytotoxic impact on healthy cells. The associated substantial systemic side effects could be suppressed by the use of ligand/receptor-mediated systems that improve target specificity [42]. A lower concentration of an active drug with improved bioavailability can be achieved by changing the surface receptor-mediated drug delivery mechanism with a nanoengineered delivery system [43].

Folate Receptor

Since the folate receptor is differentially expressed in several cancer types, folic acid plays the role of a malignant cell-targeting ligand [44]. Numerous researches have indicated that folic acid-coated nanoparticles can help in tumor-selective medication absorption. The folate receptors (FRs) are membrane-bound glycosylphosphatidylinositol (GPI)-anchored glycoproteins that transport folate into cancerous cells through endocytosis [45]. FRs are consistently overexpressed in most cancer tissues, including epithelial, ovarian, prostate, cervical, breast, liver, brain, and colorectum. One of the most promising and intensively investigated cancer markers for the advancement of selective drug delivery systems is the incidence of FR overexpression in human cancer. Folic acid-conjugated liposomes improved daunorubicin's anti-cancer efficacy by boosting folate receptor-mediated drug absorption, according to *Xiong et al.* [46].

Mannose Receptor (MR)

It is a powerful endocytic carbohydrate-binding receptor also known as the cluster of differentiation 206 (CD206) [47]. In inflammatory conditions, MR is upregulated on the exterior area of macrophages and dendritic cells (DCs). This transmembrane receptor is made up of C-type lectin-like domains (CTLD), FNII domains (fibronectin type II), and R-type cysteine-rich domains (CRD) [48]. Mannose receptors express through macrophages in the human body as they bind specifically with mannosylated substances present on pathogens to mediate their endocytosis. Mannosylated molecules and carbohydrates were found on the surfaces of yeasts, gram-negative and positive bacteria, mycobacteria, and parasites. The receptor's job is to recognize and engulf the pathogens linked to it, then transport them to lysosomes for destruction *via* phagocytic pathways. *Xiong et al.,* formulated mannosylated liposomes with paclitaxel (PTX) that exhibit better CT26 cell uptake capability and tumor suppression levels due to MR targeting effectiveness with decreased toxicity [49]. *Ye et al.* prepared amphiphilic-cyclodextrin nanoparticles containing doxorubicin with multivalent mannose for identifying overexpressed MR on breast cancer cells (MDA-MB-231). The prepared nanoparticles efficiently invaded MR and inhibit the activity of breast cancer cells *in vivo* with lesser harmful effects [50].

Breast Cancer Targeting

It is one of the frequently diagnosed cancer in women and is dependent upon a variety of molecular characteristics. Drug resistance and the tendency of breast cancer to metastasize to numerous organs account for the majority of breast cancer deaths [51]. It has been well recognized that an ATP-binding cassette (ABC) family protein is known to primarily affect drug tolerance in a wide range of cancers, and its increased expression is associated with increased chemotherapy resistance. The breast cancer diagnosis is based on cancer's histology and molecular characteristics while locoregional treatment and systemic therapy are the two basic components of effective management [52]. MDR is a significant barrier in breast cancer prognosis and causation, owing to enhanced expression of proteins such as P-glycoprotein, *etc.* [53]. HER-2 positive breast cancer is one of the frequently encountered breast cancer that strikes one of every five women, with a bad prognosis and rapid growth because of excessive expression of HER-2 on the breast tumor's surface. The following section addresses the various drug delivery platforms employed in the breast cancer therapy paradigm -systemic, localized, and receptor-based. Approaches for systemic drug administration include organic drug delivery, inorganic drug delivery, localized drug delivery (Fig. **8.4**).

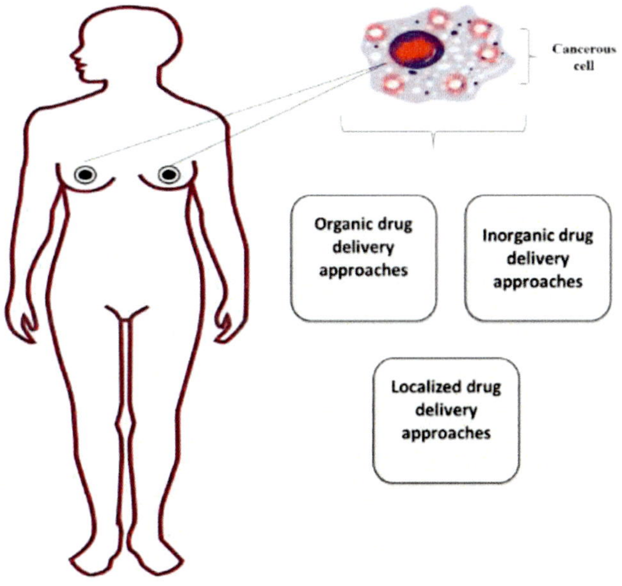

Fig. (8.4). Breast cancer therapeutics methods.

Organic Drug Delivery Approaches

Coated Nano-liposomes

On many malignant sites, chemotherapeutic drug delivery methods based on nanocarriers operate well. The medicaments are most commonly delivered as organic and inorganic particles. In breast cancer, encapsulating anticancer drugs in nano-scale packaging is the safest technique to reduce side effects and improve medicine absorption. The coated nano-liposomal formulations produced from marine and plant sources can be utilized as a controlled release product for breast cancer [22]. Liposomes boost curcumin bioavailability while the chitosan covering extends its circulation time, according to Hasan M. *et al.* 2020. The nanoliposomes coated with chitosan enhanced their size, and surface charges were changed *i.e*; negative to positive, leading to enhanced curcumin entrapment efficiency. The experiments revealed considerable improvement when condensed liposome formulations were lined with curcumin or encapsulated with chitosan.

Dendrimers

In 1978, Vogtle identified the first dendrimer-based nanotechnology platforms for medication delivery [54]. Dendrimers are 3D highly branched, spherical macromolecules with low polydispersity indices and 1–100 nm in diameter. They have three unique domains: a core nucleus, a hyperbranched mantle, and a corona with reactive functional groups on the periphery. Various anticancer drugs have been incorporated into dendrimers to prevent breast cancer [55]. Dendrimers of various sorts have been effectively built for medication delivery [56]. *Finlay et al.* developed a PAMAM-RNA dendrimer system to treat advanced breast cancer by targeting the TWIST1 transcription factor, which is frequently expressed excessively. The siRNA-loaded PAMAM dendrimers were readily absorbed by TNBC cells, resulting in significant suppression of TWIST1-related target genes. As a result, the dendrimers' ability to deliver siRNA to a xenograft orthotopic tumor model was critical. After surgery, siRNA stayed in the tumor for more than four hours. TWIST1 has the perspective of being a clinically beneficial method for metastatic breast cancer treatment. It could be utilized as an adjuvant treatment to prevent active tumors from migrating or invading, as well as chemoresistance [17].

Drug Delivery Based on Inorganic Compounds: Gold Nanoparticles

Chemotherapy has made use of gold nanoparticles (GNPs). Because of their smaller area (about 130 nm) and selectivity, they tend to accumulate in cancerous cells. GNP coating can be used as a cancer biomarker, a probe for transmission electron microscopy, and an antibacterial agent [53]. Michael Faraday presented the first research analysis on GNP synthesis in the nineteenth century, describing the refining of colloidal gold *via* the conversion of aurochloric acid by phosphorus. Several techniques were employed in the twentieth century, such as TEM and AFM allowed direct imaging of GNPs, and monitoring of parameters like size and surface coating was refined [57]. *Balakrishnan et al.* confirmed that AuNPs-Qu-5 reduce breast cancer cell propagation, invasion, angiogenesis, and metastasis by targeting the EGFR/VEGFR-2 signaling pathway. This research looked at how AuNPs-Qu-5 treatment suppressed various proteins, like N-cadherin, Akt, p-GSK3, Snail, p-PI3K, *etc.* [18]. *Jiang et al.* created gold nanoparticles with trastuzumab with a diameter range from 2 to 100 nm. According to the findings, they appear to target HER-2-positive SK-BR-3 breast cancer cells. AuNPs with diameters of 40 to 50 nm are endocytosed by cells, but AuNPs with smaller diameters are liable to detach from the plasma membrane [19].

Approaches to Localize Therapeutic Agents: Nanofibers

Depending on the location and stage of the tumor, anticancer medicines, radiation, or surgery are presently utilized to treat persistent breast cancer. Localized medication administration, as opposed to systemic medications, has a stronger effect as a treatment option for early-stage malignancies [58].

Nanofibers are fibers with lengths ranging from a few 10 to 1000 nm [59]. Their production processes involve phase separation, prototype synthesis, self-assembly, electrospinning, and mechanical drawing [60]. Nanofibers can be fabricated using a variety of polymers and therefore have distinct tensile strength and chemical properties [61]. *Sapountzi et al.* created polyvinyl alcohol/ polyethyleneimine nanofibers on the exterior of gold electrodes for enzyme-based glucose identification using an electrospinning process. On the nanofibers, the enzyme glucose oxidase was immobilized. Nanofibers covered with gold nanoparticle coats may enhance conductivity. Researchers also affirmed that employing the combination of metal nanoparticles and electrospun nanofibers enhances thermal tolerance, mechanical efficiency, *etc.* The nanosensor showed excellent glucose selectivity, operating and storage stability, and minimal glucose detection limit [20].

Brain Cancer Targeting

The brain, a three-pound organ encased within the skull that controls memory, adaptive motor skills, and many other processes, is the most significant and powerful organ having three parts- cerebrum, cerebellum, brain stem, and four lobes that make cerebrum are frontal, parietal, occipital and temporal [62].

Encephalitis, neurological disorders, multiple sclerosis, stroke, and tumors are only a few of the conditions that cause brain activity to decline. The BBB brings forth an obstacle for delivering the active molecules developed for brain illnesses (Fig. **8.5**). Anticancer drug products administered intravenously fail to get to the brain parenchyma, therefore targeted delivery of drugs in the brain tumor is not an easy feat. Alternative clinical techniques for these illnesses are difficult to develop [63]. Numerous barriers around the CNS impede the disposition of the anticancer agents to the tumor site in the brain [64].

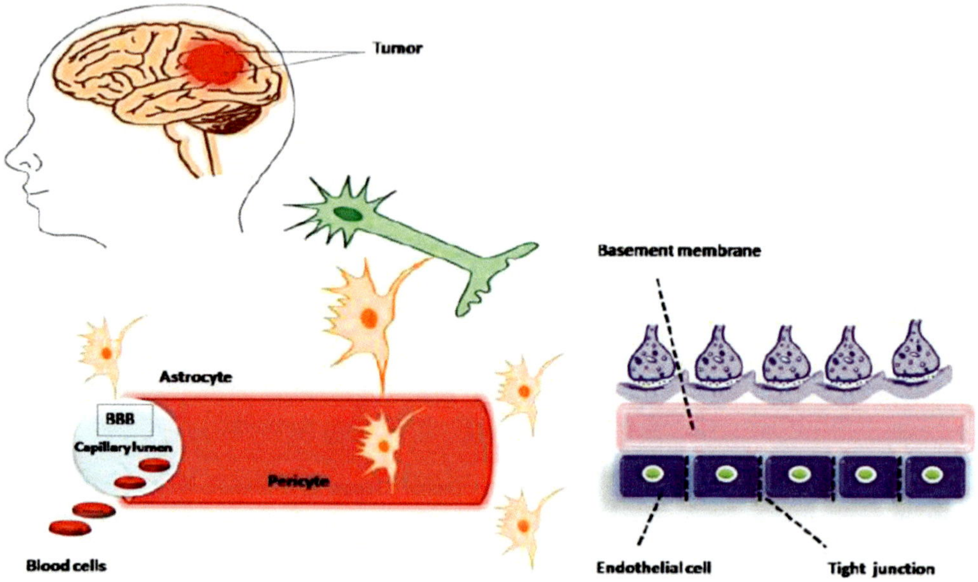

Fig. (8.5). Brain drug delivery and blood-brain barrier.

Lipid Drug Conjugation for Brain Delivery

Shinde G et al. explored the possibility to develop nanoparticles for delivering 5-fluorouracil (5-FU) for brain cancer treatment. *In vitro* release patterns in their investigation demonstrated immediate release in starting, afterward persistent release for up to 48 hours. On human glioma cell lines, anticancer potential of blank stearic acid nanoparticles, lipid–drug conjugated (LDC) nanoparticles, and 5-FU solution was compared and LDC-NPs were found to cause higher cytotoxicity in U373 MG cells than in other cells. LDC was discovered to have larger quantities in the bloodstream, but 5-FU showed predominant localization in tissue rather than systemic circulation. The $t_{1/2}$ for LDC indicates a ninefold increase, whereas MRT produces a 12-fold increase over pure 5-FU, showing that LDC circulates for a longer time. After 3 hours, the maximal concentration in the brain was two-fold higher with improved LDC formulation, and the efficacy of 5-FU in LDC nanoparticles, for treating brain tumors is increased [65].

Intra-arterial Drug Delivery

The goal of the intra-arterial (IA) dosage form is to enhance the amount of a drug that reaches the vascular area by avoiding first-pass metabolism [66]. Although some of the drugs may travel through CNS quickly, their shorter retention time may result in decreased efficacy. IA treatment has not yet resulted in a better prognosis for patients with brain cancer. The BBB delivery has been iatrogenically disrupted before systemic chemotherapy delivery, which has resulted in improved efficacy [67]. Combining IA chemotherapy with BBBD enhances the number of active molecules in the brain parenchyma, according to preclinical investigations [68]. Drugs are delivered directly through an artery near the tumor in intra-arterial medication delivery [69]. After the targeted region has been cannulated, the medicine is administered into the blood vessel. Osmotic BBBD with drugs like mannitol supplemented by IA chemotherapy is the most commonly utilized technique. Numerous researches have been carried out to look into the utilization of intra-arterial medication administration in glioblastoma (GBM) patients. The survival rate was estimated from about 4.5 to 10 months after treatment with nimustine, bevacizumab, rituximab, and carboplatin in conjunction with additional standard chemotherapy. Toxicity and a lack of medication efficacy appear to be impeding the application of intra-arterial medication administration in brain tumors [70].

Receptor-mediated Endocytosis

Several receptors are found in BBB such as transferrin, insulin, vascular permeability factor, and amino acid receptors. Receptor-mediated endocytosis is the primary method for the agents to travel past the blood-brain barrier (BBB) [71]. The Tf receptor (TfR) is a membrane glycoprotein in BBB which is among the key targets for the distribution of therapeutics to the CNS tumor. *Sun et al.,* developed PAMAM-PEG-Tf/TMZ TMZ/transferrin (Tf) nanoparticles that permeate the BBB and kills glioma tumor cells. The prepared nanoparticles generate somewhat extended mean survival time (MST) in mice with gliomas [16].

Nose to Brain Delivery

The blood-brain barrier (BBB) and blood-cerebrospinal fluid (CSF) barrier are two main physiological barriers impeding the transmission of drug molecules to the CNS. Nasal administration however permits more drugs to penetrate the brain. The nasal cavity is split into two sections (respiratory and olfactory), each of which is susceptible to drug absorption into the brain or bloodstream [72]. The two nerve cells olfactory and trigeminal present in the nose helps the medication to enter directly into the brain avoiding BBB [73]. Because of its proximity to the cerebrospinal fluid (CSF) and direct neuronal attachment to the brain, the olfactory area has aroused researchers' interest for potential nose-to-brain transmission [74]. *Bonferroni et al.*, created polymeric nano-micelles packed with geraniol, an acyclic monoterpene, using chitosan oleate, as an amphiphilic polymer. Geraniol is an anticancer and neuroprotective compound found in aromatic plant essential oils. The nano-emulsions were tested *in vitro*, and the formulation containing 2% (w/w) chitosan oleate had viscosity outcomes consistent with oral and nasal administration to rats, as well as a mean diameter of the dispersed phase of roughly 800 nm. When compared to formulations containing coarse geraniol emulsion, *in vivo* tests on rats confirmed that oral administration of this formulation resulted in a considerable increase in geraniol bioavailability as well as an improvement in its ability to reach the CNS from the bloodstream [21].

Cervical Cancer

Cervical cancer is observed in women and would be the fourth foremost cause of cancer globally. With a fatality rate of 27.6 per 100,000 inhabitants, Eastern Africa is the most afflicted region in the country [75]. The treatment for cervical cancer varies based on the stage. Although cancer in the initial stages can be treated with radiotherapy or surgery, concomitant chemotherapy and pelvic irradiation are frequently used for locally advanced stage cancer [76]. All cervical malignancies are caused by human papillomaviruses (HPVs). More than 100 distinct types of HPV have been found since Zur Hausen identified the link between HPVs and cervical cancer in the 1970s [77]. Only 12 types of HPV have been linked to cancer thus far, but this number could rise as more study is done. HPV16 and HPV18 are responsible for over 70% of cervical malignancies. There are various treatment options available after a cervical cancer diagnosis, many of which are dependent upon the cancer stage and the patient's overall condition. The route of administration and equipment type utilized is used to classify drug distribution systems (Fig. **8.6**).

Systemic Drug Delivery Systems

Because of their structure, variable composition, and surface changes, the entrapment of chemotherapy agents in nanosystems has received much interest. The most commonly employed structures for targeting delivery include nanoparticles, liposomes, micelles, and dendrimers. These particles typically range in size from 10 to 150 nanometers, assuring higher tumor aggregation. The kidneys would quickly clear particles less than 10 nm, whereas macrophage cells would recognize and destroy particles larger than 150 nm [79]. Drug specificity has been shown to improve, systemic drug toxicity has been reduced, absorption rates have increased, and active drugs have been protected from biological and chemical degradation using nanoscale drug delivery devices [80].

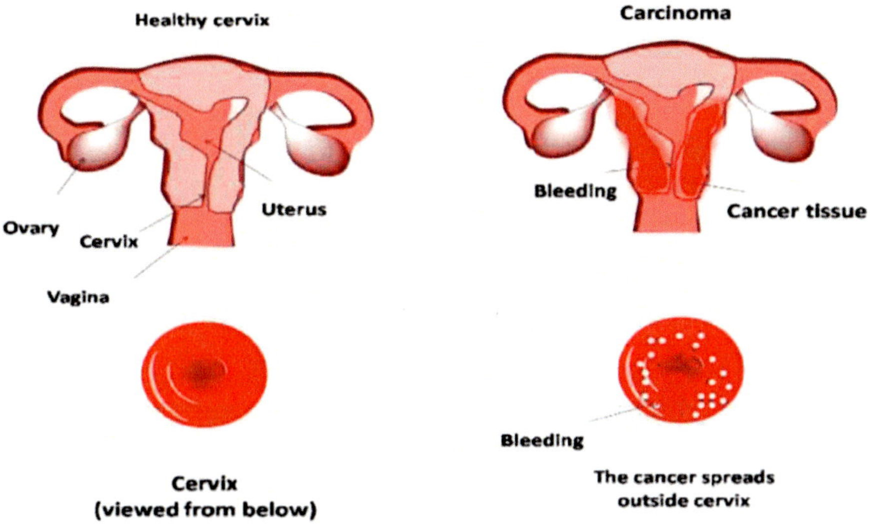

Fig. (8.6). Cervical cancer location and spread.

Polymeric Nanoparticles

Biodegradable polymeric NPs have piqued the interest of researchers as carriers for anticancer drugs because of their excellent drug loading potential, enhanced absorption, self-stability, favorable biodistribution. While the stealth polymers that come with these NPs let them circulate longer, their dense covering of polymers may prevent target cancer cells from taking anticancer medications [81]. Because of their small size, NPs have been utilized as special instruments with various advantages, including quick penetration across cell membranes, reduced off-target effects, enhanced drug kinetics, and lysosomal escape following endocytosis [82]. Cisplatin (CDDP) is a potent anti-cancer medication; however, it has been limited in its use due to its inability to target cervical cancer tissue. *Cheng et al.* fused CDDP into fluorescein PEG amine grafted-aldehyde Hyaluronic acid (HA) nanoparticles to enhance their specificity for cervical cancer by acidic pH response to the tumor [83]. While HA is utilized in nanocarriers as a targeting moiety, a large amount can collect in the liver and be further removed promptly. The tests revealed that the NPs may internalize and induce death in tumor cells, confirming CDDP biocompatibility and targeting cervical tumors. Significant CDDP-Cy5.5-PEG-g-A-HA aggregation was seen *in vivo* at the cervical tumor location, indicating greater CDDP targeting. A recent study used the conjunction of paclitaxel and carboplatin, subsequently coated with folic acid which allows targeting cervical cancer cells. These bi-functional NPs enhance cell viability and tumor inhibition due to their pH-sensitive drug release and receptor recognition characteristics [84]. *Sarisozen et al.* examined the efficacy of combination products (paclitaxel and curcumin) comprising of transferrin-modified polyethylene glycol phosphatidylethanolamine (PEG-PE) based polymeric micelles *in vivo* model of ovarian cancer cell *via* confocal imaging and flow cytometry to test cytotoxicity and cellular aggregation. Micelles penetrate far deeper into spheroids, allowing them to produce more cytotoxic agents and hence increase cytotoxicity. The system's relevance for cervical cancer treatment is demonstrated by the *in vivo* data [85].

Dendrimers

Dendrimers are highly monodisperse circular, extremely symmetric, also exceedingly branching macromolecules having a precise form, comprising charge over the surface [86]. They are especially versatile because of their structure, which allows for the adhesion and appearance of foreign matters at their edge. The pharmaceutical compound loaded into the cavities of dendrimers for hydrophobic interactions or hydrogen bonding, or conjugation to the polymer can all be employed [87]. They are typically multifunctional due to their layout, which enables the marginal linking of the antigen molecules [24]. To achieve the confined therapeutic efficacy of peptide-based cervical cancer vaccinations, polyacrylate star polymer associated with HPV E7 protein was used. After single vaccination, these conjugates demonstrated mitigation of tumor formation and obliterate E7-expressing TC-1 tumors in mice [88]. *Mekuria et al.* evaluated the activity of doxorubicin dendrimer conjugated with IL-6 antibody in HeLa cells, the outcome of the proposed work shows better cellular internalization, higher drug incorporation, better release characteristics, and enhanced cytotoxicity than RGD (arginyl-glycyl-aspartic acid) peptide-conjugated dendrimers. It is most likely due to the higher density of multivalent ligands on the substrate of IL6-conjugated dendrimers, which results in improved drug delivery *via* receptor-mediated endocytosis [89].

Localized Drug Delivery System

The advantages of targeted medication delivery to the cervix over systemic delivery include restricting the widespread movement of anti-cancer drugs that ensures reduction in loss of medicament and adverse effects, at the same time the retention of a large concentration of the therapeutic agent in the cervix, will increase the effectiveness of the therapy [58]. When the disease has spread to distant organs, localized medication carriers may be ineffective, signaling the necessity for more systemic therapy. Recent studies, however, reveal that only about 20% of individuals have distant metastases, highlighting the significance of targeted drug carriers for controlling cervical cancer [24]. Many recent studies on localized delivery strategies for several anticancer agents are being reported where the drug is administered through the vaginal route using specialized devices. Xu X et al., 2019 produced peptide cationic lipid (CDO14) with resveratrol liposomes using thin film with ultrasonic dispersion approach to achieve a synergistic inhibiting effect on the tumor gene p53. Localized delivery enhances the overall quality of patients' lives by allowing them to reduce the frequency of hospital visits and hospitalizations while cutting healthcare expenditures worldwide [78].

Scaffolds/nanofibers

Scaffolds are polymeric materials injected or implanted into the body for the delivery of medications, genes, and cells. Various examples of polymeric scaffolds include 3D structure matrix, thermosensitive hydrogel, microsphere, *etc*[90]. Drug delivery is one of the many uses for nanofibers, particularly in local chemotherapy. Electrospinning in drug delivery has several appealing properties, including good encapsulation performance, the convenience of service, cost-effectiveness, high loading power, and simultaneous distribution of numerous medicines [91]. To make the scaffold, natural polymers including alginate, collagen, gelatin, vitamins, fibrins, and albumin, as well as synthetic polymers like polyglycolide and polyvinyl alcohol, can be employed [92]. *Keskar et al.* formulated a cisplatin-loaded poly (ethylene-co-vinyl acetate) device akin to vaginal contraceptives. The device disintegrates in a biphasic manner, and the system release the drug in a regulated manner, initially higher release was observed later on a linear slower release phase. The device shows better outcomes in both HPV +ve and HPV-ve cases, followed by *in vitro* testing. According to the data, a distribution mechanism is a favorable tool for the diagnosis of cervical cancer [24]. *In vivo* trials of the device showed greater antitumor effectiveness and improved systemic protection than IV injections at the same drug stage, demonstrating the advantages of targeted delivery over systematic delivery [24].

Hydrogels

Hydrogels are prepared from hydrophilic polymers that entrap the drug agents inside the matrix and release the drug out of the polymeric matrix that tends to swell [93]. It can be applied in the vagina that helps to maintain pH, moisture and provide antimicrobial action [94]. *Perez et al.,* formulated paclitaxel loaded poly-N-isopropyl acrylamide (NIPA), tert-butyl 2-acrylamidoethyl carbamate (2AAECM), and N-hydroxyethyl acrylamide (HEAA) gel employing a microemulsion polymerization technique. The produced formulations were tested against cancer cell lines for cytotoxicity and cellular uptake utilizing the MTT assay and coumarin-6, respectively (MCF-7, T47D, and HeLa). Nanogel containing coumarin-6 was quickly taken up (in 2 hours) and gathered intracellularly, according to the findings (after 48 h) [25]. *Jaiswal et al.,* created a magnetic nanoparticle of iron oxide comprising of poly- (N-isopropyl acrylamide)-chitosan-based nano hydrogel using poly (N-isopropyl acrylamide)-chitosan. The *in vitro* anticancer activity and drug delivery profile were tested using a model drug doxorubicin. In terms of doxorubicin release, the developed system responded well to both stimuli. Furthermore, when the cervical cancer (HeLa) cell line was exposed to an AC magnetic field while the hydrogel contained nanoparticles were heated, the number of malignant cells was significantly reduced [26].

Prostate Cancer

The prostate gland represents the most common site for cancer occurrence accounting for 15% of all male malignancies. Cancer of the prostate leads to prostate enlargement and constriction of the urethra leading to the problem of painful urination and even bleeding (Fig. **8.7**). Prostate adenocarcinoma accounts for roughly 20% of cancer-related deaths in the Western world [95]. Roughly 70% of new prostate cancer cases diagnosed are in developed countries and also it has spread to underdeveloped countries and has become a major health concern. Variations in lifestyle, diet, environmental variables, and genetic variants have all contributed to a rise in prostate cancer cases [96].

Androgen receptor (AR) is a light-dependent transcription factor that has been linked to prostate cancer in several studies [97]. The androgen receptor (AR) shows a prompt target for the management of prostate cancer. Many negative health issues have been linked to disruptions in the AR signaling pathway, including prostate cancer, poor reproductive health, and under virilized male syndrome. Prostate cancer is currently treated by blocking the androgen AR axis by lowering androgen levels and reducing AR function. Early-stage localized disease can be successfully treated with radical surgery or radiation; nevertheless, androgen restriction (AD) is used to treat the majority of locally progressed and all metastatic diseases and causes tumor reduction and a metabolic response for 14-20 months without really extending survival [98]. Furthermore, the available conventional therapy options are insufficient to treat prostate cancer Conventional treatment for prostate cancer comes with several drawbacks. It has been discovered that anticancer drugs accumulate poorly at the target region and that rapid clearance or drug resistance occurs. Aside from that, it has a slew of negative consequences on regular cells and tissues. These are the main reasons why traditional chemotherapy has lost its effectiveness. Nanotechnology has facilitated the production of various nanocarriers for the delivery of appropriate chemotherapeutics in the body [99].

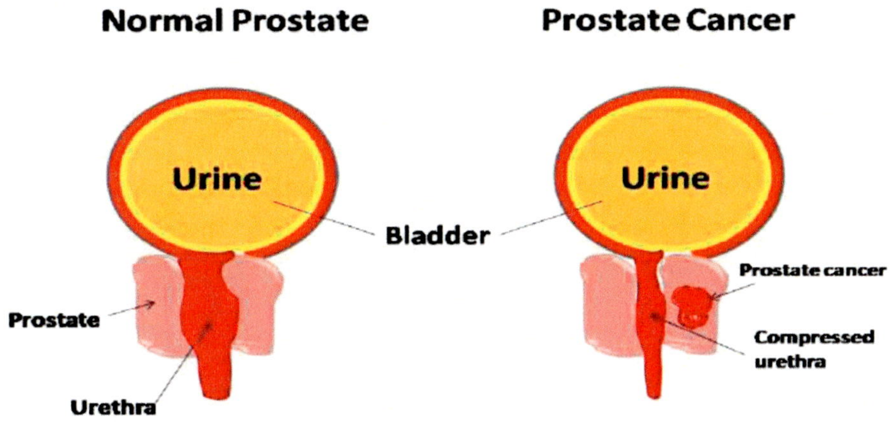

Fig. (8.7). Prostate cancer.

Mesoporous Silica Nanoparticles (MSNPs)

According to the findings, gonadotropin-releasing hormone GnRH analog-conjugated targeted MSNPs could be a viable technique for delivering target drugs to all hormone-dependent cancer cells. *Tambe P. et al.,* prepared Doxorubicin (DOX) loaded mesoporous silica nanoparticles (MSNPs) coupled with polyethylene glycol and an agonist of (GnRH). PEG-triptorelin was utilized to create improved MSNPs to deliver the DOX in a targeted manner. Targeted MSNPs were simply internalized in MCF-7 and LNCaP cancer cells and displayed considerable cytotoxicity. Furthermore, apoptosis studies revealed the manner of action as well as the early and late stages of apoptosis. Finally, the created versatile nanocarriers have advantageous properties, such as effective drug incorporation and better cancer cell targeting [27]. According to *Li K. et al.,* Docetaxel (DOC) and DOX co-delivery nanoparticles (DDC NPs) showed good localized delivery and impeding prostate cancer cells (PCA) *in vitro* and *in vivo.* DDC NPs exhibited a similar effect on apoptotic initiation, cytotoxicity, and antimigration as compared to the drug combinations. The synthetically generated DDC NPs increased drug accumulation in tumor tissues while reducing nonspecific accumulation in normal organs; consequently, the NPs efficiently increased the therapeutic impact besides toxicity reduction [28].

Androgen Signaling By Heat Shock Protein 90

Current medication aims to produce AR antagonist activity. Androgens are a significant promoter of prostate tumor growth. This form of the action takes advantage of AR's need for hormone activation, whereas current measures fail to work in castrate-resistant prostate cancer (CRPC), even though CRPC is still ligand/AR-dependent [100]. Testosterone and dihydrotestosterone (DHT) are the ligands of androgen, and the AR controls the transcription of androgen-sensitive genes by binding to endogenous androgenic ligands. Heat Shock Protein 90 (Hsp90) attaches to the AR in the absence of androgens, and when androgen attaches to the AR, Hsp90 releases the AR, exposing the Nuclear Localization Signal (NLS) [101].

CYP17A1, a 17–20 lyase and 17- hydroxylase of the cytochrome P450 family that transforms pregnanes into steroid hormones is irreversibly inhibited by abiraterone acetate [102]. As a result, it can limit prostate cancer growth by blocking the generation of androgen in the testis and adrenal glands, as well as in prostate cancers. The main negative effects are caused by increased mineralocorticoid levels as a result of CYP17A1 inhibition. Food and Drug Administration (FDA) approved Abiraterone acetate in 2011 for CRPC late-stage patients who had docetaxel, and then one year later for usage before docetaxel therapy. It is presently being evaluated alongside various treatments, and it was just approved by the FDA [103]. Clinical trials of other CYP17A1 inhibitors have failed to meet their primary endpoints. Darolutamide is a second-generation competitive oral AR antagonist [104]. A significant binding to the AR LBD has been discovered, which translates to substantial anti-tumor efficacy. Darolutamide, an oral AR antagonist has a lower blood-brain barrier penetration than other AR antagonists, which may lead to a better side-effect profile. Darolutamide is now being studied in phase 3 studies in nmCRPC with metastases free survival (MFS) as the key endpoint and in mHSPC with darolutamide along with regular ADT plus docetaxel.

Alpha Therapy Targeted Approach

The discharge of particles, such as alpha and beta particles, can be used to classify radionuclides. The specificity of targeting and inherent properties of the particle absorbed, such as probable range, appropriate length of traversing in tissue, and amount of energy transmitted, have an impact on the treatment efficacy of some of these radionuclides [105]. Surprisingly, radium-223 (^{223}Ra) is the first radiopharmaceutical drug to show enhanced survival in castration-resistant prostate cancer patients, with only minor adverse effects due to localized dose deposition [106]. According to the report of the ALSYMPCA trial, the Food and

Drug Administration (FDA) approved Xofigo ($^{223}RaCl_2$, previously Alpharadin) from Bayer Healthcare for clinical usage in 2013. Radium-223 dichloride is one of the intravenous targeted alpha treatments (TAT). It binds to hydroxyapatite, a significant component of bone, and is specifically used up in osteoblastic bone metastases [107]. In clinical settings, radium-223 is explored a lot and possesses calcium mimicking property and therefore can be employed to develop bone and bring forth strong and local cytotoxic effects on cancerous cells as well tumor microenvironment [108]. Radium-223 inhibits osteoblastic activity due to tumor, pathological bone formation, and tumor development in murine tumor models. The abnormal bone metabolic activity in PC xenograft models is reduced by Radium-223 by suppressing the numerous osteoblasts and osteoclasts. Under *in vitro* studies, T-cell mediated lysis of lung, breast, and prostate cancer may be enhanced by Radium-223 by inciting the immunogenic cell death [109]. Furthermore, recent studies have confirmed it to be effective in various forms of tumor and therefore, it can be used along with immunotherapies to confer even better clinical intervention [109]. Various clinical studies are undergoing with radium-223 dichloride in combination with several agents includes enzalutamide, docetaxel, olaparib, niraparib, pembrolizumab, atezolizumab, and sipuleucel-T.

Clinical Studies For Various Types of Cancer

A review of clinical studies in the recent past involving different screening parameters related to nano-formulation in cancer treatment has been summarized using a narrative approach. The parameters selected during screening included, "the completed interventional trial" and anticancer drug and nanoparticle were the main search criteria, followed by "phase of a clinical trial" it belongs and last was its "NCT number" as references to the specific trial. The role of nano-formulation for targeting chemotherapy medicines and their combination for cancer treatment is being continuously examined under various trials, a summary of the recent clinical trials involving nanocarriers for the treatment of different cancers is presented here and the compilation includes the findings of clinical trials in which cancer patients were subjected to either nanocarrier containing a single drug or a combination of standard nanocarriers. The exact search term combination used in the Clinical database search was: "cancer", "nanocarriers", "brain cancer", "breast cancer", "cervical cancer", "prostate cancer", and "lung cancer". Out of the 39 clinical trials included in this review, 15 trials "Has no results" and are compiled in Table **8.3** while other trials reported as "Has results" are discussed here.

Brain Cancer Trials

A phase I trial is being conducted to discern tumor drug levels and efficacy of Ferumoxytol Magnetic Resonance Imaging to estimate tumor-associated macrophages and envisage patient's response to the therapy with Nanoliposomal Irinotecan (Nal-IRI) (MM-398) in the reported research (NCT01770353). This research aims to learn more about MM-398's biodistribution and to see whether Ferumoxytol can be used as a tumor imaging agent. To measure tumor levels of irinotecan and SN-38, two tumor samples were collected up to 72 hours following the initial MM-398 IV injection. On October 2, 2019, the most recent primary outcome measure was submitted, which occurred throughout Cycle 1 of the MM-398 and the Pilot phase's treatment period (an active metabolite). The preliminary core biopsy was performed based on FMX-MRI in the tumor area showing maximum signal alterations on either the T2 or T1 sequences. The subsequent core biopsy was collected from the field showing minimum signal change on FMX-MRI, avoiding necrosis regions.

Table 8.3. Clinical trials study for different types of cancer.

Title	Drug/Nanoparticle	Phase	Last Updated	NCT Number
	Brain Cancer			
Liposomal Doxorubicin in Treating Children with Refractory Solid	Doxorubicin HCl liposome	I	April 28, 2015	NCT00019630
Nanosuspension of BP31510 (Ubidecarenone, USP) for Intravenous Injection into Patients with Solid Tumours	BP31510 monotherapy and in combination with chemotherapy	I	November 8, 2019	NCT01957735
Recurrent Grade 4 Malignant Brain Tumours: A Safety and Efficacy Study	TP-38 as drug	II	May 23, 2011	NCT00104091
Efficacy and Safety Panzem NCD in Glioblastoma Research	Panzem Nanocrystal Colloidal Dispersion	II	December 10, 2008	NCT00306618
	Breast Cancer			
Paricalcitol with Chemotherapy in the Treatment of Metastatic Breast Cancer in Women	Docetaxel, ixabepilone, paricalcitol, and paclitaxel albumin stabilized nanoparticle formulations	I	May 30, 2017	NCT00637897
In a Phase II study, Abraxanea was administered weekly as a single drug in the first-line treatment of metastatic breast cancer.	Nanoparticles of Paclitaxel Albumin for Injectable Suspension	II	May 11, 2012	NCT00251472
An Early Phase testing of Abraxane in conjunction with Phenelzine Sulphate in Patients with Metastatic Breast Cancer	Nanoparticle albumin-bound paclitaxel and Phenelzine Sulphate	I	November 13, 2019	NCT03505528
PK/PD Clinical Trial of Nanogen Pegfilgrastim (Pegcyte) in Breast Cancer Patients	Pegfilgrastim	I	December 19, 2017	NCT03376503

(Table 3) cont.....

Title	Drug/Nanoparticle	Phase	Last Updated	NCT Number
Prostate Cancer				
Magnetic Nanoparticle Thermoablation-Retention and Maintenance in the Prostate: A Phase 0 Study in Men	Magnetic Nanoparticle Injection	Early Phase 1	May 10, 2017	NCT02033447
Rapamycin Nanoparticles with Albumin-Bound Rapamycin in the Treatment of mTOR Mutated Advanced Cancer Patients	Nanoparticle albumin-bound Rapamycin	Early Phase 1	June 6, 2019	NCT02646319
Lapatinib and Paclitaxel are used to treat patients with advanced solid tumors	Lapatinib & paclitaxel	I	July 2, 2014	NCT00313599
Cervical cancer				
Rapamycin Nanoparticles with Albumin-Bound Rapamycin in the Treatment of Advanced Cancer Patients with mTOR Mutations	Nanoparticle albumin-bound Rapamycin	Early Phase 1	June 6, 2019	NCT02646319
Colorectal Cancer				
FOLFOXIRI Compared with FOLFIRI for Metastatic Colorectal Cancer	FOLFIRI and FOLFOXIRI	III	March 11, 2015	NCT01219920
A study collating adjuvant oral UFT/LV to 5-FU/l-LV in Stage III colorectal cancer was carried out (JCOG-020--MF)	5-FU+l leucovorin, UFT+ Leucovorin	III	September 22, 2016	NCT00190515
For patients with stage II/III colon cancer, 3 months of FOLFOX-4 vs. 6 months of FOLFOX-4 and Bevacizumab as adjuvant therapy	FOLFOX (Oxaliplatin, 5-Fluorouracil, Lederfolin)	III	November 26, 2014	NCT00646607

(Source: website- **http://clinicaltrials.gov/**).

Breast Cancer Trials

A trial updated on August 15, 2017, asserted the use of a combination of pertuzumab and Herceptin for the treatment of HER2-positive breast cancer. This included the testing efficiency and safety of four neoadjuvant regimens in patients (especially, females) with inflammation in a specific area, or early-stage HER2 positive breast cancer. Both patients can receive appropriate chemotherapy as per standard of care during the entire pre-and post-surgery phase, as well as any surgery and/or radiotherapy that may be needed. The duration of trial medication is expected to be 3-12 months, with a sample size of 100-500 people. The hypothesis of a Phase II study (NCT00629499) called Nanoparticle Albumin-Bound (Nab) Paclitaxel/Cyclophosphamide in Early-Stage Breast Cancer was last updated on September 9, 2013. Toxicity due to treatment, survival of patient, and recurrence of disease are the current major outcome criteria for adjuvant Nab-Paclitaxel utilizing a weekly dose protocol in this trial. Although the study's primary aim is not efficacy, patients' progression-free survival will be monitored. On December 4, 2018, another Phase II study, incorporated the combination of Nab-Paclitaxel, and Bevacizumab, followed by Bevacizumab and Erlotinib in Metastatic Breast Cancer (NCT00733408), was published. Erlotinib hydrochloride works by inhibiting a few of the enzymes that are vital for cell development. This research looks at erlotinib and bevacizumab as a replacement treatment after Nab-paclitaxel and bevacizumab, and how they can better control cancer progression with biological therapies. In a Phase II analysis (NCT00407888), Doxorubicin Hydrochloride, Cyclophosphamide, and Filgrastim were used to treat breast cancer of individuals who underwent surgery previously, followed by Nab-Paclitaxel which may or may not be given with Trastuzumab. The last time this trial was updated on August 31, 2017. The purpose is to investigate how well a combination of doxorubicin hydrochloride, cyclophosphamide, and filgrastim, enhanced with Nab-Paclitaxel and trastuzumab, for the management of breast cancer in patients who had already had surgery.

Cervical Cancer Trials

Phase II study (NCT00309959) updated on January 8, 2019, focused upon ABI-007 for the management of persistent or recurrent cervical cancer. This phase II trial is examining the effectiveness of ABI-007 in treating women with chronic or persistent cervical cancer. ABI-007 and other chemotherapy medications work in a variety of ways to stop tumor cells from developing, either by destroying them or by preventing their division. This is an open-label, multicenter study.

Colon/colorectal Cancer Trials

Phase IV trial (NCT00577031) comprises a combination of Avastin (Bevacizumab) with XELOX for controlling the colon or rectal cancer, also known as OBELIX Study, that was last updated on August 18, 2015. In patients who have a stable condition or a full or partial response to Avastin, therapy should be continued. The period of research therapy is anticipated to be until the onset of illness. In patients with metastatic colon or rectum cancer, this single-arm research would assess the effectiveness and safety of a first-line Avastin and XELOX (oxaliplatin + Xeloda) treatment.

CONCLUSION

Perhaps with the creation of nanocarriers, NPs' adaptability allows them to boost pharmacological synergy while maintaining meticulous control over the spatial and temporal disposition of the drug, which aids in lowering the chances of drug resistance and targeting many forms of cancer. Numerous biocompatible nanoscale carriers have been examined and coupled with a variety of active medicinal components. Researchers have looked into many forms of nanocarriers, which have helped them to overcome the constraints of traditional chemotherapy by boosting the solubility of the free medication and lowering the toxicity to healthy tissues. The development of nanocarriers has helped to overcome the limitation of anticancer medications; nonetheless, new problems have emerged. Although the safety of these nanoparticles is still unknown, the recent findings intensely imply that nanomaterials have a potential scope of being employed in the treatment of solid tumors.

CONSENT FOR PUBLICATION

Not applicable.

CONFLICT OF INTEREST

The authors declare no conflict of interest, financial or otherwise.

ACKNOWLEDGEMENT

Declared none.

REFERENCES

[1] Stahl M, Kohrman N, Gore SD, Kim TK, Zeidan AM, Prebet T. Epigenetics in cancer: A hematological perspective. PLoS Genet 2016; 12(10): e1006193. [http://dx.doi.org/10.1371/journal.pgen.1006193] [PMID: 27723796]

[2] Callow AD. Cardiovascular disease 2005 — the global picture. Vascul Pharmacol 2006; 45(5): 302-7. [http://dx.doi.org/10.1016/j.vph.2006.08.010] [PMID: 17074537]

[3] Ahuja R, Panwar N, Meena J, Singh M, Sarkar DP, Panda AK. Natural products and polymeric nanocarriers for cancer treatment: A review. Environ Chem Lett 2020; 18(6): 2021-30. [http://dx.doi.org/10.1007/s10311-020-01056-z]

[4] Liang XJ, Chen C, Zhao Y, Wang PC. Circumventing tumor resistance to chemotherapy by nanotechnology. Methods Mol Biol 2010; 596: 467-88. [http://dx.doi.org/10.1007/978-1-60761-416-6_21] [PMID: 19949937]

[5] Bandopadhyay S, Manchanda S, Chandra A, *et al.* Overview of different carrier systems for advanced drug delivery. Drug Delivery Systems. Academic Press 2020; pp. 179-233. [http://dx.doi.org/10.1016/B978-0-12-814487-9.00005-3]

[6] Dang Y, Guan J. Nanoparticle-based drug delivery systems for cancer therapy. Smart Materials in Medicine 2020; 1: 10-9. [http://dx.doi.org/10.1016/j.smaim.2020.04.001] [PMID: 34553138]

[7] Silva F, Cabral Campello MP, Paulo A. Radiolabeled gold nanoparticles for imaging and therapy of cancer. Materials (Basel) 2020; 14(1): 4. [http://dx.doi.org/10.3390/ma14010004] [PMID: 33375074]

[8] Conte C, Mastrotto F, Taresco V, *et al.* Enhanced uptake in 2D- and 3D- lung cancer cell models of redox responsive PEGylated nanoparticles with sensitivity to reducing extra- and intracellular environments. J Control Release 2018; 277: 126-41.
[http://dx.doi.org/10.1016/j.jconrel.2018.03.011] [PMID: 29534890]

[9] Rizzo LY, Theek B, Storm G, Kiessling F, Lammers T. Recent progress in nanomedicine: Therapeutic, diagnostic and theranostic applications. Curr Opin Biotechnol 2013; 24(6): 1159-66.
[http://dx.doi.org/10.1016/j.copbio.2013.02.020] [PMID: 23578464]

[10] Liu W, Zhu Y, Wang F, *et al.* Galactosylated chitosan-functionalized mesoporous silica nanoparticles for efficient colon cancer cell-targeted drug delivery. R Soc Open Sci 2018; 5(12): 181027.
[http://dx.doi.org/10.1098/rsos.181027] [PMID: 30662725]

[11] Salehi B, Selamoglu Z, S Mileski K, *et al.* Liposomal cytarabine as cancer therapy: From chemistry to medicine. Biomolecules 2019; 9(12): 773.
[http://dx.doi.org/10.3390/biom9120773] [PMID: 31771220]

[12] Kanapathipillai M, Brock A, Ingber DE. Nanoparticle targeting of anti-cancer drugs that alter intracellular signaling or influence the tumor microenvironment. Adv Drug Deliv Rev 2014; 79-80: 107-18.
[http://dx.doi.org/10.1016/j.addr.2014.05.005] [PMID: 24819216]

[13] Haley B, Frenkel E. Nanoparticles for drug delivery in cancer treatment. Urol Oncol 2008; 26(1): 57-64.
[http://dx.doi.org/10.1016/j.urolonc.2007.03.015] [PMID: 18190833]

[14] Kang MJ, Oh YJ, Shim YS, *et al.* The usefulness of circulating levels of leptin, kisspeptin, and neurokinin B in obese girls with precocious puberty 2018; 34: 627-30.
[http://dx.doi.org/10.1080/09513590.2017.1423467]

[15] Handali S, Moghimipour E, Rezaei M, *et al.* A novel 5-Fluorouracil targeted delivery to colon cancer using folic acid conjugated liposomes. Biomed Pharmacother 2018; 108: 1259-73.
[http://dx.doi.org/10.1016/j.biopha.2018.09.128] [PMID: 30372827]

[16] Sun T, Wu H, Li Y, *et al.* Targeting transferrin receptor delivery of temozolomide for a potential glioma stem cell-mediated therapy. Oncotarget 2017; 8(43): 74451-65.
[http://dx.doi.org/10.18632/oncotarget.20165] [PMID: 29088799]

[17] Finlay J, Roberts CM, Lowe G, Loeza J, Rossi JJ, Glackin CA. RNA-based TWIST1 inhibition *via* dendrimer complex to reduce breast cancer cell metastasis. BioMed Res Int 2015; 2015: 1-12.
[http://dx.doi.org/10.1155/2015/382745] [PMID: 25759817]

[18] Balakrishnan S, Bhat FA, Raja Singh P, *et al.* Gold nanoparticle-conjugated quercetin inhibits epithelial-mesenchymal transition, angiogenesis and invasiveness *via* EGFR/VEGFR-2-mediated pathway in breast cancer. Cell Prolif 2016; 49(6): 678-97.
[http://dx.doi.org/10.1111/cpr.12296] [PMID: 27641938]

[19] Han J, Li J, Jia W, *et al.* Photothermal therapy of cancer cells using novel hollow gold nanoflowers. Int J Nanomedicine 2014; 9: 517-26.
[PMID: 24549034]

[20] Chen C, Tang Y, Vlahovic B, Yan F. Electrospun polymer nanofibers decorated with noble metal nanoparticles for chemical sensing. Nanoscale Res Lett 2017; 12(1): 451.
[http://dx.doi.org/10.1186/s11671-017-2216-4] [PMID: 28704979]

[21] Miele D, Rossi S, Sandri G, *et al.* Chitosan oleate salt as an amphiphilic polymer for the surface modification of poly-lactic-glycolic acid (PLGA) nanoparticles. Preliminary studies of mucoadhesion and cell interaction properties. Mar Drugs 2018; 16(11): 447.
[http://dx.doi.org/10.3390/md16110447] [PMID: 30445668]

[22] Hasan M, Elkhoury K, Belhaj N, *et al.* Growth-inhibitory effect of chitosan-coated liposomes encapsulating curcumin on MCF-7 breast cancer cells. Mar Drugs 2020; 18(4): 217.

[http://dx.doi.org/10.3390/md18040217] [PMID: 32316578]

[23] Xu X, Liu A, Bai Y, *et al.* Co-delivery of resveratrol and p53 gene *via* peptide cationic liposomal nanocarrier for the synergistic treatment of cervical cancer and breast cancer cells. J Drug Deliv Sci Technol 2019; 51: 746-53.
[http://dx.doi.org/10.1016/j.jddst.2018.05.008]

[24] Ordikhani F, Erdem Arslan M, Marcelo R, *et al.* Drug delivery approaches for the treatment of cervical cancer. Pharmaceutics 2016; 8(3): 23.
[http://dx.doi.org/10.3390/pharmaceutics8030023] [PMID: 27447664]

[25] Pérez E, Fernández A, Olmo R, Teijón JM, Blanco MD. pH and glutathion-responsive hydrogel for localized delivery of paclitaxel. Colloids Surf B Biointerfaces 2014; 116: 247-56.
[http://dx.doi.org/10.1016/j.colsurfb.2014.01.004] [PMID: 24491841]

[26] Jaiswal MK, Pradhan A, Banerjee R, Bahadur D. Dual pH and temperature stimuli-responsive magnetic nanohydrogels for thermo-chemotherapy. J Nanosci Nanotechnol 2014; 14(6): 4082-9.
[http://dx.doi.org/10.1166/jnn.2014.8662] [PMID: 24738355]

[27] Tambe P, Kumar P, Paknikar KM, Gajbhiye V. Decapeptide functionalized targeted mesoporous silica nanoparticles with doxorubicin exhibit enhanced apoptotic effect in breast and prostate cancer cells. Int J Nanomedicine 2018; 13(13): 7669-80.
[http://dx.doi.org/10.2147/IJN.S184634] [PMID: 30538451]

[28] Li K, Zhan W, Chen Y, Jha RK, Chen X. Docetaxel and doxorubicin codelivery by nanocarriers for synergistic treatment of prostate cancer. Front Pharmacol 2019; 10(10): 1436.
[http://dx.doi.org/10.3389/fphar.2019.01436] [PMID: 31920642]

[29] Ashford M, Fell J. Targeting drugs to the colon: Delivery systems for oral administration. J Drug Target 1994; 2(3): 241-57.
[http://dx.doi.org/10.3109/10611869408996806] [PMID: 7812693]

[30] Langman M, Boyle P. Chemoprevention of colorectal cancer. Gut 1998; 43(4): 578-85.
[http://dx.doi.org/10.1136/gut.43.4.578] [PMID: 9824590]

[31] Akala EO, Elekwachi O, Chase V, Johnson H, Lazarre M, Scott K. Organic redox-initiated polymerization process for the fabrication of hydrogels for colon-specific drug delivery. Drug Dev Ind Pharm 2003; 29(4): 375-86.
[http://dx.doi.org/10.1081/DDC-120018373] [PMID: 12737531]

[32] Reddy JRK, Jyothsna MV, Saleem TSM, *et al.* Review on : Pulsatile drug delivery systems. J Pharm Sci Res 2009; 4: 109-15.

[33] Derakhshankhah H, Izadi Z, Alaei L, *et al.* Colon cancer and specific ways to deliver drugs to the large intestine. Anticancer Agents Med Chem 2017; 17(10): 1317-27.
[PMID: 28270073]

[34] Jain A. Colon targeting using pH sensitive materials. Adv Res Gastroenterol Hepatol 2017; 8: 1-3.

[35] Rudolph M, Klein S, Beckert TE, Petereit H, Dressman JB. A new 5-aminosalicylic acid multi-unit dosage form for the therapy of ulcerative colitis. Eur J Pharm Biopharm 2001; 51(3): 183-90.
[http://dx.doi.org/10.1016/S0939-6411(01)00134-5] [PMID: 11343881]

[36] Liu F, Moreno P, Basit AW. A novel double-coating approach for improved pH-triggered delivery to the ileo-colonic region of the gastrointestinal tract. Eur J Pharm Biopharm 2010; 74(2): 311-5.
[http://dx.doi.org/10.1016/j.ejpb.2009.11.008] [PMID: 19932177]

[37] Varum FJO, Hatton GB, Freire AC, Basit AW. A novel coating concept for ileo-colonic drug targeting: Proof of concept in humans using scintigraphy. Eur J Pharm Biopharm 2013; 84(3): 573-7.
[http://dx.doi.org/10.1016/j.ejpb.2013.01.002] [PMID: 23348235]

[38] Philip A, Philip B. Colon targeted drug delivery systems: A review on primary and novel approaches. Oman Med J 2010; 25(2): 70-8.

[http://dx.doi.org/10.5001/omj.2010.24] [PMID: 22125706]

[39] Ashford M, Fell J, Attwood D, Sharma H, Woodhead P. An evaluation of pectin as a carrier for drug targeting to the colon. J Control Release 1993; 26(3): 213-20. [http://dx.doi.org/10.1016/0168-3659(93)90188-B]

[40] Barclay TG, Day CM, Petrovsky N, Garg S. Review of polysaccharide particle-based functional drug delivery. Carbohydr Polym 2019; 221: 94-112. [http://dx.doi.org/10.1016/j.carbpol.2019.05.067] [PMID: 31227171]

[41] Song Q, Jia J, Niu X, *et al.* An oral drug delivery system with programmed drug release and imaging properties for orthotopic colon cancer therapy. Nanoscale 2019; 11(34): 15958-70. [http://dx.doi.org/10.1039/C9NR03802G] [PMID: 31418432]

[42] Si XY, Merlin D, Xiao B. Recent advances in orally administered cell-specific nanotherapeutics for inflammatory bowel disease. World J Gastroenterol 2016; 22(34): 7718-26. [http://dx.doi.org/10.3748/wjg.v22.i34.7718] [PMID: 27678353]

[43] Kunjiappan S, Pavadai P, Vellaichamy S, *et al.* Surface receptor-mediated targeted drug delivery systems for enhanced cancer treatment: A state-of-the-art review. Drug Dev Res 2021; 82(3): 309-40. [http://dx.doi.org/10.1002/ddr.21758] [PMID: 33170541]

[44] Shia J, Klimstra DS, Nitzkorski JR, *et al.* Immunohistochemical expression of folate receptor α in colorectal carcinoma: Patterns and biological significance. Hum Pathol 2008; 39(4): 498-505. [http://dx.doi.org/10.1016/j.humpath.2007.09.013] [PMID: 18342661]

[45] Weitman SD, Lark RH, Coney LR, *et al.* Distribution of the folate receptor GP38 in normal and malignant cell lines and tissues. Cancer Res 1992; 52(12): 3396-401. [PMID: 1596899]

[46] Xiong S, Yu B, Wu J, Li H, Lee RJ. Preparation, therapeutic efficacy and intratumoral localization of targeted daunorubicin liposomes conjugating folate-PEG-CHEMS. Biomed Pharmacother 2011; 65(1): 2-8. [http://dx.doi.org/10.1016/j.biopha.2010.10.003] [PMID: 21177069]

[47] Taylor P, Gordon S, Martinezpomares L. The mannose receptor: Linking homeostasis and immunity through sugar recognition. Trends Immunol 2005; 26(2): 104-10. [http://dx.doi.org/10.1016/j.it.2004.12.001] [PMID: 15668126]

[48] East L, Isacke CM. The mannose receptor family. Biochim Biophys Acta, Gen Subj 2002; 1572(2-3): 364-86. [http://dx.doi.org/10.1016/S0304-4165(02)00319-7] [PMID: 12223280]

[49] Xiong M, Lei Q, You X, *et al.* Mannosylated liposomes improve therapeutic effects of paclitaxel in colon cancer models. J Microencapsul 2017; 34(6): 513-21. [http://dx.doi.org/10.1080/02652048.2017.1339739] [PMID: 28705043]

[50] Shi Y, Ye P, Long X. Differential expression profiles of the transcriptome in breast cancer cell lines revealed by next generation sequencing. Cell Physiol Biochem 2017; 44(2): 804-16. [http://dx.doi.org/10.1159/000485344] [PMID: 29176322]

[51] Carty NJ, Foggitt A, Hamilton CR, Royle GT, Taylor I. Patterns of clinical metastasis in breast cancer: An analysis of 100 patients. Eur J Surg Oncol 1995; 21(6): 607-8. [http://dx.doi.org/10.1016/S0748-7983(95)95176-8] [PMID: 8631404]

[52] Im SA, Lu YS, Bardia A, *et al.* Overall survival with ribociclib plus endocrine therapy in breast cancer. N Engl J Med 2019; 381(4): 307-16. [http://dx.doi.org/10.1056/NEJMoa1903765] [PMID: 31166679]

[53] Anniebell S, Gopinath SCB. Polymer conjugated gold nanoparticles in biomedical applications. Curr Med Chem 2018; 25(12): 1433-45. [http://dx.doi.org/10.2174/0929867324666170116123633] [PMID: 28093984]

[54] Pandita D, Poonia N, Kumar S, Lather V, Madaan K. Dendrimers in drug delivery and targeting: Drug-dendrimer interactions and toxicity issues. J Pharm Bioallied Sci 2014; 6(3): 139-50. [http://dx.doi.org/10.4103/0975-7406.130965] [PMID: 25035633]

[55] Alven S, Aderibigbe B. Combination therapy strategies for the treatment of malaria. Molecules 2019; 24(19): 3601. [http://dx.doi.org/10.3390/molecules24193601] [PMID: 31591293]

[56] Tomalia DA, Reyna LA, Svenson S. Dendrimers as multi-purpose nanodevices for oncology drug delivery and diagnostic imaging. Biochem Soc Trans 2007; 35(1): 61-7. [http://dx.doi.org/10.1042/BST0350061] [PMID: 17233602]

[57] Faraday M. X. The Bakerian Lecture. Experimental relations of gold (and other metals) to light. Philos Trans R Soc Lond 1857; 147: 145-81. [http://dx.doi.org/10.1098/rstl.1857.0011]

[58] Wolinsky JB, Colson YL, Grinstaff MW. Local drug delivery strategies for cancer treatment: Gels, nanoparticles, polymeric films, rods, and wafers. J Control Release 2012; 159(1): 14-26. [http://dx.doi.org/10.1016/j.jconrel.2011.11.031] [PMID: 22154931]

[59] Rošic R, Kocbek P, Pelipenko J, Kristl J, Baumgartner S. Nanofibers and their biomedical use. Acta Pharm 2013; 63(3): 295-304. [http://dx.doi.org/10.2478/acph-2013-0024] [PMID: 24152893]

[60] Goonoo N, Bhaw-Luximon A, Jhurry D. Drug loading and release from electrospun biodegradable nanofibers. J Biomed Nanotechnol 2014; 10(9): 2173-99. [http://dx.doi.org/10.1166/jbn.2014.1885] [PMID: 25992453]

[61] Jayakumar R, Prabaharan M, Nair SV, Tamura H. Novel chitin and chitosan nanofibers in biomedical applications. Biotechnol Adv 2010; 28(1): 142-50. [http://dx.doi.org/10.1016/j.biotechadv.2009.11.001] [PMID: 19913083]

[62] Mukhtar M, Bilal M, Rahdar A, *et al.* Nanomaterials for diagnosis and treatment of brain cancer: Recent updates. Chemosensors (Basel) 2020; 8(4): 117. [http://dx.doi.org/10.3390/chemosensors8040117]

[63] Bhowmik A, Khan R, Ghosh MK. Blood brain barrier: A challenge for effectual therapy of brain tumors. BioMed Res Int 2015; 2015: 1-20. [http://dx.doi.org/10.1155/2015/320941] [PMID: 25866775]

[64] Meng J, Agrahari V, Youm I. Advances in targeted drug delivery approaches for the central nervous system tumors: The inspiration of nanobiotechnology. J Neuroimmune Pharmacol 2017; 12(1): 84-98. [http://dx.doi.org/10.1007/s11481-016-9698-1] [PMID: 27449494]

[65] Shinde G, Shiyani S, Shelke S, Chouthe R, Kulkarni D, Marvaniya K. Enhanced brain targeting efficiency using 5-FU (fluorouracil) lipid–drug conjugated nanoparticles in brain cancer therapy. Prog Biomater 2020; 9(4): 259-75. [http://dx.doi.org/10.1007/s40204-020-00147-y] [PMID: 33252721]

[66] Ashby LS, Shapiro WR. Intra-arterial cisplatin plus oral etoposide for the treatment of recurrent malignant glioma: A phase II study. J Neurooncol 2001; 51(1): 67-86. [http://dx.doi.org/10.1023/A:1006441104260] [PMID: 11349883]

[67] Fortin D, Desjardins A, Benko A, Niyonsega T, Boudrias M. Enhanced chemotherapy delivery by intraarterial infusion and blood-brain barrier disruption in malignant brain tumors. Cancer 2005; 103(12): 2606-15. [http://dx.doi.org/10.1002/cncr.21112] [PMID: 15880378]

[68] Remsen LG, Trail PA, Hellström I, Hellström KE, Neuwelt EA. Enhanced delivery improves the efficacy of a tumor-specific doxorubicin immunoconjugate in a human brain tumor xenograft model. Neurosurgery 2000; 46(3): 704-9. [http://dx.doi.org/10.1097/00006123-200003000-00034] [PMID: 10719867]

[69] Joshi S, Ellis JA, Ornstein E, Bruce JN. Intraarterial drug delivery for glioblastoma mutiforme. J Neurooncol 2015; 124(3): 333-43.
[http://dx.doi.org/10.1007/s11060-015-1846-6] [PMID: 26108656]

[70] Happold C, Roth P, Wick W, *et al.* ACNU-based chemotherapy for recurrent glioma in the temozolomide era. J Neurooncol 2009; 92(1): 45-8.
[http://dx.doi.org/10.1007/s11060-008-9728-9] [PMID: 18987781]

[71] Barar J, Rafi MA, Pourseif MM, Omidi Y. Blood-brain barrier transport machineries and targeted therapy of brain diseases. Bioimpacts 2016; 6(4): 225-48.
[http://dx.doi.org/10.15171/bi.2016.30] [PMID: 28265539]

[72] Wu H, Hu K, Jiang X. From nose to brain: Understanding transport capacity and transport rate of drugs. Expert Opin Drug Deliv 2008; 5(10): 1159-68.
[http://dx.doi.org/10.1517/17425247.5.10.1159] [PMID: 18817519]

[73] Savale S, Mahajan H. Nose to brain: A versatile mode of drug delivery system. Asian J Biomater Res 2017; 3(16): 16-38.

[74] Bahadur S, Pathak K. Physicochemical and physiological considerations for efficient nose-to-brain targeting. Expert Opin Drug Deliv 2012; 9(1): 19-31.
[http://dx.doi.org/10.1517/17425247.2012.636801] [PMID: 22171740]

[75] Major I, McConville C. Vaginal drug delivery for the localised treatment of cervical cancer. Drug Deliv Transl Res 2017; 7(6): 817-28.
[http://dx.doi.org/10.1007/s13346-017-0395-2] [PMID: 28597123]

[76] Lorusso D, Petrelli F, Coinu A, Raspagliesi F, Barni S. A systematic review comparing cisplatin and carboplatin plus paclitaxel-based chemotherapy for recurrent or metastatic cervical cancer. Gynecol Oncol 2014; 133(1): 117-23.
[http://dx.doi.org/10.1016/j.ygyno.2014.01.042] [PMID: 24486604]

[77] Petry KU. HPV and cervical cancer. Scand J Clin Lab Invest 2014; 74(sup244): 59-62.
[http://dx.doi.org/10.3109/00365513.2014.936683] [PMID: 25083895]

[78] McConville C. The use of localised vaginal drug delivery as part of a neoadjuvant chemotherapy strategy in the treatment of cervical cancer. Gynecol Obstet Res 2015; 2(1): 26-8.
[http://dx.doi.org/10.17140/GOROJ-2-106]

[79] Kijanka M, Dorresteijn B, Oliveira S, van Bergen en Henegouwen PMP. Nanobody-based cancer therapy of solid tumors. Nanomedicine (Lond) 2015; 10(1): 161-74.
[http://dx.doi.org/10.2217/nnm.14.178] [PMID: 25597775]

[80] Ma Y, Zheng Y, Liu K, *et al.* Nanoparticles of poly (lactide-co-glycolide)-da-tocopheryl polyethylene glycol 1000 succinate random copolymer for cancer treatment. Nanoscale Res Lett 2010; 5(7): 1161-9.
[http://dx.doi.org/10.1007/s11671-010-9620-3] [PMID: 20596457]

[81] Sun L, Wu Q, Peng F, Liu L, Gong C. Strategies of polymeric nanoparticles for enhanced internalization in cancer therapy. Colloids Surf B Biointerfaces 2015; 135: 56-72.
[http://dx.doi.org/10.1016/j.colsurfb.2015.07.013] [PMID: 26241917]

[82] de Jong WH, Borm PJA. Drug delivery and nanoparticles: Applications and hazards. Int J Nanomedicine 2008; 3(2): 133-49.
[http://dx.doi.org/10.2147/IJN.S596] [PMID: 18686775]

[83] Cheng C, Meng Y, Zhang Z, Li Y, Zhang Q. Tumoral Acidic pH-Responsive *cis* - Diaminodichloroplatinum-incorporated Cy5.5-PEG- *g* -A-HA nanoparticles for targeting delivery of CDDP against cervical cancer. ACS Appl Mater Interfaces 2018; 10(32): 26882-92.
[http://dx.doi.org/10.1021/acsami.8b07425] [PMID: 30024147]

[84] Jin KT, Lu ZB, Chen JY, *et al.* Recent trends in nanocarrier-based targeted chemotherapy: Selective delivery of anticancer drugs for effective lung, colon, cervical, and breast cancer treatment. J

Nanomater 2020; 2020: 1-14.
[http://dx.doi.org/10.1155/2020/9184284]

[85] Sarisozen C, Abouzeid AH, Torchilin VP. The effect of co-delivery of paclitaxel and curcumin by transferrin-targeted PEG-PE-based mixed micelles on resistant ovarian cancer in 3-D spheroids and *in vivo* tumors. Eur J Pharm Biopharm 2014; 88(2): 539-50.
[http://dx.doi.org/10.1016/j.ejpb.2014.07.001] [PMID: 25016976]

[86] Kesharwani P, Banerjee S, Gupta U, *et al.* PAMAM dendrimers as promising nanocarriers for RNAi therapeutics. Mater Today 2015; 18(10): 565-72.
[http://dx.doi.org/10.1016/j.mattod.2015.06.003]

[87] Wang AZ, Langer R, Farokhzad OC. Nanoparticle delivery of cancer drugs. Annu Rev Med 2012; 63(1): 185-98.
[http://dx.doi.org/10.1146/annurev-med-040210-162544] [PMID: 21888516]

[88] Liu TY, Hussein WM, Jia Z, *et al.* Self-adjuvanting polymer-peptide conjugates as therapeutic vaccine candidates against cervical cancer. Biomacromolecules 2013; 14(8): 2798-806.
[http://dx.doi.org/10.1021/bm400626w] [PMID: 23837675]

[89] Mekuria SL, Debele TA, Chou HY, Tsai HC. IL-6 antibody and RGD peptide conjugated poly(amidoamine) dendrimer for targeted drug delivery of HeLa cells. J Phys Chem B 2016; 120(1): 123-30.
[http://dx.doi.org/10.1021/acs.jpcb.5b11125] [PMID: 26670944]

[90] Langer R. Biomaterials in drug delivery and tissue engineering: One laboratory's experience. Acc Chem Res 2000; 33(2): 94-101.
[http://dx.doi.org/10.1021/ar9800993] [PMID: 10673317]

[91] Hu X, Liu S, Zhou G, Huang Y, Xie Z, Jing X. Electrospinning of polymeric nanofibers for drug delivery applications. J Control Release 2014; 185(1): 12-21.
[http://dx.doi.org/10.1016/j.jconrel.2014.04.018] [PMID: 24768792]

[92] Garg T, Singh O, Arora S, Murthy RSR. Scaffold: A novel carrier for cell and drug delivery. Crit Rev Ther Drug Carrier Syst 2012; 29(1): 1-63.
[http://dx.doi.org/10.1615/CritRevTherDrugCarrierSyst.v29.i1.10] [PMID: 22356721]

[93] Bahram M, Hoseinzadeh F, Farhadi K, Saadat M, Najafi-Moghaddam P, Afkhami A. Synthesis of gold nanoparticles using pH-sensitive hydrogel and its application for colorimetric determination of acetaminophen, ascorbic acid and folic acid. Colloids Surf A Physicochem Eng Asp 2014; 441: 517-24.
[http://dx.doi.org/10.1016/j.colsurfa.2013.09.024]

[94] Caramella CM, Rossi S, Ferrari F, Bonferoni MC, Sandri G. Mucoadhesive and thermogelling systems for vaginal drug delivery. Adv Drug Deliv Rev 2015; 92: 39-52.
[http://dx.doi.org/10.1016/j.addr.2015.02.001] [PMID: 25683694]

[95] Siegel RL, Miller KD, Jemal A. Cancer statistics, 2017. CA Cancer J Clin 2017; 67(1): 7-30.
[http://dx.doi.org/10.3322/caac.21387] [PMID: 28055103]

[96] Mirzaei M, Mirzadeh M, Mirzaei M. Mortality rate and years of life lost due to prostate cancer in Yazd province, Iran: A 10-year study. Sultan Qaboos Univ Med J 2018; 17(4): 424.
[http://dx.doi.org/10.18295/squmj.2017.17.04.008] [PMID: 29372084]

[97] Dai C, Heemers H, Sharifi N. Androgen signaling in prostate cancer. Cold Spring Harb Perspect Med 2017; 7(9): a030452.
[http://dx.doi.org/10.1101/cshperspect.a030452] [PMID: 28389515]

[98] Pagliarulo V. Androgen deprivation therapy for prostate cancer.Molecular & Diagnostic Imaging in Prostate Cancer. 2018; pp. 1-30.

[99] Barani M, Sabir F, Rahdar A, Arshad R, Kyzas GZ. Nanotreatment and nanodiagnosis of prostate cancer: Recent updates. Nanomaterials (Basel) 2020; 10(9): 1696.

[http://dx.doi.org/10.3390/nano10091696] [PMID: 32872181]

[100] Moore TW, Mayne CG, Katzenellenbogen JA. Minireview: Not picking pockets: Nuclear receptor alternate-site modulators (NRAMs). Mol Endocrinol 2010; 24(4): 683-95.
[http://dx.doi.org/10.1210/me.2009-0362] [PMID: 19933380]

[101] Kargbo RB. PROTAC compounds targeting androgen receptor for cancer therapeutics: Prostate cancer and Kennedy's disease. ACS Med Chem Lett 2020; 11(6): 1092-3.
[http://dx.doi.org/10.1021/acsmedchemlett.0c00236] [PMID: 32550986]

[102] Scott LJ. Abiraterone acetate: A review in metastatic castration-resistant prostrate cancer. Drugs 2017; 77(14): 1565-76.
[http://dx.doi.org/10.1007/s40265-017-0799-9] [PMID: 28819727]

[103] Rydzewska LHM, Burdett S, Vale CL, *et al.* Adding abiraterone to androgen deprivation therapy in men with metastatic hormone-sensitive prostate cancer: A systematic review and meta-analysis. Eur J Cancer 2017; 84: 88-101.
[http://dx.doi.org/10.1016/j.ejca.2017.07.003] [PMID: 28800492]

[104] Fizazi K, Albiges L, Loriot Y, Massard C. ODM-201: A new-generation androgen receptor inhibitor in castration-resistant prostate cancer. Expert Rev Anticancer Ther 2015; 15(9): 1007-17.
[http://dx.doi.org/10.1586/14737140.2015.1081566] [PMID: 26313416]

[105] Volkert WA, Goeckeler WF, Ehrhardt GJ, Ketring AR. Therapeutic radionuclides: Production and decay property considerations. J Nucl Med 1991; 32(1): 174-85.
[PMID: 1988628]

[106] Parker C, Nilsson S, Heinrich D, *et al.* Alpha emitter radium-223 and survival in metastatic prostate cancer. N Engl J Med 2013; 369(3): 213-23.
[http://dx.doi.org/10.1056/NEJMoa1213755] [PMID: 23863050]

[107] Wilson JM, Parker C. The safety and efficacy of radium-223 dichloride for the treatment of advanced prostate cancer. Expert Rev Anticancer Ther 2016; 16(9): 911-8.
[http://dx.doi.org/10.1080/14737140.2016.1222273] [PMID: 27501059]

[108] Suominen MI, Fagerlund KM, Rissanen JP, *et al.* Radium-223 inhibits osseous prostate cancer growth by dual targeting of cancer cells and bone microenvironment in mouse models. Clin Cancer Res 2017; 23(15): 4335-46.
[http://dx.doi.org/10.1158/1078-0432.CCR-16-2955] [PMID: 28364014]

[109] Malamas AS, Gameiro SR, Knudson KM, Hodge JW. Sublethal exposure to alpha radiation (223Ra dichloride) enhances various carcinomas' sensitivity to lysis by antigen-specific cytotoxic T lymphocytes through calreticulin-mediated immunogenic modulation. Oncotarget 2016; 7(52): 86937-47.
[http://dx.doi.org/10.18632/oncotarget.13520] [PMID: 27893426]

CHAPTER 9

Nanoemulsion: A Potential Carrier for Topical Drug Delivery

Karthikeyan Kesavan[1,*], **Parasuraman Mohan**[1], **Sunil K Jain**[1], **Olivia Parra-Marín**[2] and **Selvasankar Murugesan**[3]

[1] *Department of Pharmacy, Guru Ghasidas Vishwavidyalaya (A Central University), Bilaspur, Chhattisgarh, India*

[2] *Departamento de Biología Molecular y Biotecnología, Instituto de Investigaciones Biomédicas, Universidad Nacional Autónoma de México, Ciudad Universitaria, 04510, Ciudad de México, Mexico*

[3] *Mother and Child Health Department, SIDRA Medicine, Doha, Qatar*

Abstract: Nanoemulsions (NEs) are stable nanocarrier systems consisting mainly of oil and water, which are stabilized by surfactant with cosurfactant. Due to their typical size, nano-emulsions are transparent or translucent, and minute droplet size makes them stable against sedimentation or creaming. The nanoemulsion system may be in the form of oil-in-water (O/W) or water-in-oil (W/O). The recent literature revealed that NEs as a colloidal carrier system has been confirmed to be a valuable strategy to improve the bioavailability of topically applied drugs. NE has been proposed as a viable alternative to conventional topical dosage forms due to the ability to overcome the skin/ocular barriers faced after administration. Better permeation rate, improved therapeutic efficacy and reduction of dose, non–specific toxicity, and targeted drug delivery system can improve drug effectiveness when drugs are incorporated into NEs. In recent years, research studies have focused more on ion nanoemulsion systems using a mixture of surfactants to solve critical factors, such as solubility, stability, and drug delivery applications. This chapter outlines the recent development in nanoemulsion as a delivery system to study topical drug delivery.

Keywords: Nanocarrier, Nanoemulsion, Ocular, Skin, Topical drug delivery.

INTRODUCTION

Oil and water are immiscible liquids for blending two phases; the phases are miscible with the addition of the third substance like an emulsifier [1]. Uniting the combination of these phases requires energy contribution to make up dissimilar contacts with in water-oil systems that can restore similar phase

* **Corresponding author Karthikeyan Kesavan:** Department of Pharmacy, Guru Ghasidas Vishwavidyalaya (A Central University), Bilaspur, Chhattisgarh, India; E-mails: **kesavanmpharm@gmail.com**; **k7_76@rediffmail.com**

Akhlesh K. Jain & Keerti Mishra (Eds.)

systems like water-water and oil-oil connections. The immiscible oil and interfacial water tension are as high as 30-50 dynes/cm [2]. The reduction of interfacial tension to the addition of a surface-active agent or surfactant, or emulsifier can be utilized based on a polar head (water-loving) and non-polar tail (oil-loving) groups with the ability to absorb the oil-water interface [3]. The lower concentration of surface-active agent adsorbs at the oil-water interface, expands the interfacial area, or diminishes the interfacial tension [2]. A stable emulsion system is formed by a minute amount of suitable surface active agent added and mechanically mixed with oil and water components. The consequence of the biphasic dispersion system shows that oil globules coated with a surface-active agent are promptly distributed throughout the distribution medium. These emulsified systems are opaque or milky because the globule diameter ranges from 0.1 to 1 micron [3]. As a general rule, the class of emulsion systems is formed based on the type of emulsifier used [4]. W/O type of emulsion is generated by the surfactant used in the system that is more soluble in the oil phase than water, and *vice versa*. In another way, the continuous phase of the emulsion system is in which the surface-active agents are predominantly soluble. The emulsified system is called emulsions, nanoemulsions, submicron emulsions, or mini emulsions. There are numerous identical properties among these systems. Nevertheless, every emulsified system has its physical properties and thermodynamic stability for making a specific application compared with other systems [5].

The emulsified systems have three main compositions: aqueous phase, oily phase, and a combination of surface-active agents. An appropriate emulsifying agent is vital for the system to formulate a stable emulsion from the discontinuous and continuous phases. There are fundamental emulsions like oil-in-water (O/W) emulsion, in which oil droplets are dispersed into the continuous water phase, and water-in-oil (W/O) emulsion, wherein water droplets are dispersed into the continuous oil phase. The multiple types of emulsion, like oil-in-water-in-oil (O/W/O) or water-in-oil-in-water (W/O/W) emulsion, are formed by the overlap of O/W and W/O types of emulsion in which minute globules are within larger ones [6, 7]. Significant differences exist among the systems like emulsion, nanoemulsion, and microemulsions. Emulsions appear to be milky, and their globule size ranges between 100 nm and 1mm [8]. The systems are thermodynamically unstable due to physical contact between the oil and water phase.

Conversely, emulsions are kinetically stable systems because the statement of the energy formation is more significant than zero. The surface-active agent is tightly adsorbed between the oil /water interface, so the system is kinetically stable [9]. Expressly, the microemulsion is noted as thermodynamically stable, isotropic, clear, and usually has a globule size less than 100 nm in diameter and is commonly close to the matching micelles system [10]. Low energy input is required to form the microemulsion, and an immense amount of surfactant is needed to form the system compared to nanoemulsion.

A nanoemulsion with globule size in the nanometric scale (less than 1 micron) is denoted as nano, submicron, mini, or ultrafine emulsions [11 - 13]. The term nano-emulsion is preferred because it provides a nanoscale size range of droplets and avoids misapprehension when compared with microemulsion, which alters their physicochemical properties and leads to superior kinetic stability. The different instability processes such as flocculation and coalescence are insignificant in the form of nano-emulsified systems. The formulation requires a high-speed homogenizer with high energy inputs, and a lower amount of surfactant is sufficient [14 - 17]. The choice of nanocarrier system is widely used for topical delivery systems like liposomes, niosomes, transferosomes, ethosomes, solid lipid nanoparticles (SLN) and nanostructured lipid carriers (NLC) [18 - 21]. Even though nanoemulsion systems have numerous pharmaceutical applications in the field of pharmaceutics, cosmetics, *etc.*, it likewise assumes an imperative part as reaction initiation for many polymer dispersions and nanoparticle synthesis, owing to the smaller size globule, reasonably long-term stability, and effective solubilization capacity, acting as a medium for active pharmaceutical substance, improving the therapeutic efficiency, minimizing the drug dose, and by this means side effects and toxicity. The presence of surfactants in the emulsified system has to alter the membrane fluidity that helps to enhance the absorption of active drug molecules [22].

The nanoemulsions system is used for parenteral, oral, ocular, and topical administration [23 - 26]. Nanoemulsion offers significant advantages in topical drug delivery systems, including (i) less surfactant concentration leads to offer minor skin irritation, (ii) adequate penetration capacity, and (iii) high drug-loading efficiency, and topical administration may be beneficial when compared to oral administration to avoid chemical or enzymatic degradation from the gastrointestinal tract and first-pass metabolic effect of drug molecule [15, 27 - 29]. It is an ideal route of drug administration because of various apparent benefits compared to parenteral and oral routes in which patient compliance and therapeutic drug efficacy are considered in the report. This system is most pertinent for encapsulating poorly soluble drugs with superior stability [30, 31]. It is mainly suitable for topical drug delivery to circumvent systemic side effects, and it acts as potential cargo for the delivery of drugs to the specific site of action [32, 33].

Moreover, due to the smaller droplet size, the system has advantages such as good rheological properties, excellent colloidal stability, and a low sedimentation rate.

For the past two decades, researchers have been focusing on nanoemulsion systems by utilizing different types of surface-active agents to sort the issues like the solubility of a drug molecule with delivery applications, improve the drug specificity and site of action, and improve the bioavailability of drugs through a biological membrane. This review aims to summarize the recently developed nanoemulsion formulation examined concerning their use in the topical route (ocular/skin) of administrations.

Components of a Nanoemulsion

Oil/lipids

The oil/lipid phase plays a significant function in formulating nanoemulsions to solubilize drug substances. In the formulation of the O/W type of emulsion, the amount of oil/lipid may contain in the range of 2 to 20%w/w, depending on the site of application [34]. The broad range of oil/lipid and the combination has been explored in Table 1 and 2. Generally, oils used in nanoemulsions like soybean oil, rice-bran oil, coconut oil, cottonseed oil, sesame oil and safflower oil [35, 36]. D-α-Tocopherol (vitamin E) has been extensively used as a vehicle to formulate nanoemulsion [37]. Fatty acids like Oleic acid and ethyl oleate are used as vehicles in the oral, topical, and parenteral formulations of nanoemulsion [38]. The esters of fatty acids oils (isopropyl myristate, isopropyl palmitate), triacetin (glyceryl triacetate), and Sefsol 218 (propylene glycol mono ethyl ether) can also be used to make nanoemulsion [3].

Surfactants and co-surfactants

Surfactant moieties are mainly incorporated in nanoemulsion to stabilize the formulation by lowering the interfacial tension and preventing globule agglomeration. These moieties readily adsorbed on the oil-water interface to stabilize globules by electro-steric interaction—a frequently used surfactant in nanoemulsions, such as phosphatidylcholine formed from egg yolk or soybean. For parenteral nanoemulsion preparation, cremophor EL (Polyoxyl-35 castor oil) and sodium deoxycholate (bile salt) are commonly used as a surfactant [39].Tween (Polyoxyethylene sorbitan monolaurate) 20, 40, 60, and 80 [40], Span (Sorbitan monolaurate) 20, 40, 60, and 80 [41], and Solutol HS-15 (polyoxyethylene-660-hydroxy stearate) are generally used [42]. Generally, co-surfactants are incorporated to complement surfactants like ethanol, propylene glycol, polyethylene glycol, transcutol IP, glycerin, ethylene glycol, and propanol.

Preservatives, Antioxidants, and Chemoprotectants

Preservatives are an essential component system to preserve the product for a prolonged storage period. The ideal characteristics of preservatives should meet the following criteria as stability on heat and storage, compatibility with other excipients used in the product; minimum quantity is required to produce broad-spectrum antimicrobial activity, and the selected preservative should be effective on both aqueous, and oil phase and does not have any toxicity, *etc.*, The different preservatives used in an emulsified system include acid and its derivatives *viz.*, benzoic acid, sorbic acid, propionic acid and dehydroacetic acid. The class of alcohols like chlorobutanol and phenoxy-2-ethanol are commonly used as a vehicle in the formulation of the ophthalmic product, and quaternary ammonium compounds can act as a broad spectrum preservative for an extensive choice of formulations [38]. The main components of the emulsified system contain oils/fats, which are readily oxidized on exposure to atmospheric conditions. Therefore, an antioxidant substance is required to diminish the oxidation process to safeguard the product [43]. The different classes of antioxidants are recommended to prevent oxidative degradation of formulation by substituting either reducing agents like ascorbic acid and sodium bisulfite or blocking agents such as butylated hydroxy toluene, tocopherols, *etc.*, or synergists, *e.g.*, ascorbic acid, citric acid, tartaric acid, *etc.*, the transparent system of nanoemulsion which implies that easily penetration of visible and UV rays photodegradation of components system.

Mechanisms of Emulsion Formation

Oil, water, emulsifier, and energy power are essential for nanoemulsion formulation. It may be calculated from the necessity of energy desired to the expansion of interface, $\Delta A\gamma$ (where ΔA is the enlarged surface of interface from the total bulk oil with area $A1$ generates a vast number of globules with area $A2$; $A2 >> A1$, γ is denoted as interfacial tension). As γ is positive, the energy is increased, and the expansion of interfacial area ultimately is positive; this power of energy can not be compensated by the little entropy of dispersion $T\Delta S$ (which is additionally positive), and hence the sum of free energy developed in nanoemulsion formation; ΔG is positive, $\Delta G = \Delta A\gamma - T\Delta S$. Accordingly, the nanoemulsion formation is non-spontaneous, and power is mandatory for the formation of minute globule size. Whereas the formation of macro emulsion is straightforward, and thus, a sophisticated instrument like Silverson Mixer is used to prepare the emulsion system. Since the submicron range of globule size is not an easy process to produce, it is necessary for the high quantity of emulsifier and energy. The principles of Laplace pressure P (The pressure variation from in and outside of the globule) indicated that the formation of nanoemulsion requires a high amount of energy.

$$P = \gamma(\frac{1}{R1} + \frac{1}{R2})$$

R1 and R2 are the radii of curvature of the drop.

For a sphere-shaped drop, $R1 = R2 = R$ and,

$$P = \frac{2\gamma}{R}$$

The size reduction of globule size into minute ones should be effectively deformed, and this way of deformation will increase the *p*-value. This will be revealed that the sphere-shaped globules converted into a prolate ellipsoid. Spherical-shaped globules have a single radius of curvature Ra, in the case of the prolate ellipsoidal structure containing two radii of curvature Rb1 and Rb2. Therefore, a high-stress level is necessary to deform from high curvature to low curvature. While the stress is permeated mainly by the encircling liquid through agitation, vigorous agitation is required to produce potent stress; this will play an essential function in forming smaller droplet sizes. Surfactants play a significant role in the development of nanoemulsions. By reducing the interfacial tension, *p* is minimized, and in the same way, the need for stress to reduce droplet size is also minimized. The newly formed droplets can be stabilized by surfactants. Numerous processes take place throughout the emulsification step, specifically droplet size reduction, surface-active agents adsorption, and collision of droplets. It could be a valid reason for coalescence during the emulsification process, and each of these processes often happens within a short period throughout the emulsification process [44]. The emulsification method revealed that the dynamic process and microsecond time were taken to attain these events. Two important factors that are essential to consider are emulsion formation hydrodynamics and interfacial science.

Preparation of Nanoemulsion

Nanoemulsion can be formulated by high-energy emulsification techniques, including high-pressure homogenization, microfluidization, and ultrasonication or low-energy emulsification techniques, like solvent diffusion method and phase inversion temperature (PIT) or spontaneous emulsification technique (Fig. **9.1**).

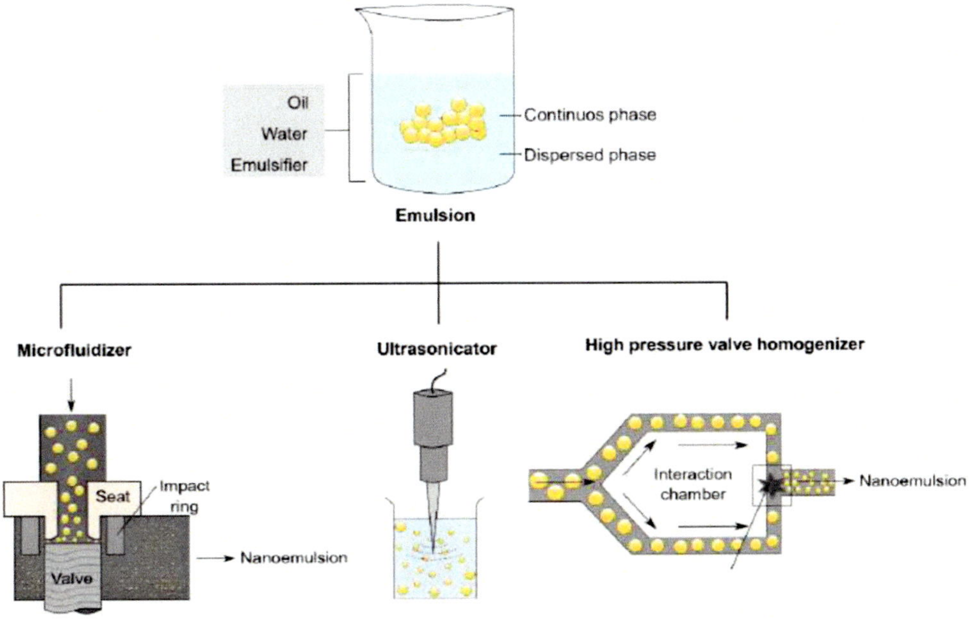

Fig. (9.1). Different methods of preparation of nanoemulsion.

High Energy Emulsification Method

This method uses high-energy producing mechanical devices to generate potent disruptive forces for size reduction. A high amount of energy is required to rupture the intermolecular force of attraction, hydrogen bonding, and Van der Waals forces between high surface tension liquids and low surface tension liquids [45]. The potential energy is given by shear stress, and powerful ultrasonic waves are used to break the larger droplets into nano-sized droplets [46]. A high-shear mixer employed a high-speed rotor, *i.e.*, powered by an electrical motor device to produce a high flow rate of liquids with shear. During this process, fluid feels a higher impact on the border of the rotor than compared with the axis of the rotor; the difference in velocity generated shear force. Moreover, the stator is known as a fixed stationary rotor and retains a very nearer clearance opening to the rotor. Due to this construction of the system, the material experienced on high shear of force *via* the larger droplets converts into smaller-sized droplets, leaving the rotor smoothly [47].

The ultrasonic waves used to form bubbles are disintegrated and simultaneously produce a considerable amount of energy into the system formed into minute droplets of internal phase with uniform distribution [48, 49]. The high-pressure homogenization technique generated potent turbulence action along with high shear stream on the oil and water system under high pressure. The frequently formed turbulence wave on this system's dispersed phase changed into minute droplets that may be less than 100 nm. The droplet size is controlled by maintaining a dynamic equilibrium between breakage and coalescence. Due to this reason, the droplets are uniform in size and improved consistency with an enhanced shelf life of the product [50].

Low Energy Emulsification Methods

The primary function of these methods is that energy consumption is maintained within the system to produce very fine droplets. This emulsification method is based on changing the preparation parameters, such as temperature and composition of ingredients that may influence the hydrophile-lipophile balance (HLB) of the formulation. The formed product is flexible; thus, the encapsulated drug molecule is preserved without damage or breakage of the dispersed system. This method consumes less energy and is more suitable for large-scale production [51]. This method includes spontaneous emulsification [52], phase inversion [53], and the less utilized catastrophic phase inversion method [54].

Spontaneous Emulsification

Spontaneous emulsification is similar to that of the nanoprecipitation technique. The preparation procedure involved two phases: the aqueous phase consisting of hydrophilic surfactant and an oil phase consisting of a drug molecule, oil, oil-soluble surfactant, and partially water-miscible organic solvent. The prepared organic phase is added drop-wise into an aqueous phase with slow stirring to form an O/W nanoemulsion. To further explain, the oil phase is solubilized with the help of a water-miscible solvent like acetone which is emulsified into an aqueous phase containing surfactant solution. Again the addition of solvent acetone into the organic medium and water shift towards each other. Due to these reasons, minute droplets of oil are formed, eventually coated by surface-active agents. Applying convection current constantly with the help of a magnetic stirrer leads to the formation of oil droplets distributed into the bulk phase. So, the newly formed surface by solvent diffusion is instantaneously enclosed by adjacent surfactant moiety. To formulate nano-scale droplets, it is essential to use a vast amount of water-miscible components in the organic phase containing oil before mixing [47].

Phase Inversion Method

Nanoemulsion prepared by phase inversion temperature (PIT) method changes explicitly in the aqueous/oil solubility of surface-active agents by modifying temperature variations in the system. It may be possible to convert the W/O type of emulsion to O/W emulsion through an intermediatory bicontinuous phase of the system. In this method, the exact amount of oil, water, and surfactant components are heated to a programmed temperature called PIT, then cooled instantly. The temperature changes from low to a higher level can lead to the formation of opening and reversal interfacial arrangement as a reason for phase inversion. Simultaneously, this process is continued, and the interfacial structure closes once again, entrapping oil or water [55].

Catastrophic inversion is known as the transition of the spontaneous curvature radius, formed by altering the quantity portion of the phase. By gradually adding an aqueous phase into the oil phase, water droplets are produced in a dispersion oil phase.

Catastrophic inversion is the transition of an instinctive radius of a curve that can be produced by altering the quantity portion of the phase. Enhancing the volume fraction ratio of water alters the instinctive curve of the surfactant primarily to stabilize the W/O nanoemulsion, which changes into O/W at the inversion point. The surfactant used in this procedure is excellent because it forms a flexible monolayer at the oil-water interface, bringing about a bicontinuous nanoemulsion at this inversion point [56].

Characterization of Emulsions

The characterization of nanoemulsion is an essential parameter to ensure the product quality, which falls within the suitable size of droplets. This is because the viscosity of nanodispersion and charge on the globule surface are stable during the expiration period. Commonly used analytical techniques to characterize nanoemulsion include globule size determination, polydispersity index, surface charge measurement, viscosity, surface tension determination, nuclear magnetic resonance (NMR), differential scanning calorimetry, *etc.*; these essential characterization techniques will be discussed in the forthcoming section.

Particle Size Determination

The various sophisticated methods can be used to determine the particle size of the nanoemulsion. Some of the most commonly used methods are photon correlation spectroscopy, hydrodynamic chromatography, field flow fractionation, spectroturbidimetry, sensing zone, sedimentation and electron microscopy.

Photon Correlation Spectroscopy

The photon correlation spectroscopy (PCS) is known as dynamic light scattering (DLS) technology or quasi-elastic light scattering (QELS); this technique can measure the particle size and the distribution of samples in the range of nanometer to micron size [57 - 59]. Size measurement is based on the principle of Brownian movement; it states that particles present in the sample solution undergo random movement. The velocity of individual particle movement is based on their size, where smaller-sized particles have a greater velocity of movement than larger particles. The principle of Brownian movement depends on the velocity of spherical particles dispersed in a liquid medium with defined viscosity at a constant temperature is directly proportional to the diameter of the particles described as per the stokes-Einstein equation:

$$D_{\circ} = \frac{kT}{3\pi\eta d}$$

Where D_o is the diffusion coefficient, η is the viscosity of the suspending medium, and d is the diameter of the particle. The instrumentation for photon correlation spectroscopy comprises principally of a light source, which is either argon or helium-neon laser, the spectroscopy comprising of an optical system for the dispersing angle and limiting the number of coherence areas, a detector (generally a photomultiplier), a signal analyzer which is a digital autocorrelation and a computer for preparing and showing the information. Instruments, for example, Nicomp® particle sizer (Particle Sizing Systems, CA) and Malvern Zetasizer Nanoseries® (Malvern Instruments, UK), are accessible for estimation of globule size. The measured diameter in this method is known as hydrodynamic diameter. The Z-average is calculated by the mean hydrodynamic diameter and is measured by the concept of ISO 13321, the international standard on dynamic light scattering [60, 61].

Polydispersity Index

The polydispersity index value is used to predict particle size and system distribution. The photon correlation spectroscopic technique can be used to determine the polydispersity index of nanodispersion. The polydispersity index is nothing but the average diameter of particles distributed in the system.

Electron Microscopy Techniques

Scanning electron microscopy and transmission electron microscopy are the essential methods for the characterization of nanoemulsion. The Microscopic technique permits the determination of the system's particle size, shape, and distribution nature. Furthermore, the topography of SEM gives information about the surface morphology, whereas the TEM image shows the internal structure of the emulsified system, and the microstructure transition level also is obtained.

Scanning Electron Microscopy

The surface morphological characterization of the emulsified system can be determined by scanning electron microscopy by fixation procedure with osmium peroxide and coating of dried samples with gold particles; the samples are added to the surface of a polycarbonate plate and dried the samples at 25 °C and then dried up to critical point drier. The dried samples are layered on gold and made into 5nm size. The prepared samples are placed in proper position and passed through a beam of electrons that act as a source of energy ranging from a couple of 100 eV to 50 Kev and is focused on the prepared sample specimen by using the deflection coil system as the electron fell on the surface of sample particle and interacted with each other to the emission of electrons and photons. The SEM images of the emitted electrons are subsequently formed on a cathode ray tube [62, 63].

Transmission Electron Microscopy

In this technique, the energy source is used as a beam of electrons, and this operation requires a vacuum while the gas nature of the molecule deflects the electrons. The electron gun is fixed in a top position of a microscopic column and followed by the main components of electromagnetic lenses that are used to focus the beam of electron on the sample cell. The TEM image is formed based on the shaft of electrons interacting with the prepared sample substance, *i.e.*, scattering of electrons. The improved resolution of the TEM image was obtained based on an acceleration voltage of the electrons used in this method. In this process, a short wavelength of electrons is formed by increasing the system's voltage. Conversely, enhancing the acceleration voltage leads to less contrast as the scattering of electrons is reduced at higher velocity [64]. Generally, the TEM image of the colloidal system can be performed in the voltage range of 80 and 200 Kv [65].

Zeta Potential Determination

Surface charge determination is an important parameter determining the physical stability and surface charge of nanoemulsion. Generally, a higher surface charge is essential to stabilize the dispersion system. Zeta potential value is constrained by different kinds of variables like the surface charge of particles, the number of counter ions present in the solution, the polarity of the solvent, and temperature. Zeta potential can be determined by several instruments like Malvern zeta sizer, Nicomp particle sizer, and electrophoretic light scattering. The electrokinetic mobility μ of zeta potential can be used to compute with the help of the Smoluchowski equation [66, 67].

$$\mu = \zeta\varepsilon / \eta$$

Where η is the viscosity of the liquid, and ε is the permittivity.

Viscosity Determination

Viscosity is characterized as estimating the functional stress per unit area necessary to maintain an actual flow or shear rate. As a rule, viscosity is the struggle to fluid flow, while fluidity is known as the coefficient of viscosity or reciprocal of viscosity. The viscosity of the liquids mainly depends on the thickness of the liquids [68]. Two sorts of viscosity may be precise dynamic viscosity or absolute viscosity μ and kinematic viscosity *v*. Kinematic viscosity, defined as the ratio of dynamic viscosity and density of the fluid. The kinematic viscosity is the viscosity owing to the force of gravity. They are connected by the expression $\mu = pv$ where *p* is the density of the liquid [69]. Various methods such as falling or rolling ball, rotational, capillary tube, orifice, and surface viscosity techniques measure viscosity.

Nanoemulsion as a skin delivery

The skin is the principal organ in the human body, which comprises three main layers, primarily the outermost epidermis layer, inner dermis layer, hypodermis, or subcutaneous fatty layer [70]. The outer epidermis layer shields the skin to provide protective properties. Despite its shallow thickness, it depends on the skin location, varying from 0.02 mm to 5mm. The epidermis layer comprises the stratified squamous epithelial layer, the keratinocytes squamous layer arranged in four different strata: stratum corneum, granular layer, spinous layer, and basal layer (Fig. **9.2**).

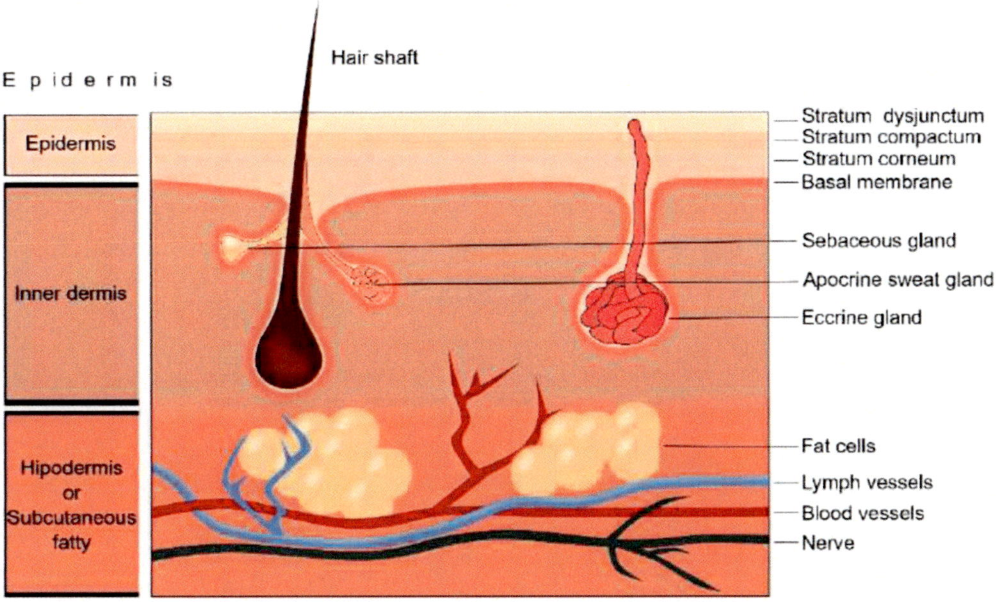

Fig. (9.2). Structure of the skin.

The uppermost crystalline nature of the stratum corneum (SC) is the main barrier to the delivery of drugs to a deeper layer of skin tissue. However, the excipient used in formulation to loosen the stratum corneum (SC) layer helps permeate the drug substance [71]. The stratum corneum is an outermost part of the epidermis, which acts as the chief barrier to skin function. The brick-like corneocyte cells are embedded in a lamellar arrangement formed on mortar-shaped rigid intercellular lipids known as desmosome-linked epithelial cells. The exclusive feature of this layer represents the essential rate-limiting step for the permeation of drug molecules larger than 500 Da [72].

The dermis layer is 1-2mm thick, is directly beneath the viable epidermis, and offers mechanical strength to the skin. The dermis consists of collagen, elastins, and glycosaminoglycans, which are jointly known as the extracellular matrix and fibroblast extent up to the extracellular matrix. The dermis layer comprises pilosebaceous glands, sweat glands, dermal adipose cells, mast cells, and infiltrating leucocytes [70]. The active drug molecule is transported *via* the stratum corneum layer principally by a passive diffusion process through three potential transcellular, intercellular, and appendageal routes [73]. The transdermal drug delivery system passive diffusion process is most prominently suitable for the movement of active drug molecules *via* the skin barriers. The two sophisticated diffusional pathways are used to transport active drug molecules passing through the skin layers *via* transappendageal and transepidermal routes (Fig. **9.3**). The transappendageal route is nothing but the transport of drug molecules across the skin shunts, such as sweat glands and hair follicles associated with sebaceous glands. The drug penetration through this route is significantly low due to logically small areas like 0.1-1% [70]. Recent research proved that the pilosebaceous units might contribute fundamentally to topical drug delivery by performing as a modest resistance transport system for nanoparticles entering the stratum corneum [74, 75]. This route is generally used to transport ions and large polar compounds.

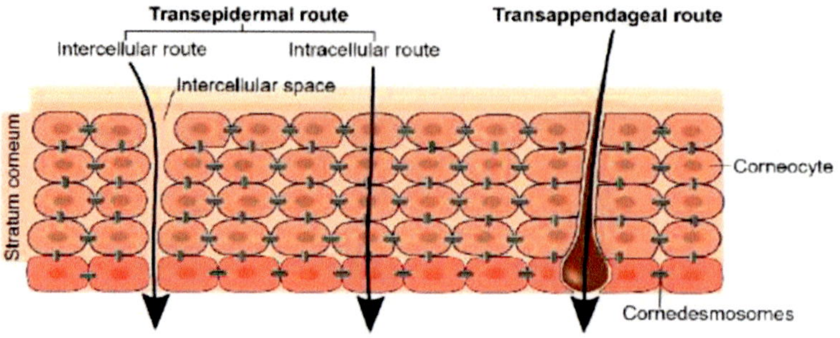

Fig. (9.3). Diagrammatic representation of percutaneous absorption of the drug in skin delivery.

However, the main pathway of drug penetration into the skin layer is believed as a transepidermal pathway. This pathway is classically divided into the transcellular and intercellular modes of drug permeation. The Intercellular path is nothing but transporting drug molecules *via* the corneocytes and lipid matrix present in the skin layer. The intercellular is known as crossing the drug molecule in between the lipid corneocytes. The extensive literature on skin layer and function showed that most of the drug molecules permeated through a tortuous but continuous intercellular route [76]. Highly polar components can cross the skin layer *via* the transcellular route due to their aqueous environment present in corneocytes of hydrated keratin corneocytes. In recent years, researchers demonstrated that emulsified system has been concluded as an elegant approach to improving the topical delivery of either hydrophilic and lipophilic drugs as compared to conventional dosage forms or other colloidal nanocarriers [77, 78]. Numerous factors may influence the skin permeation of an active component from the colloidal system, such as droplet size, the partition coefficient of the drug molecule in the system, the presence of the component at the interface, use of another component in the formulation that may influence the skin penetration rate, site or pathway of absorption [10, 79].

The active drug molecule has the essential qualities required for diffusion through the stratum corneum, such as a molecular weight less than or equal to 500 Da, lipophilic (log 1-3), and water-soluble [80]. The small drug molecule then can be moved preferentially through the intercellular route. The numerous factors that govern the diffusion rate of drug molecules *via* the stratum corneum barriers are molecular weight, lipophilicity, aqueous solubility, hydrogen bond formation, polymorphic form, and other physicochemical properties [81]. The nanocarrier transporting *via* appendages such as sweat glands, pilosebaceous units, and hair follicles are instigated either from the dermis or the subcutaneous fat tissue. These are the crucial discontinuities of the skin layer.

The altered physiological function of the skin layer is an essential factor in affecting the permeation of active drug molecules. As revealed, there is limited data on skin permeation of nanoparticles through the diseased skin layer. The topical delivery of the nanocarriers system is generally used for the local action of diseased skin. However, the skin barrier's diseased condition modulates nanoparticle permeation is unknown. The known scientific reason is that nanoparticles might go through these lesions more proficiently owing to an altered stratum corneum, inflammation and improved keratinocyte turnover [82]. The surface layer of the stratum corneum is regarded as a moving, continuously renewable barrier. This upward movement might assist in providing a mechanism to prevent foreign particles from invading the body and protect from pathogens, cancerous cells, or solid particulate material [83].

The low surfactant content of nanoemulsion considerably reduces the irritation of the skin on the topical application; the smaller droplet size of nanoemulsion offered uniform spreading ability of the skin, excellent occlusiveness, visual qualities, and skin feel smoothness [84, 52]. NEC has widely been used in the field of the food industry, pharmaceutical and cosmetic pharmaceuticals, and for therapeutic purposes such as inflammation, anti-aging, moisturization, etc [85]. Furthermore, Nanoemulsion has specifically been used to manage chronic skin diseases such as atopic dermatitis or dry skin, to afford skin guard and hydration, devoid of irritating or deteriorating the skin barrier [86]. The number of mechanisms proposed enhances the permeation of nanoemulsion into the skin. Firstly they offered enhanced solubilization ability for both hydrophilic and lipophilic active pharmaceutical ingredients, strengthening the drug loading capacity and dose significance of the formulation. Secondly, nanosize offers high surface area and excellent skin contact; due to this, coupled properties offer to enhance perfect attachment with the stratum corneum layer of skin. Third, nanoemulsion composition contains oil and surfactant generally offering permeation enhancing ability on skin layer of the lipid nature stratum corneum.

Non- Steroidal anti-inflammatory drug

Non-steroidal anti-inflammatory drug (NSAID) is extensively used to relieve pain and is generally administered orally with intolerable adverse effects like dyspepsia and gastrointestinal bleeding. Topical routes have gained importance to avoid this adverse effect. NEs have been an attractive strategy to improve the drug permeation rate into the skin layer and enhance the anti-inflammatory action of NSAIDs [85]. Sakeena *et al.*, formulated ketoprofen-loaded oil-in-water nanoemulsion for transdermal delivery using spontaneous emulsification. Palm oil esters utilized in developing nanoemulsion formulation and the *in vitro* release profile demonstrated a satisfactory drug release rate through the methyl acetate cellulose membrane [87].

Salim *et al.*, a newly developed topical drug delivery of Ibuprofen using palm kernel oil esters along with different kinds of hydrocolloid gums such as gellan gum, xanthan gum, and carrageenan by phase inversion composition method. The formed, modified nanoemulsion showed 4.40 times improved permeability of ibuprofen than that of emulsion formed without hydrocolloid gum [29]. In one study, the indomethacin-loaded nanoemulsions system was prepared using different oil components (Triacetin, capryol 90 and labrafil), surfactant (Tween 80 and pluronic F127), and co-surfactants (transcutol and propylene glycol). The result revealed that the formulation containing Pluronic F127 showed the smallest particle diameter, and the maximum viscosity was observed. They found that the drug solubility has been amplified up to 610-fold compared with water [88].

Aceclofenac is a nonsteroidal anti-inflammatory drug-specific used in the treatment of rheumatoid arthritis and osteoarthritis. However, the oral administration of dosage form produced various side effects like gastrointestinal ulcers and bleeding on chronic use, which results in an anemic condition. To circumvent this problem, the researchers developed an aceclofenac-loaded nanoemulsion consisting of triacetin (13.6%), cremophore EL (23.9%), PEG 400 (7.9%), and distilled water (54.6%). The nanoemulsion produced higher *in vitro* permeability and *in vivo* anti-inflammatory activity than the commercially available nanogel formulation [89], and similar -anti-inflammatory activity was studied by an aspirin-loaded nanoemulsion system prepared by a microfluidizer technology. The investigation discovered that formed nanoemulsions showed two-fold improved anti-inflammatory potential when contrasted with aspirin nanosuspension and accordingly proposes a conceivable technique to reduce the adverse reactions based on the high-dose level of aspirin [90].

Mou *et al.*, studied that 5% camphor, 5% menthol, and 5% methyl salicylate loaded into a hydrogel-thickened nanoemulsion system (HTN) which showed high penetration rates with 138.0±6.5 µg cm^{-2} h^{-1} of camphor, 63.6±3.3 µg cm^{-2} h^{-1} of menthol, and 53.8±3.2 µg cm^{-2} h^{-1} of methyl salicylate and this result assured HTN as a topical dosage form for treating arthritis, minor joint and muscle pain [91]. Esmaeili *et al.* designed an O/W nanoemulsion consisting of Eugenol for the management of inflammation by using the different proportions of 2% Eugenol, 14% Tween 20, and 14% isopropyl alcohol in water. The formed nanoemulsion indicated enhanced anti-inflammatory properties compared to the commercially existing piroxicam gel. Additionally, the evaluated nanoemulsion with and without piroxicam recommended that piroxicam diminish the anti-inflammatory result of eugenol in the preparation [92].

Alvarado *et al.*, formulated nanoemulsion for dermal application in the mixture of natural or synthetic pentacyclic triterpenes with predictable anti-inflammatory properties. The formed NEs clearly noted that the active principle retained a high concentration on the surface of the skin as compared deeper layer of tissue, which is an added advantage for topical drug delivery. The result demonstrated that nanoemulsion-loaded natural triterpenes proved better to treat inflammation than nanoemulsion-loaded synthetic triterpenes [15]. Baspinara and Borcherta developed a positive and negative charged nanoemulsion of prednicarbate with a high-pressure homogenization method. They proved that the formed positively charged nanoemulsion has more interacted with a negative charge of skin surface to an enhanced penetration rate of prednicarbate. Simultaneously negatively charged nanoemulsion showed a higher release rate than positively charged nanoemulsion. The results showed that prednicarbate-loaded positively charged nanoemulsion is proof that its local action could be beneficial for the treatment of atopic dermatitis [93].

Local Anaesthetics

Negi *et al.* described biocompatible lidocaine and prilocaine-loaded nanoemulsion by high-pressure homogenization method for a better topical delivery system of local anesthetic agents. They found that greater penetration rates and an elevated concentration of the drugs in the skin layer were achieved compared to that of available marketed cream and formulated nanoemulsion systems showed better biocompatibility with the skin layer [94].

Antimicrobial

Hussain *et al.*, developed Amphotericin B-loaded nanoemulsion (NEs) for topical delivery consisting of lipids with different proportions of Peceol, Captex, Capmul, Miglyol 829, and Labrasol along with surfactants like Cremophor RH40, Tween-80, Cremophor-EL, Propylene glycol. A slow spontaneous titration technique prepared the system. The *in-vitro* studies of nanoemulsion displayed a sustained release pattern was achieved and an improved flux value (21.62 ± 1.6 μg/cm²/h) as evaluated to the Amphotericin B drug solution and Fungisome without showing toxicity. The researchers concluded that optimized formulation showed a good therapeutic response with superior activity and productivity for topically treating a wide range of fungal diseases [30]. Another research group, Hussain *et al.*, demonstrated a topical nanoemulsion drug delivery system of amphotericin B with various amounts of sefsol-218 oil, polysorbate 80 (Tween80) as surfactant, and polyethylene glycol-400 (PEG-400), propylene glycol (PG) as cosurfactant by using phase titration method for NEs preparations. The researchers concluded that the maximum flux rate of 17.85 ± 0.5 mg/cm²/h than drug solution (5.37 ± 0.01 mg/cm²/h) and Fungisome (7.97 ± 0.01 mg/cm²/h).The physical-chemical stability studies revealed that a nanoemulsion is an option for sustained delivery of amphotericin B for topical treatment of microbial diseases [71].

Further, a new research group has explored the development of Amphotericin B nanoemulsion synthesized from Capmul PG8 (CPG8), Labrasol, and polyethylene glycol-400 for the delivery of sustained release. The nanosized emulsion has been employed to treat cutaneous infections caused by candida albicans and aspergillus niger and proved to have better antifungal efficacy than a commercial product of fungisome or drug solution [95]. Yu *et al.* developed metronidazole-loaded nanoemulsion permeated into the deeper layer of skin and confined in epidermal/dermal tissue and drug released up to 24 h for the betterment of topical treatment for rosacea when contrasted with that of commercially available metronidazole gel [96].

For instance, Borges *et al.* formulated a dapsone-loaded nanoemulsion for the management of acne and leprosy. The nanosystem was prepared by using isopropyl myristate or n-methyl-pyrrolidone as an oil component. The result exhibited that use of n-methyl-pyrrolidone gave a more noteworthy nanoemulsion area and superior solubility of dapsone, and better *in-vitro* release profile data was achieved as compared with that of NEs formulated by using isopropyl myristate. The researchers again concluded that the oil phase used methyl pyrrolidone nanoemulsion showed an enhanced permeation rate when contrasted with the oil phase used as an isopropyl myristate [97]. Kaur *et al.*, formulated clobetasol propionate (CP) and calcipotriol (CT) loaded nanoemulsion-based gel for the treatment of psoriasis. The nanosystem is composed of Capmul MCM C8 EP, and Cremophor RH 40/Labrafil11 1944 CS used as oil and surfactant/co-surfactant, respectively. The outcome of this formulation confirmed the enhanced antipsoriatic activity of NEs as compared with free drug solutions or commercially existing products and insignificant skin disturbance in spite of increased penetration into the skin [98].

Mattos *et al.* investigated the utilization of nanoemulsion synthesized from medium-chain triglycerides alongside soybean lecithin or sorbitan monooleate surfactant and polysorbate 20 or polysorbate 80) co-surfactant by spontaneous emulsification strategy for the delivery of antileishmanial agent (Chalcones) against *Leishmania amazonensis* for the topical treatment of cutaneous leishmaniasis and showed greater stability of the nanosystem established by the antileishmanial assay by *Leishmania amazonensis* designed for 24 hours and 60 days after the formulation of the nanoemulsion. Pentyl gallate (PG) is an n-alkyl ester of gallic acid used as an -herpes activity but characterized as low aqueous solubility due to limited use of therapeutic applications [99]. Kelmann *et al.* formulated nanoemulsions to ensure penetration of the skin and inhibit herpes simplex virus (HSV)-1 replication. The drug-loaded oil/water nanoemulsion was developed using castor oil, medium-chain triglycerides (MCT), and estimated *in vitro* antiviral activity against HSV-1. In acute dermal toxicity and risk of dermal sensitization experiments, pentyl gallate-loaded nanoemulsion could penetrate into a more profound layer of the dermis, with higher physicochemical characteristics, stability, safe, and antiherpes activity [100].

Anticancer Drug

Shakeel *et al.* investigated the use of lesser HLB value surfactant moiety chosen to prepare nanoemulsion with an active 5-fluoro uracil (5-FU) for topical treatment of skin cancer and adopted by oil phase titration method of preparation. They found higher drug penetration, lower-sized droplet, a narrow range of polydispersity index, and accepted *in vitro* cytotoxicity results on melanoma cancer cells. For this reason, 5-FU loaded nanoemulsion is better efficacious than free 5-FU [101]. The recent research on the nanoemulsion system for topical (skin) use is summarized in Table **9.1**.

Table 9.1. Recent studies on nanoemulsion systems for the treatment of skin diseases.

Drug	Oil	Surfactant and Cosurfactant	Result	Reference
Ketoprofen	Palm oil esters	Tween 80	Showed a better *in-vitro* release and suitable physicochemical properties.	[85]
Ibuprofen	Palm kernel oil esters	Tween 80	Illustrated superior permeability of ibuprofen as compared to that of emulsion prepared without hydrocolloid gum.	[29]

(Table 1) cont.....

Drug	Oil	Surfactant and Cosurfactant	Result	Reference
Indomethacin	Triacetin, capryol 90 and labrafil	Tween 80, pluronic F127 & transcutol, propylene glycol	Showed prolonged systemic effect was observed up to 32 h.	[88]
Aceclofenac	Isopropyl myristate (IPM), oleic acid, castor oil, ethyl oleate,	Tween 80 and Cremophore El and PEG 400.	Exhibited a better *in-vitro* permeation rate and *in-vivo* anti-inflammatory activity when compared with a commercial product.	[89]
Aspirin	Soybean oil	Polysorbate 80	An improved anti-inflammatory activity occurred as compared to that of aspirin suspension.	[90]
Mixture of camphor, menthol, methyl Salicylate.	Soybean oil	Soybean lecithin, Tween 80 poloxamer407 and propylene glycol	Showed an improved permeation rate and efficient treatment of arthritis.	[91]
Eugenol and Piroxicam	Eugenol	Tween 20 and isopropyl alcohol	Demonstrated a superior anti-inflammatory activity as compared to piroxicam gel.	[92]
Oleanolic and ursolic acids	Castor oil	Labrasol and transcutol-P, propylene glycol.	Exhibited high ability to penetration into the skin layer and showed superior anti-inflammatory effect.	[15]
Prednicarbate	Eutanol® G (octyldodecanol), Myristic acid	Tween 80	Showed a better permeation rate when compared with negatively charged nanoemulsion of prednicarbate.	[93]
Lidocaine and Prilocaine	Olive oil, Soybean oil	Tween 20, Tween 80 and propylene glycol	Proved a greater permeation rate and high concentration of drugs retained on skin layer as compared with commercial cream.	[94]
Amphotericin B	Peceol	Labrasol and Propylene glycol	Exhibited better *in-vitro* release and an enhanced flux rate was observed.	[30]
Amphotericin B	Propylene glycol mono caprylic ester (sefsol-218)	Polysorbate 80 (Tween 80), polyethylene glycol-400 (PEG-400) and propylene glycol (PG)	Confirmed highest flux rate when compared with drug solution and Fungisome.	[71]

(Table 1) cont.....

Drug	Oil	Surfactant and Cosurfactant	Result	Reference
Amphotericin B	Capmul PG8 (CPG8),	Labrasol, Tween-80, Polyethylene glycol 400 (PEG-400)	Displayed better permeation and superior antifungal activity.	[95]
Metronidazole	Labrafil	Cremophor EL and tetraethylene glycol	Permeated into a deeper layer of skin and retained in dermal layers up to 24 h and improves the treatment of rosacea.	[96]
Dapsone	Isopropyl myristate, Methyl pyrrolidone	Tween 80, Span 20	Showed an enhanced permeation rate.	[97]
Clobitasol propionate and calcipotriol	Capmul MCM C8 EP	Cremophor RH 40 and Labrafil 11 1944 CS	Illustrated superior anti-psoriatic activity than the existing preparations.	[98]
Chalcones	Medium chain triglycerides(MCT)	Soybean lecithin, sorbitan monooleate and polysorbate 20, polysorbate 80.	Revealed a superior antileishmanial activity.	[99]
Pentyl Gallate	Castor oil, medium chain triglycerides (MCT)	Soybean lecithin (SL), polysorbate 80 (PL80), vitamin E	Showed better permeation and superior antiherpes activity.	[100]
5-Fluorouracil	Propylene glycol monolaurate (Lauroglycol-90)	Transcutol-HP (diethylene glycol monoethyl ether) and Isopropyl alcohol.	Demonstrated a better therapeutic efficacy compared with free 5-FU.	[101]

Nanoemulsion as Ocular Drug Delivery

The eye is a ball-shaped organ; it is covered by three-layer, such as the outer layer consisting of the hairy sclera, the center vascular coat, and the uvea (iris, ciliary body choroid), and the interior layer consisting of nervous tissue, the retina. The specific structure of the eye is composed of three compartments like

(i) the former compartment, which is located in between the iris and the cornea,

(ii) the posterior compartment, placed between the lens and the iris; and

(iii) the vitreous compartment, expanding from the lens to the retina.

The role of aqueous humor is to maintain the intraocular pressure between the former and posterior chambers of an eye. While the vitreous chamber is filled with vitreous humor as a function of the ciliary processes of the ciliary body. Anatomically eye can be divided into two portions such as the anterior portion consists of (iris, cornea, ciliary body, and crystalline lens) and the posterior portion (vitreous humor, retina, retinal pigmented epithelium, and choroid) [102, 103] (Fig. **9.4**). Topical administration of ocular dosage form is the most suitable method to deliver medicament to anterior segment compared to posterior one. The different barrier systems should affect the delivery of drugs to the anterior static portion (corneal stroma, corneal epithelium, and blood-aqueous barrier), active part (lymph flow, conjunctival blood flow, and tear drainage), and metabolic hurdles [104, 105].

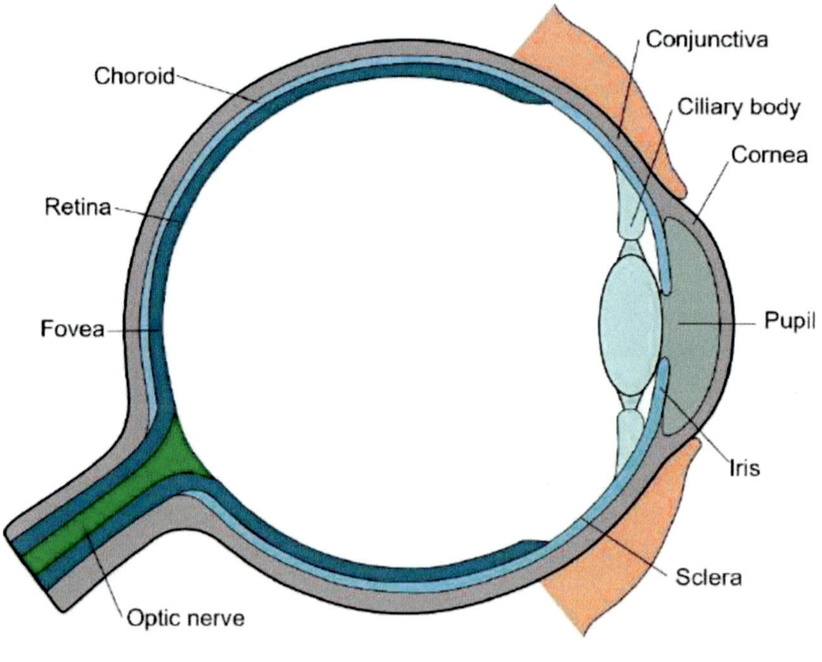

Fig. (9.4). Stucture of eye.

The topical route of drug administration to the anterior segment of ocular delivery offers various advantages such as non-invasiveness, restricted entry of the drug into the systemic circulation, avoidance of first-pass metabolism, simplicity of administration, and a nearly low dose enough, best patient compliance route [106]. However, after topical instillation into existing formulations like solutions, emulsions, suspensions are rapidly drained out, communication with tear components, tear production rate, and quick removal dosage owing to reflex blinking actions is the main reason that needs to be optimized to achieve the better ocular bioavailability of drug substance.

The rate of normal tear formation (0.5-2.2 μL/min) and tear turnover, the retention period of the medicament with the ocular surface is a reasonably short time (1-2 min), the continuous blinking action of eye preocular administered conventional dosage form is eliminated *via* the lacrimal fluid [104]. Approximately 75% of the ophthalmic liquid dosage form vanishes *via* nasolacrimal elimination or systemic absorption *via* conjunctiva; for this reason, ocular drug availability is deficient. Due to the above-mentioned reasons, only a fraction of the drug substance is successful in crossing the cornea while applied to the corneal epithelium [107].

The cornea is a primary static obstacle that significantly limits the drug permeation into intraocular tissue. This construction is highly based on vascular tissue; the corneal layer is consequently layered as the epithelium, Bowman's layer, stroma, Descemet's membrane, and endothelium. The corneal epithelium is an important barrier to the delivery of drugs to ocular tissues, which controls the permeation of drugs explicitly [108]. It consists of single cells of the basal layer and non-keratinized layer, mainly 4-5 celles, laminated squamous epithelial cells, which collectively jointly form a rigid junction (zonula occludens), and it acts as an effectual layer to prevent the loss of fluid and pathogen diffusion. The lipophilic nature of the epithelial tisssue acts as a barrier for most hydrophilic drug moiety absorption and is also called a rate-limiting barrier for hydrophilic drug substances [109]. The corneal transport of drug molecules passed through the paracellular and transcellular pathways.

Water-soluble drugs or low molecular weight compounds (less than 350 MW) generally permeated through the paracellular route, whereas lipid-soluble drugs pass through the transcellular pathway. The hydrophilic nature of stroma and arrangement of collagen fiber within the cell prevents the permeation of lipophilic molecules. The lipoidal nature of the endothelium layer act as a barrier between the stroma and aqueous humor. It does not act as a significant barrier to the trans-corneal diffusion of most drugs [108, 110, 111]. The trans-corneal penetration is delayed due to the binding of drug molecule on the corneal layer and slowly delivering of drug molecule into aqueous humor when the level of drug concentration decreases than the distribution drug from aqueous humor to intraocular tissue like iris-ciliary body, lens, vitreous and choroids-retina and primarily the elimination pathway of aqueous humor turnover and venous blood flow in the anterior uvea [112].

The vascularised thin layer of conjunctiva contained goblet cells that secrete mucin that coated the eyelids' inner surface and enveloped the anterior portion of the sclera. It extended up to the cornea [108]. The conjunctiva is a leakier epithelium than the corneal layer, which is expected to have a superior permeation ability of hydrophilic drug substances transported *via* paracellular pathways [113, 114]. The sclera is a fibrous tissue and is more permeable to drug molecules as compared with cornea and conjunctiva. The fibrous nature of the sclera helps to improve drug absorption and to deliver drugs across; it has become an intelligent way to manage retinal disorders based on this less invasive character compared to the intravitreous strategy [115]. The sclera is a hydrophilic fibrous tissue, so hydrophilic drugs readily penetrate *via* scleral matrix pores freely, in contrast to lipophilic drugs. The permeation of drug molecules in the scleral layer is controlled by particle size and charge of the active drug moiety [116].

The two main barriers present in the intraocular environment are blood-aqueous barriers and blood-retinal barriers, which impede the delivery and targeting of ocular therapeutic efficiently. Drugs administered through the systemic route reach the intraocular tissues of the anterior segment and the RPE or the retinal vasculature after crossing these blood-aqueous barriers and blood-retinal barriers, respectively [117]. The blood-aqueous barrier (BAB) is positioned in the anterior segment of the eye. It consists of the endothelial cells in the uvea, non-pigmented epithelial cells of the ciliary body, which mainly includes the iris epithelium and iris vessel endothelium with tight junctions that control both active and passive transport of water-soluble drugs from the systemic circulation into the aqueous humor [118, 119]. The blood-retinal barrier (BRB) situated in the posterior portion of the eye is a further subdivision of the inner and outer BRB. The inner layer of BRB is highly formed by the tight junction between retinal capillary endothelial cells, and its barrier looks like a blood-brain barrier (BBB). The outer BRB consists of retinal pigment epithelial (RPE) cells connected through tight junctions. The inside BRB is a highly efficient rate-limiting barrier to transport drugs from the blood into the retina [120, 121].

Anti-inflammatory Drugs

Ibrahim *et al.*, developed a submicron emulsion containing prednisolone acetate molecule with different proportions of oil such as castor oil, soybean oil, and ethyl oleate along with the apposite concentration of Tween 80; Pluronic F68 could be used as a cosurfactant for the preparation ocular nanoemulsions. As indicated by the physicochemical properties of the emulsified system, Pluronic F68 was the most appropriate choice of cosurfactant for the formulation of an autoclavable nanoemulsion system [122]. They prepared a submicron emulsion containing active indomethacin moiety using phospholipids and lauroamphodiacetate as an amphoteric surfactant. The result showed that formed submicron emulsion is more stable in acidic pH, and the corneal permeability coefficient of indomethacin was up to 3.8 times greater than that of the commercially available product [123].

Akhtera *et al.*, formulated a novel polymeric mucoadhesive chitosan-coated NEs of cyclosporine A (Cy-A) for the treatment of cornea transplant rejection and keratoconjunctivitis sicca (so-called dry eye disease), and various *in-vitro*, *in-vivo* studies of mucoadhesive immunosuppressant proved better entrapment efficiency, enhanced corneal retention period and conjunctival bioavailability [124]. Panatieri *et al.*, studied the active molecule of 5-methoxy-6,7-methylenedioxycoumarin extract obtained from *Pterocaulon balansae* loaded nanoemulsion composed of medium-chain triglycerides and egg lecithin, through which spontaneous emulsification method. This result recommended that the formed oil-in-water nanoemulsion is purposeful for the topical management of ocular keratitis caused by *Acanthamoeba* [125].

Patel *et al.*, demonstrated on newly formulated positively charged nano emulsified *in-situ* gel of loteprednol elaborate (LE) using Capryol 90, tween 80, and transcutol P along with thermosensitive polymers. The developed *in-situ* gel nanoformulations showed higher C_{max} delayed T_{max} extended residence time and enhanced bioavailability up to 2.54- fold improved compared to the commercially existed formulation for the management of different kinds of inflammatory diseases and improved patient compliance [126]. Tayel *et al.*, formulated *in situ* gellan gum-based nanoemulsion (NE) gel of Terbinafine hydrochloride (T-HCl) for treating ocular fungal keratitis. The formulation contains a different ratio of oils, surfactant, and cosurfactant to produce the thermodynamically stable nanoemulsion. The NE-based gel showed pseudoplastic; a mucoadhesive and controlled release pattern was achieved [127].

Antiglaucoma Drugs

Ammar and coworkers developed *in situ* gel nanoemulsion of dorzolamide hydrochloride to improve the ocular duration of action and bioavailability. This formulation contains a different ratio of oil, surfactant, and co-surfactant. These researchers further confirmed that formulated *in-situ* gel nanoemulsion showed better therapeutic efficacy compared to drug solution alone or marketed product of dorzolamide hydrochloride [128]. Sznitowska *et al.*, demonstrated *O,O*^{1}-dipivaloyl (1, 2-ethylene) bispilocarpic acid diester of Pilocarpine was incorporated into the oil phase containing soybean oil, egg lecithin and glycerol. These emulsified systems produced sustained release patterns, and reduced prodrug ocular irritation potential when compared to Pilocarpine HCl solution [129]. Ammar *et al.*, demonstrated the nanoemulsion containing an antiglaucoma drug dorzolamide hydrochloride using a different concentration of oil, surfactant, and cosurfactant to produce O/W type and formed formulation revealed to be stable, prolonged duration of action, and better drug bioavailability was achieved as compared to that of marketed available conventional eye drops [130].

An adrenergic-blocking agent like timolol is used as an intraocular pressure-lowering agent for the treatment of glaucoma. Unfortunately, some severe side effects on cardiovascular, respiratory, and central nervous systems to the ocular administration of timolol. Gallarate *et al.* investigated the ocular administration of nanoemulsion containing timolol maleate, or Hydrophobic ion pairing of timolol with AOT can improve corneal permeation. Retention property of drug in both solutions and emulsions of *ex vivo* corneal irritation test based on opacity measurement showed decreased corneal opacity was observed when compared drug solutions [131]. Mahboobian *et al.*, investigated the development of the nanoemulsion containing brinzolamide using different types and concentrations of oil (triacetin and CapryolTM 90), surfactant (Cremophor RH 40, Brij 35, Labrasol, and tyloxapol), and co-surfactant (Transcutol P) adapted with spontaneous emulsification method. The pharmacodynamic result showed that the optimized NEs have been able to reduce the IOP in contrast to that of commercially available Brinzolamide ophthalmic suspension [132].

Morsi *et al.* reported their study on acetazolamide-loaded nanoemulsion from isopropyl myristate, oleic acid, peanut oil, cremophor EL, tween 80, transcutol P, and different concentration of water content (39% or 59%). An *in-vitro* study showed that nanoemulsions with higher water content (59%) achieved the fastest drug release pattern. Therapeutic efficacy confirmed that nanoemulsion containing peanut oil along with 39% water content revealed better and prolonged intraocular pressure reducing effect was reached as compared to commercially available brinzolamide eye drops (Azopt) or oral acetazolamide tablet (cidamex) [133].

Miscellaneous Drugs

Liu *et al.* prepared cyclodextrin containing nanoemulsions with lutein as an active principle. The macular pigment of Lutein is used as an eye tonic. The formed 2% HEβCD modified nanoemulsion showed 9.2-fold enhanced lutein accumulation compared to lutein suspension alone. The nanoemulsion showed superior drug loading efficiency and a lower cytotoxicity effect on retinal cells. These researchers further concluded that the partition coefficient value of lutein was improved in the porcine sclera [134]. Ying *et al.* demonstrated that surface-modified submicron emulsion contains coumarin - 6 as a model drug and a fluorescent marker. Chitosan-coated positively charged nanoemulsions were formulated by high-pressure homogenization method and poloxamer 407, used as

a surface modifier, to improve the lipid emulsion retention time on the surface of ocular tissue. The authors concluded that surface-modified submicron emulsion is a suitable vehicle for hydrophobic drug delivery to the posterior ocular segment [135]. Table **9.2** illustrates the recent investigation on the nanoemulsion system to treat ocular diseases.

Table 9.2. Recent studies on nanoemulsion systems for the treatment of ocular diseases.

Drug	Oil	Surfactant and cosurfactant	Result	Ref.
Prednisolone acetate	Castor oil, soybean oil, Ethyl oleate.	Tween 80, Pluronic F68.	Emulsion containing Pluronic F68 displayed better physicochemical properties.	[122]
Indomethacin	Medium chain triglyceride (MCT)	Lauroamphodiacetate (Miranol), Glycerin.	Corneal permeability coefficient was improved compared with a commercial product.	[123]
Cyclosporine A	Oleic acid, Olive oil, Castor oil, Safsol 218, Ispropylmyristate,, Labrafac PG, Soyabean oil, Triacetin.	Tween 20, Tween80, Cremophore EL, Labrasol & Propylene glycol, PEG 200, PEG 400 and Transcutol P.	Showed improved ocular residence time due to mucoadhesive nature	[124]
5-methoxy-6,7 methylenedioxycoumarin	Medium chain triglyceride	Egg lecithin (Lipoid E-80)	Showed efficient management of keratitis caused by Acanthamoeb.	[125]
Loteprednol etabonate	Capryol 90	Tween 80 & Transcutol P	Better drug bioavailability than the existing commercial products.	[126]
Terbinafine hydrochloride	Isopropyl myristate, Miglyol 812	Tween80, Cremophor EL, and polyethylene glycol 400.	Displayed an improved mean residence time and superior ocular bioavailability.	[127]
Dorzolamide hydrochloride	Isopropyl myristate (IPM), Miglyol 812 (capric triglyceride), Triacetin(glycerol triacetate)	Poloxamer 407 AND propylene glycol, Transcutol, and Miranol.	Showed superior therapeutic efficacy when compared with dorzolamide eye drops.	[128]

(Table 2) cont.....

Drug	Oil	Surfactant and cosurfactant	Result	Ref.
Pilocarpine Prodrug	Medium chain Triglycerides, soybean oil	Egg phospholipids, and Miranol MHT as emulgators glycerol.	Showed reduced irritant effect.	[129]
Dorzolamide hydrochloride	Isopropyl myristate, Miglyol 812, and triacetin.	Tween 80, Cremophor EL, and propylene glycol, triacetin, Transcutol P, Miranol C2M.	Higher therapeutic potential as compared to commercial eye drops.	[130]
Timolol maleate	soya oil (capryc-caprylic triglyceride)	soya lecithin, Tween80 and Pluronic® F68	Improve the corneal permeation and retention of drug	[131]
Brinzolamide	Triacetin and CapryolTM 90	Cremophor RH 40, Brij 35, Labrasol, tyloxapol, and Transcutol P	Reduced intraocular pressure more effectively than brinzolamide suspension.	[132]
Acetazolamide	Isopropyl myristate, oleic acid, peanut oil	Cremophor EL, Tween80,transcutol P and water.	Prolonged intraocular pressure-lowering effect than marketed eye drops.	[133]
Lutein	corn oil	Diethylene glycol monoethyl ether (Transcutol), Span 20, Pluronic F68	Enhanced lutein accumulation as compared to lutein suspension.	[134]
Coumarin-6	Medium chain triglyceride (MCT, Triester F-810),castor oil	Egg phosphatidylcholine (EPC), hydrogenated Soy L-α phosphatidylcholine (HSPC)	Improve the bioavailability of coumarin-6 to inner plexiform layer of retina.	[135]

Stability Issues

The stability of a pharmaceutical emulsified system is defined as the dosage form remaining stable and effective within specified limits for a pressured duration of time. The first stage of any stability assessment preparation is to specify the value of established parameters such as physical stability, chemical stability, and microbial stability. The next step is to assess the set parameters [136]. Nanoemulsions are thermodynamically unstable, showing coalescence and flocculation if not considerable energetic barriers to globule interactions are present. The emulsion is susceptible to instability phenomena similar to Ostwald ripening and coalescence. The globule dimension is not identical, and concentration gradients force mass exchange, thus suggesting modification in the globule dimension [137]. The emulsified systems are subjected to an elevated temperature to study the degradation products obtained from the dosage forms. As per ICH guidelines for stability study, the emulsified system was subjected to a stress test and accelerated stability test for the quality of product characterization. Centrifugation and freeze-thaw cycles of the emulsion are the methods for including stress tests. The characterization of the emulsion can be performed before and after the examination.

Physical Instability

There are principally different ways in which the structure of dispersion of minute globules into a continuous medium can modify consequent physical instability. The instability of emulsified system can occur from modification in globule diameter leading to creaming and coalescence or hydrolysis of emulgent, change in pH, or oxidation of the oil component [138] (Fig. **9.5**).

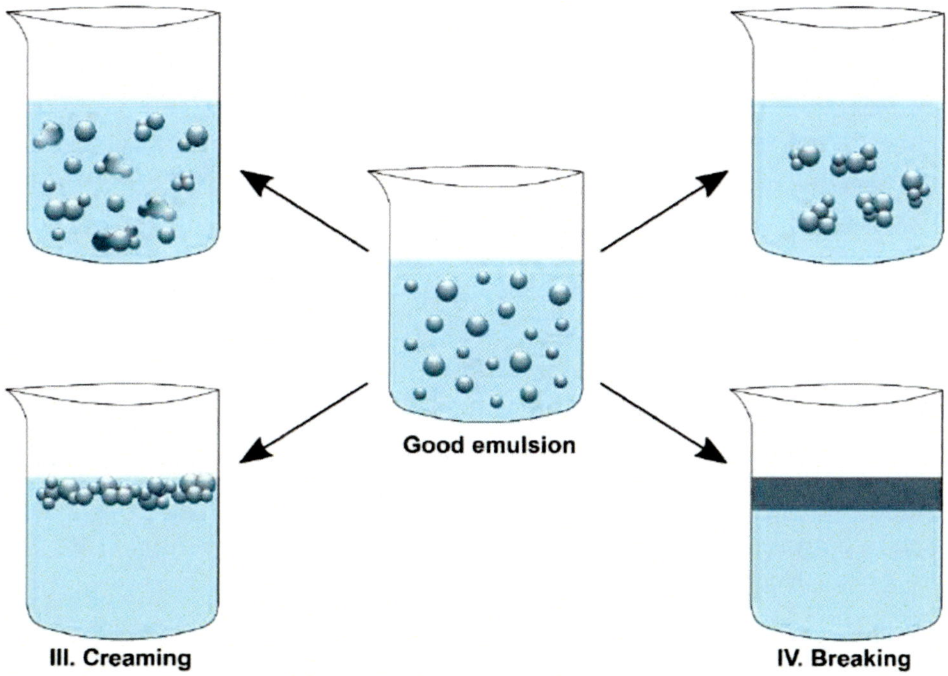

Fig. (9.5). Physical instability of nanoemulsion.

Creaming

Creaming is the process of upward motion of dispersed globules concerning dispersion medium. If the dispersed globule is denser than the dispersion medium, the globules are settled down quickly; this phenomenon is generally known as downward creaming. This process occurs typically due to outside force fields, generally centrifugal or electrostatic gravitational, involving the system. The rate of the creaming process can be minimized by maintaining the densities of the two phases equally [139].

Flocculation

The main principle of formation flocculation is the existence of attractive forces between the droplets. Flocculation is the process of increasing the aggregation of droplets within the emulsion, and there is no modification in globule size or distribution.

Coalescence

As in the type of O/W emulsion, the oil dispersions are nonuniform in size. Due to the more potent cohesive force, the smaller globules combined with larger ones, the internal phase can cause coalescence readily. Accordingly, a moderately coarse dispersion of uniformly sized particles should have the best stability.

Ostwald Ripening

Ostwald ripening is one of the primary stability issues of nanoemulsion formulation. The different ratios of solubility of active principle in tiny and larger droplets may occur [11]. Ostwald ripening is the expense of smaller droplets combined with the formation of larger droplets (*i.e.*, phase separation). This instability problem can be minimized by incorporating another disperse phase substance, which is insoluble in the dispersion medium. The interfacial tension reduction between the O/W interface minimizes Ostwald ripening [140, 141].

Phase Inversion

Phase inversion is a phenomenon that modifies emulsion type from o/w to w/o emulsion and *vice versa*. This inversion may occur due to changes in temperature or concentration of a substance present in the system or by adding other substances to the system.

Chemical Instability

The chemical instability of an emulsion may occur due to the Inactivation of drug molecules. The number of degradation pathways involved in the deactivation of drug molecules, are dehydration, hydrolysis, oxidation, isomerization, elimination, racemization, photodegradation, and complex interaction with drug and excipient. The inactivation pathway mainly depends on the nature of the drug substance.

Regulatory Strategy for Assessment of Emulsion Stability

The stability studies of the emulsion system can be conducted as per the International Conference on Harmonization (ICH) rules of technical specification for the registration of a pharmaceutical product for human use. This guideline comprises accent testing, and longstanding and intermediary or quick stability studies. In addition, accent testing on drug molecules based on the probable degradation products, which can establish the degradation mechanism of roadways and inherent instability of the drug molecule and authenticate the stability-point out analytical technique, can be used.

ICH guidelines suggested an accent test protocol based on a single lot of the drug product. The batch of products integrates the impact of temperature in 10°C enlargements up to 50°C, 60°C, *etc.*, which can be used for accelerated stability testing with 75% RH or greater and can be used for stability studies. The testing is also carried out on the receptiveness of drug molecule hydrolysis across an extensive space of pH values when in a solution form. Photostability assessment is an essential class of accent testing [142]. Accelerated stability studies can be performed at varying temperature and humidity ranges which include at 40 °C ± 2 °C/75% RH± 5% RH for the least period of 6 months, and longstanding stability studies at 25 °C ± 2 °C/60% RH ± 5% RH or 30 °C ± 2 °C/65% RH ± 5% RH for 12 months on at least three prime batches [143].

Recent Patents on Nanoemulsion for Topical (ocular/skin) Therapeutics

Numerous scientists filed patents on nanoemulsion as a topical (ocular/skin) delivery system. We investigated the only few recently filed patents in the nanoemulsion system in topical (ocular/skin) drug delivery. Lee *et al.*, explored an ophthalmic nanoemulsion for delivering cyclosporine for the potential healing property of dry eye syndrome, employing the composition of 0.02-0.3 w/v % of cyclosporine, 0.1 to 2.5 w/v % of vegetable oil act as a non-aqueous solvent, a hydrophilic and hydrophobic emulsifier used in the ratio of 0.1 -5.0 w/v %, was patented. The particle size of nanoemulsion was found to be in the range of 1 nm to 100 nm. The nanoemulsion showed minimizing foreign body sensation and visual disturbance as compared with the corresponding restasis™ product [144].

Simonnet *et al.* patented the nanoemulsion composition that contains oily phase components dispersed into the aqueous phase, and the used surfactant has solid at a temperature of less than or equal to 45°C such as ethoxylated fatty ethers and ethoxylated fatty esters. Moreover, the selection of the oil phase has a molecular weight more significant than 400; and the oil globule has a diameter less than that of 100 nm. The compositions were especially useful for various topical routes like skin, hair, scalp, mucous membranes, and eyes [145]. The same research group patented the O/W nanoemulsion containing anionic surfactants such as phosphoric acid fatty esters and oxyethylene derivatives. In the non-aqueous phase containing oil components having a molecular weight of greater than 400 and oil globules having a diameter of less than 100 nm, the composition of nanoemulsion is exclusively useful in topical, dermatological and cosmetic ophthalmic drug delivery [146]. Simonnet *et al.* developed the new nanoemulsion composition that includes a 1-80% oil phase; the aqueous phase contains one cationic surfactant such as 0.1% -0.4% of cetylpyridinium chloride or 0.05%-1.6% of benzalkonium chloride, 0.1-50% of organic solvent, and water. The average globule diameter was found in less than that of 3 microns. The improved composition displayed used for the treatment of acne or inhibiting the growth of Propionibacterium acnes [147].

Chaudhary and Naithani prepared nanoemulsion containing the blend of lemon juice and rose water as active principles of the aqueous phase incorporated into selected essential oils, such as tulsi oil, lavender oil, tea tree oil, bergamot oil, rosemary oil, jojoba oil, clove oil, and mentha oil along with non-ionic surfactant and co-surfactant. The formed nanoemulsion showed superior therapeutic activity in treating acne and other skin disorders [148]. Baker *et al.* investigated nano-emulsion of terbinafine hydrochloride to treat onychomycosis caused by a fungal, yeast, or mold. Nanoemulsions were formulated with varying composition of 1%-80% oil, 0.1%-50% organic solvent, 0.001%-10% surfactant, 0.0005% -1% of a chelating agent. The average droplet diameter of nanoemulsion has less than that of 1000 nm. Nanoemulsion with key components such as ceteareth-20, ceteareth-12, glyceryl stearate, Cetearyl alcohol, and cetyl palmitate was developed [149]. Gesztesi *et al.* prepared cosmetic products that impart an opaque coloration, along with other benefits such as better absorption of the components *via* skin layer, improved softness, velvetiness, and moisturizing outcome observed for 24 hours. The nanoemulsion showed improved bactericidal action without the incorporation of preservatives. The average diameter of the oil globule was obtained in the range of 50 to 200 nm) [150].

Schmid and Burmeister applied for a patent of 5-aminolevulinic acid nanoemulsion composition containing lipid phase along with emulsifier soybean lecithin. The formed nanoemulsion size ranges from 10 to 200 nm. This formulation is used for photodynamic therapy and photo diagnostic findings of proliferative cells [151]. Baker *et al.* developed an O/W type of antimicrobial nanoemulsion comprised of quaternary ammonium compound that acts as an active principle along with surfactant, ethanol, glycerol, and polyethylene glycol as co-surfactant, detergent, colorant, and flavoring. The nanoemulsion principle was primarily used to protect the foodstuffs from pathogenic microbes [152].

CONCLUSION

Nanoemulsion has been established as a flexible vehicle for topical (skin/ocular) delivery of different drug molecule categories. It has been considered an intelligent way to resolve solubility and bioavailability-related problems and may be an effective therapeutic dosage form compared to different semisolid forms. The surface characteristic of nanoemulsion is vital for improving their contact with ocular/skin surface and plays a vital role in drug transport. The topical delivery of positively charged carriers is beneficial because this charge supports intensive adsorption to the negatively charged (skin/ocular) surface. Therefore, it enhances the retention time and bioavailability of drug molecules.

Similarly, mucoadhesive coating on nanoemulsion has also proven a promising outcome in managing ocular diseases. These systems represent an intelligent approach to surmounting barriers (skin/ocular). The nanoemulsions can interact with the topical (skin/ocular) membranes and deliver the drug efficiently.

CONSENT FOR PUBLICATION

Not applicable.

CONFLICT OF INTEREST

The authors declare no conflict of interest, financial or otherwise.

ACKNOWLEDGEMENT

Declared none.

REFERENCES

[1] Bourrel M, Salager JL, Schechter RS, Wade WH. A correlation for phase behavior of nonionic surfactants. J Colloid Interface Sci 1980; 75(2): 451-61. [http://dx.doi.org/10.1016/0021-9797(80)90470-1]

[2] Holmberg K, Dinesh OS, Milan JS. Handbook of applied surface and colloid chemistry. New York:

Wiley-Blackwell 2002.

[3] Wormuth KR, Kaler EW. Microemulsifying polar oils. J Phys Chem 1989; 93(12): 4855-61. [http://dx.doi.org/10.1021/j100349a035]

[4] Rosen MJ, Joy TK. Surfactants and interfacial phenomena. 4th ed., USA: John Wiley & Sons 2012. [http://dx.doi.org/10.1002/9781118228920]

[5] Rao J, McClements DJ. Formation of flavor oil microemulsions, nanoemulsions and emulsions: influence of composition and preparation method. J Agric Food Chem 2011; 59(9): 5026-35. [http://dx.doi.org/10.1021/jf200094m] [PMID: 21410259]

[6] Date AA, Nagarsenker MS. Parenteral microemulsions: An overview. Int J Pharm 2008; 355(1-2): 19-30. [http://dx.doi.org/10.1016/j.ijpharm.2008.01.004] [PMID: 18295991]

[7] Tamilvanan S. Oil-in-water lipid emulsions: implications for parenteral and ocular delivering systems. Prog Lipid Res 2004; 43(6): 489-533. [http://dx.doi.org/10.1016/j.plipres.2004.09.001] [PMID: 15522762]

[8] Ranade VV, John BC. Drug delivery systems. 3rd ed., New York: CRC Press 2011. [http://dx.doi.org/10.1201/b10846]

[9] McClements DJ. Nanoemulsions versus microemulsions: terminology, differences, and similarities. Soft Matter 2012; 8(6): 1719-29. [http://dx.doi.org/10.1039/C2SM06903B]

[10] Lawrence MJ, Rees GD. Microemulsion-based media as novel drug delivery systems. Adv Drug Deliv Rev 2000; 45(1): 89-121. [http://dx.doi.org/10.1016/S0169-409X(00)00103-4] [PMID: 11104900]

[11] Solans C, Solé I. Nano-emulsions: Formation by low-energy methods. Curr Opin Colloid Interface Sci 2012; 17(5): 246-54. [http://dx.doi.org/10.1016/j.cocis.2012.07.003]

[12] Ganta S, Talekar M, Singh A, Coleman TP, Amiji MM. Nanoemulsions in translational research-opportunities and challenges in targeted cancer therapy. AAPS PharmSciTech 2014; 15(3): 694-708. [http://dx.doi.org/10.1208/s12249-014-0088-9] [PMID: 24510526]

[13] Gupta A, Eral HB, Hatton TA, Doyle PS. Nanoemulsions: formation, properties and applications. Soft Matter 2016; 12(11): 2826-41. [http://dx.doi.org/10.1039/C5SM02958A] [PMID: 26924445]

[14] Anton N, Vandamme TF. Nano-emulsions and micro-emulsions: clarifications of the critical differences. Pharm Res 2011; 28(5): 978-85. [http://dx.doi.org/10.1007/s11095-010-0309-1] [PMID: 21057856]

[15] Alvarado HL, Abrego G, Souto EB, *et al.* Nanoemulsions for dermal controlled release of oleanolic and ursolic acids: *In vitro, ex vivo* and *in vivo* characterization. Colloids Surf B Biointerfaces 2015; 130: 40-7. [http://dx.doi.org/10.1016/j.colsurfb.2015.03.062] [PMID: 25899842]

[16] Pawar KR, Babu RJ. Lipid materials for topical and transdermal delivery of nanoemulsions. Crit Rev Ther Drug Carrier Syst 2014; 31(5): 429-58. [http://dx.doi.org/10.1615/CritRevTherDrugCarrierSyst.2014010663] [PMID: 25271559]

[17] Gupta S, Bansal R, Gupta S, Jindal N, Jindal A. Nanocarriers and nanoparticles for skin care and dermatological treatments. Indian Dermatol Online J 2013; 4(4): 267-72. [http://dx.doi.org/10.4103/2229-5178.120635] [PMID: 24350003]

[18] Schreier H, Bouwstra J. Liposomes and niosomes as topical drug carriers: dermal and transdermal drug delivery. J Control Release 1994; 30(1): 1-15. [http://dx.doi.org/10.1016/0168-3659(94)90039-6]

[19] Cevc G, Blume G. New, highly efficient formulation of diclofenac for the topical, transdermal administration in ultradeformable drug carriers, Transfersomes. Biochim Biophys Acta Biomembr 2001; 1514(2): 191-205.
[http://dx.doi.org/10.1016/S0005-2736(01)00369-8] [PMID: 11557020]

[20] Bhalaria MK, Naik S, Misra AN. Ethosomes: a novel delivery system for antifungal drugs in the treatment of topical fungal diseases. Indian J Exp Biol 2009; 47(5): 368-75.
[PMID: 19579803]

[21] Souto EB, Wissing SA, Barbosa CM, Müller RH. Development of a controlled release formulation based on SLN and NLC for topical clotrimazole delivery. Int J Pharm 2004; 278(1): 71-7.
[http://dx.doi.org/10.1016/j.ijpharm.2004.02.032] [PMID: 15158950]

[22] Gupta S, Kesarla R, Omri A. Formulation strategies to improve the bioavailability of poorly absorbed drugs with special emphasis on self-emulsifying systems. ISRN Pharm 2013; 2013: 1-16.
[http://dx.doi.org/10.1155/2013/848043] [PMID: 24459591]

[23] Shen Q, Wang Y, Yi Zhang . Improvement of colchicine oral bioavailability by incorporating eugenol in the nanoemulsion as an oil excipient and enhancer. Int J Nanomedicine 2011; 6: 1237-43.
[http://dx.doi.org/10.2147/IJN.S20903] [PMID: 21753875]

[24] Araújo FA, Kelmann RG, Araújo BV, Finatto RB, Teixeira HF, Koester LS. Development and characterization of parenteral nanoemulsions containing thalidomide. Eur J Pharm Sci 2011; 42(3): 238-45.
[http://dx.doi.org/10.1016/j.ejps.2010.11.014] [PMID: 21130164]

[25] Hagigit T, Abdulrazik M, Valamanesh F, Behar-Cohen F, Benita S. Ocular antisense oligonucleotide delivery by cationic nanoemulsion for improved treatment of ocular neovascularization: An *in-vivo* study in rats and mice. J Control Release 2012; 160(2): 225-31.
[http://dx.doi.org/10.1016/j.jconrel.2011.11.022] [PMID: 22138070]

[26] Abdulkarim M, Abdullah GZ, Chitneni M, *et al.* Topical piroxicam *in vitro* release and *in vivo* anti-inflammatory and analgesic effects from palm oil esters-based nanocream. Int J Nanomedicine 2010; 5: 915-24.
[http://dx.doi.org/10.2147/IJN.S13305] [PMID: 21116332]

[27] Sonneville-Aubrun O, Simonnet JT, L'Alloret F. Nanoemulsions: a new vehicle for skincare products. Adv Colloid Interface Sci 2004; 108-109: 145-9.
[http://dx.doi.org/10.1016/j.cis.2003.10.026] [PMID: 15072937]

[28] Mason TG, Wilking JN, Meleson K, Chang CB, Graves SM. Nanoemulsions: formation, structure, and physical properties. J Phys Condens Matter 2006; 18(41): R635-66.
[http://dx.doi.org/10.1088/0953-8984/18/41/R01]

[29] Salim N, Basri M, Rahman MB, Abdullah DK, Basri H. Modification of palm kernel oil esters nanoemulsions with hydrocolloid gum for enhanced topical delivery of ibuprofen. Int J Nanomedicine 2012; 7: 4739-47.
[PMID: 22973096]

[30] Hussain A, Singh S, Webster TJ, Ahmad FJ. New perspectives in the topical delivery of optimized amphotericin B loaded nanoemulsions using excipients with innate anti-fungal activities: A mechanistic and histopathological investigation. Nanomedicine 2017; 13(3): 1117-26.
[http://dx.doi.org/10.1016/j.nano.2016.12.002] [PMID: 28007632]

[31] Ahmed M, Ramadan W, Rambhu D, Shakeel F. Potential of nanoemulsions for intravenous delivery of rifampicin. Pharmazie 2008; 63(11): 806-11.
[PMID: 19069240]

[32] McNeill SC, Potts RO, Francoeur ML. Local enhanced topical delivery (LETD) of drugs: does it truly exist? Pharm Res 1992; 9(11): 1422-7.
[http://dx.doi.org/10.1023/A:1015854728278] [PMID: 1475228]

[33] Pradhan M, Singh D, Singh MR. Novel colloidal carriers for psoriasis: Current issues, mechanistic insight and novel delivery approaches. J Control Release 2013; 170(3): 380-95. [http://dx.doi.org/10.1016/j.jconrel.2013.05.020] [PMID: 23770117]

[34] Choudhury S, Dasgupta S, Patel DK, Ramani YR, Ghosh SK, Mazumder B. Advanced Nanomaterials and Nanotechnology.Nanoemulsion as a Carrier for Topical Delivery of Aceclofenac. Berlin, Heidelberg: Springer 2013; pp. 1-19.

[35] Ghosh V, Mukherjee A, Chandrasekaran N. Eugenol-loaded antimicrobial nanoemulsion preserves fruit juice against, microbial spoilage. Colloids Surf B Biointerfaces 2014; 114: 392-7. [http://dx.doi.org/10.1016/j.colsurfb.2013.10.034] [PMID: 24252231]

[36] Abd-Elsalam KA, Khokhlov AR. Eugenol oil nanoemulsion: antifungal activity against Fusarium oxysporum f. sp. vasinfectum and phytotoxicity on cottonseeds. Appl Nanosci 2015; 5(2): 255-65. [http://dx.doi.org/10.1007/s13204-014-0398-y]

[37] Morais Diane JM, Burgess J. Vitamin E nanoemulsions characterization and analysis. Int J Pharm 2014; 465(1-2): 455-63. [http://dx.doi.org/10.1016/j.ijpharm.2014.02.034] [PMID: 24560639]

[38] Ali MS, Alam MS, Alam N, Siddiqui MR. Preparation, characterization and stability study of dutasteride loaded nanoemulsion for treatment of benign prostatic hypertrophy. Iran J Pharm Res 2014; 13(4): 1125-40. [PMID: 25587300]

[39] Zhang T, Dong D, Lu D, Wang S, Wu B. Cremophor EL-based nanoemulsion enhances transcellular permeation of emodin through glucuronidation reduction in UGT1A1-overexpressing MDCKII cells. Int J Pharm 2016; 501(1-2): 190-8. [http://dx.doi.org/10.1016/j.ijpharm.2016.01.067] [PMID: 26850314]

[40] Jo YJ, Kwon YJ. Characterization of β-carotene nanoemulsions prepared by microfluidization technique. Food Sci Biotechnol 2014; 23(1): 107-13. [http://dx.doi.org/10.1007/s10068-014-0014-7]

[41] Jadhav C, Kate V, Payghan SA. Investigation of effect of non-ionic surfactant on preparation of griseofulvin non-aqueous nanoemulsion. J Nanostructure Chem 2015; 5(1): 107-13. [http://dx.doi.org/10.1007/s40097-014-0141-y]

[42] Scheller KJ, Williams SJ, Lawrence AJ, Jarrott B, Djouma E. An improved method to prepare an injectable microemulsion of the galanin-receptor 3 selective antagonist, SNAP 37889, using Kolliphor® HS 15. MethodsX 2014; 1: 212-6. [http://dx.doi.org/10.1016/j.mex.2014.09.003] [PMID: 26150955]

[43] Lante A, Friso D. Oxidative stability and rheological properties of nanoemulsions with ultrasonic extracted green tea infusion. Food Res Int 2013; 54(1): 269-76. [http://dx.doi.org/10.1016/j.foodres.2013.07.009]

[44] Tadros T, Izquierdo P, Esquena J, Solans C. Formation and stability of nano-emulsions. Adv Colloid Interface Sci 2004; 108-109: 303-18. [http://dx.doi.org/10.1016/j.cis.2003.10.023] [PMID: 15072948]

[45] Shakeel F, Shafiq S, Haq N, Alanazi FK, Alsarra IA. Nanoemulsions as potential vehicles for transdermal and dermal delivery of hydrophobic compounds: an overview. Expert Opin Drug Deliv 2012; 9(8): 953-74. [http://dx.doi.org/10.1517/17425247.2012.696605] [PMID: 22703228]

[46] Sutradhar KB, Amin ML. Nanoemulsions: increasing possibilities in drug delivery. Eur J Nanomed 2013; 5(1): 97-110.

[47] Rai VK, Mishra N, Yadav KS, Yadav NP. Nanoemulsion as pharmaceutical carrier for dermal and transdermal drug delivery: Formulation development, stability issues, basic considerations and applications. J Control Release 2018; 270: 203-25.

[http://dx.doi.org/10.1016/j.jconrel.2017.11.049] [PMID: 29199062]

[48] Sugumar S, Ghosh V, Nirmala MJ, Mukherjee A, Chandrasekaran N. Ultrasonic emulsification of eucalyptus oil nanoemulsion: Antibacterial activity against Staphylococcus aureus and wound healing activity in Wistar rats. Ultrason Sonochem 2014; 21(3): 1044-9. [http://dx.doi.org/10.1016/j.ultsonch.2013.10.021] [PMID: 24262758]

[49] Laxmi M, Bhardwaj A, Mehta S, Mehta A. Development and characterization of nanoemulsion as carrier for the enhancement of bioavailability of artemether. Artif Cells Nanomed Biotechnol 2015; 43(5): 334-44. [http://dx.doi.org/10.3109/21691401.2014.887018] [PMID: 24641773]

[50] Hsieh CW, Li PH, Lu IC, Wang TH. Preparing glabridin-in-water nanoemulsions by high pressure homogenization with response surface methodology. J Oleo Sci 2012; 61(9): 483-9. [http://dx.doi.org/10.5650/jos.61.483] [PMID: 22975782]

[51] Solè I, Maestro A, González C, Solans C, Gutiérrez JM, Gutiérrez JM. Optimization of nano-emulsion preparation by low-energy methods in an ionic surfactant system. Langmuir 2006; 22(20): 8326-32. [http://dx.doi.org/10.1021/la0613676] [PMID: 16981744]

[52] Bouchemal K, Briançon S, Perrier E, Fessi H. Nano-emulsion formulation using spontaneous emulsification: solvent, oil and surfactant optimisation. Int J Pharm 2004; 280(1-2): 241-51. [http://dx.doi.org/10.1016/j.ijpharm.2004.05.016] [PMID: 15265563]

[53] Fernandez P, André V, Rieger J, Kühnle A. Nano-emulsion formation by emulsion phase inversion. Colloids Surf A Physicochem Eng Asp 2004; 251(1-3): 53-8. [http://dx.doi.org/10.1016/j.colsurfa.2004.09.029]

[54] Ostertag F, Weiss J, McClements DJ. Low-energy formation of edible nanoemulsions: Factors influencing droplet size produced by emulsion phase inversion. J Colloid Interface Sci 2012; 388(1): 95-102. [http://dx.doi.org/10.1016/j.jcis.2012.07.089] [PMID: 22981587]

[55] Singh Y, Meher JG, Raval K, *et al.* Nanoemulsion: Concepts, development and applications in drug delivery. J Control Release 2017; 252: 28-49. [http://dx.doi.org/10.1016/j.jconrel.2017.03.008] [PMID: 28279798]

[56] Yu L, Li C, Xu J, Hao J, Sun D. Highly stable concentrated nanoemulsions by the phase inversion composition method at elevated temperature. Langmuir 2012; 28(41): 14547-52. [http://dx.doi.org/10.1021/la302995a] [PMID: 22985401]

[57] Filipe V, Hawe A, Jiskoot W. Critical evaluation of Nanoparticle Tracking Analysis (NTA) by NanoSight for the measurement of nanoparticles and protein aggregates. Pharm Res 2010; 27(5): 796-810. [http://dx.doi.org/10.1007/s11095-010-0073-2] [PMID: 20204471]

[58] Jornada DS, Fiel LA, Bueno K, *et al.* Lipid-core nanocapsules: mechanism of self-assembly, control of size and loading capacity. Soft Matter 2012; 8(24): 6646-55. [http://dx.doi.org/10.1039/c2sm25754h]

[59] Rahimian S, Fransen MF, Kleinovink JW, *et al.* Polymeric nanoparticles for co-delivery of synthetic long peptide antigen and poly IC as therapeutic cancer vaccine formulation. J Control Release 2015; 203: 16-22. [http://dx.doi.org/10.1016/j.jconrel.2015.02.006] [PMID: 25660830]

[60] Frisken BJ. Revisiting the method of cumulants for the analysis of dynamic light-scattering data. Appl Opt 2001; 40(24): 4087-91. [http://dx.doi.org/10.1364/AO.40.004087] [PMID: 18360445]

[61] Mailer AG, Clegg PS, Pusey PN. Particle sizing by dynamic light scattering: non-linear cumulant analysis. J Phys Condens Matter 2015; 27(14)145102 [http://dx.doi.org/10.1088/0953-8984/27/14/145102] [PMID: 25788443]

[62] Calderilla-Fajardo SB, Cázares-Delgadillo J, Villalobos-García R, Quintanar-Guerrero D, Ganem-Quintanar A, Robles R. Influence of sucrose esters on the *in vivo* percutaneous penetration of octyl methoxycinnamate formulated in nanocapsules, nanoemulsion, and emulsion. Drug Dev Ind Pharm 2006; 32(1): 107-13.
[http://dx.doi.org/10.1080/03639040500388540] [PMID: 16455609]

[63] Hatziantoniou S, Deli G, Nikas Y, Demetzos C, Papaioannou GT. Scanning electron microscopy study on nanoemulsions and solid lipid nanoparticles containing high amounts of ceramides. Micron 2007; 38(8): 819-23.
[http://dx.doi.org/10.1016/j.micron.2007.06.010] [PMID: 17693092]

[64] Kuntsche J, Horst JC, Bunjes H. Cryogenic transmission electron microscopy (cryo-TEM) for studying the morphology of colloidal drug delivery systems. Int J Pharm 2011; 417(1-2): 120-37.
[http://dx.doi.org/10.1016/j.ijpharm.2011.02.001] [PMID: 21310225]

[65] Klang V, Matsko NB, Valenta C, Hofer F. Electron microscopy of nanoemulsions: An essential tool for characterisation and stability assessment. Micron 2012; 43(2-3): 85-103.
[http://dx.doi.org/10.1016/j.micron.2011.07.014] [PMID: 21839644]

[66] Hunter RJ. Zeta Potential in Colloid Science. 1st ed., New York: Academic Press 1981.

[67] Sze A, Erickson D, Ren L, Li D. Zeta-potential measurement using the Smoluchowski equation and the slope of the current–time relationship in electroosmotic flow. J Colloid Interface Sci 2003; 261(2): 402-10.
[http://dx.doi.org/10.1016/S0021-9797(03)00142-5] [PMID: 16256549]

[68] Fujii M, Büyüktimkin S, Büyüktimkin N, Rytting JH. Enhancement of skin permeation of miconazole by phospholipid and dodecyl 2-(N,N-dimethyl amino)propionate (DDAIP). Int J Pharm 2002; 234(1-2): 121-8.
[http://dx.doi.org/10.1016/S0378-5173(01)00951-6] [PMID: 11839443]

[69] Peira E, Carlotti ME, Trotta C, Cavalli R, Trotta M. Positively charged microemulsions for topical application. Int J Pharm 2008; 346(1-2): 119-23.
[http://dx.doi.org/10.1016/j.ijpharm.2007.05.065] [PMID: 17618070]

[70] Montenegro L, Lai F, Offerta A, *et al.* From nanoemulsions to nanostructured lipid carriers: A relevant development in dermal delivery of drugs and cosmetics. J Drug Deliv Sci Technol 2016; 32: 100-12.
[http://dx.doi.org/10.1016/j.jddst.2015.10.003]

[71] Hussain A, Samad A, Nazish I, Ahmed FJ. Nanocarrier-based topical drug delivery for an antifungal drug. Drug Dev Ind Pharm 2014; 40(4): 527-41.
[http://dx.doi.org/10.3109/03639045.2013.771647] [PMID: 23627443]

[72] Shahzad Y, Louw R, Gerber M, du Plessis J. Breaching the skin barrier through temperature modulations. J Control Release 2015; 202: 1-13.
[http://dx.doi.org/10.1016/j.jconrel.2015.01.019] [PMID: 25616160]

[73] Ghaffarian R, Muro S. Models and methods to evaluate transport of drug delivery systems across cellular barriers. J Vis Exp 2013; 80(80)e50638
[http://dx.doi.org/10.3791/50638] [PMID: 24192611]

[74] Papakostas D, Rancan F, Sterry W, Blume-Peytavi U, Vogt A. Nanoparticles in dermatology. Arch Dermatol Res 2011; 303(8): 533-50.
[http://dx.doi.org/10.1007/s00403-011-1163-7] [PMID: 21837474]

[75] Manca ML, Manconi M, Nacher A, *et al.* Development of novel diolein–niosomes for cutaneous delivery of tretinoin: Influence of formulation and *in vitro* assessment. Int J Pharm 2014; 477(1-2): 176-86.
[http://dx.doi.org/10.1016/j.ijpharm.2014.10.031] [PMID: 25455770]

[76] Wartewig S, Neubert RHH. Properties of ceramides and their impact on the stratum corneum structure: a review. Part 1: ceramides. Skin Pharmacol Physiol 2007; 20(5): 220-9.

[http://dx.doi.org/10.1159/000104420] [PMID: 17587886]

[77] Azeem A, Talegaonkar S, Negi LM, Ahmad FJ, Khar RK, Iqbal Z. Oil based nanocarrier system for transdermal delivery of ropinirole: A mechanistic, pharmacokinetic and biochemical investigation. Int J Pharm 2012; 422(1-2): 436-44.
[http://dx.doi.org/10.1016/j.ijpharm.2011.10.039] [PMID: 22057087]

[78] Lallemand F, Daull P, Benita S, Buggage R, Garrigue JS. Successfully improving ocular drug delivery using the cationic nanoemulsion, novasorb. J Drug Deliv 2012; 2012: 1-16.
[http://dx.doi.org/10.1155/2012/604204] [PMID: 22506123]

[79] Kreilgaard M. Influence of microemulsions on cutaneous drug delivery. Adv Drug Deliv Rev 2002; 54(1) (Suppl. 1): S77-98.
[http://dx.doi.org/10.1016/S0169-409X(02)00116-3] [PMID: 12460717]

[80] Dhote V, Bhatnagar P, Mishra PK, Mahajan SC, Mishra DK. Iontophoresis: a potential emergence of a transdermal drug delivery system. Sci Pharm 2012; 80(1): 1-28.
[http://dx.doi.org/10.3797/scipharm.1108-20] [PMID: 22396901]

[81] Park CW, Son DD, Kim JY, *et al.* Investigation of formulation factors affecting *in vitro* and *in vivo* characteristics of a galantamine transdermal system. Int J Pharm 2012; 436(1-2): 32-40.
[http://dx.doi.org/10.1016/j.ijpharm.2012.06.057] [PMID: 22771734]

[82] Prow TW, Grice JE, Lin LL, *et al.* Nanoparticles and microparticles for skin drug delivery. Adv Drug Deliv Rev 2011; 63(6): 470-91.
[http://dx.doi.org/10.1016/j.addr.2011.01.012] [PMID: 21315122]

[83] Langbein L, Grund C, Kuhn C, *et al.* Tight junctions and compositionally related junctional structures in mammalian stratified epithelia and cell cultures derived therefrom. Eur J Cell Biol 2002; 81(8): 419-35.
[http://dx.doi.org/10.1078/0171-9335-00270] [PMID: 12234014]

[84] Solans C, Izquierdo P, Nolla J, Azemar N, Garcia-Celma MJ. Nano-emulsions. Curr Opin Colloid Interface Sci 2005; 10(3-4): 102-10.
[http://dx.doi.org/10.1016/j.cocis.2005.06.004]

[85] Wu Y, Li YH, Gao XH, Chen HD. The application of nanoemulsion in dermatology: an overview. J Drug Target 2013; 21(4): 321-7.
[http://dx.doi.org/10.3109/1061186X.2013.765442] [PMID: 23600746]

[86] Silva HD, Cerqueira MÂ, Vicente AA. Nanoemulsions for food applications: development and characterization. Food Bioprocess Technol 2012; 5(3): 854-67.
[http://dx.doi.org/10.1007/s11947-011-0683-7]

[87] Sakeena MH, Elrashid SM, Muthanna FA, *et al.* Effect of limonene on permeation enhancement of ketoprofen in palm oil esters nanoemulsion. J Oleo Sci 2010; 59(7): 395-400.
[http://dx.doi.org/10.5650/jos.59.395] [PMID: 20513974]

[88] El-Leithy ES, Ibrahim HK, Sorour RM. *In vitro* and *in vivo* evaluation of indomethacin nanoemulsion as a transdermal delivery system. Drug Deliv 2015; 22(8): 1010-7.
[http://dx.doi.org/10.3109/10717544.2013.844742] [PMID: 24188427]

[89] Dasgupta S, Dey S, Choudhury S, Mazumder B. Topical delivery of aceclofenac as nanoemulsion comprising excipients having optimum emulsification capabilities: preparation, characterization and *in vivo* evaluation. Expert Opin Drug Deliv 2013; 10(4): 411-20.
[http://dx.doi.org/10.1517/17425247.2013.749234] [PMID: 23316798]

[90] Subramanian B, Kuo F, Ada E, *et al.* Enhancement of anti-inflammatory property of aspirin in mice by a nano-emulsion preparation. Int Immunopharmacol 2008; 8(11): 1533-9.
[http://dx.doi.org/10.1016/j.intimp.2008.06.009] [PMID: 18625344]

[91] Mou D, Chen H, Du D, *et al.* Hydrogel-thickened nanoemulsion system for topical delivery of lipophilic drugs. Int J Pharm 2008; 353(1-2): 270-6.

[http://dx.doi.org/10.1016/j.ijpharm.2007.11.051] [PMID: 18215479]

[92] Esmaeili F, Rajabnejhad S, Partoazar AR, *et al.* Anti-inflammatory effects of eugenol nanoemulsion as a topical delivery system. Pharm Dev Technol 2016; 21(7): 887-93. [http://dx.doi.org/10.3109/10837450.2015.1078353] [PMID: 26365132]

[93] Baspinar Y, Borchert HH. Penetration and release studies of positively and negatively charged nanoemulsions—Is there a benefit of the positive charge? Int J Pharm 2012; 430(1-2): 247-52. [http://dx.doi.org/10.1016/j.ijpharm.2012.03.040] [PMID: 22486953]

[94] Negi P, Singh B, Sharma G, Beg S, Katare OP. Biocompatible lidocaine and prilocaine loaded-nanoemulsion system for enhanced percutaneous absorption: QbD-based optimisation, dermato-kinetics and *in vivo* evaluation. J Microencapsul 2015; 32(5): 419-31. [http://dx.doi.org/10.3109/02652048.2015.1046513] [PMID: 26066775]

[95] Hussain A, Singh VK, Singh OP, Shafaat K, Kumar S, Ahmad FJ. Formulation and optimization of nanoemulsion using antifungal lipid and surfactant for accentuated topical delivery of Amphotericin B. Drug Deliv 2016; 23(8): 3101-10. [http://dx.doi.org/10.3109/10717544.2016.1153747] [PMID: 27854145]

[96] Yu M, Ma H, Lei M, Li N, Tan F. *In vitro/in vivo* characterization of nanoemulsion formulation of metronidazole with improved skin targeting and anti-rosacea properties. Eur J Pharm Biopharm 2014; 88(1): 92-103. [http://dx.doi.org/10.1016/j.ejpb.2014.03.019] [PMID: 24704200]

[97] Borges VR, Simon A, Sena ARC, Cabral LM, de Sousa VP. Nanoemulsion containing dapsone for topical administration: a study of *in vitro* release and epidermal permeation. Int J Nanomedicine 2013; 8: 535-44. [PMID: 23411489]

[98] Kaur A, Katiyar SS, Kushwah V, Jain S. Nanoemulsion loaded gel for topical co-delivery of clobitasol propionate and calcipotriol in psoriasis. Nanomedicine 2017; 13(4): 1473-82. [http://dx.doi.org/10.1016/j.nano.2017.02.009] [PMID: 28259803]

[99] de Mattos CB, Argenta DF, Melchiades GdeL, *et al.* Nanoemulsions containing a synthetic chalcone as an alternative for treating cutaneous leshmaniasis: optimization using a full factorial design. Int J Nanomedicine 2015; 10: 5529-42. [PMID: 26366075]

[100] Kelmann RG, Colombo M, De Araújo Lopes SC, *et al.* Pentyl gallate nanoemulsions as potential topical treatment of herpes labialis. J Pharm Sci 2016; 105(7): 2194-203. [http://dx.doi.org/10.1016/j.xphs.2016.04.028] [PMID: 27290627]

[101] Shakeel F, Haq N, Al-Dhfyan A, Alanazi FK, Alsarra IA. Chemoprevention of skin cancer using low HLB surfactant nanoemulsion of 5-fluorouracil: a preliminary study. Drug Deliv 2015; 22(4): 573-80. [http://dx.doi.org/10.3109/10717544.2013.868557] [PMID: 24350612]

[102] Siggers JH, Ethier CR. Fluid mechanics of the eye. Annu Rev Fluid Mech 2012; 44(1): 347-72. [http://dx.doi.org/10.1146/annurev-fluid-120710-101058]

[103] Yellepeddi VK, Palakurthi S. Recent advances in topical ocular drug delivery. J Ocul Pharmacol Ther 2016; 32(2): 67-82. [http://dx.doi.org/10.1089/jop.2015.0047] [PMID: 26666398]

[104] Ali J, Fazil M, Qumbar M, Khan N, Ali A. Colloidal drug delivery system: amplify the ocular delivery. Drug Deliv 2016; 23(3): 710-26. [PMID: 24892625]

[105] Zafar A, Ahmad J, Addo RT, Akhter S. Progress of Controlled Drug Delivery Systems in Topical Ophthalmology: Focus on Nano and Micro Drug Carriers.Ocular Drug Delivery: Advances, Challenges and Applications. Cham: Springer 2016; pp. 131-63. [http://dx.doi.org/10.1007/978-3-319-47691-9_9]

[106] Cholkar K, Patel SP, Vadlapudi AD, Mitra AK. Novel strategies for anterior segment ocular drug delivery. J Ocul Pharmacol Ther 2013; 29(2): 106-23.
[http://dx.doi.org/10.1089/jop.2012.0200] [PMID: 23215539]

[107] Natarajan JV, Chattopadhyay S, Ang M, *et al.* Sustained release of an anti-glaucoma drug: demonstration of efficacy of a liposomal formulation in the rabbit eye. PLoS One 2011; 6(9)e24513
[http://dx.doi.org/10.1371/journal.pone.0024513] [PMID: 21931735]

[108] Almeida H, Amaral MH, Lobão P, Sousa Lobo JM. Applications of poloxamers in ophthalmic pharmaceutical formulations: an overview. Expert Opin Drug Deliv 2013; 10(9): 1223-37.
[http://dx.doi.org/10.1517/17425247.2013.796360] [PMID: 23688342]

[109] Ghate D, Edelhauser HF. Ocular drug delivery. Expert Opin Drug Deliv 2006; 3(2): 275-87.
[http://dx.doi.org/10.1517/17425247.3.2.275] [PMID: 16506953]

[110] Lee VHL. Mechanisms and facilitation of corneal drug penetration. J Control Release 1990; 11(1-3): 79-90.
[http://dx.doi.org/10.1016/0168-3659(90)90122-A]

[111] Champalal KD, Sushilkumar P. Current status of ophthalmic *in-situ* forming hydrogel. Int J Pharm Bio Sci 2012; 3(3): 372-88.

[112] Gonzalez-Mira E, Nikolić S, Calpena AC, Egea MA, Souto EB, García ML. Improved and safe transcorneal delivery of flurbiprofen by NLC and NLC-based hydrogels. J Pharm Sci 2012; 101(2): 707-25.
[http://dx.doi.org/10.1002/jps.22784] [PMID: 22012873]

[113] Hosoya K, Lee VHL, Kim KJ. Roles of the conjunctiva in ocular drug delivery: a review of conjunctival transport mechanisms and their regulation. Eur J Pharm Biopharm 2005; 60(2): 227-40.
[http://dx.doi.org/10.1016/j.ejpb.2004.12.007] [PMID: 15939235]

[114] Järvinen K, Järvinen T, Urtti A. Ocular absorption following topical delivery. Adv Drug Deliv Rev 1995; 16(1): 3-19.
[http://dx.doi.org/10.1016/0169-409X(95)00010-5]

[115] Kang-Mieler JJ, Osswald CR, Mieler WF. Advances in ocular drug delivery: emphasis on the posterior segment. Expert Opin Drug Deliv 2014; 11(10): 1647-60.
[http://dx.doi.org/10.1517/17425247.2014.935338] [PMID: 24975820]

[116] Kim YC, Chiang B, Wu X, Prausnitz MR. Ocular delivery of macromolecules. J Control Release 2014; 190: 172-81.
[http://dx.doi.org/10.1016/j.jconrel.2014.06.043] [PMID: 24998941]

[117] Kompella UB, Kadam RS, Lee VHL. Recent advances in ophthalmic drug delivery. Ther Deliv 2010; 1(3): 435-56.
[http://dx.doi.org/10.4155/tde.10.40] [PMID: 21399724]

[118] Weng Y, Liu J, Jin S, Guo W, Liang X, Hu Z. Nanotechnology-based strategies for treatment of ocular disease. Acta Pharm Sin B 2017; 7(3): 281-91.
[http://dx.doi.org/10.1016/j.apsb.2016.09.001] [PMID: 28540165]

[119] Urtti A. Challenges and obstacles of ocular pharmacokinetics and drug delivery. Adv Drug Deliv Rev 2006; 58(11): 1131-5.
[http://dx.doi.org/10.1016/j.addr.2006.07.027] [PMID: 17097758]

[120] Cunha-Vaz J. The blood-ocular barriers. Surv Ophthalmol 1979; 23(5): 279-96.
[http://dx.doi.org/10.1016/0039-6257(79)90158-9] [PMID: 380030]

[121] van Bekkum DW. Use of ionizing radiation in transplantation. Transplant Proc 1974; 6(4) (Suppl. 1): 59-65.
[PMID: 4155159]

[122] Ibrahim SS, Awad GAS, Geneidi A, Mortada ND. Comparative effects of different cosurfactants on

sterile prednisolone acetate ocular submicron emulsions stability and release. Colloids Surf B Biointerfaces 2009; 69(2): 225-31.
[http://dx.doi.org/10.1016/j.colsurfb.2008.11.034] [PMID: 19157802]

[123] Muchtar S, Abdulrazik M, Frucht-Pery J, Benita S. Ex-vivo permeation study of indomethacin from a submicron emulsion through albino rabbit cornea. J Control Release 1997; 44(1): 55-64.
[http://dx.doi.org/10.1016/S0168-3659(96)01503-9]

[124] Akhter S, Anwar M, Siddiqui MA, *et al.* Improving the topical ocular pharmacokinetics of an immunosuppressant agent with mucoadhesive nanoemulsions: Formulation development, *in-vitro* and *in-vivo* studies. Colloids Surf B Biointerfaces 2016; 148: 19-29.
[http://dx.doi.org/10.1016/j.colsurfb.2016.08.048] [PMID: 27591567]

[125] Panatieri LF, Brazil NT, Faber K, *et al.* Nanoemulsions containing a coumarin-rich extract from Pterocaulon balansae (Asteraceae) for the treatment of ocular Acanthamoeba keratitis. AAPS PharmSciTech 2017; 18(3): 721-8.
[http://dx.doi.org/10.1208/s12249-016-0550-y] [PMID: 27225384]

[126] Patel N, Nakrani H, Raval M, Sheth N. Development of loteprednol etabonate-loaded cationic nanoemulsified *in-situ* ophthalmic gel for sustained delivery and enhanced ocular bioavailability. Drug Deliv 2016; 23(9): 3712-23.
[http://dx.doi.org/10.1080/10717544.2016.1223225] [PMID: 27689408]

[127] Tayel SA, El-Nabarawi MA, Tadros MI, Abd-Elsalam WH. Promising ion-sensitive *in situ* ocular nanoemulsion gels of terbinafine hydrochloride: Design, *in vitro* characterization and *in vivo* estimation of the ocular irritation and drug pharmacokinetics in the aqueous humor of rabbits. Int J Pharm 2013; 443(1-2): 293-305.
[http://dx.doi.org/10.1016/j.ijpharm.2012.12.049] [PMID: 23333217]

[128] Ammar HO, Salama HA, Ghorab M, Mahmoud AA. Development of dorzolamide hydrochloride *in situ* gel nanoemulsion for ocular delivery. Drug Dev Ind Pharm 2010; 36(11): 1330-9.
[http://dx.doi.org/10.3109/03639041003801885] [PMID: 20545523]

[129] Sznitowska M, Zurowska-Pryczkowska K, Janicki S, Järvinen T. Miotic effect and irritation potential of pilocarpine prodrug incorporated into a submicron emulsion vehicle. Int J Pharm 1999; 184(1): 115-20.
[http://dx.doi.org/10.1016/S0378-5173(99)00106-4] [PMID: 10425357]

[130] Ammar HO, Salama HA, Ghorab M, Mahmoud AA. Nanoemulsion as a potential ophthalmic delivery system for dorzolamide hydrochloride. AAPS PharmSciTech 2009; 10(3): 808-19.
[http://dx.doi.org/10.1208/s12249-009-9268-4] [PMID: 19536653]

[131] Gallarate M, Chirio D, Bussano R, *et al.* Development of O/W nanoemulsions for ophthalmic administration of timolol. Int J Pharm 2013; 440(2): 126-34.
[http://dx.doi.org/10.1016/j.ijpharm.2012.10.015] [PMID: 23078859]

[132] Mahboobian MM, Foroutan SM, Aboofazeli R. Brinzolamide-loaded nanoemulsions: *in vitro* release evaluation. Iran J Pharm Sci 2016; 12(3): 75-93.

[133] Morsi NM, Mohamed MI, Refai H, El Sorogy HM. Nanoemulsion as a novel ophthalmic delivery system for acetazolamide. Int J Pharm Pharm Sci 2014; 6(11): 227-36.

[134] Liu CH, Lai KY, Wu WC, Chen YJ, Lee WS, Hsu CY. In vitro scleral lutein distribution by cyclodextrin containing nanoemulsions. Chem Pharm Bull (Tokyo) 2015; 63(2): 59-67.
[http://dx.doi.org/10.1248/cpb.c14-00318] [PMID: 25748776]

[135] Ying L, Tahara K, Takeuchi H. Drug delivery to the ocular posterior segment using lipid emulsion *via* eye drop administration: Effect of emulsion formulations and surface modification. Int J Pharm 2013; 453(2): 329-35.
[http://dx.doi.org/10.1016/j.ijpharm.2013.06.024] [PMID: 23796836]

[136] Schachat A. New treatments for age-related macular degeneration. Ophthalmology 2005; 112(4): 531-2.
[http://dx.doi.org/10.1016/j.ophtha.2005.01.018] [PMID: 15808239]

[137] Shams N, Ianchulev T. Role of vascular endothelial growth factor in ocular angiogenesis. Ophthalmol Clin North Am 2006; 19(3): 335-44.
[PMID: 16935208]

[138] Garrett KL, Shen WY, Rakoczy PE. *In vivo* use of oligonucleotides to inhibit choroidal neovascularisation in the eye. J Gene Med 2001; 3(4): 373-83.
[http://dx.doi.org/10.1002/jgm.197] [PMID: 11529667]

[139] Gatto B, Cavalli M. From proteins to nucleic acid-based drugs: the role of biotech in anti-VEGF therapy. Anticancer Agents Med Chem 2006; 6(4): 287-301.
[http://dx.doi.org/10.2174/187152006777698178] [PMID: 16842232]

[140] Capek I. Degradation of kinetically-stable o/w emulsions. Adv Colloid Interface Sci 2004; 107(2-3): 125-55.
[http://dx.doi.org/10.1016/S0001-8686(03)00115-5] [PMID: 15026289]

[141] Ee SL, Duan X, Liew J, Nguyen QD. Droplet size and stability of nano-emulsions produced by the temperature phase inversion method. Chem Eng J 2008; 140(1-3): 626-31.
[http://dx.doi.org/10.1016/j.cej.2007.12.016]

[142] Kelmann RG, Kuminek G, Teixeira HF, Koester LS. Carbamazepine parenteral nanoemulsions prepared by spontaneous emulsification process. Int J Pharm 2007; 342(1-2): 231-9.
[http://dx.doi.org/10.1016/j.ijpharm.2007.05.004] [PMID: 17582711]

[143] Lund Walter. The pharmaceutical codex: principles and practice of pharmaceutics. 12th ed., London: Pharmaceutical Press 1994.

[144] Lee JY, Shin YJ, Sang-Rok RYU. Ophthalmic nanoemulsion composition containing cyclosporine and method for preparing same. US Patent 2016.

[145] Simonnet JT, Sonneville O, Legret S, L'Oreal SA. Nanoemulsion based on ethoxylated fatty ethers or on ethoxylated fatty esters and its uses in the cosmetics, dermatological and/or ophthalmological fields. US Patent 6,375,960 2002.

[146] Simonnet JT, Sonneville O, Legret S, L'Oreal SA. Nanoemulsion based on phosphoric acid fatty acid esters and its uses in the cosmetics, dermatological, pharmaceutical, and/or ophthalmological fields. US Patent 6,274,150 2001.

[147] Simonnet J, Ciotti S, Baker JR. Methods of treating acne using nanoemulsion compositions, WO. Patent 2017023751A2 2017.

[148] Chaudhary M, Naithani V. Topical herbal formulation for treatment of acne and skin disorders. US Patent 8,268,367 2012.

[150] Gesztesi JL, Santos LM, Hennies PDT, Macian KA. Oil-in-water nanoemulsion, a cosmetic composition and a cosmetic product comprising it, a process for preparing said nanoemulsion. US Patent 8,956,597 2015.

[151] Schmid HW, Burmeister G. Nano-emulsion of 5-aminolevulinic acid. US Patent 6,559,183 2003.

[152] Baker JR, Hamouda T, Shih A, Myc A. Non-toxic antimicrobial compositions and methods of use. US Patent 6,559,189 2003.

CHAPTER 10

Lipoidal Carrier as Drug Delivery System

Bina Gidwani[1], Priya Namdeo[2], Sakshi Tiwari[2], Atul Tripathi[4], Ravindra Kumar Pandey[1], Shiv Shankar Shukla[1], Veenu Joshi[3], Vishal Jain[2], Suresh Thareja[5] and **Amber Vyas[2,*]**

[1] *Columbia Institute of Pharmacy, Raipur (C.G), India*

[2] *University Institute of Pharmacy, Pt. Ravishankar Shukla University, Raipur (C.G), India*

[3] *Center of Basic Science, Pt. Ravishankar Shukla University, Raipur (C.G), India*

[4] *People's Institute of Pharmacy & Research Centre, Bhopal, (M.P.), India*

[5] *Department of Pharmaceutical Sciences and Natural ProductsCentral University of Punjab Bathinda, Punjab-151001, India*

Abstract: The delivery system plays a vital role in managing the pharmacokinetics and pharmacodynamics of a drug. The size of the carrier system contributes to its pharmacological action. Lipid-based carriers refer to the formulations containing a dissolved or suspended drug in lipidic excipients. Lipoidal systems as carriers are achieving heights due to their significant lipid nature and the size of particles in the delivery system. The micro/nano-sized lipid-based carriers possess versatility in improving the physic-chemical properties of drugs. Also, they are biocompatible and can be administered through all possible routes. Lipid-based drug delivery carrier systems of new and existing formulations can be commercialized to achieve the desired range of product specifications. Solubility of the drug in various lipids is a key factor in the development of the delivery system. Lipids as functional excipients are compatible with solid, liquid, and semi-solid dosage forms. Besides improving/enhancing the solubility and bioavailability, lipids provide multiple broad-based applications in the pharmaceutical delivery system.

Keywords: Bioavailability, BCS Class, Cancer, Carriers, Delivery system, Lipids, Micro/nano, Pharmacokinetics, Pharmacodynamics, Solubility, Liposomes, Solid Lipid Nanoparticles, Nanostructured lipid carrier, Lipid-drug conjugate, Liposphere, Topical, Oral, Parenteral, Pulmonary, Protein/peptide.

INTRODUCTION

Lipoidal carrier is a versatile delivery platform, which has achieved a lot of attention in the current era. Lipoidal carriers are systems with significant

[*] **Corresponding author Amber Vyas:** University Institute of Pharmacy, Pt. Ravishankar Shukla University, Raipur, Chhattisgarh, India; Tel: 9926807999; E-mail: **ambervyas@gmail.com**

Akhlesh K. Jain & Keerti Mishra (Eds.)

biopharmaceutical and technological benefits, making them suitable for effective & optimum therapeutic delivery of drugs. These carriers are based on the concept that ingested fats (lipids) improving lipophilic drug absorption. Monoglycerides, diglycerides, and triglycerides are the most widely accepted lipid excipients, followed by oils containing different combinations of glycerides, sphingolipids, & phospholipids [1]. Typically, the most common use of lipoidal carrier has been to boost the solubility of aqueous insoluble drugs, particularly those classified as Biopharmaceutics Classification System (BCS) Class II & IV [2]. The lipoidal carriers have several unique features that include effective encapsulation of lipophilic and hydrophilic drug candidates, enhanced bioavailability of drug-loaded in the carrier, prolonging of circulation period, targeted distribution to cells and/or organs, increased therapeutic efficacy along with reducing toxicity by modifying the drug pharmacokinetics and biodistribution [3].

When these amphiphilic building blocks are exposed to water, they create highly organized assemblies of one or more concentric lipid bilayers. Carrier particles can be made from a variety of building blocks of amphiphilic drugs [4]. The use of lipoidal carriers for drug delivery emerged in the early 1960s when fatty emulsions were provided *via* parenteral administration of nutrition [5]. In 1965, the first closed bilayer phospholipid system was discovered, thus, encouraging experts worldwide to produce significant technical innovations in the delivery of the lipoidal carrier; as a result, a large number of clinical trials have been conducted [6]. There are several licensed & commercialized lipid-based drug preparations; however, due to the unique features of the lipoidal carrier system, overcoming the delivery of drugs is a challenge for pharmaceuticals with considerable formulating obstacles [7].

Lipoidal carrier-based delivery systems are a broad category of products that can incorporate a drug that has been suspended or dissolved in lipidic excipients. Lipids are fatty acid esters, which are lipophilic hydrocarbon chains connected to a hydrophilic group such as polyalcohol, polyglycerol, and glycerol. The lipoidal carrier system consists of the simple drug in oil to a more complex preparation that is meant to emulsify spontaneously when exposed to an aqueous medium [8]. The temperature, *i.e.*, melting point of lipids, typically increases with molecular weight (hydrocarbon chain length) & decreases with fatty acid unsaturation. Lipids are insoluble in water and are frequently characterized by their fatty acid composition, solubility for non-polar organic solvents, melting temperature & Hydrophilic-Lipophilic Balance (HLB). Lipoidal carriers, including liposomes, submicron lipid emulsions & lipid microspheres, are strongly desired and are now being researched in several ways, with several items being commercially accessible [9].

Need for Lipoidal Carrier System [10]

• If conventional preparations deliver poor bioavailability (Fig. **10.1** shows the reasons for poor bioavailability), a Lipoidal Carrier System is essential.

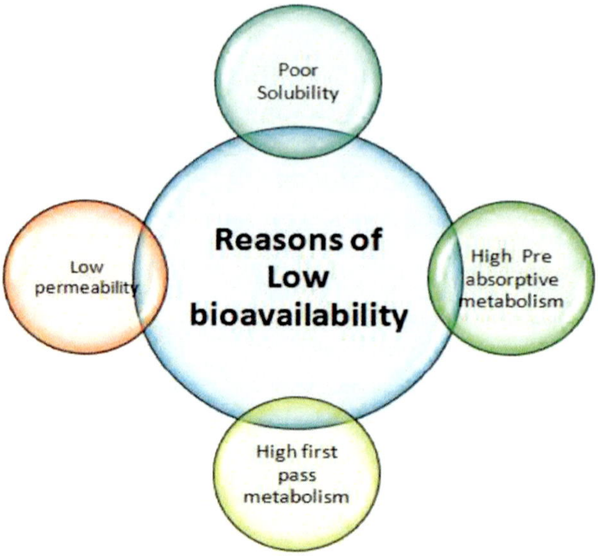

Fig. (10.1). Reasons for low bioavailability.

• Lipoidal Carrier Systems are versatile; they involve the usage of lipids & lipid-based technology in pharmaceutical preparations designed for a wide range of administration routes such as oral, parenteral, transdermal, ophthalmic, *etc.*

• To modify local or systemic drug distribution by solubility, penetration, absorption, circulation & metabolism.

• To develop physiologically & chemically stable preparations that provide an effective and safe method of delivering pharmaceuticals at the targeted location for absorption or activity.

• Improving taste, general consumer acceptability, dose frequency, and/or toxicity to achieve patient compliance barriers [11].

Advantages of lipoidal Carrier System [12, 13]

While dealing with poorly soluble molecules, there are several advantages of using a lipoidal carrier system:

• Reducing the amount by enhancing oral bioavailability, resulting in cost reductions in pharmaceutically active ingredients (API) costs.

• Controlled and targeted drug release

• Stability of drugs in the formulation

• Good Biocompatibility and Low toxicity

• Opportunities for delivering drugs that are lipid-soluble & water-soluble

• Significant reduction/elimination of intra and inter-subject variability caused by drug molecule delivery in a "solubilized" state (overcomes the limitation of absorption due to rate of dissolution)

• By boosting lymphatic transport, it is likely to reduce hepatic first-pass metabolism

• Enhance the content uniformity of dosage form for low portion compounds

• Relying on the finalized lipoidal carrier system content, the dosage can be incorporated in soft gel shells, hard shell capsules, or used as a liquid pre-concentrate offering for dose titration

Disadvantages of lipoidal Carrier System [13]

There are occasions, unless mitigated, when the lipoidal carrier system is not the ideal formulation approach;

• Physicochemical property complexity

• The greatest difficulty is the stability of API and manufacturing

• A few inadequately water-soluble drugs have minimal solubility in lipids

• Processing in the gastrointestinal tract before absorption

• Lack of understanding of the *in-vivo* activity & effect of co-administered lipids/drugs

• There is a lack of predictive *in-vivo* and *in-vitro* test methods

• Compatibility challenges of shell -Excipients

• Post-dosing uncontrolled medication precipitation

The lipoidal carrier system is a complex, formulation-dependent approach with a wide range of lipid excipient availability & a lot of considerations in selecting appropriate lipid combinations of lipids, surfactants, & cosolvents to be used.

Ideal Characters

The following are the primary considerations influencing the selection of excipients for lipid-based compositions (shown in Fig. **10.2**.).

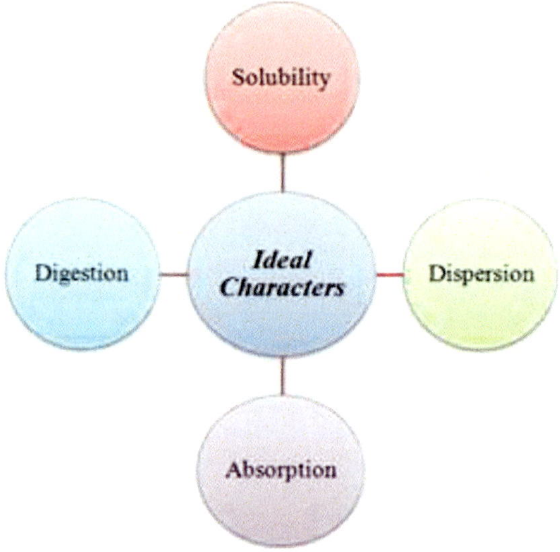

Fig. (10.2). Ideal characters for lipoidal-based compositions.

Various factors that influence the selection of excipients for lipoidal carrier preparations are:

• Solvent capacity

• Miscibility

• Digestibility and digested products' fate

• Information, expertise, toxic effects, and irritation- Regulatory Concerns

• Chemical stability, Purity

• Capsule compatibility

- Morphological features at ambient temperature (*i.e.*, melting point)
- Capability to facilitate formulation self-dispersion-Self dispersibility
- Cost of products

Solubility

Although lipids are the most important component of the composition, a hydrophilic cosolvent, as well as one or more surfactants, may be needed to boost dispersion & enhance solubilization capabilities. The hydrophilic-lipophilic balance (HLB) value is used to classify surfactants, with the lower value (≤10), indicating higher lipophilicity & higher hydrophilicity indicating a higher value (≥10). As a guideline, the preliminary step for the development of a formulation is that the lipids that are mostly used in oral dosage forms have an existing "required HLB" value that is the ideal HLB for the surfactant combination required to incorporate the oil in water [14 - 16]. Depending on their HLB values, different emulsifiers can be utilized for the different plans relying upon their HLB values, as portrayed in Table **10.1**.

Table 10.1. Emulsifier Used in lipid-based delivery [13].

Common Name/Type	Examples
Low HLB* (<10) *emulsifier	
Phosphatidylcholine and phosphatidylcholine/solvent mixtures	Phosphatidylcholine, phosphatidylcholine in propylene glycol, phosphatidylcholine in medium chain triglycerides, and phosphatidylcholine in safflower oil/ethanol
Unsaturatedpolyglycolizedglycerides	Oleoyl macrogolglycerides, linoleoyl Macrogolglycerides
Sorbitan esters	Sorbitan monooleate, sorbitan monostearate, sorbitan monolaurate, and sorbitanmonopalmitate
High HLB* (>10) *emulsifier	
Polyoxyethylene sorbitan esters	Polysorbate 20, polysorbate 40, polysorbate 60, and polysorbate 80
polyoxyl castor oil derivatives	Polyoxyl 35 castor oil, polyoxyl40 hydrogenated castor oil
Polyoxyethylene Polypropylene block copolymer	Poloxamer 188, poloxamer 407

(Table 1) cont.....

Common Name/Type	Examples
Saturated polyglycolized glycerides	Lauroylmacrogolglycerides, stearoyl Macrogolglycerides
PEG-8 Caprylic/capric Glycerides	Caprylocaproylmacrogolglycerides
Vitamin E derivative	Tocopherol PEG succinate

Dispersion

Formulations of adequate drug candidate solubility should be tested in aqueous mediums for emulsification and dispersion capabilities. For the screening step, a microscopic analysis of the preparation after it has been dissolved in water might be used. Complete mixing at the water/formulation interface, in conjunction with diffusion & stranding processes, suggests that emulsification is efficacious. An additional criterion is a minimum of drug deposition following complete mixing of the formulation with an aqueous system. The particle size of emulsion droplets can be measured using laser light scattering or alternative techniques that help in choosing acceptable formulations. The drawing of ternary phase graphs is a common method for determining the kind of structures produced by emulsification & characterizing the behavior of preparation along a diluted path [16].

Digestion

Some functions of gastrointestinal lipases might have a significant impact on the activity of lipoidal carrier-dependent preparations within the GI tract & when designing, it should be considered into account. Non-dispersible yet digestible lipids like triglycerides have previously been reported to be degraded into mono-/diglycerides & fatty acids *via* lipases, which emulsify any surplus oil. As a result, the existence of significant quantities of surfactants may not be required to ensure the formation of the appropriate small particulate sizes & broad surface areas for the release of the drug. Pouton proposed a classification system concerning lipid-based preparations in 2000, focusing on formulation ingredients and relying on digestion to enhance dispersion [17].

Absorption

In general, the eventual aim of any oral lipid-based preparation is efficient drug uptake by intestinal mucosal membranes. For a lipoidal carrier-based drug Composition, these reactions take place in the intestinal environment [16]. The components are first distributed to produce lipid or emulsion droplets, accompanied by lipolysis & by bile acid-solubilization of digestive products, resulting in the formation of mixed colloidal micelles. The drug is predicted to ultimately dissociate chiefly from oil droplets of emulsion & Micelles containing bile salts that will be ingested by the mucosa of the intestinal lining.

TYPES OF LIPIDS USED FOR CARRIER SYSTEM

Triglycerides

Triglyceride vegetable oils are the most commonly utilized excipients in lipoidal carrier-based drug delivery. As they are fully absorbed & digested, this is a class of lipids that offers no safety concerns [18]. Long-chain triglycerides (LCT), medium-chain triglycerides (MCT), and short-chain triglycerides (SCT) are the three different types of triglycerides [19].The ability of a drug as a solvent is mostly determined *via* the optimal ester group concentration. MCT has a solvent capacity greater than LCT and is less susceptible to oxidation [20]. The ratios of each fatty acid in oils derived from various vegetable sources vary. A natural vitamin E water-soluble derivative is D-α-tocopheryl polyethylene glycol succinate (Vitamin E TPGS, or simply TPGS) obtained as a result of the esterification of Vitamin E succinate with polyethylene glycol (PEG). It serves as an absorption booster for drugs that are poorly aqueous soluble. Refined edible oils include pure triglycerides [21 - 23].

Mixed Glycerides and Polar Oils

Partial vegetable oil hydrolysis gives rise to mixed glycerides. The level of hydrolysis and the chemical composition of the resulting mixed glycerides are determined by the beginning material (triglyceride). Mixed Glycerides of medium chains do not oxidize, have a higher solvent efficiency, and facilitate emulsification. The excipients that are polar oily also boost the formulation's solvent capacity and dispersibility. Polar oils include Sorbitantrioleate (Span85). Aside from that, oleic acid is employed in several commercial items [23, 24].

Cosolvents

Cosolvents are used in the majority of marketed medicinal formulations to improve the solubilization mechanism [15, 24]. Ethanol, propylene glycol, polyethylene glycols (PEG)-400 & glycerol are some of the most often used cosolvents. The solvent capacity of drug preparation is increased, which may be related to their use and to promote the system's dispersion containing aqueous-soluble surfactants in a high concentration. In addition, these cosolvents show considerable practical issues, containing solubilized solvent drug precipitate; as a result, there is a decrease insolvent capacity after dilution [25]; some cosolvents are incompatible with oils and solvents with lower molecular weight having incompatibilities with capsule shells.

Water-Insoluble Surfactants

There is a class with moderate hydrophilic-lipophilic equilibrium (HLB of 8–12), which adsorb at oil-water interfaces. Contingent upon the level of ethoxylation, these have limited solvency in water. They can frame emulsions whenever exposed to shear and are at times referred to as 'dispersible' in water. These compounds can create micelles yet can not self-emulsify because of their inadequately hydrophilic nature. Water-insoluble surfactants with HLB values between 11 and 11.5 are oleate esters, including polyoxyethylene(20) sorbitan-trioleate (Tween-85) and polyoxyethylene(20) glyceryl tri oleate (Tagot-TO). A combination of Tween-80 & Span-80 with an average HLB value of 11 is not functionally equivalent to Tween-85. The former comprises both water-insoluble & water-soluble molecules, whereas the latter is mostly made up of water-insoluble molecules [17, 26, 27].

Water-soluble Surfactants

These are the most frequent surfactants utilized in the development of self-emulsifying medication delivery systems [28, 29]. By dissolving in distilled water over their basic micellar concentration, materials having HLB values of 12 or more can create micellar solutions at low concentrations. Polyethylene glycols (PEG) and hydrolyzed vegetable oils can be combined to create these materials. Then again, alcohol can also be induced to react using ethylene oxide to form alkyl ether ethoxylate, which is a normally utilized surfactant (*e.g.*, cetostearyl liquor ethoxylate 'cetomacrogol'). Polysorbates are formed when sorbitan esters react with ethylene oxide (predominantly ether ethoxylates) [30].

Cremophor RH60 and RH40 (ethoxylated hydrogenated castor oil) are instances of this kind, produced through the hydrogenation of components from vegetable oils. Cremophor EL (ethoxylated castor oil) is a widely used non-hydrogenated oil. Cremophor is known to improve absorption by blocking efflux pumps, although the mechanism of inhibition is unknown [21, 31, 32]. This could be referred to as an on-specific conformational shift caused by surfactant molecule penetration into the membrane, adsorption onto the surface of the efflux pumps, or association of molecules with intracellular spaces of efflux pump [33, 34].

Additives

Different lipid dissolvable anti-oxidants, for example, α-tocopherol, propyl gallate, β-carotene, butylated hydroxyanisole (BHA), or butylated hydroxyl toluene (BHT) can be utilized to shield the preparation from oxidation [35].

MECHANISM OF LIPOIDAL CARRIERS IN IMPROVED DRUG DELIVERY

Lipids have increasingly sparked the interest of researchers as carriers for aqueous-insoluble drug administration. Many factors influence drug absorption from lipid carrier preparations, including particle size, rate of dispersion, drug precipitation, and level of emulsification in dispersion [17, 28, 36]. For the lipoidal carrier system to be productive, an appropriate lipid carrier development approach and a sensible drug-delivery mechanism must be chosen.

Topical Delivery

The drug delivery method utilized to deliver drugs *via* the skin ought to be nontoxic & non-irritant, particularly on damaged skin or inflamed and capable of adjusting the release (prolonged delivery, skin penetration). Lipid carriers are more suitable for topical distribution than conventional formulations because of their qualities like particles of small size, utilization of biocompatible fatty acids, & the potential for film formation. Smaller particle sizes aid in skin particle adhesion, allowing for proper contact among particles with skin to increase absorption of drugs *via* skin. The utilization of biocompatible lipids does not cause aggravation or poisonousness of dose form after administration. The structural similarities of these lipids towards skin lipids aid in drug molecule penetration. Due to the enhanced stability & sustained release of the drug as a result of encapsulation into the lipid core, it is possible to achieve greater concentrations just at the site of application and better penetration. Occlusion caused by the development of a lipid film on the skin leads to skin hydration and enhanced uptake of loaded active ingredients [37].

Oral Delivery

Poor water solubility, limited intestinal permeability, first-pass metabolism, as well as the efflux process all contribute to lower oral bioavailability. These goals can be achieved by increasing the period of residence, boosting solubility and permeability, thereby improving the absorption and lymphatic circulation of drugs through the lipoidal carrier. Adherence to the mucosal surfaces (with the large surface area) of smaller lipid particles, as well as slowed motility of the gastrointestinal (GI) tract caused by the existence of lipid, increases lipid particle exposure to GI media, this leads to a longer period of residency and hence uptake. Bile acids as well as contents delivered into the intestine to respond to lipid stimulation, wherein the drug is distributed, lead to improved lipophilic compound solubility. Endocytosis of lipidic particles into enterocytes (caveolae-dependent or clathrin-mediated) or nanoparticle ingestion by M cells at Peyer's patches results in increased drug intake (Fig. **10.3**). Due to their reduced size, carriers enter lymphatic systems, avoiding exposure to the liver and thus metabolism. The simultaneous release of efflux inhibitors *via* co-encapsulation or the addition of excipients with Pg-P inhibiting action (either oils or surfactants) in the formulation causes efflux pump inhibition and boosts the plasma concentration of the drug. Surface alteration of the particle with certain ligands can improve mucosal contact, penetration, and absorption, which improves the drug's pharmacokinetics and bioavailability [38].

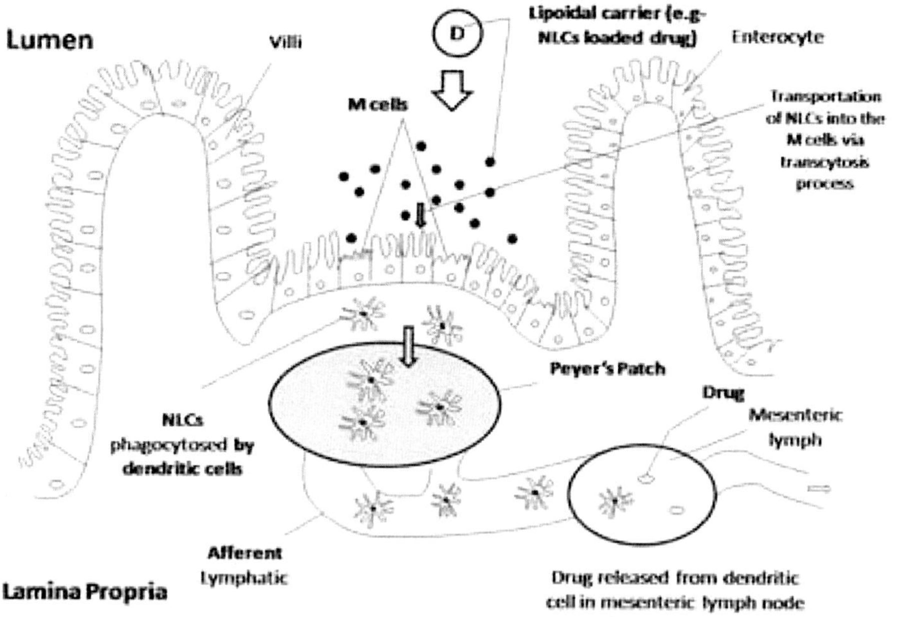

Fig. (10.3). M cell transport of lipoidal Carrier System (nanostructured lipid carriers) to lymphatic vessels is depicted in a schematic cross-section of Peyer's patch [40].

Pulmonary Delivery

For localized therapy of respiratory disorders, pulmonary administration is recommended, but it can be used instead of the oral route for increasing the bioavailability of drugs that undergo first-pass metabolism. Due to its vast surface area, readily permeable membrane, thin alveolar epithelium, & broad vasculature, which allows for faster drug absorption, the pulmonary route is a desirable mode of administration for systemic delivery. Size, size distribution & contact duration with the mucosal surface are factors that influence drug distribution & penetration in the respiratory tract. The smaller particle size of nanocarriers allows for better drug permeation and increased adhesion to mucosal surfaces. Long-term drug release allows for enhanced drug exposure & enhanced medication delivery [39].

Ophthalmic Delivery

The principal hurdles that limit drug availability in ocular delivery include poor permeability *via* the cornea, short retention duration, and drug elimination by nasolacrimal drainage. Due to their wide surface area offered by their tiny size and mucoadhesion capabilities, lipid carriers can solve these obstacles & exhibit promising outcomes in drug delivery *via* the ocular route [41].

MICRO AND NANO-CARRIERS AS LIPID-BASED SYSTEM

Lipoidal carrier systems (some of the carriers are shown in Fig. **10.4**) have innovative nanoscale properties that are essential for clinical applications.

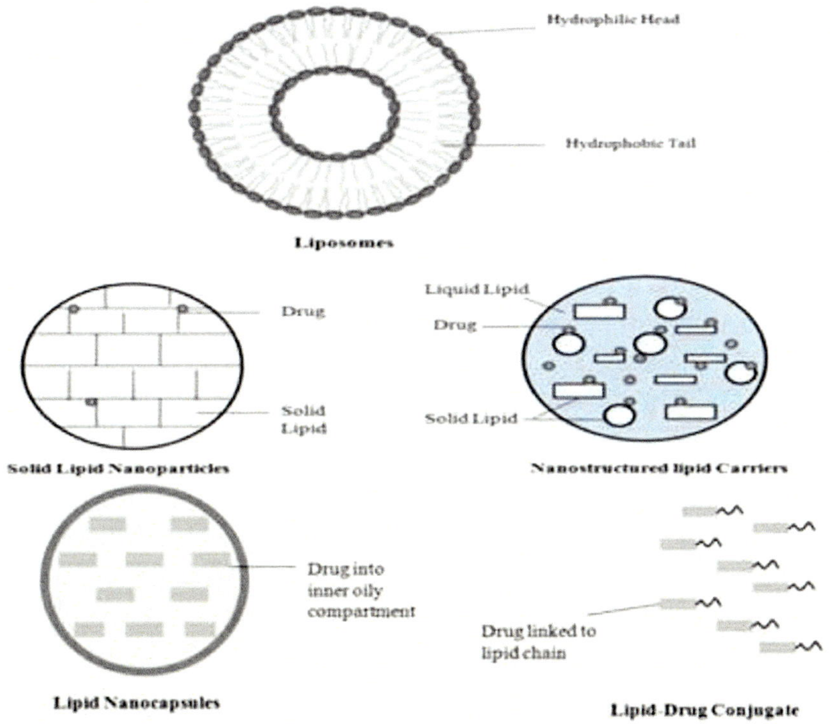

Fig. (10.4). Some examples of Lipoidal Nano/microcarrier.

Lipid nano, as well as microparticles, are interesting for clinical uses due to critical & unique characteristics like a significantly greater surface-to-mass ratio over other colloidal particles that have the potential to bind, permeate, & deliver substances. The following are some potential systems of the lipoidal carrier for controlled delivery of drugs:

1. Liposome

2. Solid lipid nanoparticles

3. Nanostructured lipid carriers

4. Lipid-drug conjugate

5. Lipid nanocapsules

6. Solid lipid microparticles

7. Lipid microspheres (lipospheres)

8. Submicron lipid emulsions

Liposome

Liposomes are novel in terms of delivering biologically active compounds due to their versatile ability. Bangham, with his colleagues, revealed them for the first time in 1961." Liposome" is a Greek word, formed by combining "lipos" (fat) with "soma" (body) [42]. Liposomes are aqueous-centered structures surrounded by a lipid bilayer that acts as a wall, isolating the inner aqueous core from the outer bulk. When lipids were exposed to water, the hydrophobic portions of the molecule began to self-associate with the solvent, most commonly as the type of liposomes [43]. They are spherical vesicles having a size ranging from 30 nm to several micrometers. Depending on the application, many forms of liposomes can be manufactured using various methods [44].

Advantages

1. Improved drug effectiveness and therapeutic index

2. Improved stability by encapsulation

3. Non-toxic, biocompatible, fully biodegradable, & non-immunogenic for systemic & non-systemic delivery

4. Lower the encapsulated agent's toxicity (amphotericin B)

5. The ability to pair with site-specific ligands to facilitate active targeting [43]

Solid Lipid Nanoparticles (SLNs)

The most well-known type of nanosphere in the SLNs comprises primarily solid lipids having a mean diameter of 50 to 1000 nm with a photon correlation spectroscopy [45]. Solid lipid(s), water, and surfactant(s) are common ingredients. Triglycerides (*e.g.*, tristearin), partial glycerides, steroids (*e.g.*, cholesterol), fatty acids (*e.g.*, stearic acid), and waxes (*e.g.*, cetyl palmitate) are all examples of lipids. To stabilize lipid dispersions, all kinds of surfactants (in terms of charge and molecular weight) have been utilized [46]. SLNs were developed in 1990 and have historically been thought to be potential carrier systems of the drug because nanocarriers are stable physicochemically & efficiently produced on a large scale, with comparatively low raw material prices and processing. SLNs production is mostly, but not entirely, based on solidified nanoemulsion technology. In the preparation of nanoemulsions, high-pressure homogenization (HPH), ultrasonication, & high shear homogenization are used [47, 48].

Advantages

When compared to certain other approaches, SLNs have numerous advantages, including ease of production, high-scale creation, minimal expense, great delivery profile, incredible physical stability, production without organic solvent, chemical variability, negligible toxicity of lipid carrier, being inexpensive, easier to obtain approval & biodegradability of fats [10].

Nanostructured Lipid Carriers (NLCs)

NLCs are small particles differentiated by a solid fatty core composed of a blend of both lipids, *i.e.*, solid & liquid. Whereas this emerging lipoidal carrier matrix has a melting point lower than the initial solid lipid, it remains solid at body temperature. Relying on the technique of preparation & composition of the lipid mixture, many forms of NLCs are formed, including amorphous, imperfect, and multiple-type NLCs. Small quantities of oils change lipid crystallization in imperfect form. The lipid matrix in the amorphous form is solid and not crystalline (amorphous state) –it can be achieved by combining specific lipids, such as isopropyl myristate and hydroxyoctacosanyl hydroxystearate. The solid lipid matrix of the multiple types contains small oil compartments. This form combines a solid lipid with a considerable oil amount. The main concept is that by offering the lipid matrix, a specific nanostructure, the active drug payload is raised while the release of entrapped components throughout storage is minimized" [49]. High-pressure homogenization can make NLC, as well as the technique, could be altered for producing lipid nanoparticle dispersions, which can have solid concentrations ranging around 30 80% [50].

Lipid-Drug Conjugate (LDC)

LDC is a type of nanoparticle that contains drugs that are attached to nanoparticles. To solve the hydrophilic compound loading issue of SLN & NLC, lipid-drug conjugate (LDC) nanoparticles were produced. "An insoluble drug-lipid conjugate bulk is created by the common approach either through covalent linking (*e.g.*, esters or ethers) or through salt production" (*e.g.*, with a fatty acid). The resulting LDC is then used to make a nanoparticles preparation utilizing High-pressure homogenization and an aqueous surfactant solution" [49, 51].

Advantages

- Enhance the loading of drugs into lipid carriers, enhance the efficiency of drugs for oral delivery, chemotherapeutic drugs delivery can be enhanced, reduce drug resistance, increase brain penetration, improve gene-drug delivery, and accomplish extended release of the drug & minimize GI enzymatic or pH-dependent breakdown

- Targeted/ controlled release of drug and its conjugated molecule kinetics

- Several active pharmaceutical compounds have advanced instability & bioavailability

Lipid Nanocapsules (LNC)

Lipidic core-shell nanostructured materials are also known as lipid nanocapsules(LNC). The external shell comprises a mixture of solid lipids, emulsifying agents, and an oil-based core [52]. Whereas multiple-type NLCs are composed of a matrix of solid-lipid with numerous oil-based compartments within which pharmaceutical drugs try to partition, LNCs have only one drug-containing oil-based core covered by a thin barrier surface (core-shell nanostructure). Proceeding further to lipids microparticles is another excellent lipoidal carrier system.

Solid Lipid Microparticles (SLM)

"SLM is composed similarly to SLN, with larger (>1000 nm) particle size, that means their areas of application and routes of delivery may differ" [49, 53]. In simple terms, by comparison to SLN, even after their tremendous potential as nanocarriers, SLM has yet to achieve widespread application. The major limitation of their parenteral delivery systems utilization is that they are not appropriate for I.V. delivery due to size considerations. Furthermore, its application in pulmonary drug administration appears to be beneficial.

Lipospheres

Lipospheres are water-dispersible lipid-based solid particles with size particles ranging from 0.01 to 100 m in diameter. They are made up of solid hydrophobic lipids containing a lot of active drug moiety dispersed or solubilized inside a matrix of solid fat stabilized by an external coat of phospholipid molecules [54 - 56]. Improved drug stability in the formulation, high-drug load, controlled particle size, Freeze dry and recovery qualities, well-controlled drug release, and no carrier toxicity. Lipospheres prevent hydrolysis of drug candidates and confirm shelf life, facilitating good bioavailability and extended plasma levels [57]. The lipospheres allow controlled delivery of anti-inflammatory drugs, local anesthetics, antibiotics, and anticancer medicines. The liposphere-encapsulated vaccinations were delivered with an adjuvant effect [58].

Submicron Lipid Emulsions

Lipid emulsions (LEs), which are submicron particulates with sizes ranging from 100 to 300 nm and were originally used as an intravenous delivery of both calories & essential fatty acids (FAs), were effectively turned into parenteral pharmaceutical products. For parenteral delivery of weakly water-soluble medicines, LEs demand has been on the rise, and poorly absorbing drugs orally for bioavailability improvements [59, 60]. Due to their excellent biocompatibility, enhanced pharmacokinetics, & pharmacodynamics, LEs are a valuable tool in innovative drug delivery systems [61].

APPLICATIONS IN NUMEROUS FIELDS

The applications are classified into two basic categories, therapeutic applications, and drug delivery routes, and in the second half of the applications, other applications are also described, including cancer therapy, crossing the blood-brain barrier, gene therapy, protein and peptide delivery, antioxidant and vitamin delivery (Fig. **10.5**). These are addressed in wider context below:

Therapeutic Applications

Topical Application

Dermal administration offers considerable promise using lipid micro and nano-carrier, and the quick time-to-market makes it particularly desirable to be used in pharmaceutical products [62]. The capacity to maintain chemically unstable components from chemical breakdown, control drug release, and produce self-adhesive lipid coatings just on the surface of the skin, offering a potentially occlusive impact, are all significant benefits of epidermal therapeutics of lipid carriers [63].

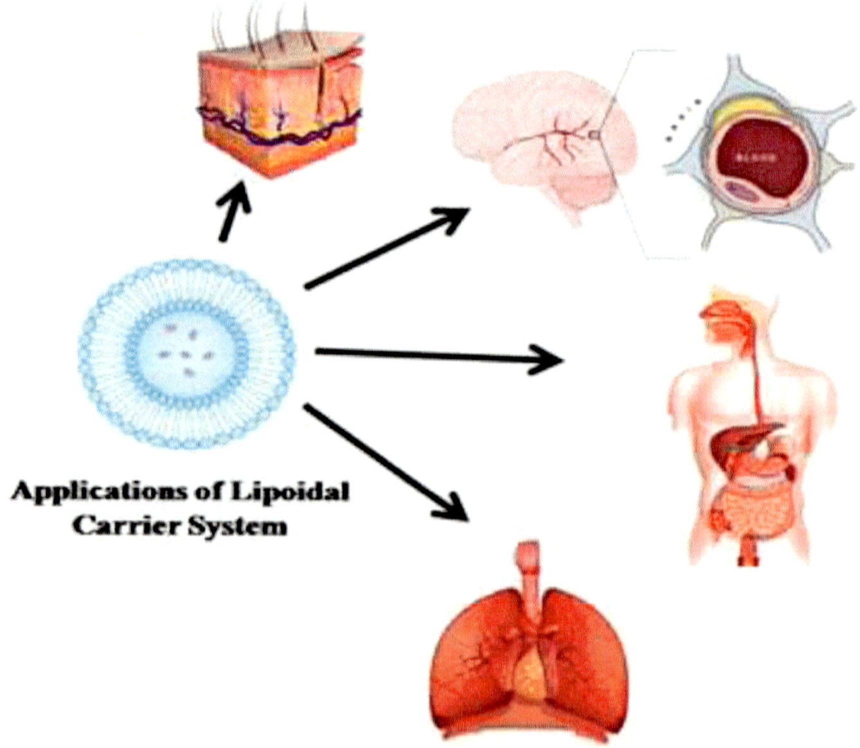

Fig. (10.5). Applications of Lipoidal carrier system.

Parenteral Application

Their molecule size and helpful goals imply that lipoidal nano/microcarriers can be utilized for all parenteral purposes: from intramuscular and subcutaneous, involving the organization from the intra-articular to intravenous [1]. Lipid nano and microcarrier, due to their tiny size, could be infused *via* intravenous route&

utilized to reach the target organs for delivering the drug. Ultimately, intravenously administered colloidal particles are eliminated from the bloodstream by the spleen and liver. By covering the surface of lipid nanoparticles with polyethylene glycol (PEG), "stealth" lipid nanoparticles that can avoid the reticuloendothelial system (RES), can be produced.

Oral Application

Aqueous dispersions or transformation into solid formulations of lipid-micron and nano-carrier can be taken orally, including tablets, capsules, powders in cachets, or pellets are preferred. Particle aqueous dispersions in the tablet production process can be employed as granulation fluid. On the other hand, it can be transformed into a powder (*e.g.*, freeze-drying or spray-drying) & for filling hard capsules of gelatine or introduced to a tableting powder mixture. Drying in a spray dryer can be the most effective option for converting lipoidal particle dispersions, as it is cheaper to produce powders [45].

Lipid micro- & nanoparticles, when delivered orally, can contribute to the solubilization of the drug in the GI tract. In addition, they can keep solubilizing poorly soluble materials & improve solute-solvent interactions, particularly when combined with endogenous solubilizers like phospholipids or bile acids. Furthermore, their shielding action, combined with its controlled and/or sustained release features, protects drugs (particularly macromolecules) from degrading prematurely and enhances their stability in GIT [38]. Additionally, the nanosized carrier can be absorbed by M cells of Peyer's patches, allowing the nanocarrier to avoid first-pass effect metabolism & reach lymphatic circulation. Reduced side effects (*e.g.*, Non-steroidal anti-inflammatory- gastrointestinal toxicity) & flavor concealing are two more key targets for oral lipoidal carrier delivery [64].

Pulmonary Application

Lipoidal micro/nanocarriers are especially interesting for pulmonary applications because they have high aerosolization capabilities & when nebulized as liquid preparations, it has good stability. For this application, the solid form of SLM produced (*i.e.*, using spray-drying) because of their aerodynamic size, is a suitable approach. Appropriate lipid carrier design should prevent them from accumulating in the bronchial areas. However, even if bronchial clearance is efficient and may result in the concentration of drugs under therapeutic values, the retention of lipid particles in the lungs contributes to the extended release of drugs. Increased bioavailability of drug & prolonged pharmacological efficacy can therefore be attained, resulting in lower dosage & prolonged dose intervals. As a result, lipid carriers may be capable of delivering several benefits in both the localized serious airway problems and systemic delivery of the drug. Furthermore, various investigations have shown that pulmonary delivery of lipid matrices has a minimal toxicity potential. Unfortunately, there have been no long-term investigations on the consequences of frequent pulmonary delivery [39].

Other Applications

Cancer Therapy

The use of nanocarriers to administer anticancer drug administration is justified for a variety of pharmacological reasons. Frequently, a tumor is accompanied by faulty, leaking vascularisation caused by poorly controlled angiogenesis. Due to enough improved permeability & retention (EPR) effect, submicron-sized particulate materials can selectively extravasate further into the tumor and also be sustained there. Using an adequately designed lipid carrier, EPR-effect-based passive tumor targeting can be accomplished, which can prevent complement opsonization & subsequent removal by the RES. For this reason, a "long-circulating", lipid carrier is created with smaller sizes particles & hydrophilic surfaces (hydrophilic polymers cover them) [65].

Furthermore, surface-engineered nanocarriers could be used for targeted delivery to boost cancer cell-specific cytotoxic effects. This can be accomplished by taking advantage of variations in the receptors &surface antigens of cancerous & normal cells. Ultimately, multidrug resistance (MDR) is a significant barrier to anticancer medication therapy. P-glycoprotein (P-gp) is mostly connected to MDR, which functions as a cellular efflux pump from the cell for several medicines (antibiotics, anticancer agents, *etc.*). Lipid carriers may aid in the treatment of MDR as they transport entrapped medications into cancer cells using endocytosis, thus avoiding the P-glycoprotein drug ejection *via* the efflux mechanism [65, 66].

Crossing the Blood-Brain Barrier

Lipoid carriers' system has often been suggested as carriers capable of getting across the blood-brain barrier (BBB). The BBB regulates the transfer of certain chemicals across the brain & blood circulation. Due to the close connections among endothelial cells, passive solute diffusion *via* the paracellular pathway is relatively modest. Lipoidalmicro/Nanocarrier has the potential to be efficient in terms of brain uptake approach on several levels, as they are capable -of (i) maintaining drugs from being chemically broken down in biological secretions, (ii) improving bloodstream persistence and, as a result, indirectly favor brain translocation, & (iii) effectively stimulating endothelial cells, resulting in endocytosis, and also receptor-mediated active targeting is possible. While simple lipoidal nanocarriers have been utilized as BBB crossing carriers, attention is now shifting toward specialized nanocarriers that increase contact efficiency between particles and endothelial cells [67].

Gene Therapy

Lipoidal carrier-based gene therapy works best with non-viral vectors. Genetic material (plasmid DNA, pDNA) is injected into targeted cells to boost protein production or using a small interfering RNA (siRNA) or antisense oligonucleotides (ASO) to quiet faulty genes by inhibiting transcription and/or translation. Nucleic acids exposed to enzymes are easily absorbed in body fluid. In addition, as there is a negatively loaded surface on nucleic acids and cell membranes, cell internalization does not occur naturally, and therapeutic response is ineffectual. The most efficient carriers are viral vectors, but they do not include a DNA limit, and non-viral vectors are safer, cheaper, and replicable. Positively charged lipids are required (that may electrostatically attach nucleic acids) for nanocarriers as a non-viral vector in gene delivery. This is helpful for transfection as condensation enhances the mobility of nucleic acids, shields it against environmental enzymes, and permits contact with cationic surfaces having negative charges [68].

Protein and Peptide Delivery

Protein administration using lipoidal nano- and microparticles is a common practice. Despite their low availability, reduced transfer across cell membranes, and poor circulation stability, peptides, and proteins have not yet been used for medical purposes. Most peptides and proteins are supplied *via* injection, as their short half-life requires frequent dosages that are expensive, unpleasant, & poorly accepted by patients. Significant work has been devoted to developing needle-free delivery options for these biomacromolecules, with the majority using the oral approach. However, administration methods such as buccal, pulmonary, nasal, and transdermal have also been studied. Delivery of Protein and peptide may be boosted by lipoidal nano/microparticles, because of lipids' absorption &stabilizing -improving properties. Even though peptide and protein antigens tend to be unstable in mucosal regions, considerable research has been conducted in the field of vaccine composition using lipid carriers [69].

Delivery of Antioxidant and Vitamin

Lipoidal micro-and nanoparticles have potential possibilities to protect against the degradation of antioxidants and vitamins (They are frequently oxygen & light-sensitive). They can also enhance the entry of nutrients into the skin. Micro/nanoparticles may be seen as a successful way of improving the potency of antioxidants given topically. Certain beauty products with antioxidant-loaded nanocarriers are already on the market [70]. Moreover, upon oral treatment, antioxidants are usually characterized by limited bioavailability. The trapping into nanocarriers may aid in increasing intestinal absorption and, as a result, improving pharmacokinetics [71].

Diagnostics Delivery

Essential preclinical research in the diagnostic field has recently been conducted employing lipid nanoparticles designed for magnetic resonance imaging (MRI) with positive contrast. $MnCl_2$, gadolinium(III) diethylenetriaminepentaacetic acid (Gd-DTPA), and the manganese(II) equivalent (Mn-DTPA) are among these systems. Lipid nanoparticles were also linked with Alexa FluorTM 488 and several other near-infrared dyes (NiR). Furthermore, in cancer therapy, a novel approach is gaining popularity: the coupling of therapeutic drugs & diagnostic instruments in certain multimodal theranostic nanoparticles [72, 73].

PATENTS IN LIPIODOL SYSTEM

Table **10.2** summarizes the primary types of lipoidal carriers that are the aspect of patent applications. Key quality criteria for identifying patents concerned with varieties of lipoidal Carrier Systems; patents published or registered between 2013 and 2019.

Table 10.2. Overview of the Patents of the lipoidal carrier system.

S.No.	Lipoidal Carrier	Title	Patent Number	Ref.
1.	SLNs	Solid lipid nanoparticles composition for skin whitening effect comprising MHY498 and preparation method thereof	KR101860555B1	[74]
2.	SLNs	Curcumin solid lipid particles and methods for their preparation and use	US10166187B2	[75]
3.	SLNs	Cosmetic composition aimed at the sustained release of substances that repel insects	WO2017143421	[76]
4.	SLNs	Application of solid lipid nanoparticles as antidepressant drug carrier	CN105919973A	[77]
5.	SLNs	Spinosin solid lipid nanoparticles and preparation method and application thereof	CN103845307B	[78]
6.	SLNs	Roxithromycin topical delivery to stop hair loss or for acne treatment	WO2014077712	[79]
7.	NLCs	Nanostructured lipid carriers and stable emulsions and uses thereof	WO2018232257A9	[80]

S.No.	Lipoidal Carrier	Title	Patent Number	Ref.
8.	NLCs	Nanostructured lipid carriers, methods, and uses thereof	WO2018002853A1	[81]
9.	NLCs	Nanostructured carriers for guided and targeted on-demand substance delivery	US patent 20170119891	[82]
10.	NLCs	Preparation of nanostructured lipid carriers (NLCs) method and products made	CN102283809B	[83]
11.	NLCs	A method for producing nano lipid formulation for skincare and/ or repair and a nano lipid formulation of the same	WO2015105407	[84]
12.	NLCs	A composition for treating leukemia	WO2014123406	[85]
13.	LNC	Improvement of the dissolution profile of benznidazolewithincreased bioavailability	WO2015039199	[86]
14.	LNC	Avermectin delivery for acne rosacea treatment	US20130034612	[87]
15.	LNC	Lipid nanocapsules, the method for preparing same, and use thereof as a drug	WO2011036234	[88]
16.	LDC	Polymer - cyclodextrin - lipid conjugates	US10064954	[89]
17.	Sub-micron emulsion	Microemulsion & sub-micron emulsion process & compositions	US 20150258023	[90]
18.	Sub-micron emulsion	Preparation of submicron-sized nanoparticles *via* dispersion lyophilization	USOO8722091	[91]
19.	Liposome	Liposome comprising synthetic receptor-phospholipid conjugate, and composition, for functional material transfer, which can be bonded to the synthetic receptor and which comprises as active ingredient ligand having functional material bonded thereto	WO2017213328	[92]
20.	Liposome	Method for inclusion of the drug in membrane vesicle through cell modification using membrane fusogenic liposome and drug delivery method using same	WO2015060504	[93]
21.	Liposome	Neuroprotective liposome compositions and methods for treatment of stroke	WO2017213328	[94]

CONCLUSION

Utilizing a lipoidal carrier system has revolutionized the delivery of certain older medications with severe side effects that are now considered safe for use. Considering GRAS excipients and their historical experience of use in various nutritional and medicinal products, the utilization of lipid drug carrier systems has recently gained popularity. A lipoidal carrier system has the potential benefit over polymer-based methods, including improved drug penetration, fewer adverse reactions, controlled release of the drug, and site-specific delivery.

For nearly 25 years, scientists have been studying lipid nano- and microparticles. Patent work has surged; at the same time, the need for nanotechnology for curing diseases as an advanced tool has expanded, which has significant commercial applications, including solvent-free preparation procedures for biocompatible materials. Many lipid compositions offer good stability, high carrier capability, the ability to incorporate both lipophilic & hydrophilic compounds, and the ability to administer by a variety of channels, including oral, parenteral, dermal, and pulmonary approaches. Lipids & lipid micro and nanocarriers are potential delivery strategies for dermal delivery of drugs; inventions have been filed demonstrating a variety of benefits given by such delivery mechanisms, including chemical stabilization and enhanced drug permeation through the skin.

The lipoidal carrier system for oral delivery of the drug is the most common & effective therapy, although BCS class II and IV drugs have various bioavailability difficulties. Lipoidal-based carriers can be taken orally as an aqueous dispersion or turned into conventional pharmaceutical formulations like powders in sachets, tablets, capsules, or pellets. The capacity to insert medicines into lipid nanocarriers provides a new concept in the delivery of drugs that might be employed for both active and passive drug targeting. Additionally, some drug delivery issues can be viewed as possibilities for lipid nanocarriers. First and foremost, lipid nanoparticles are believed to be an intriguing method for defeating the BBB as a result of the overall composition of lipids and the simplicity of functioning. Second, several aspects associated with the usage of nanocarriers can improve cancer treatment. With the advancement and curiosity in lipoidal carrier-based drug delivery methods demonstrated by pharmaceutical formulation researchers, the market is expected to be flooded with lipid carrier system products shortly.

FUTURE POTENTIAL OF INNOVATIVE LIPOIDAL PARTICULATE DELIVERY SYSTEMS OF DRUG

The lipoidal carrier delivery system is now one of the most exciting fields of research. Lipoidal Carrier-based nanoparticles will provide a dynamic foundation for pharmaceuticals whose key problems are solubility and/or bioavailability. These systems concentrate on producing and stabilizing micro and nano-drug particles to enhance the *in vivo* dissolution surface area & consequently, the dissolution rate and the drug plasma or tissue levels. Due to its physicochemical features, this system will have a promising potential to overcome the problems associated with drug delivery. The drug's lipid nano and microcarrier formulation will develop effective nanotechnology purposes, particularly when targeted release is necessary, just like cancer therapy. Tremendous study in this area in the previous two decades was carried out, several patents have previously been filed, and dozens of clinical trials have been completed; the development of nanomedicine and micro/nano-drug delivery systems is undoubtedly the direction that will persist for the platform of production and innovation for future decades. Further research will be performed on drug loading, particle uniformity, and release capacity. Pharmaceutical experts' attention will be focused in the future on *in vivo* research of these lipoidal carrier systems and evaluating their mechanism of action. More research is needed on the physicochemical stability of pharmaceuticals compound in lipoidal carrier-based systems and their interactions.

CONSENT FOR PUBLICATION

Not applicable.

CONFLICT OF INTEREST

The authors declare no conflict of interest, financial or otherwise.

ACKNOWLEDGEMENTS

The authors acknowledge the Department of Science and Technology, New Delhi, India (DST/NM/NT/2018/20 and DST/INSPIRE Fellowship/2019/IF190329) for providing financial assistance for the successful completion of this work.

REFERENCES

[1] Wissing SA, Kayser O, Müller RH. Solid lipid nanoparticles for parenteral drug delivery. Adv Drug Deliv Rev 2004; 56(9): 1257-72. [http://dx.doi.org/10.1016/j.addr.2003.12.002] [PMID: 15109768]

[2] Shah VP, Amidon GL. G.L. Amidon, H. Lennernas, V.P. Shah, and J.R. Crison. A theoretical basis for a biopharmaceutic drug classification: the correlation of *in vitro* drug product dissolution and *in vivo* bioavailability, Pharm Res 12, 413-420, 1995--backstory of BCS. AAPS J 2014; 16(5): 894-8. [http://dx.doi.org/10.1208/s12248-014-9620-9] [PMID: 24961917]

[3] Patra JK, Das G, Fraceto LF, *et al.* Nano based drug delivery systems: recent developments and future prospects. J Nanobiotechnology 2018; 16(1): 71. [http://dx.doi.org/10.1186/s12951-018-0392-8] [PMID: 30231877]

[4] Lombardo D, Kiselev MA, Magazù S, Calandra P. Amphiphiles Self-Assembly: Basic Concepts and Future Perspectives of Supramolecular Approaches. Adv Condens Matter Phys 2015; 2015: 1-22. [http://dx.doi.org/10.1155/2015/151683]

[5] Jaiswal P, Gidwani B, Vyas A. Nanostructured lipid carriers and their current application in targeted drug delivery. Artif Cells Nanomed Biotechnol 2016; 44(1): 27-40. [http://dx.doi.org/10.3109/21691401.2014.909822] [PMID: 24813223]

[6] Bulbake U, Doppalapudi S, Kommineni N, Khan W. Liposomal Formulations in Clinical Use: An Updated Review. Pharmaceutics 2017; 9(4): 12. [http://dx.doi.org/10.3390/pharmaceutics9020012] [PMID: 28346375]

[7] Duan Y, Dhar A, Patel C, *et al.* A brief review on solid lipid nanoparticles: part and parcel of contemporary drug delivery systems. RSC Advances 2020; 10(45): 26777-91. [http://dx.doi.org/10.1039/D0RA03491F] [PMID: 35515778]

[8] Hauss DJ. Oral lipid-based formulations. Adv Drug Deliv Rev 2007; 59(7): 667-76. [http://dx.doi.org/10.1016/j.addr.2007.05.006] [PMID: 17618704]

[9] Kalepu S, Manthina M, Padavala V. Oral lipid-based drug delivery systems – an overview. Acta Pharm Sin B 2013; 3(6): 361-72.https://doi.org/https://doi.org/10.1016/j.apsb.2013.10.001 [http://dx.doi.org/10.1016/j.apsb.2013.10.001]

[10] Attama AA, Momoh MA, Builders PF. Lipid nanoparticulate drug delivery systems: a revolution in dosage form design and development. Recent Adv Nov Drug Carr Syst 2012; pp. 107-40.

[11] Patel A, Cholkar K, Mitra AK. Recent developments in protein and peptide parenteral delivery approaches. Ther Deliv 2014; 5(3): 337-65. [http://dx.doi.org/10.4155/tde.14.5] [PMID: 24592957]

[12] Erdine S, De Andrés J. Drug delivery systems. Pain Pract 2006; 6(1): 51-7. [http://dx.doi.org/10.1111/j.1533-2500.2006.00059.x] [PMID: 17309710]

[13] Shrestha H, Bala R, Arora S. Lipid-Based Drug Delivery Systems. J Pharm (Cairo) 2014; 2014: 1-10. [http://dx.doi.org/10.1155/2014/801820] [PMID: 26556202]

[14] Constantinides PP. Lipid microemulsions for improving drug dissolution and oral absorption: physical and biopharmaceutical aspects. Pharm Res 1995; 12(11): 1561-72. [http://dx.doi.org/10.1023/A:1016268311867] [PMID: 8592652]

[15] Strickley RG. Solubilizing excipients in oral and injectable formulations. Pharm Res 2004; 21(2): 201-30. [http://dx.doi.org/10.1023/B:PHAM.0000016235.32639.23] [PMID: 15032302]

[16] Cannon JB, Long MA. 11 Emulsions, Microemulsions, and Lipid-Based Drug Delivery Systems for Drug Solubilization and Delivery—Part II: Oral Applications. Water-Insoluble Drug Formula 2018.

[17] Pouton CW. Lipid formulations for oral administration of drugs: non-emulsifying, self-emulsifying and 'self-microemulsifying' drug delivery systems. Eur J Pharm Sci 2000; 11 (Suppl. 2): S93-8. [http://dx.doi.org/10.1016/S0928-0987(00)00167-6] [PMID: 11033431]

[18] Pouton CW, Porter CJH. Formulation of lipid-based delivery systems for oral administration: Materials, methods and strategies. Adv Drug Deliv Rev 2008; 60(6): 625-37. [http://dx.doi.org/10.1016/j.addr.2007.10.010] [PMID: 18068260]

[19] Cao Y, Marra M, Anderson BD. Predictive relationships for the effects of triglyceride ester concentration and water uptake on solubility and partitioning of small molecules into lipid vehicles. J Pharm Sci 2004; 93(11): 2768-79. [http://dx.doi.org/10.1002/jps.20126] [PMID: 15389678]

[20] Kaukonen AM, Boyd BJ, Porter CJH, Charman WN. Drug solubilization behavior during *in vitro* digestion of simple triglyceride lipid solution formulations. Pharm Res 2004; 21(2): 245-53. [http://dx.doi.org/10.1023/B:PHAM.0000016282.77887.1f] [PMID: 15032305]

[21] Collnot EM, Baldes C, Wempe MF, *et al.* Influence of vitamin E TPGS poly(ethylene glycol) chain length on apical efflux transporters in Caco-2 cell monolayers. J Control Release 2006; 111(1-2): 35-40. [http://dx.doi.org/10.1016/j.jconrel.2005.11.005] [PMID: 16410030]

[22] Collnot EM, Baldes C, Wempe MF, *et al.* Mechanism of inhibition of P-glycoprotein mediated efflux by vitamin E TPGS: influence on ATPase activity and membrane fluidity. Mol Pharm 2007; 4(3):

465-74.
[http://dx.doi.org/10.1021/mp060121r] [PMID: 17367162]

[23] Griffin BT, O'Driscoll CM. A comparison of intestinal lymphatic transport and systemic bioavailability of saquinavir from three lipid-based formulations in the anaesthetised rat model. J Pharm Pharmacol 2010; 58(7): 917-25.
[http://dx.doi.org/10.1211/jpp.58.7.0006] [PMID: 16805951]

[24] Strickley RG. Currently marketed oral lipid-based dosage forms: drug products and excipients. Drugs Pharm Sci 2007; 170: 1.

[25] Yalkowsky SH. Solubility and solubilization in aqueous media. American Chemical Society 1999.

[26] Wakerly MG, Pouton CW, Meakin BJ, Morton FS. Self-emulsification of vegetable oil-nonionic surfactant mixtures: a proposed mechanism of action 1986.
[http://dx.doi.org/10.1021/bk-1986-0311.ch018]

[27] Pouton CW. Formulation of self-emulsifying drug delivery systems. Adv Drug Deliv Rev 1997; 25(1): 47-58.
[http://dx.doi.org/10.1016/S0169-409X(96)00490-5]

[28] Pouton CW. Formulation of poorly water-soluble drugs for oral administration: Physicochemical and physiological issues and the lipid formulation classification system. Eur J Pharm Sci 2006; 29(3-4): 278-87.
[http://dx.doi.org/10.1016/j.ejps.2006.04.016] [PMID: 16815001]

[29] Hauss DJ. Oral lipid-based formulations: enhancing the bioavailability of poorly water-soluble drugs. CRC Press 2007; Vol. 170.
[http://dx.doi.org/10.3109/9781420017267]

[30] Rowe RC, Sheskey P, Quinn M. Handbook of pharmaceutical excipients. Libros Digitales-Pharmaceutical Press 2009.

[31] Cuiné JF, Charman WN, Pouton CW, Edwards GA, Porter CJH. Increasing the proportional content of surfactant (Cremophor EL) relative to lipid in self-emulsifying lipid-based formulations of danazol reduces oral bioavailability in beagle dogs. Pharm Res 2007; 24(4): 748-57.
[http://dx.doi.org/10.1007/s11095-006-9194-z] [PMID: 17372700]

[32] Grove M, Müllertz A, Pedersen GP, Nielsen JL. Bioavailability of seocalcitol. Eur J Pharm Sci 2007; 31(1): 8-15.
[http://dx.doi.org/10.1016/j.ejps.2007.01.007] [PMID: 17383165]

[33] Shono Y, Nishihara H, Matsuda Y, *et al.* Modulation of intestinal P-glycoprotein function by cremophor EL and other surfactants by an *in vitro* diffusion chamber method using the isolated rat intestinal membranes. J Pharm Sci 2004; 93(4): 877-85.
[http://dx.doi.org/10.1002/jps.20017] [PMID: 14999725]

[34] Hugger ED, Novak BL, Burton PS, Audus KL, Borchardt RT. A comparison of commonly used polyethoxylated pharmaceutical excipients on their ability to inhibit P□glycoprotein activity *in vitro.* J Pharm Sci 2002; 91(9): 1991-2002.
[http://dx.doi.org/10.1002/jps.10176] [PMID: 12210046]

[35] Gibson L. Lipid-based excipients for oral drug delivery. Drugs Pharm Sci 2007; 170: 33.

[36] Jannin V, Musakhanian J, Marchaud D. Approaches for the development of solid and semi-solid lipid-based formulations. Adv Drug Deliv Rev 2008; 60(6): 734-46.
[http://dx.doi.org/10.1016/j.addr.2007.09.006] [PMID: 18045728]

[37] Cannon JB. Lipids in transdermal and topical drug delivery. Am Pharm Rev 2014; •••: 17.

[38] Harde H, Das M, Jain S. Solid lipid nanoparticles: an oral bioavailability enhancer vehicle. Expert Opin Drug Deliv 2011; 8(11): 1407-24.
[http://dx.doi.org/10.1517/17425247.2011.604311] [PMID: 21831007]

[39] Weber S, Zimmer A, Pardeike J. Solid Lipid Nanoparticles (SLN) and Nanostructured Lipid Carriers (NLC) for pulmonary application: a review of the state of the art. Eur J Pharm Biopharm Off J Arbeitsgemeinschaft Fur Pharm Verfahrenstechnik eV 2014; 86: 7-22. [http://dx.doi.org/10.1016/j.ejpb.2013.08.013]

[40] Darwis Y, Ali Khan A, Mudassir J, Mohtar N. Advanced drug delivery to the lymphatic system: lipid-based nanoformulations. Int J Nanomedicine 2013; 8: 2733-44. [http://dx.doi.org/10.2147/IJN.S41521] [PMID: 23926431]

[41] Pignatello R, Carbone C, Puglia C, Offerta A, Bonina FP, Puglisi G. Ophthalmic applications of lipid-based drug nanocarriers: an update of research and patenting activity. Ther Deliv 2015; 6(11): 1297-318. [http://dx.doi.org/10.4155/tde.15.73] [PMID: 26608630]

[42] Bozzuto G, Molinari A. Liposomes as nanomedical devices. Int J Nanomedicine 2015; 10: 975-99. [http://dx.doi.org/10.2147/IJN.S68861] [PMID: 25678787]

[43] Akbarzadeh A, Rezaei-Sadabady R, Davaran S, *et al.* Liposome: classification, preparation, and applications. Nanoscale Res Lett 2013; 8(1): 102. [http://dx.doi.org/10.1186/1556-276X-8-102] [PMID: 23432972]

[44] Wagner A, Vorauer-Uhl K. Liposome technology for industrial purposes. J Drug Deliv 2011; 2011: 1-9. [http://dx.doi.org/10.1155/2011/591325] [PMID: 21490754]

[45] Müller RH, Mäder K, Gohla S. Solid lipid nanoparticles (SLN) for controlled drug delivery - a review of the state of the art. Eur J Pharm Biopharm 2000; 50(1): 161-77. [http://dx.doi.org/10.1016/S0939-6411(00)00087-4] [PMID: 10840199]

[46] Mehnert W, Mäder K. Solid lipid nanoparticles. Adv Drug Deliv Rev 2012; 64: 83-101. [http://dx.doi.org/10.1016/j.addr.2012.09.021] [PMID: 11311991]

[47] Battaglia L, Gallarate M. Lipid nanoparticles: state of the art, new preparation methods and challenges in drug delivery. Expert Opin Drug Deliv 2012; 9(5): 497-508. [http://dx.doi.org/10.1517/17425247.2012.673278] [PMID: 22439808]

[48] Mishra D, Dhote V, Mishra P. Solid lipid nanoparticles: a promising colloidal carrier. Nov Carriers Drug Deliv 2014; pp. 278-301.

[49] Battaglia L, Gallarate M, Panciani PP, *et al.* Techniques for the preparation of solid lipid nano and microparticles. Appl Nanotechnol Drug Deliv 2014; 1: 51-75. [http://dx.doi.org/10.5772/58405]

[50] Müller RH, Radtke M, Wissing SA. Nanostructured lipid matrices for improved microencapsulation of drugs. Int J Pharm 2002; 242(1-2): 121-8. [http://dx.doi.org/10.1016/S0378-5173(02)00180-1] [PMID: 12176234]

[51] Olbrich C, Gessner A, Kayser O, Müller RH. Lipid-drug-conjugate (LDC) nanoparticles as novel carrier system for the hydrophilic antitrypanosomal drug diminazenediaceturate. J Drug Target 2002; 10(5): 387-96. [http://dx.doi.org/10.1080/1061186021000001832] [PMID: 12442809]

[52] Anton N, Benoit JP, Saulnier P. Design and production of nanoparticles formulated from nano-emulsion templates—A review. J Control Release 2008; 128(3): 185-99. [http://dx.doi.org/10.1016/j.jconrel.2008.02.007] [PMID: 18374443]

[53] Jaspart S, Piel G, Delattre L, Evrard B. Solid lipid microparticles: formulation, preparation, characterisation, drug release and applications. Expert Opin Drug Deliv 2005; 2(1): 75-87. [http://dx.doi.org/10.1517/17425247.2.1.75] [PMID: 16296736]

[54] Benita S. Microencapsulation: methods and industrial applications. CRC Press 2005. [http://dx.doi.org/10.1201/9781420027990]

[55] Maniar M, Hannibal D, Amselem S, Xie X, Burch R, Domb A. Characterization of lipospheres: Effect of carrier and phospholipid on the loading of drug into the lipospheres. Pharm Res 1991; 8: 175-85.

[56] Bekerman T, Golenser J, Domb A. Cyclosporin nanoparticulate lipospheres for oral administration. J Pharm Sci 2004; 93(5): 1264-70.
[http://dx.doi.org/10.1002/jps.20057] [PMID: 15067702]

[57] Mohammadi-Samani S, Ghasemiyeh P. Solid lipid nanoparticles and nanostructured lipid carriers as novel drug delivery systems: applications, advantages and disadvantages. Res Pharm Sci 2018; 13(4): 288-303.
[http://dx.doi.org/10.4103/1735-5362.235156] [PMID: 30065762]

[58] Yalavarthi PR, Dudala TB, Mudumala NL, *et al.* A perspective overview on lipospheres as lipid carrier systems. Int J Pharm Investig 2014; 4(4): 149-55.
[http://dx.doi.org/10.4103/2230-973X.143112] [PMID: 25426435]

[59] Xiong F, Wang H, Chen YJ, Geng KK, Gu N, Zhu JB. Characterization, biodistribution and targeting evaluation of breviscapine lipid emulsions following intravenous injection in mice. Drug Deliv 2011; 18(2): 159-65.
[http://dx.doi.org/10.3109/10717544.2010.528068] [PMID: 21028951]

[60] Zheng J, Tang Y, Sun M, *et al.* Characterization, pharmacokinetics, tissue distribution and antitumor activity of honokiol submicron lipid emulsions in tumor-burdened mice. Pharmazie 2013; 68(1): 41-6.
[PMID: 23444779]

[61] Zhang X, Wu B. Submicron Lipid Emulsions: A Versatile Platform for Drug Delivery. Curr Drug Metab 2015; 16(3): 211-20.
[http://dx.doi.org/10.2174/1389200216031508l2124221] [PMID: 26279328]

[62] Benson HAE, Grice JE, Mohammed Y, Namjoshi S, Roberts MS. Topical and Transdermal Drug Delivery: From Simple Potions to Smart Technologies. Curr Drug Deliv 2019; 16(5): 444-60.
[http://dx.doi.org/10.2174/1567201816666190201143457] [PMID: 30714524]

[63] Müller RH, Radtke M, Wissing SA. Solid lipid nanoparticles (SLN) and nanostructured lipid carriers (NLC) in cosmetic and dermatological preparations. Adv Drug Deliv Rev 2002; 54 (Suppl. 1): S131-55.https://doi.org/https://doi.org/10.1016/S0169-409X(02)00118-7
[http://dx.doi.org/10.1016/S0169-409X(02)00118-7] [PMID: 12460720]

[64] Fricker G, Kromp T, Wendel A, *et al.* Phospholipids and lipid-based formulations in oral drug delivery. Pharm Res 2010; 27(8): 1469-86.
[http://dx.doi.org/10.1007/s11095-010-0130-x] [PMID: 20411409]

[65] Wong H, Bendayan R, Rauth A, Li Y, Wu X. Chemotherapy with anticancer drugs encapsulated in solid lipid nanoparticles. Adv Drug Deliv Rev 2007; 59(6): 491-504.
[http://dx.doi.org/10.1016/j.addr.2007.04.008] [PMID: 17532091]

[66] Battaglia L, Ugazio E. Lipid Nano- and Microparticles: An Overview of Patent-Related Research. J Nanomater 2019; 2019: 1-22.
[http://dx.doi.org/10.1155/2019/2834941]

[67] Gastaldi L, Battaglia L, Peira E, *et al.* Solid lipid nanoparticles as vehicles of drugs to the brain: Current state of the art. Eur J Pharm Biopharm 2014; 87(3): 433-44.
[http://dx.doi.org/10.1016/j.ejpb.2014.05.004] [PMID: 24833004]

[68] Pozo-Rodriguez A, del , Delgado D, Gascon MAS. Recent Pat Drug Deliv Formul 2011; 5: 214-26.
[http://dx.doi.org/10.2174/187221111797200515] [PMID: 21834776]

[69] Almeida A, Souto E. Solid lipid nanoparticles as a drug delivery system for peptides and proteins. Adv Drug Deliv Rev 2007; 59(6): 478-90.
[http://dx.doi.org/10.1016/j.addr.2007.04.007] [PMID: 17543416]

[70] Montenegro L. Lipid-Based Nanoparticles as Carriers for Dermal Delivery of Antioxidants. Curr Drug

Metab 2017; 18(5): 469-80.
[http://dx.doi.org/10.2174/1389200218666170222152038] [PMID: 28228079]

[71] Nunes S, Madureira R, Campos D, *et al.* Solid lipid nanoparticles as oral delivery systems of phenolic compounds: Overcoming pharmacokinetic limitations for nutraceutical applications. Crit Rev Food Sci Nutr 2015; 57(9): 00.
[http://dx.doi.org/10.1080/10408398.2015.1031337] [PMID: 26192708]

[72] Bhaskar S, Tian F, Stoeger T, *et al.* Multifunctional Nanocarriers for diagnostics, drug delivery and targeted treatment across blood-brain barrier: perspectives on tracking and neuroimaging. Part Fibre Toxicol 2010; 7(1): 3.
[http://dx.doi.org/10.1186/1743-8977-7-3] [PMID: 20199661]

[73] Shah MR, Imran M, Ullah S. Nanostructured lipid carriers. In: Technol MN, Ed. Shah MR, Imran M, Ullah SBT-L-BN for DD and D. William Andrew Publishing 2017; pp. 37-61.
[http://dx.doi.org/10.1016/B978-0-323-52729-3.00002-0]

[74] Wook E, Hae-young J. Solid lipid nanoparticles composition for skin- whitening effect comprising MHY498 and preparation method thereof. KR10186055B1. 2018.

[75] Diorio C, Lokhnauth J. Curcumin solid lipid particles and methods for their preparation and use. Patent US10166187B2

[76] Paula CAD, Dias AMR. Nanoscale system for the sustained release of active cosmetic and/or repellent substances. Patent WO2017143421 2017.

[77] Shilong W, Rongrong Z XH. Application of solid lipid nanoparticles as antidepressant drug carriers. CN105919973A 2016.

[78] Yanqing Z, Junbo X, Ting Z, *et al.* Spinosin solid lipid nanoparticles and preparation method and application thereof. CN103845307B 2015.

[79] Krysxtof C, Wosicka H. Solid lipid nanoparticles of roxithromycin for hair loss or acne. Patent WO2014077712 2014.

[80] Fox CB, Khandhar AP, Van Hoeven N, *et al.* Nanostructured lipid carriers and stable emulsions and uses thereof. WO2018232257A9 2019.

[81] Seabra CL, Nunes CD. Nanostructured lipid carriers, methods and uses thereof. WO2018002853A1 2018.

[82] Lal R, Landon PB. Nanostructured carriers for guided and targeted on-demand substance delivery. The United States Patent Application 20170119891 2017.

[83] Ismail R, Qiuhong L, Linan HL, Hassan HA, Yunmei Z, Basili MH, *et al.* Preparation of nanostructured lipid carriers (NLC) method and products made. Chinese patent CN102283809B 2016.

[84] Ujang Z, Ab Rashid AH, Suboh SK, Ahmad Z, Othman MNDM. A method for producing nano lipid formulation for skincare and/or repair and a nano lipid formulation of the same. International patent WO2015105407A1 2015.

[85] Abdullah RM, Rahman HS, Abdul AB, Wun HCKY. A composition for treating leukemia International patent WO2014123406A1 2014.

[86] Mosqueira CCF, Oliveira LT. Micro- and nanostructured pharmaceutical and veterinary compositions, containing benznidazole and derivatives thereof, which form micro and nanostructures in the gastrointestinal tract, and biologicals uses thereof. Patent WO2015039199

[87] Mallard C, Baudonnet L. Dermatological compositions comprising avermectin nanocapsules. Patent S20130034612 2013.

[88] Roger E, Lagarce F. Lipid nanocapsules, method of preparing same, and use thereof as a drug. Patent WO2011036234 2014.

[89] Wu N, North Brunswick N. POLYMER - CYCLODEXTRIN - LIPID CONJUGATES. Patent US10

064954 2018.

[90] LARM MG HR, *et al.* Microemulsion & sub-micron emulsion process & compositions. Patent US20150258023 2015.

[91] Brynjelsen S, Doty M, Kipp JE, Jayswal N NK. Preparation of submicron-sized nanoparticles via dispersion lyophilization. USOO8722091 2014.

[92] Park JH KH. Liposome comprising synthetic receptor-phospholipid conjugate, and composition, for functional material transfer, which can be bonded to the synthetic receptor and which comprises as active ingredient ligand having functional material bonded thereto. WO201721 2017.

[93] Park JH, Lee J KJ. Method for inclusion of the drug in membrane vesicle through cell modification using membrane fusogenic liposome and drug delivery method using same. WO2015060504 2015.

[94] Huang SL, Klegerman ME, Geng YJ, *et al.* Neuroprotective liposome compositions and methods for treatment of stroke. WO2014026117 2014.

CHAPTER 11

Liposomal Drug Delivery

Unnati Batra[1], **Tejashree Waghule**[1], **Ranendra N. Saha**[1] and **Gautam Singhvi**[1,*]

[1] *Department of Pharmacy, Birla Institute of Technology and Science (BITS), Pilani, Rajasthan, India*

Abstract: Liposomes are emerging as uni or multilamellar micro particulate phospholipid bilayer sphere vesicles, which can be produced synthetically and have the ability to encapsulate any kind of drug molecule. Either hydrophilic or lipophilic drug substances can be easily entrapped in these vesicles for efficient delivery of a drug. Over the past decades, these have been under investigation to develop novel and revolutionary drug delivery aspects in the pharmaceutical field. Liposomes are based on a simple mechanism of formation of the enclosed sphere formed when amphiphilic lipid comes in contact with the aqueous layer. The advancements in liposomes have paved pathways towards efficient drug delivery through alteration in the bioavailability and bio-distribution of drugs. Classified into various types, liposomes can be prepared using various techniques involving mechanical dispersion, solvent dispersion, and detergent removal methods. The development of these liposomes has profound the advanced delivery characterization. This helps deliver the molecules at the target site, and the number of liposomal products in clinical use has now increased. Recent advances are incorporating the emergence of second-generation liposomes over conventional liposomes, which will help modulate the encapsulation efficiency and drug release from liposomes. This literature briefly focusses on various aspects of liposomes, which further relates to the growing advances and interest in this field.

Keywords: Bio-distribution, Drug delivery, Drug release, Encapsulation efficiency, Liposomes, Liposomal products, Mechanical dispersion, Multilamellar vesicles, Phospholipids, Second generation liposomes, Solvent dispersion, Targeting, Unilamellar vesicles.

INTRODUCTION

Liposomes are the simple spherical structures that can encapsulate any type of material, either hydrophilic or lipophilic, like nutrients, drugs, or any biotechnological agents. Constituting lipid bilayer obtained from phospholipids

* **Corresponding author Gautam Singhvi:** Department of Pharmacy, Birla Institute of Technology and Science (BITS), Pilani, Rajasthan, India; Tel: +919314490535; E-mail: **gautam.singhvi@pilani.bits-pilani.ac.in**

Akhlesh K. Jain & Keerti Mishra (Eds.)

which are non-toxic natural lipids, form concentric spaces for entrapment of the formerly stated substances [1, 2]. Not new as emerging vesicles that need to be established for their roles in drug delivery, these were discovered and described around 60 years ago by British hematologist Alec D Bangham, which were later published after 3-4 years. The idea of naming them was created from the idea of these spheres being fat bodies comprising lipids. Lipo means "fat," and soma represents "body," and this states its composition of phospholipids [3, 4].

The discovery of the liposomes was attributed to Bangham and R.W. Horne when they were testing the new electron microscope they received at Babraham Institute in Cambridge. During this study, they added a negative stain to the phospholipid. Along with the simple plasmalemma, they observed the cell membrane structure, which was the first of its kind. They studied the integrity of the lipid bilayer and further worked on it to find out what that bilayer was. Sooner they recognized the layer as an integrated bilayer lipid that can release its content upon treatment with the surfactants. In the next year, Weissmann, who was of the Babraham Institute, in a meeting with Bangham, named the structure of one of its special kind as "Liposome." This was somewhat influenced by the word lysosome, on which the people were already working. Bangham called these structures "Multilamellar smectic mesophases" or "Banghasomes." This all led to the beginning of the liposome industry, which today has spread its legs almost to every area of drug delivery and its processes [5].

The assembly of liposomes was nothing but just a simple observation of the natural cell membrane which is comprised of the bilayered lipid. These observations led to the development in this field that enhanced its usage in various fields. The composite structure includes the lipids arranged in such a way that they form a bilayer with the hydrophilic head of the lipid molecules facing outside in the region of the aqueous state [6]. The lipophilic tails of the lipid molecules of two individual layers face inwards towards each other, forming a bilayer of lipid molecules. The two layers are just oppositely overlapping each other. They are in the formation in such a way that the circular position of these structures leads to the development of concentric space. Fig. (**11.1**) below illustrates the complete structure of liposomes and the drug entrapment in liposomes [7, 8].

The physicochemical nature of liposomes states the amphipathic nature that inculcates their strong tendency to strengthen the structure. These inclusive properties enhance the structuring of lipid layers and act as a barrier to the permeation of the entrapped molecules. The occurrence of the hydrophilic layer provides the stability of this structural organization to remain in contact with the dispersion media and inner substance. The latter only emerges out of the vesicle on the changes in the solution or dispersion, pH, temperature, or ultimately diffusion of the membrane [9, 10]. The concentric space thus formed can be utilized as a loading area for any type of molecule to deliver them to the targeted site of action. In addition to this, they can easily add up with different bilayer membranes and can diffuse their content easily, making it a way much easier to deliver drugs into the biological system [11]. Many approaches are now coming up, which are easing the content delivery through liposomes by just inculcating the simple phenomenon of the pH or charge systems of the fluids which need to be delivered at the targeted site [5].

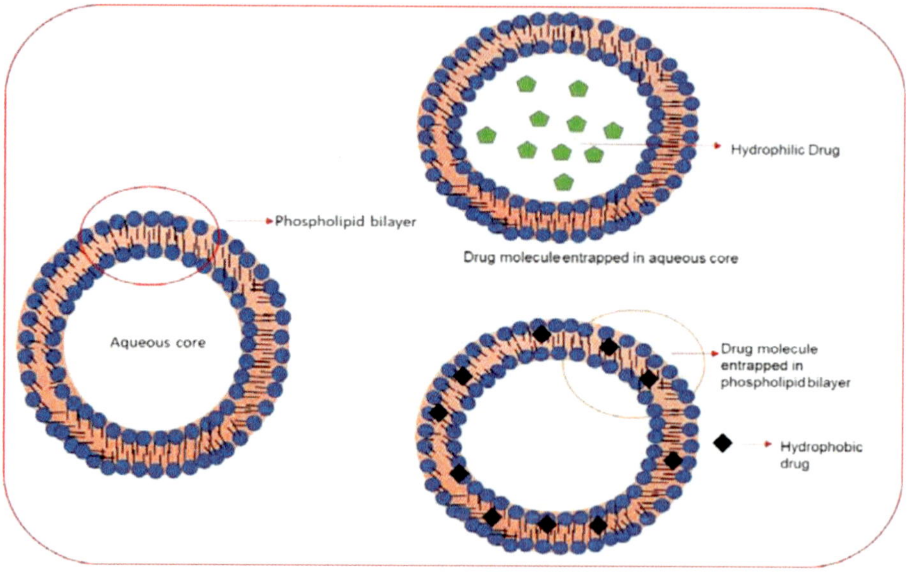

Fig. (11.1). Structure of liposomes and entrapment of drug molecules.

Some advantages of liposomes include an increase in efficiency of the targeted drug delivery, site avoidance effect, passive targeting to the desired site of action, improvised pharmacokinetic parametric effects on the human body, flexibility of coupling with certain kinds of site-specific ligands, increase in the therapeutic efficiency of drugs, and most importantly increasing stability of the molecule being administered by encapsulation [1]. The applications of liposomes are emerging as a variety of drug delivery in oral systems, sustained-release drug delivery systems, immunological adjuvants, site-specific targeting in gene delivery, tailored drug release, and recent advances in anti-HIV, and anticancer drug delivery. In addition to this, they have been into the delivery of fabrics to the dying industry, nutritional supplements to the food industry, and cosmetics to the skin. The list is increasing with the upsurge in the studies going on liposomes. These have now been one of the greatest achievements in the area of clinical applications as compared to conventional approaches that were earlier used for drug delivery [2, 10].

CATEGORIZATION OF LIPOSOMES

Liposomes can be classified based on various aspects as discussed below [2]:

Based on morphology (Lamellarity)

- Unilamellar vesicles
    - Small Unilamellar Vesicles (SUV)
    - Medium Unilamellar Vesicles (MUV)
    - Large Unilamellar Vesicles (LUV)
- Oligolamellar vesicles (OLV)
- Multilamellar vesicles (MLV)
- Multivesicular Vesicles (MVV)

Based on Composition and Application

- Conventional Liposomes
- Fusogenic Liposomes
- pH-Sensitive Liposomes
- Cationic Liposomes
- Stealth Liposomes
- Immuno-Liposomes

Based on preparation methods

- Dehydration Rehydration Vesicles (DRV)
- SUVs/ OLVs made by Reverse Phase Evaporation Method (REV)
- MLV made by REV
- Vesicles by Extrusion Techniques
- Frozen and Thawed MLVs
- Stable Plurilamellar Vesicles

Unilamellar liposomes are used in the studies of the biological system which reflect cell membrane structure and are in the size range of 20-100 nm for SUVs and more than 100 nm as LUVs. In contrast, Oligolamellar vesicles illustrate lamellae ranging between two to five, and those containing more than five are typically called multilamellar vesicles. The size of oligolamellar vesicles ranges from 0.1 to 1.0 μm. These structures are explained in Figs. (**11.2** and **11.3**) [2, 12, 13].

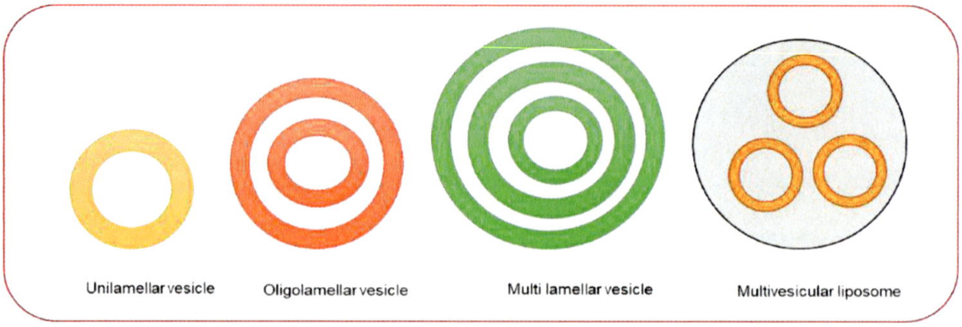

Fig. (11.2). Classification of Liposome.

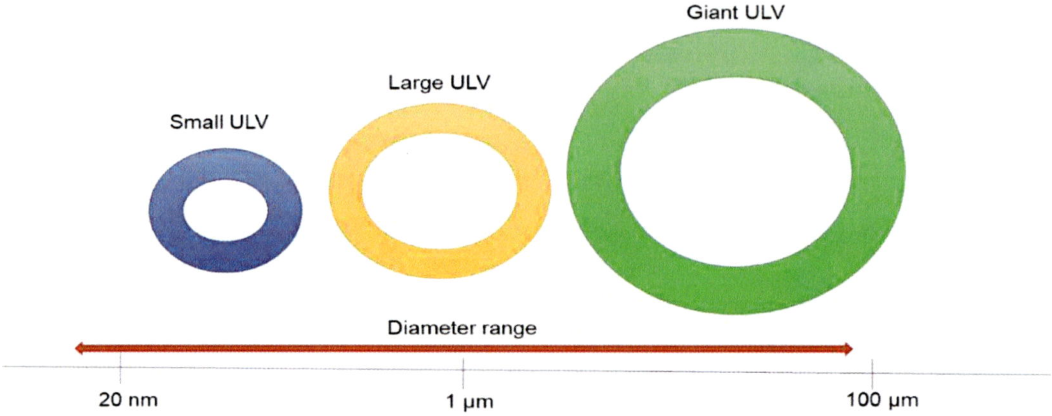

Fig. (11.3). Classification of Liposome based on size.

Conventional Liposomes are the most common type of liposomes based on lipid bilayer-based therapeutics applications. Fusogenic liposomes are another class of liposomes that are evident in the properties of being able to fuse with ease within the biological membrane, and thus, they can improvise delivery of the substances into the desired site of action. Whereas pH-sensitive liposomes are activated at certain pH and can be destined according to the pH of the target area [14, 15].

Stealth Liposomes are the emerging type of liposomes, also referred to as second-generation liposomes, which are further coated by the use of some polymers like poly hydroxyethyl L- aspargines, Polyethylene glycol (PEG) and Polyglycerol-Polyethylene glycol (H-PG-PEG). The surface coating of liposomes prevents the uptake by macrophages which are called the stealth effect. This enhances the circulation time of the liposomes in the biological system and thus helps in targeting drugs. Also, stability increases multifold if the liposomes containing lipid bilayer are coated with derivatives of PEG. Due to their application in controlling the drug release and prolonging the circulation time, these liposomes have found application in cancer therapy, gene transfection, vaccines, also in inflammations, and some respiratory diseases [16, 17].

Cationic liposomes are another type of liposomes, now emerging and extensively being used in gene delivery. This type of liposome possesses a positive charge and is easily associated with the negatively charged molecule/surface and provides targeted delivery. The most widely used concept is the use of these liposomes to deliver the DNA and RNA molecules in the gene delivery, as these molecules are negatively charged, cationic liposomes easily attach to them and deliver them across the cell membrane compared to the classical liposomes. The delivery is associated with the process of fusion of the cell membrane and the cationic liposomes, which bypasses the route responsible for the degradation of the classical liposomes. Another method of delivery involves attaching the cationic liposomes to the DNA molecules in such a way that it forms the aggregated vesicle forming a cluster, which crosses the plasma membrane. They are highly biodegradable, bioresponsive, and have high nucleic acid encapsulation efficiency [18].

ADVANTAGES OF LIPOSOMES

With the growing advances in liposomal technology, here are listed advantages of the liposomal drug delivery system [19 - 21].

- Liposomes potentially help to widen the therapeutic index of the drug and help in the case of drugs with significant toxicity.
- Reduction of the toxicity being caused by the encapsulated agent being rather provided by any other formulation.
- Variable size and tailoring of the formulation can be done.
- A good carrier for controlled and sustained release drug delivery.
- Encapsulation stability is much higher.
- This bilayer lipid particle provides an improvement in the pharmacokinetic behaviors of the drug being targeted.
- Provides selective passive targeting, which is helpful in tumor tissue and their adjoining tissues.
- Avoids the effect on the non-target site, which proves beneficial for gene targeting and anticancer therapy.
- The incorporation of both hydrophobic and lipophilic drugs enables the development of a wide range of drugs in liposomal formulation.
- Drug distribution can also be altered according to the alteration of the sizes of liposomes.
- The *in-vivo* behavior of the drug can be modified just by optimizing some formulation parameters.

- Various advances like stealth liposomes, targeted liposomes, tailored drug delivery are proving recent advances in the technology.
- These are non-toxic, flexible, and biodegradable vesicles.
- Reduced exposure of the toxic drugs to non-site tissues.
- Liposome helps in the prevention of the DNA from degenerative processes.
- Ability to load significantly large molecular weight compounds such as parts of DNA as large as chromosomes.

LIMITATIONS OF LIPOSOMES

While liposomes have sparked considerable impact in the pharmaceutical field for the delivery of the drugs based on the specification and release, they have been restricted in their industrial and biomedical applications due to several drawbacks, including the lack of stability and reduction in the quality of the drug and its formulation aspect during storage. Liposome stability is influenced by several factors, especially the lipid bilayer [22]. The limited encapsulation of molecules, rapid clearance, instability being caused on storage and transportation or as a result of time, issues with precisional reproducibility, numerous factors that need to be considered during manufacturing have imposed a greater challenge in the organization and establishment of the liposomal drug delivery in the market [23]. Liposome sterilization remains a major challenge due to its high sensitivity and proclivity for physicochemical changes. The sterilization of the liposomal formulation cannot be completed by normal gaseous or radiation sterilization, and these need to be manufactured in aseptic conditions, which are again a great challenge to impose both economically and reproducibly [24, 25].

Stability: The stability conditions directly affect the shelf life of liposomes. The instabilities can be either physical or chemical. The lipidic fusion of the molecules or oozing out of the drug from formulation lead to physical instability. Generally, the decrease of the shelf life of liposomal formulation does not account for physical instability but chemical degradation like hydrolysis and oxidation [26].

Sterilization: Since basic components of the liposomal drug delivery are prone to degradation by heat and vulnerable to procedures that involve direct application of heat, chemicals, or sometimes radiation, finding a suitable technique for sterilizing liposome formulations is a great concern. Filtration *via* sterile 0.22 μm membranes is one method for sterilizing liposome formulations. On the other hand, filtration is not appropriate for large vesicles (>0.2 μm) and does not kill viruses. Some methods cannot be applied for the sterilization of the liposomes as they facilitate degradation in the phospholipids of the liposomal content [26].

The major set of liposomal formulations in the clinical world is being targeted as parenteral drug delivery. But what remains challenging in that type of formulation is again the concerns of sterilization; suitable techniques to be included always remain a question. All the methods like steam sterilization, chemical sterilization, and radiation sterilization involve the risk of product degradation in the liposomal formulation. Although sterile filtration does not affect the stability of the product, it does impose a limitation on the product and its particle size [26, 27].

The heat sterilization method for the liposomes, which involves autoclaving, should be done under circumstances where the drug is encapsulated after the sterilization. However, various studies show that liposomes containing hydrophilic drugs can be sterilized using the autoclaving method [28].

But various advanced research has proven that conventional and earlier used sterilization methods like heat, gaseous, and radiations have been found to be unsuitable. A recent very promising study for sterilization of products like liposomes is done using Supercritical carbon dioxide, which needs to be optimized but works effectively in sterilization [24].

Rapid clearance: A significant drawback of using liposomal formulations that are ligand-based and act upon immunity has been their rapid clearance due to non-specific absorption by Reticular-Endothelial system cells. Since liposomes are cleared as quickly by RES, the production of immune liposomes conjugated with ligands has reignited interest in this area [26, 29].

Low Encapsulation Efficiency of hydrophilic drugs: The efficiency by which the lipid vesicles entrap the drug says a lot about the quality and safety of the formulation. Hydrophilic drugs are likely to leach out easily or show faster drug release from liposomes. A high dose of certain drugs can prove toxic. Liposomal delivery needs to be optimized to release the drug at a slow and constant rate. Higher lipid concentrations might be required to deliver such drugs, which can improve the product cost and lower patient compliance [26].

METHODS OF PREPARATION AND DRUG LOADING

As the development of liposomes started with the observation of natural cell membrane structure, with the advancements in liposomal studies, advances are also emerging in the field of its preparation. Numerous methods are utilized in liposomes' development, much of which is dependent on some of the following mentioned points [7, 19].

1. The properties of the substance that must be entrapped within a liposome vesicle, such as its molecular weight, solubility, log P, and shelf life.
2. Dispersion media of liposomes.

3. The intended application of liposomes and delivery site which dictates the size, polydisperse nature, and desired life of the vesicle.
4. The concentration of the entrapped material required.
5. The simulated toxicity of the material and its compatibility with the bilayer.
6. The scale-up process for production.
7. The cost, reproducibility, and applicability of the desired formulation.

Preparation of Liposomes

Preparation of Liposomes includes four general steps [14].

- Dissolution in organic solvent: Lipids are first dissolved in the organic solvent of choice.
- Drying lipids from organic solvent: The lipids are then dried, and the organic solvent is separated. This is the basic step in the start of any type of liposomes prepared from both natural and synthetic lipids.
- The aqueous dispersion of lipids: The desired media for dispersion based on the application of that particular liposome is selected, and dispersion is conducted by the use of various mechanical methods or solvent dispersion methods. This is the stage where drug loading is performed.
- Step of Purification: After the final assembly of the liposomes, they are purified subject to the applicability of the same [5, 13, 14].
- Analysis of the final product: The prepared liposomes are characterized for size, polydispersity index (PDI), surface charge, encapsulation efficiency, and lamellarity. These are discussed in detail in section 6.0 [2].

The above steps of liposomal preparation are depicted in Fig. **(11.4)** below:

Methods of Drug Loading

The liposomes are prepared and loaded with a drug or desired substances by the following two main techniques.

Passive Loading

This method involves the process of rehydration in which the drug is loaded along with the preparation of the liposomal particle. The drug is entrapped in the lipidic sphere during the continuous process of production. The passive loading method for liposomal preparation is based on co-current loading leading to the formation of liposomes. Passive equilibrium is achieved when the drug is added to the preformed liposome preparation, and simultaneous encapsulation occurs. The drug is added constantly while preparing the liposome [10]. When hydrophobic drugs are encapsulated by this method, this achieves high trapping efficiency. The biggest disadvantage of this strategy is that it requires using the organic solvent prior to the loading [7, 12]. The passive type of drug loading can be of three types.

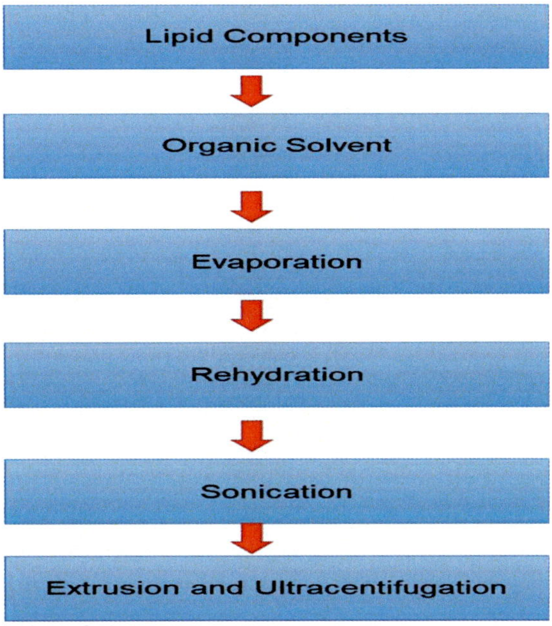

Fig. (11.4). Steps for Preparation of Liposome.

Mechanical Dispersion Method

- Sonication: It is an extensively used method for passive drug loading of liposomes. Probe sonication and Bath sonication are the two most widely used techniques. Low encapsulation efficiency is the major drawback of sonication.
- Freeze thawed liposomes: In this method, the liposomes are rapidly frozen and then thawed for the passive entrapment of the drug.
- French Pressure Cell Extrusion: Liposomes are passed through a small orifice. This method recalls entrapped solutes significantly longer than sonication and is widely used for unstable products.
- Membrane Extrusion: Liposomal dispersion is extruded through a polycarbonate filter to obtain small uniform vesicles.
- Micro Emulsification

Solvent Dispersion Method

- Ether Injection: The lipids are subjected to the solvent, either ether or ether methanol mixture, and then added dropwise to an aqueous solution with the entrapping material at the selected temperature and reduced pressure. Solvent evaporation under vacuum leads to the formation of liposomes.
- Ethanol Injection: Lipids dissolved in ethanol are injected instantaneously to an

excess of buffer, but the dispersion formed by this method is not homogenous [30, 31].

- Reverse Phase Evaporation Method: This method enhanced the advantage of the liposomal technology by incorporating a large amount of entrapping material when compared to the lipid ratio. This occurs by the process of formation of inverted micelles, which are shaped upon sonication and filled with a buffered aqueous phase. Slow elimination leads to the formation of viscous gel, and with time, this gel collapse, and the excess of the lipids forms the actual lipid bilayer Phospholipids are dissolved in organic solvents further the aqueous phase is added to the solution. The mixing of two phases leads to the formation of a two-phase system. An inverted phase solution is formed upon vigorous shaking, which is evaporated to form LUVs [12].

Detergent Removal Methods

- Dialysis: Solubilization of lipids at their critical micelle concentration (CMC) is utilized in this approach of drug loading. When the surfactant reaches the CMC, micelle formation starts, and the process of detachment is exaggerated by dialyzing unit. As detergent is detached, micelles combine to form phospholipid bilayer and then finally combine to form liposomes [32].

Gel Permeation Chromatography

This chromatography is used to separate particles based on size. The separation of monomers occurs through the use of the concept that liposomes do not penetrate in the gel-packed column pores, which subsequently result in the separation. This method requires pretreatment [20].

Active Loading

This method of drug loading is based on the loading of the drug actively after the complete formation of the liposome. First, the liposome is prepared through general steps which do not include drug loading [7, 12, 19]. This is also referred to as remote loading of liposomes [13]. The final product is loaded with the drug by the efficient process of the pH gradient in which the drug is transferred to the core of the liposome leading to entrapment of the drug. In the pH gradient method, the change in the pH from the outside environment to the inner core affects the process of drug entry which entraps the drug at respective pH. The other process by which it is done is loading by the use of agents which helps to deliver the drug inside the core. Sahil *et al.* demonstrated the Stealth property of the Doxorubicin Hydrochloride which is demonstrated by the process of active loading with the help of ammonium sulfate [16, 33]. Both passive and active drug loading methods are indicated in Figs. **(11.5)** and **(11.6)** below.

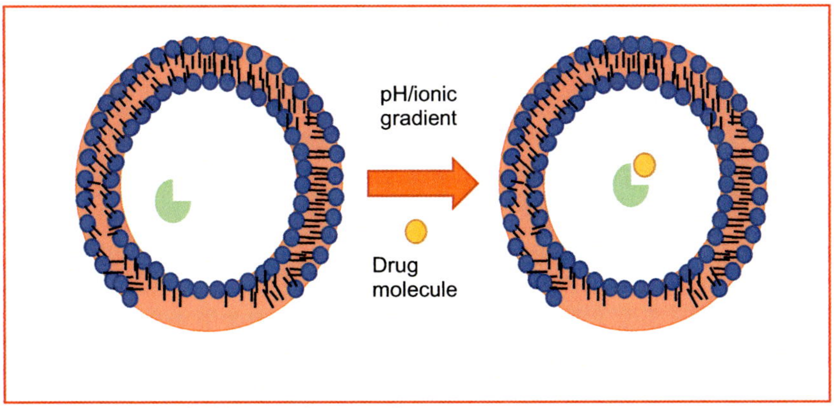

Fig. (11.5). Active drug loading in liposomal preparation.

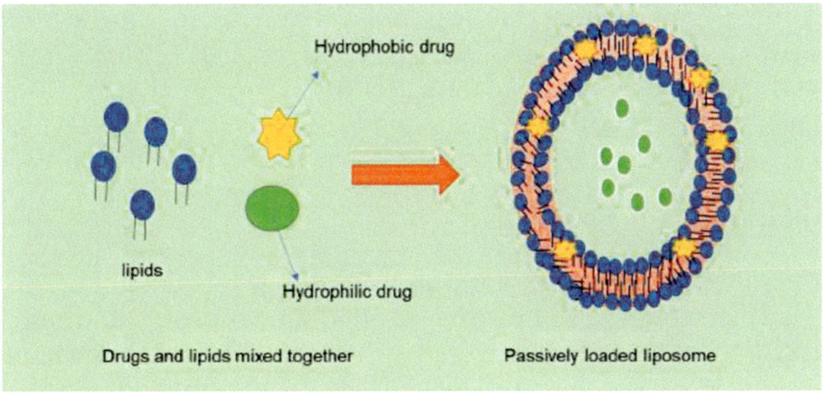

Fig. (11.6). Passive drug loading in a liposomal preparation.

CHARACTERIZATION OF LIPOSOMES

After the liposomes are prepared, they are characterized based on various parameters. These include visual appearance, structure, shape, size distribution, lamellarity of the liposomes, the efficiency of encapsulation, drug release characteristics, zeta potential, and their stability [34]. They are detailed as follows [10].

Size and Size Distribution

With respect to liposomes, size distribution is usually studied through dynamic light scattering which is reliable for the determination of homogenous mass. Mainly electron microscopy is utilized for the characterization of the size of the liposomes. Negative staining and freeze fracturing are the most commonly used methods but due to some reasons, they are prone to change in the sample while processing of sample preparation. In lieu of this, cryoelectronic microscopy can be used as the substitute for the determination of the size and the particle distribution of the liposomal preparation. This involves direct observation in electron beams and is done on frozen samples which makes it more effective [19].

Zeta Potential

The zeta potential is a term given to the difference of the potential between the mobile particles' electric double layer (EDL) and the slipping plane's dispersant layer, which is present thereof [35]. The key content that determines the overall charge on the membrane of the liposome is the phospholipid composition of liposomes (positively and negatively charged phospholipids) [19, 34].

Lamellarity Determination

A variety of spectroscopic techniques and electron microscopy are utilized for the determination of the exact lamellarity of the liposomes. Usually, it is done using Nuclear Magnetic Resonance Imaging (NMR). The lamellarity of the vesicles is determined by the help of Electronic Spin Resonance techniques which help in the determination of voluminous nature and hence reflect the lamellarity [19, 35].

Encapsulation Efficiency (EE)

The entrapment calculation is done on the basis of the amount of the drug that is loaded in the vesicles, compared to the amount of the drug which was theoretically to be loaded in the vesicle; therefore, the total amount of drug in the system as well as the free drug needs to be determined. This will directly influence the bioavailability and other pharmacokinetic parameters of the drug [19, 34].

In a study, the liposomal suspension was formulated, which was then added to the double amount of ethanol. This process effectively disrupts the primary layer of the liposome, which leads to the release of the entrapped content of the liposome. Also, the method involved the use of a marker molecule suitable to the drug candidate. This solution, after filtering, was measured for the drug content with the appropriate method with respect to the drug properties. In this study, calcein was used as a marker for the drug. This was detected using fluorescence. The encapsulation efficiency was determined by the following formula **(1)** as given by [36, 37].

$$Fi = \frac{Ct - Co}{Ct} * 100 \tag{1}$$

Where F_i= Encapsulation efficiency in percent; C_t= Concentration of the marker used in total inside and outside; C_o= Concentration of the marker detected outside of the membrane.

Calculation of Encapsulation efficiency (EE) without the use of a marker is done by the following equation **(2)**:

EE= amount of drug entrapped/ Total amount of drug added *100 **(2)**

Drug Release

The *in vivo* conditions and sink conditions are maintained to evaluate the drug release studies of the liposomal drug formulations. A suitable buffer system is used as release media which can be according to specifications. The study is conducted at 37 °C for evaluation of parenteral products. Different types of *in vitro* release studies can be performed with respect to the specific molecular weight cut-off patterns, which include- the dialysis membrane method dialysis bag method, which are soaked under the reciprocating conditions in the release media. Liposomal dispersion containing dialysis bag is immersed in the release media. Aliquots are taken at specific intervals of time. The cumulative amount of drug released at different time points is calculated [19, 38].

Stability

The stability of liposomes is a major issue. Stability can be characterized as physical, chemical, and biological. It is the major indicator of liposomal efficacy and its storage conditions. Physical stability is indicative of consistency in the size and size ratio of liposomes. Chemical stability describes the liposomes that are not prone to oxidation or hydrolysis type of reactions. But the biological stability of the liposomes is rather limited compared to the other stabilities that are again affected when tested under *in-vivo* conditions. In the presence of poorly soluble salts (at optimum pH) and antioxidants, highly charged cationic liposomes can be effective in a fluid state. The addition of cryoprotectants improves the stability of freeze-dried liposomes greatly [9].

Physical Stability

The addition of antioxidants and chelating agents in the liposomal formulation provides physical stability. Aggregation and coalescence are the signs of instability in liposomes. Changes in the particle size of the formulation can be detected using the Zetasizer, which can depict the physical stability of the formulation. Encapsulation efficiency and holding of the drug without leakiness also resemble the physically stable product [39].

Chemical Stability

There are two pathways in terms of chemical stability that can reduce the liposomes' shelf life, namely, oxidative and hydrolytic pathways. The phospholipids in an aqueous state need to be checked for these pathways. Other major types of chemical instability may be due to the effect of pH, ionic strength, temperature, which are process variables and need to be controlled during the fabrication. The other variables are the length of the lipidic chain in liposomes and the effect of aggregation [39].

PARAMETERS AFFECTING *IN-VIVO* BEHAVIOR OF LIPOSOME

The most important parameters that affect the pharmacological advances of the liposomes are surface characterization which involves fluidity, surface charge, and size. Other factors like the preparation method also play a great role in the drug's release kinetics and final *in vivo* behavior [29]. The liposomal formulations can be managed in terms of the content and quality of the drug, cellular uptake, charge density, and fluidity of the bilayer membrane. The direct effect of these parameters influences the physiological and biological effects of the liposomal delivery of the drug. Simultaneously these parameters also provide the way to influence the *in vivo* behavior by knowing the extent of its property relating to the effect [4].

Bilayer Membrane Fluidity

The existence of different phases of the lipids in the terms of their glass transition temperature provides the different states of lipids. The lower temperature with respect to the glass transition temperature particularly forms a well-ordered solid-state arrangement of the lipid molecules which completely neglects the fluidity of the membrane thus formed [40]. Depending on the length and complexity of the lipids being used, an alteration in the glass temperature leads to a change in the fluidity of the lipid bilayer membrane which can be utilized in the formation of the characterized lipid for targeted delivery [41]. These bilayers and their fluidity directly influence the interaction of the lipids and the drug molecule to the biological membrane. The lipids with higher glass transition temperature appear to have less uptake by the biological membrane. An increase in the temperature above the individual glass transition temperature leads to increased lipid bilayer fluidity [29]. Membrane fluidity directly influences the *in-vivo* release of the drug. The ordered state of the bilayer membrane affects the flow of drugs out from the lipid vesicle in a slow manner where they are used as controlled delivery devices. The exceptionally high fluidic nature of the lipid membrane leads to the *in vivo* release of the drug at a very fast rate [32].

Surface Charge

The nature of lipid decides the surface charge of liposomes which ultimately affects the *in vivo* behavior of the drug entrapped within [7]. Neutral liposome does not interact significantly with the cells and biological membrane. However, the association of liposomes and biological cell membranes may be aided by a huge amount of electrostatic charge. The membranes of the biological cells which possess negative surface charge significantly take up the positively charged liposomes through coated pit endocytosis. This provides improved permeation of the drug through the stratum corneum when administered topically. Charged liposomes are easily cleared from the plasma and influence the plasma circulation of liposomes when administered parenterally [13].

Method of Preparation

Preparation using different methods affects the formulation of liposomes and influences the characteristics like hydration of the surface, surface charge, and liposome size. These factors affect the encapsulation efficiency of the liposomes and the mechanism with which it interacts with the biological cells. An example may include the hydration technique, which is the simplest of all the liposomal preparation methods but has poor encapsulation efficiency. Also, a decrease in the size of the liposome decreases the encapsulation efficiency of the drug [12, 29].

RECENT MODIFICATIONS IN LIPOSOMAL DRUG DELIVERY

Even though this new knowledge of liposomal drug delivery emerging in the recent past has helped researchers develop novel anticancer drugs and related therapy, successful cancer control has proven to be a challenge. The main bottlenecks are early detection of disease signs, off-target drug delivery that causes unintended damage to healthy tissues, and tumor cell drug resistance [42].

To keep up with developments in analytical methods used in science, quality by design-based tactic known as Formulation by Design (FbD) is being investigated extensively by emerging scientists for a deeper understanding of drug delivery and its growth and unmistakable universal acceptance. The industrial scale-up for the production of liposomes in the manufacturing field demands the usage to be stable, effective, and safe, which should be reproducible. These, in a way, pave some challenges to the liposomal drug delivery aspects. But the, technological intervention has created the methodologies that focus on these aspects for suitable drug delivery [43, 44].

For the treatment of pulmonary diseases, various pulmonary delivery systems such as pressurized metered-dose inhalers (pMDIs), soft mist inhalers (SMI), dry powder inhalers (DPI), and nebulizers have been planned, created, and studied [45].

The other aspect of the recent development of liposomal drug delivery is magnetic gels. These have a combination of properties of hydrogels and magnetic nanoparticles, which are taken into a single piece of drug delivery element. They are emerging as the efficient and the most demanding piece for drug release. They allow control over functions that suit the biomedical need resembling the on-demand and tailored drug release of the product suiting to the drug formulation [46].

Drug targeting through liposomes is accomplished by the use of ligands that are attached to the vesicular lipid molecules. The ligand binds to particular receptor sites, causing the lipid vesicles to congregate at those locations. This technique helps in minimizing the absorption and distribution of the liposomes in the reticular endothelial system RES (liver, spleen, and bone marrow) [41].

The idea of site-specific delivery was first presented by Paul Ehrlich, entails delivering a greater fraction of the drug to the target site, thereby minimizing absorption by normal tissues not requiring the therapeutic delivery. Liposomes have been used to achieve drug targeting that is both passive and active [41].

Passive targeting of liposome drug delivery takes advantage of certain cells' natural ability to phagocyte foreign microparticulates, including liposomes, such as Kupffer cells in the liver and circulating macrophages in the RES. Drug and immune stimulator formulations in conventional liposome (CL) shapes have been successfully used to target cells. By coupling specific antibodies to vesicles, active targeting of liposome-encapsulated drugs can be achieved (immunoliposomes). Diphtheria toxin (DT) immunoliposomes have been shown to protect against the non-specific toxicity of DT during cancer chemotherapy [13, 47].

APPLICATION OF LIPOSOMES AND RECENT ADVANCES

Drugs encapsulated in liposomes might alter the therapeutic molecule's real properties, potentially reducing undesired side effects and boosting treatment success. The use of liposomes as a medium, method or clinically therapeutic devices can be taken into the therapeutic and diagnostic application of the drugs entrapped in liposomes. The drugs and the variety of the elements that can be used to form liposomal drug delivery can act as a tool, reagent, interfaces for studies, recognition procedures, *etc.* The interaction of liposomes with cells and their fate *in vivo* after administration are crucial factors in determining the benefits and disadvantages of liposomal drug carriers [10]. The fourth potential interaction is the exchange of bilayer constituents such as cholesterol and lipid: membrane-bound compounds with cell membrane components [48].

Liposomal vesicles greatly impact the drug delivery of the therapeutic targeting ensuring a way of drug delivery. Today liposomes are utilized in a number of ways as drug carriers in a variety of clinical applications like immunological treatments, benign and malignant tumors therapy, gene delivery, and anti-viral therapies. Furthermore, these are utilized as a drug carrier to obtain a sustained and controlled release of drug [8].

Liposomes form vesicles with a diameter of approximately 25-500 nm and around 5 nm of thickness in water. Hydrophilic drugs are easily incorporated in the aqueous region of the liposomal formulation while lipophilic drugs can be easily incorporated in the lipidic part of the liposomes [49]. The proportion of parts that are hydrophilic and those that are hydrophobic of lipid particles can be adjusted to alter the morphology of vesicles.

The following are advantages of the liposomes acting as drug carriers:

1. They help to increase the solubilization power of lipophilic drugs.
2. Simultaneously they increase the stability of the drug *in vivo*.
3. They assist in controlling the release time of drugs from the liposomal packets.
4. These types of carriers tend to decrease the uptake of therapeutic agents by normal tissues, which in turn decreases the side effects being caused by the molecule.

In a study, TAT peptide was taken by both conventional and PEGylated liposomes. The resultant localization of TAT peptide remained inside the cell for the first few hours, and complete disintegration occurred in the next 9 hours. The drug carriers, including the TAT Peptide, showed as a promising carrier for non-endocytic intracellular drug delivery which can also carry DNA as entrapped in the vesicle [50].

Celecoxib was found as an efficient means of cancer treatment and enhancing the efficiency of anticancer medicines in the treatment of skin tumors when applied topically. The study focused on creating an efficient celecoxib topical formulation that could facilitate drug skin delivery and provide in-depth penetration through the skin layers. As drug carriers, three types of vesicular formulations have been studied: liposomes with a surfactant, transfersomes, ethosomes with appropriate edge activators, and liposomes without a surfactant. The stratum corneum is thought to be the most important limiting stage in drug penetration through the skin. Due to their established success in improving skin penetration and clinical effectiveness of a number of medications, liposomes have been widely used as a safe and effective technique for delivering effective topical drug administration [51].

Liposomes have been shown to improve the permeation of the drug, stabilizing the formulation and establish the local deposition into the skin and deeper tissues, as well as the duration of their release. It can also provide a moist condition on the wound skin's upper layer due to liposomes' successful closure as epidermic cells, resulting in the treatment of wounds [52]. Cysteine protease is a higher proteolytic activity enzyme derived from the Papaya fruit that encourages skin exfoliation and softens skin by removing fibrosis. However, contributing to the high molecular weight and hydrophilic nature, it is not suitable for topical use. To address these disadvantages, liposomes were used to encapsulate the papain enzyme and found a major area in the development of wound healing devices using liposomes [19].

Amoxicillin (alpha-amino-hydroxybenzylpenicillin) belongs to the penicillin family of antibiotics and is utilized to treat bacterial infections of various organs. To get the desired therapeutic results, Amoxicillin needs to be given in higher doses as the drug is poorly soluble in water. Amoxicillin has a short half-life and reduced absorption in the small intestine, resulting in low colonic absorption. Liposomes are one of the most important encapsulation technologies because of their high water stability, highly biocompatible with human cells, highly flexible as drug carriers, and strong ability to entrap any kind of drug molecule with high encapsulation efficiency [53].

Due to the histology and pathophysiology of cancer tissue and the significant differences between it and normal tissue, cancer tissue is thought to be a good target for drug delivery systems. For example, the tumor vasculature is characterized by leaky vasculature and reduced lymphatic drainage [5, 54]. Once the anticancer drug delivery systems access the extracellular spaces, the active drug can be released by a variety of channels, such as the pH difference between the blood (7.4) and the extracellular spaces of cancer cells (4-5 acidic pH), which can affect acid-responsive polymers. Another mechanism is in which anticancer drugs containing polymers are exposed to lysosomal enzyme degradation [6].

For large biological molecules like nucleic acid, oligonucleotides, and interfering RNA, liposomal drug delivery is investigated as delivery vectors for these therapeutics: high-molecular-weight, hydrophilic, and strongly charged nucleic acid-based materials [7, 55]. Alternatively, a range of techniques has been dedicated to developing cationic liposomal drug delivery, which ensures the neutral charge on the inner surface for the liposome and approaches gene therapy [56]. Coated cationic liposomes (CCL), lipidic nanoparticles (LNP), stable nucleic acid-lipid particles (SNALP), and liposome-polycation-hyaluronic acid particles are just a few of the options (LPD) [19, 57]. In a study by Bibi *et al.*, three patients with metastatic cancer were tested to see whether liposomes can be used as drug carriers. The fate of the liposomal formulation was tested into the bloodstream of the patients with the help of normal and tumor cell characterization using electron microscopy. The deposits of the malignant tumor cells showed a great amount of absorbed drug through the liposomal delivery. These showed a great enhancement as cancer therapy through liposomal drug carriers [58].

Doxil® was developed by Sequus Pharmaceuticals, a US-based company, in 1995. It is the first product of nano liposomal technology to be approved by the FDA. This is the liposomal formulation of Doxorubicin which is classified under the anthracycline antibiotic class. The technology associated with the liposomal production of Doxil is the PEGylation of the surface of the liposome. This PEGylation refers to the encapsulation of the drug inside the layer of Polyethylene glycol polymer, which helps to provide a stealth effect to the drug. The indications approved by the FDA for liposomes of Doxorubicin are advanced ovarian cancer, multiple myeloma, and the Kaposi's sarcoma which is linked to HIV infection. This involves active loading of the Doxorubicin by the use of Ammonium sulfate and this type of loading of the Doxorubicin leads to the attainment of approx. 1500 doxorubicin molecules in one lipid layer vesicle. The reason for Doxil preparation is associated with limitations of Doxorubicin molecule which is irritant when given through venous route. The Doxil encapsulates the drug in the lipidic bilayer and hence the side effects are also reduced [8, 59].

DaunoXome® is the product of NeXstar Pharmaceuticals, a US-based company, launched in 1996. The first therapeutic indication of this product was for Kaposi's sarcoma linked to HIV infection. This developed product consists of the anticancer drug Donorubicin in its citrate salt. This product's benefits include the fact that it is free from pyrogen and preservatives. The side effects associated with the drug are reduced and a controlled delivery is established [60, 61].

Depocyt® (Liposomal Cytarabine) is the product of SkyePharm Inc. It is the liposomal preparation of the parenteral suspension of the drug cytarabine. The main therapeutic indication of Cytarabine (Ara-C) is in the treatment of neoplastic meningitis. It encapsulates the aqueous drug suspension in the lipid membrane which is supported by multivesicular particles. The major advantage associated with this product is that it enhances the permeation of the drug. The hydrophilic type of drugs like Ara-C is limited with the permeation characteristics and hence disables the quick onset of action. With the liposomal encapsulation, the lipid vesicles created help boost the permeation of the drug from the blood-brain barrier and induce the direct effect of the drug on the site [62].

Mepact® is the product of Takeda Pharmaceutical Company Ltd. The generic name for this product is liposomal mifamurtide. It is the first-ever product approved for the non-metastatic bone tumor. The indication is now extended to infants, teenagers, and adults in the chemotherapeutic combinations by European Medicines Agency (EMA). The formulation consists of muramyl tripeptide phosphatidylethanolamine encapsulated in 100 nm multilamellar lipidic vesicles. The major advantage of this product is that it has very low variations in pharmacokinetics and the release rate can be modified. Also, encapsulation enhances the targeting of the drug which reduces the major side effects associated with the drug. The mechanistic approach behind the Mepact product formulation is that lipid provides the biosignalling in the cells which helps to target the immune cells and hence work efficiently in the body [63].

DepoDur™ (Morphine sulfate) is the liposomal formulation of the sulfate form of morphine. The approved therapeutic indication of this product is a single dose administered analgesic. It is given at the lumbar stage before surgery or after clamping of the umbilical cord. The advantage associated with DepoDur is that it leads to extended release from the formulation, which increases its efficiency [64].

Liposomes have been shown to be efficient immunological adjuvants for protein and peptide antigens up to this stage. This can activate both the types of immunity- humoral and cellular immune responses for a wide range of infectious diseases and cancers without triggering granulomas or hypersensitivity reactions at the injection site [21]. Liposomes with structural modifications, such as pH-sensitive liposomes, have an advantage over conventional adjuvants in that they enable the peptide antigen to escape from endosomes and thus associate with the MHC-I complex, inducing a cytotoxic T-lymphocyte (CTL) response. The interesting part of the lipid substances is that tailor-made immunogenicity can be produced by alteration in the lipid contents [65]. The immune system response has been shown to be controlled by manipulating the surface charge density of cationic liposomes [66].

There has been enough evidence that liposomes activate cellular immunity to a wide range of antigens from the contributing literature of the past ten years. Liposomes' immunoadjuvant activity is focused on structural characteristics that regulate vesicle fate *in vivo* [67]. Liposomes' immunoadjuvant properties are complemented by their ability to transport co-entrapped B and T-cell epitopes, obviating the need for a vehicle. Liposomes' immunoadjuvant properties are improved by their ability to serve as carriers for co-entrapped B and T-cell epitopes, obviating a requirement for a carrier protein. Recently, a method for encasing live microbial vaccines in large liposomes while preserving their viability has been developed [68, 69].

Because of the special properties of liposome technology, researchers have been working tirelessly to build novel drug delivery vehicles based on liposomes. However, liposomes have some drawbacks in biomedical applications due to their low stability, and fast release of therapeutic molecules. Due to this the impactful area is in modifying the layers of the liposomal surface by combining it with a variety of the tailored substances to get the interesting molecule. However, there isn't much information on chitosan-liposome-based systems. Chitosan as a polymer is a highly biologically active, biodegradable, and hydrophilic polymer. On the other hand, liposomes allow the efficient delivery of the drug entrapped in the vesicles due to the structure similarity to that of cellular membranes that can easily bypass all the barriers in the cells and tissues in the drug delivery [22].

Some approved liposomal products are enlisted below in Table **11.1**.

Table 11.1. List of Approved Liposomal Products.

S.No.	Name of Product	API	Indication	Company
1	Doxil	Doxorubicin	Anti-neoplastic agent or cytotoxic agent	ALZA corporation
2	DaunoXome	Daunorubicin	Acute Myeloid Leukemia	Galen Ltd.
3	DepoCyt	Cytarabine	Acute Myeloid Leukemia, Acute lymphocytic Leukemia, non-' 'Hodgkin's lymphoma	Leadiant Biosciences
4	Onivyde	Irinotecan	Colon Cancer, Small cell lung cancer	Merrimack Pharmaceuticals
5	Inflexal	Viral vector-based vaccine	Influenza Vaccine	Crucell
6	DepoDur	Morphine	Moderate to severe pain	Endo Pharmaceuticals
7	Exparel	Bupivacaine	Non-opioid Analgesic	Pacira
8	Visudyne	Verteporfin	Photosensitizer for photodynamic therapy	Intas Pharmaceutical
9	Ambisome	Amphotericin-B	Serious Fungal Infections, Leishmaniasis	Fujisawa Healthcare Inc.
10	Abelcet	Amphotericin-B	Serious Fungal Infections, Leishmaniasis	The Liposome Company

(Table 11.1) cont.....

S.No.	Name of Product	API	Indication	Company
11	Amphotec	Amphotericin-B	Serious Fungal Infections, Leishmaniasis	Sequus

REGULATORY ASPECTS

Liposomes have good prospects as gene and drug delivery mechanisms, excellent biocompatibility, and versatile properties, with the added benefit of mitigating the chances of systemic toxicity from the encapsulated drug moiety. For a very long time, liposomal formulations have been researched and developed for various medical applications, including cancer therapeutics and analgesics. Some work has also been put into evaluating the potential to cause toxicity and immune responses of these drug formulations [68].

Even though clinical use of liposomal agents has increased dramatically since 1995, there are still a number of disadvantages that restrict their scope of use. Consider combining predictive toxicological assessment with a deliberate investigation into aspects like absorption, delivery, metabolism, and excretion (ADME) and toxicokinetic profiles, the risk posed during nano manufacture, and unique nanomaterial. These efforts can be integrated into a rational regulatory decision-making infrastructure. The studies involving the acceptance of the liposomal product may include the important parameters of physicochemical properties so that risks to the safety evaluation are somewhat reduced [68, 70].

Despite decades of growth and clinical liposome drug delivery experience, liposome clinical efficiency is still hampered by certain issues and therapeutic challenges. To begin with, only a small percentage of injected doses enter their intended therapy sites through the systemic circulation. Although studies comparing the biodistribution of labeled drug versus labeled lipid for liposomes administered *in vivo* yield mixed results, most studies using covalent radiolabels on liposome components indicate that 5% of the injected dose reaches the target site. While lipid modifications can alter biodistribution profiles, liposome dose "targeting" using externally attached ligands (*e.g.*, RGD peptides, antibodies, glycans) rarely enhances specific site targeting in humans. Second, liposomes are not as immunologically inert as previously thought, considering their typical phospholipid shell composition [71].

However, the three guiding principles that were applicable when Doxil was approved are still applicable today and can be used in any liposomal delivery system. The majority of FDA-approved products are either entirely liposomal or PEG-ylated as of 2015, and none have attempted compositions with higher degrees of sophistication, such as ethosomes or pharmacosomes, implying that either more experimental research is required to show the effectiveness of such formulations, or the FDA must move with greater urgency [72].

The last 10 years have given the regulation on the liposomes from the regulatory agencies including US and European Regulatory agencies which contain the guidance papers for the liposome-based drug. The first of this kind was issued in 2002 while USFDA issued the first draught paper in 2010, which was continually revisited in February 2010 for Parenteral products based on liposomal technologies. In November 2015, revised guidelines were issued by USFDA which include a wide range of the liposomal drug delivery aspects [72].

The guidance provided by FDA does not impose a requirement in the case of liposomal products, but these are the recommendations given by the regulatory agencies to meet certain standards for the designing of the novel and existing liposomal formulations in the pharmaceutical market. These draught guidelines by USFDA also provide the basis for IVIVC studies in the case of the liposomal formulations' bioequivalence studies. The guidelines also include the test and number of tests to be done, blood sampling time points, and the analytes, along with the specification of testing. Along with these, the characterization-composition and physicochemical properties are the major parts of the regulatory requirements [34].

CONCLUSION

Liposomes are a unique drug delivery system that exhibit huge advantage in controlling the drug delivery as well as targeting the same. These are being widely used as versatile carrier for drug delivery which needs to be targeted. Liposome carriers, well known for their potential application, are worthy and prevalent carriers and have the capacity to typify hydrophilic and lipophilic drugs and ensure their desired release. There are several strategies accessible by which liposomes can be made independently or depending on the property of the particle. The liposomal drugs can be given by various routes of delivery (intravenous, oral inhalation, local delivery, ocular), each having its own advantage, which can further involve use in various treatments of different infections [73]. Several issues related to a medicating agent, such as bioavailability, and stability, can be reduced by consolidating it into liposomes. With the incorporation of various advancements in the preparation of liposomes, a lot of correlation can be formed concerning its release in the biological surrounding providing a tailored way for drug delivery. This topic is widening and enhancing day by day to its incorporation into the world of pharmaceuticals which is enriching because of active targeting as an advantage of the liposomal technology. Starting from basics like wound healing and various dermatological effects of liposomes, these have found great application in gene therapy, tailored anticancer therapy, ophthalmic preparation, vaccine, and biotechnological approaches. These are vast growing backgrounds of the medical sciences and are influencing daily the most reliable approach to treatment in every way [31].

CONSENT FOR PUBLICATION

Not applicable.

CONFLICT OF INTEREST

The authors declare no conflict of interest, financial or otherwise.

ACKNOWLEDGEMENT

Declared none.

REFERENCES

[1] Bozzuto G, Molinari A. Liposomes as nanomedical devices. Int J Nanomedicine 2015; 10: 975-99. [http://dx.doi.org/10.2147/IJN.S68861] [PMID: 25678787]

[2] Hope MJ, Bally MB, Webb G, Cullis PR. Production of large unilamellar vesicles by a rapid extrusion procedure. Characterization of size distribution, trapped volume and ability to maintain a membrane potential. BBA - Biomembr 1985; 812: 55-65. [http://dx.doi.org/10.1016/0005-2736(85)90521-8]

[3] Wang Y, Grainger DW. Lyophilized liposome-based parenteral drug development: Reviewing complex product design strategies and current regulatory environments. Adv Drug Deliv Rev 2019; 151-152: 56-71. [http://dx.doi.org/10.1016/j.addr.2019.03.003] [PMID: 30898571]

[4] Crielaard BJ, van der Wal S, Le HT, *et al.* Liposomes as carriers for colchicine-derived prodrugs: Vascular disrupting nanomedicines with tailorable drug release kinetics. Eur J Pharm Sci 2012; 45(4): 429-35. [http://dx.doi.org/10.1016/j.ejps.2011.08.027] [PMID: 21907797]

[5] Li M, Du C, Guo N, *et al.* Composition design and medical application of liposomes. Eur J Med Chem 2019; 164: 640-53. [http://dx.doi.org/10.1016/j.ejmech.2019.01.007] [PMID: 30640028]

[6] Kaye SB, Richardson VJ. Potential of liposomes as drug-carriers in cancer chemotherapy: A review. Cancer Chemother Pharmacol 1979; 3(2): 81-5. [http://dx.doi.org/10.1007/BF00254977] [PMID: 389479]

[7] Abu Lila AS, Ishida T. Liposomal delivery systems: Design optimization and current applications. Biol Pharm Bull 2017; 40(1): 1-10. [http://dx.doi.org/10.1248/bpb.b16-00624] [PMID: 28049940]

[8] Harris L, Batist G, Belt R, *et al.* Liposome-encapsulated doxorubicin compared with conventional doxorubicin in a randomized multicenter trial as first-line therapy of metastatic breast carcinoma. Cancer 2002; 94(1): 25-36. [http://dx.doi.org/10.1002/cncr.10201] [PMID: 11815957]

[9] Chonn A, Cullis PR. Recent advances in liposomal drug-delivery systems. Curr Opin Biotechnol 1995;

6(6): 698-708.
[http://dx.doi.org/10.1016/0958-1669(95)80115-4] [PMID: 8527843]

[10] Pradhan B, Kumar N, Saha S, Roy A. Liposome: Method of preparation, advantages, evaluation and its application. J Appl Pharm Res 2015; 3: 1-8.

[11] Oja CD, Semple SC, Chonn A, Cullis PR. Influence of dose on liposome clearance: Critical role of blood proteins. Biochim Biophys Acta Biomembr 1996; 1281(1): 31-7.
[http://dx.doi.org/10.1016/0005-2736(96)00003-X] [PMID: 8652601]

[12] Szoka F Jr, Papahadjopoulos D. Comparative properties and methods of preparation of lipid vesicles (liposomes). Annu Rev Biophys Bioeng 1980; 9(1): 467-508.
[http://dx.doi.org/10.1146/annurev.bb.09.060180.002343] [PMID: 6994593]

[13] Akbarzadeh A, Rezaei-Sadabady R, Davaran S, *et al.* Liposome: Classification, preparation, and applications. Nanoscale Res Lett 2013; 8(1): 102.
[http://dx.doi.org/10.1186/1556-276X-8-102] [PMID: 23432972]

[14] Maja L, Željko K, Mateja P. Sustainable technologies for liposome preparation. J Supercrit Fluids 2020; 165: 104984.
[http://dx.doi.org/10.1016/j.supflu.2020.104984]

[15] Torchilin VP. Recent advances with liposomes as pharmaceutical carriers. Nat Rev Drug Discov 2005; 4(2): 145-60.
[http://dx.doi.org/10.1038/nrd1632] [PMID: 15688077]

[16] Sahil K, Premjeet S, Ajay B, Middha A, Bhawna K. Issn 2229-3566 stealth liposomes : A review. 2011; 2: 1534-8.

[17] Rastogi M, Saha RN, Alexander A, Singhvi G, Puri A, Dubey SK. Role of stealth lipids in nanomedicine-based drug carriers. Chem Phys Lipids 2021; 235: 105036.
[http://dx.doi.org/10.1016/j.chemphyslip.2020.105036] [PMID: 33412151]

[18] Liu C, Zhang L, Zhu W, *et al.* Barriers and strategies of cationic liposomes for cancer gene therapy. Mol Ther Methods Clin Dev 2020; 18: 751-64.
[http://dx.doi.org/10.1016/j.omtm.2020.07.015] [PMID: 32913882]

[19] Ahmed KS, Hussein SA, Ali AH, Korma SA, Lipeng Q, Jinghua C. Liposome: Composition, characterisation, preparation, and recent innovation in clinical applications. J Drug Target 2019; 27(7): 742-61.
[http://dx.doi.org/10.1080/1061186X.2018.1527337] [PMID: 30239255]

[20] Lasic DD, Frederik PM, Stuart MCA, Barenholz Y, McIntosh TJ. Gelation of liposome interior A novel method for drug encapsulation. FEBS Lett 1992; 312(2-3): 255-8.
[http://dx.doi.org/10.1016/0014-5793(92)80947-F] [PMID: 1426260]

[21] Zangabad PS, Mirkiani S, Shahsavari S, *et al.* Stimulus-responsive liposomes as smart nanoplatforms for drug delivery applications. Nanotechnol Rev 2018; 7(1): 95-122.
[http://dx.doi.org/10.1515/ntrev-2017-0154] [PMID: 29404233]

[22] Kumar S, Dutta J, Dutta PK, Koh J. A systematic study on chitosan-liposome based systems for biomedical applications. Int J Biol Macromol 2020; 160: 470-81.
[http://dx.doi.org/10.1016/j.ijbiomac.2020.05.192] [PMID: 32464212]

[23] Barenholz Y. Liposome application: Problems and prospects. Curr Opin Colloid Interface Sci 2001; 6(1): 66-77.
[http://dx.doi.org/10.1016/S1359-0294(00)00090-X]

[24] Delma KL, Lechanteur A, Evrard B, Semdé R, Piel G. Sterilization methods of liposomes: Drawbacks of conventional methods and perspectives. Int J Pharm 2021; 597: 120271.
[http://dx.doi.org/10.1016/j.ijpharm.2021.120271] [PMID: 33548365]

[25] Waghule T, Dabholkar N, Gorantla S, Rapalli VK, Saha RN, Singhvi G. Quality by design (QbD) in

the formulation and optimization of liquid crystalline nanoparticles (LCNPs): A risk based industrial approach. Biomed Pharmacother 2021; 141: 111940.
[http://dx.doi.org/10.1016/j.biopha.2021.111940] [PMID: 34328089]

[26] Filion MC, Phillips NC. Major limitations in the use of cationic liposomes for DNA delivery. Int J Pharm 1998; 162(1-2): 159-70.
[http://dx.doi.org/10.1016/S0378-5173(97)00423-7]

[27] Toh MR, Chiu GNC. Liposomes as sterile preparations and limitations of sterilisation techniques in liposomal manufacturing. Asian Journal of Pharmaceutical Sciences 2013; 8(2): 88-95.
[http://dx.doi.org/10.1016/j.ajps.2013.07.011]

[28] Zuidam NJ, Lee SSL, Crommelin DJA. Sterilization of liposomes by heat treatment. Pharm Res 1993 1011 1993; 10: 1591-6.
[http://dx.doi.org/10.1023/A:1018916518515]

[29] Sharma A, Sharma US. Liposomes in drug delivery: Progress and limitations. Int J Pharm 1997; 154(2): 123-40.
[http://dx.doi.org/10.1016/S0378-5173(97)00135-X]

[30] Fendler JH, Romero A. Liposomes as drug carriers. Life Sci 1977; 20(7): 1109-20.
[http://dx.doi.org/10.1016/0024-3205(77)90481-7] [PMID: 403379]

[31] Bulbake U, Doppalapudi S, Kommineni N, Khan W. Liposomal formulations in clinical use: An updated review. Pharmaceutics 2017; 9(4): 12.
[http://dx.doi.org/10.3390/pharmaceutics9020012] [PMID: 28346375]

[32] Large DE, Abdelmessih RG, Fink EA, Auguste DT. Liposome composition in drug delivery design, synthesis, characterization, and clinical application. Adv Drug Deliv Rev 2021; 176: 113851.
[http://dx.doi.org/10.1016/j.addr.2021.113851] [PMID: 34224787]

[33] Jain R, Pradhan R, Hejmady S, Singhvi G, Dubey SK. Fluorescence-based method for sensitive and rapid estimation of chlorin e6 in stealth liposomes for photodynamic therapy against cancer. Spectrochim Acta A Mol Biomol Spectrosc 2021; 244: 118823.
[http://dx.doi.org/10.1016/j.saa.2020.118823] [PMID: 32898725]

[34] Jensen GM, Hodgson DF. Opportunities and challenges in commercial pharmaceutical liposome applications. Adv Drug Deliv Rev 2020; 154-155: 2-12.
[http://dx.doi.org/10.1016/j.addr.2020.07.016] [PMID: 32707149]

[35] Shahraki N, Mehrabian A, Amiri-Darban S, Moosavian SA, Jaafari MR. Preparation and characterization of PEGylated liposomal Doxorubicin targeted with leptin-derived peptide and evaluation of their anti-tumor effects, *in vitro* and *in vivo* in mice bearing C26 colon carcinoma. Colloids Surf B Biointerfaces 2021; 200: 111589.
[http://dx.doi.org/10.1016/j.colsurfb.2021.111589] [PMID: 33545570]

[36] Ishii F, Nagasaka Y. Simple and convenient method for estimation of marker entrapped in liposomes. J Dispers Sci Technol 2001; 22(1): 97-101.
[http://dx.doi.org/10.1081/DIS-100102684]

[37] Waghule T, Rapalli VK, Singhvi G, *et al.* Design of temozolomide-loaded proliposomes and lipid crystal nanoparticles with industrial feasible approaches: Comparative assessment of drug loading, entrapment efficiency, and stability at plasma pH. J Liposome Res 2021; 31(2): 158-68.
[http://dx.doi.org/10.1080/08982104.2020.1748648] [PMID: 32290733]

[38] Waghule T, Narayan Saha R, Singhvi G. UV spectroscopic method for estimation of temozolomide: Application in stability studies in simulated plasma pH, degradation rate kinetics, formulation design, and selection of dissolution media. Spectrochim Acta A Mol Biomol Spectrosc 2021; 258: 119848.
[http://dx.doi.org/10.1016/j.saa.2021.119848] [PMID: 33933945]

[39] Grit M, Crommelin DJA. Chemical-stability-of-liposomes-implications-for-their-physical-stability_1993_chemistry-and-physics-of-lipids. Chem Phys Lipids 1993; 64: 3-18.

[http://dx.doi.org/10.1016/0009-3084(93)90053-6] [PMID: 8242840]

[40] Arias-Alpizar G, Kong L, Vlieg RC, *et al.* Light-triggered switching of liposome surface charge directs delivery of membrane impermeable payloads *in vivo*. Nat Commun 2020; 11(1): 3638. [http://dx.doi.org/10.1038/s41467-020-17360-9] [PMID: 32686667]

[41] Alphandéry E, Grand-Dewyse P, Lefèvre R, Mandawala C, Durand-Dubief M. Cancer therapy using nanoformulated substances: Scientific, regulatory and financial aspects. Expert Rev Anticancer Ther 2015; 15(10): 1233-55. [http://dx.doi.org/10.1586/14737140.2015.1086647] [PMID: 26402250]

[42] Tian J, Chi C, Bian G, Xing D, Guo F, Wang X. PSMA conjugated combinatorial liposomal formulation encapsulating genistein and plumbagin to induce apoptosis in prostate cancer cells. Colloids Surf B Biointerfaces 2021; 203: 111723. [http://dx.doi.org/10.1016/j.colsurfb.2021.111723] [PMID: 33839474]

[43] Jain A, Hurkat P, Jain SK. Development of liposomes using formulation by design: Basics to recent advances. Chem Phys Lipids 2019; 224: 104764. [http://dx.doi.org/10.1016/j.chemphyslip.2019.03.017] [PMID: 30951713]

[44] Rapalli VK, Khosa A, Singhvi G, Girdhar V, Jain R, Dubey SK. Application of QbD principles in nanocarrier-based drug delivery systems. Pharm Qual by Des 2019; 255-96. [http://dx.doi.org/10.1016/B978-0-12-815799-2.00014-9]

[45] Mehta PP, Ghoshal D, Pawar AP, Kadam SS, Dhapte-Pawar VS. Recent advances in inhalable liposomes for treatment of pulmonary diseases: Concept to clinical stance. J Drug Deliv Sci Technol 2020; 56: 101509. [http://dx.doi.org/10.1016/j.jddst.2020.101509]

[46] Veloso SRS, Andrade RGD, Castanheira EMS. Review on the advancements of magnetic gels: Towards multifunctional magnetic liposome-hydrogel composites for biomedical applications. Adv Colloid Interface Sci 2021; 288: 102351. [http://dx.doi.org/10.1016/j.cis.2020.102351] [PMID: 33387893]

[47] Palchetti S, Caputo D, Digiacomo L, *et al.* Protein corona fingerprints of liposomes: New opportunities for targeted drug delivery and early detection in pancreatic cancer. Pharmaceutics 2019; 11(1): 31. [http://dx.doi.org/10.3390/pharmaceutics11010031] [PMID: 30650541]

[48] Guimarães D, Cavaco-Paulo A, Nogueira E. Design of liposomes as drug delivery system for therapeutic applications. Int J Pharm 2021; 601: 120571. [http://dx.doi.org/10.1016/j.ijpharm.2021.120571] [PMID: 33812967]

[49] Papahadjopoulos D. Liposomes as drug carriers. Annu Rep Med Chem 1979; 14: 250-60. [http://dx.doi.org/10.1016/S0065-7743(08)61369-X]

[50] Roces CB, Port EC, Daskalakis NN, *et al.* Rapid scale-up and production of active-loaded PEGylated liposomes. Int J Pharm 2020; 586: 119566. [http://dx.doi.org/10.1016/j.ijpharm.2020.119566] [PMID: 32622812]

[51] Bragagni M, Mennini N, Maestrelli F, Cirri M, Mura P. Comparative study of liposomes, transfersomes and ethosomes as carriers for improving topical delivery of celecoxib. Drug Deliv 2012; 19(7): 354-61. [http://dx.doi.org/10.3109/10717544.2012.724472] [PMID: 23043648]

[52] Sercombe L, Veerati T, Moheimani F, Wu SY, Sood AK, Hua S. Advances and challenges of liposome assisted drug delivery. Front Pharmacol 2015; 6: 286. [http://dx.doi.org/10.3389/fphar.2015.00286] [PMID: 26648870]

[53] Trucillo P, Ferrari PF, Campardelli R, Reverchon E, Perego P. A supercritical assisted process for the production of amoxicillin-loaded liposomes for antimicrobial applications. J Supercrit Fluids 2020; 163: 104842.

[http://dx.doi.org/10.1016/j.supflu.2020.104842]

[54] Obaid G, Samkoe K, Tichauer K, *et al.* Is tumor cell specificity distinct from tumor selectivity *in vivo*? A quantitative NIR molecular imaging analysis of nanoliposome targeting. Nano Res 2021; 14(5): 1344-54.
[http://dx.doi.org/10.1007/s12274-020-3178-x] [PMID: 33717420]

[55] Gabizon AA. Liposome circulation time and tumor targeting: Implications for cancer chemotherapy. Adv Drug Deliv Rev 1995; 16(2-3): 285-94.
[http://dx.doi.org/10.1016/0169-409X(95)00030-B]

[56] Slingerland M, Guchelaar HJ, Gelderblom H. Liposomal drug formulations in cancer therapy: 15 Years along the road. Drug Discov Today 2012; 17(3-4): 160-6.
[http://dx.doi.org/10.1016/j.drudis.2011.09.015] [PMID: 21983329]

[57] Medina O, Zhu Y, Kairemo K. Targeted liposomal drug delivery in cancer. Curr Pharm Des 2004; 10(24): 2981-9.
[http://dx.doi.org/10.2174/1381612043383467] [PMID: 15379663]

[58] Bibi S, Lattmann E, Mohammed AR, Perrie Y. Trigger release liposome systems: Local and remote controlled delivery? J Microencapsul 2012; 29(3): 262-76.
[http://dx.doi.org/10.3109/02652048.2011.646330] [PMID: 22208705]

[59] Vujaskovic Z, Kim DW, Jones E, *et al.* A phase I/II study of neoadjuvant liposomal doxorubicin, paclitaxel, and hyperthermia in locally advanced breast cancer. Int J Hyperthermia 2010; 26(5): 514-21.
[http://dx.doi.org/10.3109/02656731003639364] [PMID: 20377362]

[60] Alberts DS, Bachur NR, Holtzman JL. The pharmacokinetics of daunomycin in man. Clin Pharmacol Ther 1971; 12(1): 96-104.
[http://dx.doi.org/10.1002/cpt197112196] [PMID: 5541137]

[61] Harasym TO, Cullis PR, Bally MB. Intratumor distribution of doxorubicin following i.v. administration of drug encapsulated in egg phosphatidylcholine/cholesterol liposomes. Cancer Chemother Pharmacol 1997; 40(4): 309-17.
[http://dx.doi.org/10.1007/s002800050662] [PMID: 9225948]

[62] Angst MS, Drover DR. Pharmacology of drugs formulated with DepoFoam: A sustained release drug delivery system for parenteral administration using multivesicular liposome technology. Clin Pharmacokinet 2006; 45(12): 1153-76.
[http://dx.doi.org/10.2165/00003088-200645120-00002] [PMID: 17112293]

[63] Mirzavi F, Barati M, Soleimani A, Vakili-Ghartavol R, Jaafari MR, Soukhtanloo M. A review on liposome-based therapeutic approaches against malignant melanoma. Int J Pharm 2021; 599: 120413.
[http://dx.doi.org/10.1016/j.ijpharm.2021.120413] [PMID: 33667562]

[64] Alam M, Hartrick CT. Extended-release epidural morphine (DepoDur): An old drug with a new profile. Pain Pract 2005; 5(4): 349-53.
[http://dx.doi.org/10.1111/j.1533-2500.2005.00048.x] [PMID: 17177768]

[65] Zahednezhad F, Saadat M, Valizadeh H, Zakeri-Milani P, Baradaran B. Liposome and immune system interplay: Challenges and potentials. J Control Release 2019; 305: 194-209.
[http://dx.doi.org/10.1016/j.jconrel.2019.05.030] [PMID: 31121278]

[66] Kuznetsova DA, Gabdrakhmanov DR, Gaynanova GA, *et al.* Novel biocompatible liposomal formulations for encapsulation of hydrophilic drugs – Chloramphenicol and cisplatin. Colloids Surf A Physicochem Eng Asp 2021; 610: 125673.
[http://dx.doi.org/10.1016/j.colsurfa.2020.125673]

[67] Saraf S, Jain A, Tiwari A, Verma A, Panda PK, Jain SK. Advances in liposomal drug delivery to cancer: An overview. J Drug Deliv Sci Technol 2020; 56: 101549.
[http://dx.doi.org/10.1016/j.jddst.2020.101549]

[68] Inglut CT, Sorrin AJ, Kuruppu T, *et al.* Immunological and toxicological considerations for the design of liposomes. Nanomaterials (Basel) 2020; 10(2): 190.
[http://dx.doi.org/10.3390/nano10020190] [PMID: 31978968]

[69] Semple SC, Harasym TO, Clow KA, Ansell SM, Klimuk SK, Hope MJ. Immunogenicity and rapid blood clearance of liposomes containing polyethylene glycol-lipid conjugates and nucleic Acid. J Pharmacol Exp Ther 2005; 312(3): 1020-6.
[http://dx.doi.org/10.1124/jpet.104.078113] [PMID: 15525796]

[70] Liu M, Wen J, Sharma M. Solid lipid nanoparticles for topical drug delivery: Mechanisms, dosage form perspectives, and translational status. Curr Pharm Des 2020; 26(27): 3203-17.
[http://dx.doi.org/10.2174/1381612826666200526145706] [PMID: 32452322]

[71] Park H, Otte A, Park K. Evolution of drug delivery systems: From 1950 to 2020 and beyond. J Control Release 2022; 342: 53-65.
[http://dx.doi.org/10.1016/j.jconrel.2021.12.030] [PMID: 34971694]

[72] Zylberberg C, Matosevic S. Pharmaceutical liposomal drug delivery: A review of new delivery systems and a look at the regulatory landscape. Drug Deliv 2016; 23(9): 3319-29.
[http://dx.doi.org/10.1080/10717544.2016.1177136] [PMID: 27145899]

[73] Decker C, Schubert H, May S, Fahr A. Pharmacokinetics of temoporfin-loaded liposome formulations: Correlation of liposome and temoporfin blood concentration. J Control Release 2013; 166(3): 277-85.
[http://dx.doi.org/10.1016/j.jconrel.2013.01.005] [PMID: 23313962]

CHAPTER 12

Niosome: A Vesicular Drug Delivery Tool

Preeti Patel[1], **Ashish K. Parashar**[2], **Monika Kaurav**[3], **Krishna Yadav**[4], **Dilpreet Singh**[1], **G.D. Gupta**[1] and **Balak Das Kurmi**[1,*]

[1] *ISF College of Pharmacy, Moga-142001, (Punjab), India*

[2] *Chameli Devi Institute of Pharmacy, Indore-452020, (M.P.), India*

[3] *KIET School of Pharmacy, Ghaziabad-201206, (U.P.) India*

[4] *Raipur Institute of Pharmaceutical Education and Research (RIPER), Sarona, Raipur-492010, (C.G.), India*

Abstract: Niosomes, which are well recognized for their non-ionic surfactant characteristics, are considered to be innovative drug delivery methods since they improve the solubility and stability of medicinal compounds when administered orally. It has been shown that niosome vesicles are closed bilayer structures that may exist in aqueous fluids and are produced by the self-assembly of different types of hydrated non-ionic surfactants and amphiphile monomers in aqueous media. Because the monomers maintain a wide range of kinetic activity inside the assembly, they are referred to as liquid crystal structures in terms of thermodynamics. It is just the total of different processes for the dispersion of monomers and solvents that results in the formation of the final systems. Niosomes are made up mostly of lipid molecules and nonionic surfactants, which are the two most important components in the process of making them. Nonetheless, as the name suggests, component surfactants play a key role in the creation of niosomes, owing to the fact that non-ionic surfactants were often employed to organize niosomes during their formation. They are especially well-suited for drug delivery because they have the ability to encapsulate medicines that are both lipophilic and hydrophilic in nature. These materials are appealing for a number of drug delivery goals, including drug targeting, controlled release, and permeability enhancement, because of their chemical stability, cheap production costs, and composed of biodegradable and non-immunogenic components. Niosomal vesicular carriers can also help to minimize problems such as physical and chemical instability. This book chapter contains a brief knowledge about structural components and integrity concerning the advanced method of noisome preparation. The characterization techniques essential for noisome have also been discussed in detail. The recent examples for different applications are also included for therapy /diagnostic purposes based on the route of administration and disease state.

* **Corresponding author Balak Das Kurmi:** ISF College of Pharmacy, Moga-142001, (Punjab), India; Tel: +919754275553; E-mail: **bdkurmi@gmail.com**

Akhlesh K. Jain & Keerti Mishra (Eds.)

Keywords: Anticancer, Drug delivery, Diagnostic, Drug targeting, Lipid nanocarriers, Niosome, Non-ionic surfactant, Transdermal delivery.

INTRODUCTION

Niosomes (NS) are carriers that were discovered for the first time in the 1970s. They are made up of closed bilayer structures generated by the self-assembly of non-ionic (NIC) amphiphiles in aqueous environments. Non-ionic surfactant vesicles (NISVs) are known as niosome. Handjani Vila and co-investigators were the first to describe vesicles generated by NIC surfactants. They were first mentioned as a beauty industry characteristic, but they are now widely employed as medicine delivery methods [1]. They are composed of biocompatible, non-toxic, non-immunogenic, and non-carcinogenic materials. NISVs are formed when hydrated surfactant monomers self-assemble. In aqueous conditions, the surfactant molecules self-assemble so that the hydrophobic tails face each other, reducing the high-energy interactions between the solvent and the tails. The hydrolytic breakdown is not a problem for NISVs. They're similar to liposomes, but they have a few advantages. The main benefit is that they can be used for various pH values [2]. Chemical stability, increased oral bioavailability, lower toxicity, greater therapeutic effectiveness, and convenience of handling and storage are other benefits [3 - 5]. Because of their low cost, they are more appealing for industrial production, particularly in pharmaceutical and cosmetic applications. Furthermore, no pharmaceutically undesirable solvents are used in the preparation process [6].

Encapsulation of medicines in NS has been proven to decrease drug toxicity, enhance drug absorption, enhance the therapeutic effectiveness, stability, or activity, and extend the time removing the drug from circulation when utilised in slow-release formulations. According to the research, NS may extend the circulation of occluded medicines [7, 8] and diagnostic markers [9]. NS are microscopic lamellar structures that form with the combination of cholesterol and a NIC surfactant of either the alkyl or dialkylpolyglycerol ether class [10]. The amphiphilic nature of NIC surfactants causes them to form a confined bilayer vesicle when used in aquatic circumstances. The introduction of input, such as heat or physical agitation, results in the formation of this structure. In contrast, the hydrophobic parts of the bilayer structure are oriented away from the aqueous solvent, while the hydrophilic components of the bilayer structure remain in direct contact with the aqueous solvent. There are a variety of ways to change the features of vesicles, including changing their composition, as well as their size, lamellarity, tapped volume, surface charge, concentration, and other characteristics. Internally, a number of forces are at work, including van der Waals forces between surfactant molecules, repulsive forces resulting from electrostatic interactions between electrostatic interactions of surfactant molecules, entropic electrostatic repulsion of the head groups of surfactants, and so on. It is the responsibility of these forces to ensure that the vesicular structure of NS is sustained. It is possible to use niosomal drug delivery for a broad variety of pharmacological substances in the treatment of numerous diseases. Niosomal drug delivery is now being used in the treatment of a wide range of disorders. It may also be used as a carrier for medicines that are poorly absorbable, allowing for the development of a drug carrier for poorly absorbable medications. The transcytosis of M cells from Peyer's patches in the intestinal lymphatic tissues has the potential to enhance bioavailability by overcoming the anatomical barrier of the gastrointestinal tract, as shown in this study. The reticuloendothelial system is in charge of transporting niosomal vesicles throughout the body [11]. This type of localized drug accumulation is utilized to treat disorders such as leishmaniasis, in which parasites infiltrate the liver and spleen [12, 13]. Other systems, such as immunoglobins that do not recognize the reticuloendothelial system, can also recognize the lipid surface of this delivery system [14, 15]. Various anti-neoplastic drugs have been encapsulated in this carrier vesicle, which has reduced drug-induced harmful side effects while maintaining or, in some cases, improving anti-tumor activity [16 - 18].

It is a common practice to administer specific anti-inflammatory drugs, such as flurbiprofen and piroxicam, plant extracts, and sex hormones, such as estradiol and levonorgestrel, through an NS *via* the transdermal route in order to improve their therapeutic efficacy [10, 19, 20]. The use of NS makes it possible to develop more comprehensive drug delivery strategies. One of the accomplishments is the localised drug action that is possible due to the small size of the drugs and their low penetrability through the epithelium and connective tissue. This has the potential to keep the drug localised at the administration site, and localised drug action strengthens the efficacy or potency of the drug while at the same time reducing its systemic toxic contribution of different therapeutically active agents, according to the National Institutes of Health [21, 22]. This book chapter contains a brief knowledge about structural components and integrity concerning the advanced method of noisome preparation. The characterization techniques essential for noisome have also been discussed in detail. The recent examples for different applications are also included for therapy /diagnostic purposes based on the route of administration and disease state.

SILENT FEATURES OF NSS

NS are capable of entangling solute molecules, leading to an increase in their stiffness, and are also osmotically stable.

- NS are NIC surfactants that are biodegradable and non-immunogenic.
- NS are usually structurally flexible, allowed to tether the targeted ligand diagnostic agents, *etc.*
- NS have a deliquescent and hydrophobic structure, allowing for a wide range of drug solubility.
- The medicine is better available at the site by protecting it from the biological environment.
- NS can efficiently deliver labile and sensitive drugs by encapsulating them.
- NS can improve the solubility and oral bioavailability of sparingly soluble medicines and enhance the penetration of pharmaceuticals administered topically.

A TYPICAL NSSTRUCTURE

In its amphiphilic state, NS has the tendency to develop a vesicle, which can often be stabilised by cholesterol. A little quantity of an anionic surfactant such as dicetyl phosphate, as well as a small amount of other anionic surfactants, may also assist in vesicle stability. A network of tiny lamellar [unilamellar or multilamellar] structures, as shown in Fig. **(12.1)**, provides the foundation of the network. NIC surfactants devoid of cholesterol and a charge activator produced bilayers when mixed with a charge inducer. NS is made up of a range of surfactants in different molar ratios, which makes them quite versatile. Surfactants include sorbitan fatty acid esters and polyoxyethylene fatty acid esters, to name a few examples. Cholesterol in the bilayer helps to make it firm, which helps to reduce leaky NS.

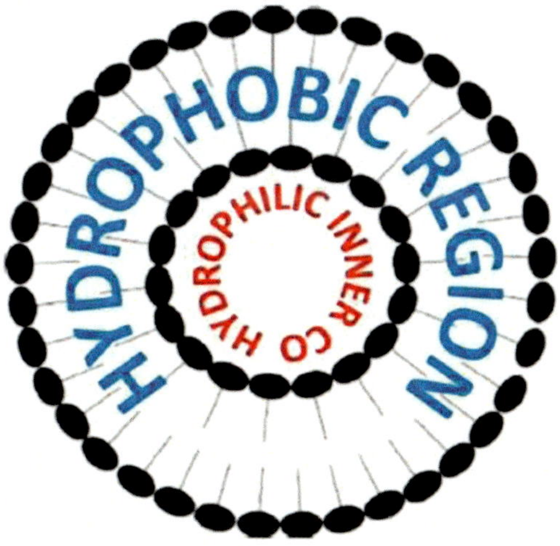

Fig. (12.1). Structure of Niosome.

However, charge causative agents charge the vesicles, which increases their size and increases the likelihood that drugs will be entrapped inside of them. It is possible to stabilise the vesicles using negative charge inducers such as dicetyl phosphate and dihexadecyl phosphate, while positive charge inducers such as stearylamine and cetylpyridinium chloride also aid in this process. Hydrophobic surfactants in NS prefer to face outwardly (toward the aqueous phase) in order to create closed bilayer structures, while NIC surfactants in NS prefer to face inward (more towards the aqueous phase) (toward each other) [10]. As a result, NS have hydrophilic inner and outer borders, with a lipophilic area in the middle of them. It is probable that changes in the vesicle's components (type, constituent, and concentration), size, surface characteristics, or volume will have an impact on the NS characteristics that follow [23].

FORMULATION COMPONENTS

There are a number of important components essential for the formulation of NS as follows:

Non-ionic Surfactants

NIC surface-active chemical is the primary component in the synthesis of NS indicated in Table **12.1**. These are used to administer medicines when the distribution's pace, timing, or position must be carefully regulated. Surface-active molecules with NIC charge are amphiphilic, having a hydrophilic [polar] head and a lipophilic (non-polar) tail [24]. Because they do not contain a significant charge on the polar head, these surfactants are more reliable, compatible, and less hazardous than anionic, cationic, and amphoteric surfactants. When these surface-active chemicals are administered to cell surfaces, the cellular surfaces are becoming less inflammatory, and haemolysis is blocked. These may be helpful as wetting agents and emulsion stabilisers and improve the permeability and solubility of solutions.

Furthermore, NIC surfactants can block p-glycoprotein, increasing the absorption and targeting of pharmaceuticals and other substances [25]. Surfactants have two distinct solubility zones: a lipophilic tail and a hydrophilic head. The head group is composed of chemical substances easily dissolved in aqueous media, such as cationic, anionic, and amphoteric compounds. Aromatic alkanes, fluorocarbons, and other non-polar groups may be found in this region. Depending on the classification, a surfactant's head group qualities are used to classify it as cationic, anionic, amphoteric, or NIC. NIC surfactants are the most often utilized surface-active agents in NS synthesis [3]. In the manufacturing of NSs, NIC surfactants such as Tween20, Tween80, Span20, and Span80 are the most widely utilized NIC surfactants. The surfactants utilized in creating NS should be biodegradable, biocompatible, and non-immunogenic, among other characteristics. They form bilayer lattices, with the polar or hydrophobic heads pointing outward toward the aqueous bulk (media). The hydrophobic head or hydrogen-bonded segments are oriented to reduce interaction with the aqueous bulk (medium). When a bilayer folds over itself, it forms vesicles that obscure the hydrocarbon/water interface, allowing the bilayer to achieve thermodynamic stability. NIC surfactants such as the ones listed below are frequently employed in the manufacturing of NS [26, 27].

Alkyl Ethers

Some of the surfactants utilized in the preparation of NS-containing drugs/chemicals, according to L'Oreal, are as follows: Surfactant-I (molecular weight (MW 473)) is a C-16 monoalkyl glycerol ether with an average of three glycerol units and a molecular weight of 473. Surfactant-I is a C-16 monoalkyl glycerol ether with an average of three glycerol units and a molecular weight of 473. MW 972, surfactant II, includes diglycerol ether, which has an average of seven glycerol units per gramme of the substance. Surfactant III is a surfactant that is ester-linked, and it is one of the most widely used [MW 393]. Alkyl glycosides and alkyl ethers having polyhydroxyl head groups may also be used as a substitute to alkyl glycerol in the preparation of NS [28, 29].

Alkyl Esters

Among this group of surfactants, sorbitan esters are the surfactants that are most commonly used in the production of NS. Researchers discovered that vesicles made with polyoxyethylene-sorbitan-monolaurate are more soluble than vesicles made with other surfactants, according to their findings. Instances include the use of polyoxyethylene (polysorbate 60) to encapsulate diclofenac sodium, which has proven to be effective [30].

Alkyl Amides

Different alkyl amides (such as galactosides and glucosides) are also helpful for preparing NS [31].

Fatty Acid and Amino Acid Compounds

In some NS preparations, long-chain fatty acids and amino acid substituent have also been used as a component [32].

Additive Agents

NS additives have been employed in niosomal formulations for various reasons, including changing biodistribution and improving drug molecule permeability and physical stability. To improve the niosomal formulation, a variety of additives have been explored. cholesterol, a natural steroid increases the (transition temperature) TC of the vesicles, giving them more stability (Fig. **12.2**) [5]. The inclusion of cholesterol within the structure of NS enhances their hydrodynamic diameter and enhances drug entrapment efficiency, allowing the amount of drug to be altered by changing the cholesterol value (Fig. **12.3**). Other features of vesicles affected by cholesterol incorporation include stiffness, membrane permeability, ease of rehydration of freeze-dried NS, and NS toxicity [33]. The HLB value of the surfactants determines the amount of cholesterol consumed. Thus, the hydrophilic head group grows when the HLB value rises above ten. To compensate for this alteration, the minimum amount of cholesterol to be added must be increased [34]. Its importance in the development of NS and the manipulation of layer characteristics cannot be overlooked, even if it does not appear to play a role in the shaping of the bilayer. By including molecules that stabilize the system against the formation of coarse aggregate prompted by repugnant steric or electrostatic forces, it is able to suppress vesicle aggregation in nonionic systems, resulting in the transition from the gel phase to the liquid phase of the system. As an outcome, the NS's nature is less leaky as a result [35].

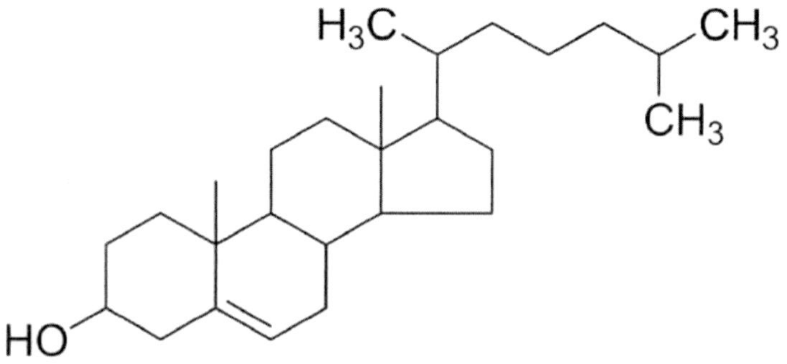

Fig. (12.2). Chemical structure of cholesterol.

Ionic compounds are another type of frequent additive. These materials prevent vesicles from sticking together and increase their stability by electrostatic repulsion. NS are made from the regulation of ionic surfactants because using more than a particular amount of these substances will hinder the production of niosome. Abdelbary and El-gendy evaluated and optimized the presence or absence of DCP in the production of gentamicin sulfate NS [36, 37].

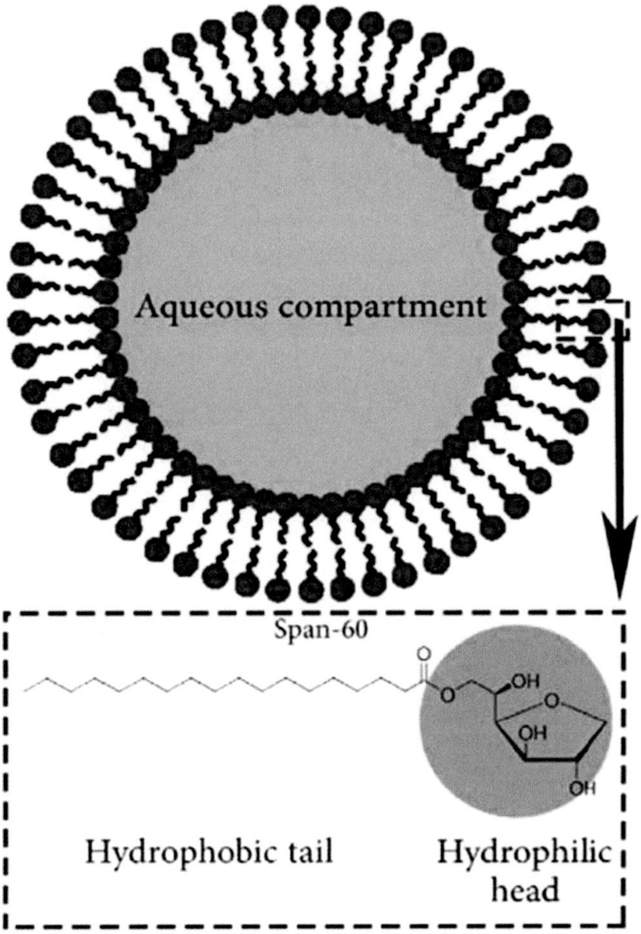

Fig. (12.3). Schematic representation of noisome prepared by sorbitonmonostearate (Span-60).

Charge Inducer Molecules

Various charge-inducing chemical entities are used in the production of NS. These molecules propagate a charge on the surface of the NS, trying to stabilize them *via* repulsive forces and stopping them from fusing. Charge-inducing molecules include molecules such as dicetyl phosphate (which is negatively charged), phosphatidic acid [which is negatively charged], stearyl amine (which is positively charged), and others [37, 38]. One such charge-inducing agent is sodium stearoyl lactate (SSL), used to prepare nisin and EDTA-loaded NS [22, 39].

Hydration Medium

In addition to the components listed above, the hydration medium is an important component in developing NS. Phosphate buffer is a hydration medium that is commonly used in research [18, 40]. The pH of the buffer, on the other hand, is determined by the solubility of the medication that is encapsulated. When Rukmani and colleagues developed zidovudine NS in phosphate buffer saline, they used the film hydration process (pH 7.4). According to their findings, increasing the volume of hydration medium increases drug leakage, whereas increasing the hydration period from 20 to 45 minutes increases drug entrapment efficiency [41].

TYPES OF NS

NS have been described in a variety of different forms throughout the literature. They can be classified according to their specific size (SUV, LUV, and so on) or the number of bilayers present (SUV, MLV, *etc.*). NS can be divided into the following subclasses based on their structure:

Vesicles [MLV]

The MLV is composed of numerous bilayers that each individually enclose the aqueous lipid compartment. The diameter of these vesicles ranges between 0.5 and 10 m in diameter. These NS are the most widely used due to the ease with which they can be manufactured and the mechanical stability they can be stored for extended periods. Lipophilic substances are effective drug carriers in these vesicles because of their high lipophilicity.

Pardakhty and co-investigators produced multilamellar vesicles (MLVs) to encapsulate human insulin using the film-hydration technique, which they reported in Science. In the presence of cholesterol, three distinct surfactants with various physical states, Span 60 (solid-state), Brij 52 (semisolid state), and Brij 92 (liquid state), were employed to produce stable niosomal suspensions: Span 60 (solid state), Brij 52 (semisolid state), and Brij 92 (liquid state) (liquid state). In this research, the mean volume diameters (dv) of produced vesicles were examined, as well as insulin entrapment efficiencies. It was found that raising the HLB value from 4.7 (Span 60) to 5.3 (Brij 52) resulted in a substantial increase in the mean volume diameter of produced vesicles [42].

Large Unilamellar Vesicles (LUV)

LUV has the aqueous phase-to-surfactants compartment and this type of NS (100–3000 nm) has a high value of component; therefore, bioactive material can be entrapped using membrane surfactants extremely economical. The film hydration method was used to prepare a Span 20-based NS loaded for Newcastle disease vaccine which is a contagious bird disease that affects many domestic and wild avian species, including turkeys [34].

Small Unilamellar Vesicles (SUV)

The separated multilamellar vesicles turn into small unilamellar vesicles (SUVs) by different techniques. The sonication, high-pressure homogenization and extrusion techniques under high pressure are commonly useful and, are used (MLV). The size of SUV ranges between 10 and 100 nanometers. SUVs have three disadvantages [1]: they are thermodynamically unstable [2], they have a tendency to coalesces, and [3] the loaded hydrophilic medicines is frequently insignificant [43].

Bola-NS

Surfactant compounds composed of two hydrophilic heads connected by one or two extended lipophilic spacers are known as bola-surfactant compounds. It was in the early 1980s that researchers discovered them in the membrane of archaebacteria [44]. Bola-NS illustrated better acceptability, and the vesicles are generated by incorporation of alpha omega-hexadecyl-bis-[1-aza-18-crown-6][Bola-surfactant]-Span 80-cholesterol (2:3:1 molar ratio) [45].

Proniosomes

Proniosomes were created by coating a water-soluble carrier with a thin layer of dry NIC surfactant and then drying the mixture [46]. The reduction of drug leakage over time is main disadvantage. On the other hand, the working with proniosomes in powder form is more convenient [47].

Apsosomes

Ascorbylpalmitate (ASP) was investigated as a vesicle-forming material in a bilayer configuration. In combination with cholesterol and a negatively charged lipid, it formed (Apsosomes) (dicetyl phosphate) [48]. The formation of apsosomes by using the film hydration method, followed by sonication, in which aqueous azidothymidine (AZT) solution was encapsulated in the aqueous regions of the bilayer. Apsosomes can be used to improve medicine transdermal penetration and minimize oxygen-related disorders [49].

Discomes

It was discovered that giant disc-shaped NS (approximately 20 microns in diameter) coexisted with spherical NS (2–5 micron) in the presence of Discomes. It has been demonstrated that certain massive discoid formations, known as discomes, can be formed under specific conditions of the phase diagram of a NIC surfactant [50]. Mechanical shaking and sonication were used by Uchegbu and co-investigators to produce NS from hexadecyldiglycerol ether [C16], cholesterol, and dicetyl phosphate, according to their findings. They discovered that the NS within the discome phase were large and that their size regularly increased after sonication [37]. Discomes are thermoresponsive NS that leak when the temperature rises above 37 degrees Celsius. There has been speculation about the potential of this type of NS as a drug delivery system for the eyes. Recent research by Abdelkader and co-investigators has demonstrated that NS discomes can be used to encapsulate naltrexone hydrochloride (NTX), a promising agent in treating diabetic complications that affect the cornea (diabetic Keratopathy). The development of NS was accomplished through the use of the reverse phase evaporation method. The NTX-entrapped NS could be entrapped up to 61.5 percent (w/w) of the NTX [51].

Elastic NS

Elastic NS can bend without losing their structure, and they can pass through smaller holes than their size. NIC surfactants, water, and ethanol are the main components of these vesicles. Their structural flexibility increases their ability to penetrate through skin layers that are still intact. Manosroiand co-investigators developed elastic NS to entrap diclofenac diethyl ammonium using Tween 61, Span 60, and ethanol, resulting in deformability index values 13.76 times higher than those of normal NS after using these materials [52].

DIFFERENT PREPARATION TECHNIQUES FOR NSDEVELOPMENT

According to the hypothesis, NS manufacturing requires particular surfactants, additives and an aquatic solvent. If the surfactant monomers are hydrated, they are aggregated by high interfacial tension between water and the lipophilic component of the surfactant form vesicles. To produce bilayers, the surfactant hydrophilic head groups tend to gaze towards the outside while the lipophilic surfactant tails tend to look towards each other. A supramolecular assembly is the outcome of two competing forces. In addition to cholesterol, chemicals such as lysine are other crucial elements in the creation of NS. There are numerous methods for preparing NS, which are further addressed on this page.

Thin Film Hydration Method

For the manufacture of NS, the thin film hydration process is a simple yet successful procedure. Surfactants and other additives like cholesterol must be dissolved using any compatible organic solvents [53]. Then this is blended in a circular bottom bottle at a particular temperature and under a vacuum. On the surface of the balloon wall, an incredibly thin layer appears when the organic solvent is evaporated [54]. The hydration of the surfactant contains the water or PBS [Phosphate-buffered saline] at a greater temperature than the temperature of the transition of the surfactant phase. Tavano and co-investigators employed a thin film hydration technique, previously reported, to include antioxidants in niosomal carriers. Tween 60 was properly weighed and dissolved with a round bottom flask in chloroform. After the solvent has evaporated at lower pressure and steady rotation [55].

The alkyl glucopyranoside NS made by Muzzalupo and co-investigators 2013 include pharmaceutical methotrexate, used in other studies by the thin film hydration technique. NS dimensions ranged from 300 to 500 nm, with low polydispersion indexes [56]. This technique creates MLVs, which have been used in several medicinal carriers, such as the manufacture and encapsulation of nimesulide-based NS, among other applications [57]minoxidil [58] Doxorubicin [18, 58], Paclitaxel [59], Resveratrol [60], Simvastatin [61], Acetaminophene [62], Antioxidants [63], salicylic acid and p-hydroxyl benzoic acid [64], insulin [42], hydroxyl camptothecin [65], glucocorticoid [66] *etc.*

"Bubble" Method

The "bubble" approach, which does not require the use of organic solvents, can be used to generate NS without the use of organic solvents. In a "bubbling unit," a round-bottomed flask with three necks is submerged in water, and a water-cooled reflux condenser and thermometer are placed on top of the flask to measure temperature. Transferring surfactants, additives, and PBS into a three-necked glass reactor is time-consuming and requires patience. The reactor is submerged in a water bath, which allows for precise temperature control of the reactor as the method shown in Fig. **(12.4)** [67].

Dehydration-Rehydration Method

The dehydration and controlled rehydration method induce the fusing of prepared vesicles, followed by rehydration steps. It was decided to alter the procedure previously described by Hope and co-investigators to create the dehydration–rehydration vesicles (DRVs). Preparation of eight millilitres of MLV dispersion, which was then frozen in liquid nitrogen and freeze-dried overnight, was accomplished using the TFH method. At 60°C, the freeze-dried bulk was rehydrated in 4 mL PBS to obtain the final product [pH 7.4]. After complete lipid hydration, the final volume of the examined NS was adjusted to 8mL in PBS using the PBS method (pH 7.4) [68 - 70]

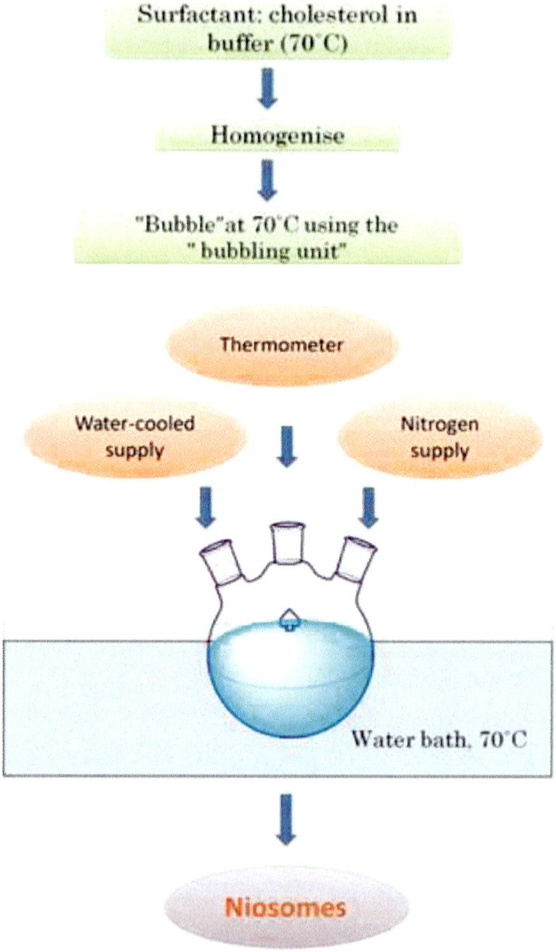

Fig. (12.4). The Bubble method of noisome preparation.

Ether Injection Method

Deamer and Bangham proposed it in 1976. In this procedure, an organic solvent having a certain ratio of surfactant and cholesterol is slowly injected into an aqueous solution phase containing the drug, which is rendered above the organic solvent's boiling point. Gradual ether evaporation produces single-layer NS [71]. NS range in size from 50 to 1000 nm, depending on reaction conditions. This method has been used to entrap drugs like Rifampicin. The entrapment efficiency of NS prepared by ether injection was higher than that of NS prepared by hand-shaking. Increasing the formulation's Cholesterol content reduced microparticle entrapment efficiency. The increasing vesicle stiffness with each fractional increase of cholesterol may explain this. The temperature and hydration time magnitude is an important parameter to obtained consistency in niosomal formulation. The higher hydration time improves NS shape and size reliability and generally it was suggested approx 45 minutes by different studies [72].

Hand-Shaking Method

Thin-film hydration yields multilamellar vesicles. To generate a thin layer on the interior wall of the flask, the components are dissolved in a compatible ratio of organic solvent. To make NS, a dry film was shaken for an hour at pH 7.4 in an aqueous solution containing the medication. Waddad and co-investigators 2013 used hand-shaking to create NS containing Morin hydrate. This study used NIC surfactants like Span 60, Span 80, and Tween 60 for different niosomal systems. Using Taguchi orthogonal array analysis, three optimal Morin hydrate [MH] NS formulations were produced. They demonstrated higher entrapment efficiency, stability, and release capability than other MH-NS [73]. Also, in another study, NS were developed by hand-shaking with sorbitan monoesters and sorbitan trioleateas nonionic surfactants [85], The co-surfactants of polyoxyethelene fatty acid esters with or without cholesterol and charged lipids like stearylamine or dicetyl phosphine also applicable for the development of NS [74].

Heating Method

In this approach, the surfactant/cholesterol mixture is treated with a medication solution in a buffer solution before being added to the mixture. NS are produced by probe sonicating the mixture at 60 degrees Celsius with a titanium probe for 3 minutes in a sonicator [35]. A polyol, such as glycerol and other additive in combinations, such as cholesterol and charge-carrying molecules, is also valuable for a hydration solution at room temperature while being exposed to a nitrogen gas atmosphere. The mixture is required for heated near to 120°C to dissolve cholesterol then the temperature reduced and the NS allowed to cool to room temperature [75].

Sonication Method

Small vesicles can be produced with this process, which is very valuable. When high-energy sonication is used, it is possible to shrink the average size of NS. Sonication can be divided into two categories: probe sonication and bath sonication. Probe sonication is preferred for small-volume suspension preparation, whereas bath sonication is preferred for large-volume dispersions preparation. The surfactant/cholesterol mixture is placed in a 10ml glass vial, and the medication solution in the buffer is added to it. This dispersion is then probe sonicated for 3 minutes at 60°C to enhance the dispersion [10]. The diallyl disulfide (DADS) formulations were used in a mouse model to see if they effectively cure widespread candid infection. Span-based niosomal formulations were created in this study by the use of a sonication technique. it is now believed that including DADS in NS can boost their therapeutic efficacy. Span 60, cholesterol, and soy lecithin were utilized in another investigation to make cefdinir NS, which were then purified using the sonication method [22].

Microfluidization Method

Using the submerged jet principle, the microfluidization approach is accomplished. This method can interact at extremely high speeds between two fluidized streams (one containing surfactant and the other containing medication). Internally, in carefully defined micro channels, the energy supplied to the system remains in the area of NS formations. The fluid collected can be recirculated by the pump until spherical vesicles are formed. The submerged jet principle is what this is known as. It leads to improved homogeneity, reproducibility, and a smaller size in the formulation of NS, among other benefits. This method resulted in unilamellar NS that were more uniform, reproducible, and smaller in size than those produced by other methods [10, 75]

Microfluidic Hydrodynamic Focusing

Making NS from two miscible liquids using microfluidic hydrodynamic focusing and diffusive mixing is demonstrated [76]. In microchannels, the miscible liquids are merged in a quick and precise manner. This procedure obtains a more appropriate size and size distribution of NS instead of those obtained using a standard method [77]. Numerous factors, including the conditions under which the microfluidic mixing occurs, the chemical structure of a surfactant, and the material used in the microchannel device, might influence how well NS are assembled. They discovered that increasing the flow rate ratio shortens the time required for diffusive mixing and results in the formation of NS of small size. When the size of the applied microchannel is increased, the diffusive mixing period rises, resulting in larger NS being formed [76].

Reverse Phase Evaporation Method

However, while the reverse-phase evaporation technique or approach has the advantage of allowing for precise control over the size of NS, it has the disadvantages of increasing drug solubility in ether and making it more challenging to remove ether from the final formulation altogether. When using this method, the most crucial issue to consider is the evaporation of the solvent from the emulsion [78]. Making an emulsion begins with preparing a cholesterol and surfactant solution in a 1:1 ratio of ether to chloroform. Then the addition of the medicine is done while both phases are being sonicated at 4 to 5 degrees Celsius. The finished dispersion was rotary evaporated at 60°C until it either had a semisolid gel-like mass or an aqueous lipid dispersion (depending on the amount of lipid present), then dried. The viscose NS suspension was diluted with PBS and cooked in a water bath at 60°C for 10 minutes before being used. The hydration process will continue indefinitely until all of the water has been completely absorbed. When an organic solvent evaporates, low-level ultraviolet radiation (LUV) is produced [79]. With the reverse phase evaporation approach, Zarei and co-investigators successfully produced paclitaxel pegylated and nonpegylated NS with Span 60 and span 20, respectively [59].

The Enzymatic Method

When surface-active agents are removed from mixed micelles or similar "open" structures by enzymatic reactions, liposomes are formed in aqueous media under mild circumstances, which can be used to deliver drugs. The procedure described here is straightforward and dependable, and it is based on well-established analytical techniques and procedures. In this technique, incubate a mixed micellar solution of $C_{16}G_2$, DCP, and polyoxy-ethylene-cholesteryl-sebacetate-diester [PCSD] with esterases, you'll get a NS dispersion, which is what you want. Using the esterases, PCSD is broken down into polyoxyethylene, sebacic acid, and cholesterol, among other things. Cholesterol, in conjunction with $C_{16}G_2$ and DCP, results in the formation of C16G2 NS [80]. In literature, a self-evolving system has been designed based on Autopoiesis linked to the investigation and study of enzyme-induced self-replicating systems such as micelles reversed to understand better the dynamic interactions between enzymes and colloidal aggregates micelles and liposomes, among other things. For chemotherapeutic applications, specific enzyme-induced decapsulation of vesicles has been documented in the literature [81]. There was a report of two unique extemporaneous enzymatic liposome fabrications using micelles made of classical amphiphilic chemicals. When the surfactant's water-interacting head group is removed through enzymatic activity, this transitions from micelle to vesicle formation [82].

Single-pass Technique

This method delivers a lipid-containing drug suspension from a porous device through a nozzle. It produces NS that are uniform in size, ranging from 50 to 500 nanometers. It is a patented method applied for liposome preparation [83].

Freeze and Thaw Method

One such technique is freeze-thaw cycles to homogenize the multilamellar liposomes to aid the formation of nano sized unilamellar liposomes. In a freeze/thaw step, LUVs (or MLVs with large fluid spaces between lamellae) are preserved, whereas MLVs change the structure. Mayer and research group Frozen and thawed multilamellar vesicles (FATMLVs) were generated by subjecting 8 mL of niosomal suspensions prepared using TFH method to five alternate cycles of freezing in liquid nitrogen for 60 s and thawing in a water bath at 60 °C for another 60 seconds [84].

FACTORS AFFECTING THE FORMATION OF NS

Preparing NS and achieving their ideal structure relies on appropriate information and a detailed grasp of the physicochemical characteristics of their components. The formation of NS is influenced by several variables. These variables can be affected by the manner of preparation, the route of administration, and the amount of material consumed. The most significant factors effects of a niosomal structure will be addressed and discussed in this chapter.

Surfactants

NIC surfactants are among the most effective polymeric nano carriers, and they play an important role in the administration of regulated, sustained, targeted, and continuous drugs. NIC amphiphiles, such as those utilized in NS, can be divided into four categories: Alkyl esters, alkyl amides, alkyl ethers, and esters of fatty acids are all types of alkyl esters [5]. The efficiency with which a medication is entrapped is typically determined by the chain length and size of the hydrophilic head group of NIC surfactants. NIC surfactants with a longer alkyl chain exhibit a greater capacity for trapping. The Tween sequence of surfactants with an extended alkyl chain and an oversized hydrophilic moiety in a 1:1 ratio with cholesterol has the highest trapping efficiency for water-soluble pharmaceuticals. The most frequently used surfactants for NS production are listed in (Fig. **12.5**). The choice of surfactant is determined by the hydrophilic-lipophilic balance [HLB] and critical packing parameter (CPP) values described below.

Hydrophilic-Lipophilic Balance (HLB) and Critical Packing Parameters (CPP)

HLB is a dimensionless surfactant parameter that acts as a time-saving guide for surfactant selection. Additionally, the HLB value of a surfactant is critical in determining the efficiency of drug entrapment. For NIC surfactants, the HLB value ranges from 0 to 20; a low HLB (b9) indicates a lipophilic surfactant, while a high HLB (N11) indicates a surfactant. Surfactants with an HLB value of between 3 and 8 are compatible with prepared bilayer surfaces and are emulsifiers for water-in-oil (W/O). Additionally, oil-in-water (O/W) emulsifiers have HLB values ranging from 8–18 [85].This parameter affects the size and concentration of the drug loading. Surfactants with an HLB value between 4 and 8 are vesicle-forming compatible. Surfactants with HLB values more than 6 cannot form vesicles; hence, cholesterol must be added to generate NS [86]. Along with the HLB number, chemical structure and a variety of other factors also influence the ability of a surfactant to form vesicles such as CPP, another dimensionless surfactant scale parameter that affects the non-spherical micelles, bilayer vesicles or inverted micelles formation.

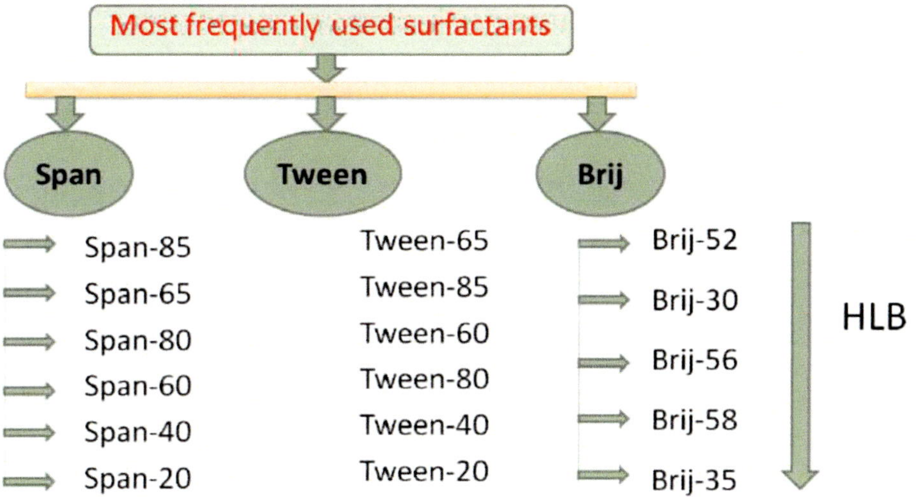

Fig. (12.5). Frequently used surfactants for NS preparation.

Quantity of surfactant and lipid

Generally, the quantity of surfactant and lipid concentrations greatly affects the various characteristic parameters of niosomal preparation such as size, charge, PDi and drug release behavior. Therefore, it should be critically optimized with respect to quality of niosomal characterizes [87].

Additive Agents Andencapsulated Drug

Incorporating additives such as surfactants and medicines into the niosomal formulation may improve the stability of NS and make it more stable. Vesicles' membrane stability, shape, and permeability are all affected by a wide range of additives. For example, increasing the stiffness of the niosomal system and decreasing the permeability of medicines across the membrane are two effects of adding cholesterol to the system. NS produced with C16G2/cholesterol/M-polyethylene glycol (PEG)-Chol show spherical vesicles with diameters ranging from 20 to 200 nm, which are surrounded by a spherical matrix [88]. Additionally, the chemical structure of the medication has an important influence in the % entrapment efficiency of the drug throughout its preparation. There are a variety of variables that affect drug entrapment, together with interaction between the drug and the nuclear membrane (NS). The chemical composition, molecular weight, and hydrophilicity and lipophilicity of the compound are all examined [89]. For instance, a water-soluble medication such as diclofenac sodium shows the greatest loading in NS when Tween 60 is used, and it's noteworthy to note that methotrexate, a hydrophobic agent, demonstrates the most trapping in NS when Span 60 is utilized The physicochemical characteristics of the encapsulated medication have an impact on the NS bilayer's charge and stiffness. The chemical attaches to surfactant head groups and produces a charge that causes mutual repulsion between surfactant bilayers, increasing vesicle size. The charge development on the bilayer inhibits vesicles from clumping [24].

Thermodynamic Feature and Geometric Features of Amphiphilic Molecule

Surfactants forming vesicles is not a coincidence. Only a limited number of surfactants and additives creates thermodynamically stable NS. Interaction energies are necessary to produce NS. The creation of NS from NIC surfactant monomers is caused by two opposing forces: strong interfacial tension between lipophilic groups and water, and repulsive forces between head groups. In various study it was suggested that the 1-10 mm size range NS are more stable than submicron NS because of low surface free energy, and they tend to decrease segregation.

Membrane Composition and Resistance of Osmotic Stress

The use of different chemicals, surfactants, and medicines stabilize NS formation. The morphology of the produced NS can be changed, as can their permeability/porousness and stability. Polyhedral NS are unaffected by adding a small amount of poly-24-oxyethylene ether solution, preventing aggregation owing to steric development [33]. Simultaneously the addition of hypertonic salt solution to niosomal suspension reduces niosomal diameter. A hypotonic salt solution causes slow release with minor enlargement of the vesicles due to inhibition of elution from the vesicles. Mechanical weakening of vesicle structure under osmotic stress speeds up release [90].

CHARACTERIZATIONS OF NS

Percent Entrapment Efficiency (% EE)

The NS's entrapment efficiency is expressed as a percentage of the drug-loaded. To determine the %EE, the unentrapped drug is first isolated with a different method, and then the separated and collected solution is analyzed for loaded drug/bioactive with suitable techniques or following that, the recovered supernatant is diluted and estimated following the drug's labeling. In addition to the manufacturing process and drug properties, the entrapment efficiency (EE) and yield of NS are also affected by the drug. The NS structure comprises the number of double layers and the size and distribution of vesicles, the efficacy of aqueous phase entrapment, and the permeability of the vesicle membrane may affect the % EE as the literature suggested.

Size, Shape and Morphology and Surface Charge

Transmission electron microscopy (TEM), scanning electron microscopy (SEM), freeze-fractured microscopy (FFM), and atomic force microscopy (AFM) are some of the techniques that can be used to detect the size, shape, and morphology of the NS. For cryoTEM investigation, liquid propane is typically used to cryofix the vesicular suspension before it is imaged with the microscope. According to some sources, glycol can also be a cryoprotectant when applied at low temperatures and pressures. According to the current scenario, the size distribution, mean surface diameter, and mass distribution of NS are all determined with the help of a laser beam-based master scaler. Additionally, the Zeta Sizer can be used to assess the zeta potential of samples in addition to size distribution and mean diameter.

ADVANTAGES OF NIOSOMAL DRUG DELIVERY SYSTEM

As the drug delivery system, NS have the following benefits:

1. NS have a higher level of patient compliance and therapeutic efficacy than traditional oily formulations.
2. Drug release is controlled and sustained in NS due to depot formation.
3. NS shape, features, size and fluidity can be adjusted as needed.
4. NS can be used to deliver a wide range of medications since they can entrap hydrophilic, lipophilic, and amphiphilic molecules.
5. NS have a greater bioavailability than other traditional formulations.
6. NS have been successfully used to target medications to specific organs.
7. NS are more stable than other liposomes formulation.

8. NS formulations are biodegradable, biocompatible and non-immunogenic to the body.
9. NS can be used to encapsulate both type of drugs such as hydrophilic as well as hydrophobic.
10. Drug penetration through the skin might be enhanced by NS.
11. NS can be administered in a variety of routes, including orally, parenterally, transdermal, ocular and pulmonary.
12. NS formulations are simple to handle, store, and transport.
13. It can protect pharmaceuticals from biological enzymes and acids, resulting in increased drug stability.
14. In the ocular medication with niosomal delivery system, penetration enhancers do not induce tissue irritation or injury.

ROUTES OF ADMINISTRATION FOR NS DELIVERY

Drug-loaded NS can be given in various ways, depending on the diseased condition, drug characteristics, and delivery site. These administration paths are briefly described below.

Intravenous

NS can be delivered *via* the intravascular route. The advantage of injecting the medicine is that it enters the systemic circulation immediately; the NS improves the drug's stability and prolongs its duration in the blood. With minimal changes, the drugs can also be administered to a specific location. The intravenous route is widely used for the delivery of NS of many drugs. Rouholamini and co-investigators, prepared Silibinin-loaded nano-niosomal coated with trimethyl chitosan formulation on miRNAs expression for breast cancer [91]. In this connection, Tavano and co-investigators, developed NS from glucuronic acid-based surfactant as new carriers for cancer treatment and incorporated doxorubicin and 5FU anticancer drugs within the vesicles for IV purposes. Akbarzadeh and co-investigators, also prepared and optimized doxycycline-loaded IV niosomal formulation to treat prostate cancer [92].

Oral

The oral route is the most preferred method of drug delivery, and NS are also delivered through this route of administration. The acidic milieu and photolytic juices, which have the potential to damage the medicine, present a challenge during oral administration of the drug. Meanwhile, it has been demonstrated that NS can successfully deliver the drug to the gastric mucosa in humans. Yaghoobian and colleagues investigated the effect of surfactant composition and surface charge of NS on the oral absorption of repaglinide, which was used as a

BCS II model drug in their study. According to the available information, the NS is supposed to increase the oral bioavailability of 17-Hydroxyprogesterone caproate and Cyclosporine-A [93].

Intramuscular

NS can also be administered *via* the intramuscular route. Sambhakar and co-investigators developed a novel NS formulation of risperidone for good biocompatibility, and Wilkhu and co-investigators developed a novel NS formulation for the delivery of subunit influenza antigen for oral and intramuscular administration.

Dermal and Transdermal

In the instance of skin diseases, the dermal route is employed to deliver medications locally. It is solely employed for local activity. This approach has the advantage of not allowing the medicine to enter the systemic circulation, resulting in fewer side effects. The medicine enters the systemic circulation *via* transdermal distribution. However, drugs confront a barrier in the skin. The vesicular system has been extremely useful in enhancing drug delivery *via* dermal and transdermal routes. NS serves as a drug reservoir, increasing the drug's penetration. NSAIDs are administered *via* a transdermal delivery system to avoid the gastric route. Catechin, propofol-loaded niosomal gel for transdermal delivery, and Annonasquamosa extract-based dermal delivery formulations were reported [94].

Ocular

When a medicine must be given in the anterior location of the eye, topical ocular administration is usually preferred. Drugs delivered in traditional forms have a bioavailability of just 1-3%, and they are subject to precorneal loss due to tear production and insufficient residence time in the conjunctival sac. The niosomal ophthalmic preparation can be successfully utilized by consideration of these criteria.

Nasal Administration

In the case of medications having a high first-pass metabolism, nasal administration is a viable alternative. However, despite the fact that diltiazem is quickly absorbed from the oral cavity, it has a bioavailability of only 30–60 percent owing to extensive first-pass processing by cytochrome P450 enzymes in the liver. Because of mucociliary clearance and airflow restriction, nasal administration has some disadvantages, including a short residence time in the nasal cavity and nasal mucosa sensitivity. All of these factors reduce drug penetration and systemic bioavailability when administered through the nasal cavity. It has been shown that nasal delivery of a niosomal new calcium channel blocker for the therapy of cardiac arrhythmias has a greater bioavailability than oral administration.

Pulmonary

The pulmonary route of administering niosomal medicines has various advantages, including enhanced mucus permeability, sustained drug delivery, targeting, and superior therapeutic outcomes. Various research groups prepared Zanamivir, ciprofloxacin-loaded, and N-Acetyl Cysteine Loaded-NS for pulmonary /Respiratory Disorders [95].

PHARMACEUTICAL APPLICATIONS OF NS

While NS are utilized in various fields, *i.e.*, medicinal, diagnostics, cosmetics, *etc.*, most applications have been in drug delivery [26, 96 - 100].

- Targeted drug delivery
- Treatment of HIV-AIDS
- Delivery of vaccine and antigen
- Delivery of anticancer drugs
- Carrier for hemoglobin
- Treatment of leishmaniasis
- Management of psoriasis
- Enhancement of bioavailability
- Delivery of proteins and peptides
- Brain targeting
- Lung diseases
- Anti-inflammatory activity
- Antimicrobial agent
- Diagnostic imaging
- Delivery of natural products
- Gene delivery system
- Glaucoma

Limitation of NS Drug Delivery System

The existence of NS toxicity research is limited, despite the fact that the toxicity of certain surfactants has been documented in a number of studies. According to these studies, ester surfactants are far less toxic than ether surfactants (because of the relative enzyme effects on the ester bond), and NIC surfactants have better compatibility with other kinds of surfactants while also generally reducing toxicity than other kinds of surfactants. As a result, the use of niosomal components as a drug carrier is limited due to the need for careful selection.

CONCLUSION

A strong technique for dealing with the issues of insolubility and poor bioavailability of medicines, NS formulations are becoming more popular. Because hydrophilic, amphiphilic, and lipophilic moieties are present in the structure, they may take medicinal compounds with a broad range of solubility. NS has the potential to address a number of disadvantages associated with alternative vesicular carriers, such as liposomal formulation, that are connected with large-scale manufacturing, sterilization, and stability. For the formation of NS, a variety of surfactants have been tested. It is possible to use niosomal drug delivery for a broad variety of pharmacological substances in the treatment of a wide range of diseases. Niosomal drug delivery is now being used in the treatment of a wide range of disorders. However, NS has the ability to encapsulate hazardous medicines, despite the fact that there is no evidence to support assertions regarding their usefulness in carrying proteins and biological.

FUTURE PROSPECTS

Since the discovery of proteins and vaccines in recent scientific studies, molecules such as these have been acknowledged as an important class of medical treatments. In recent years, there has been a significant increase and widening of interest in neuroscientific topics across a broad variety of scientific fields, with a particular focus on their use in medicine. There are several different types of NS, each with their own characteristics and applications. The information in this chapter will be useful for drug delivery research because it provides an overview of the procedures that are used in the manufacturing of NS as well as the different types and their characteristics. Although the technology being utilized in NS is still in its early phases, it has the potential to be revolutionary. As a consequence, research is being undertaken to create a technology that is appropriate for large-scale manufacturing since it has the potential to be used as a targeted medication delivery system.

CONSENT FOR PUBLICATION

Not applicable.

CONFLICT OF INTEREST

The authors declare no conflict of interest, financial or otherwise.

ACKNOWLEDGEMENTS

The authors would like to acknowledge all of their associated institutions for providing the necessary resources to compile this work.

REFERENCES

[1] Handjani-Vila RM, Ribier A, Rondot B, Vanlerberghie G. Dispersions of lamellar phases of non-ionic lipids in cosmetic products. Int J Cosmet Sci 1979; 1(5): 303-14. [http://dx.doi.org/10.1111/j.1467-2494.1979.tb00224.x] [PMID: 19467076]

[2] Fang JY, Hong CT, Chiu WT, Wang YY. Effect of liposomes and niosomes on skin permeation of enoxacin. Int J Pharm 2001; 219(1-2): 61-72. [http://dx.doi.org/10.1016/S0378-5173(01)00627-5] [PMID: 11337166]

[3] Ge X, Wei M, He S, Yuan WE. Advances of non-ionic surfactant vesicles (niosomes) and their application in drug delivery. Pharmaceutics 2019; 11(2): 55. [http://dx.doi.org/10.3390/pharmaceutics11020055] [PMID: 30700021]

[4] Vyas S, Singh R, Jain S, *et al.* Non-ionic surfactant based vesicles (niosomes) for non-invasive topical genetic immunization against hepatitis B. Int J Pharm 2005; 296(1-2): 80-6. [http://dx.doi.org/10.1016/j.ijpharm.2005.02.016] [PMID: 15885458]

[5] Rajera R, Nagpal K, Singh SK, Mishra DN. Niosomes: A controlled and novel drug delivery system. Biol Pharm Bull 2011; 34(7): 945-53. [http://dx.doi.org/10.1248/bpb.34.945] [PMID: 21719996]

[6] Niu G, Cogburn B, Hughes J. Preparation and characterization of doxorubicin liposomes. Methods Mol Biol 2010; 624: 211-9. [http://dx.doi.org/10.1007/978-1-60761-609-2_14] [PMID: 20217598]

[7] Zhang JA, Anyarambhatla G, Ma L, *et al.* Development and characterization of a novel Cremophor® EL free liposome-based paclitaxel (LEP-ETU) formulation. Eur J Pharm Biopharm 2005; 59(1): 177-87. [http://dx.doi.org/10.1016/j.ejpb.2004.06.009] [PMID: 15567316]

[8] Jacob S, Nair AB, Al-Dhubiab BE. Preparation and evaluation of niosome gel containing acyclovir for enhanced dermal deposition. J Liposome Res 2017; 27(4): 283-92. [http://dx.doi.org/10.1080/08982104.2016.1224897] [PMID: 27558522]

[9] Gao C. The investigation on the diagnosis and pathogenesis of Campylobacter-like organisms in gastric mucosal biopsy. Zhonghua Bing Li Xue Za Zhi 1987; 16(3): 216-8.

[10] Kuotsu K, Karim KM, Mandal AS, *et al.* Niosome: A future of targeted drug delivery systems. J Adv Pharm Technol Res 2010; 1(4): 374-80. [http://dx.doi.org/10.4103/0110-5558.76435] [PMID: 22247876]

[11] Jadon PS, Gajbhiye V, Jadon RS, Gajbhiye KR, Ganesh N. Enhanced oral bioavailability of griseofulvin *via* niosomes. AAPS PharmSciTech 2009; 10(4): 1186-92. [http://dx.doi.org/10.1208/s12249-009-9325-z] [PMID: 19856107]

[12] Khazaeli P, Sharifi I, Talebian E, Heravi G, Moazeni E, Mostafavi M. Anti-leishmanial effect of itraconazole niosome on *in vitro* susceptibility of Leishmania tropica. Environ Toxicol Pharmacol 2014; 38(1): 205-11. [http://dx.doi.org/10.1016/j.etap.2014.04.003] [PMID: 24956400]

[13] Hunter CA, Dolan TF, Coombs GH, Baillie AJ. Vesicular systems (niosomes and liposomes) for delivery of sodium stibogluconate in experimental murine visceral leishmaniasis. J Pharm Pharmacol 2011; 40(3): 161-5. [http://dx.doi.org/10.1111/j.2042-7158.1988.tb05210.x] [PMID: 2899143]

[14] Puras G, Martínez-Navarrete G, Mashal M, *et al.* Protamine/DNA/Niosome ternary nonviral vectors for gene delivery to the retina: The role of protamine. Mol Pharm 2015; 12(10): 3658-71. [http://dx.doi.org/10.1021/acs.molpharmaceut.5b00422] [PMID: 26334586]

[15] Nematollahi MH, Torkzadeh-Mahanai M, Pardakhty A, Ebrahimi Meimand HA, Asadikaram G. Ternary complex of plasmid DNA with NLS-Mu-Mu protein and cationic niosome for biocompatible and efficient gene delivery: A comparative study with protamine and lipofectamine. Artif Cells Nanomed Biotechnol 2018; 46(8): 1781-91. [PMID: 29081256]

[16] Parthasarathi G, Udupa N, Umadevi P, Pillai G. Niosome encapsulated of vincristine sulfate: Improved anticancer activity with reduced toxicity in mice. J Drug Target 1994; 2(2): 173-82. [http://dx.doi.org/10.3109/10611869409015907] [PMID: 8069596]

[17] Wang M, Yuan Y, Gao Y, *et al.* Preparation and characterization of 5-fluorouracil pH-sensitive niosome and its tumor-targeted evaluation: *In vitro* and *in vivo*. Drug Dev Ind Pharm 2012; 38(9): 1134-41. [http://dx.doi.org/10.3109/03639045.2011.641565] [PMID: 22182601]

[18] Hemati M, Haghiralsadat F, Yazdian F, Jafari F, Moradi A, Malekpour-Dehkordi Z. Development and characterization of a novel cationic PEGylated niosome-encapsulated forms of doxorubicin, quercetin and siRNA for the treatment of cancer by using combination therapy. Artif Cells Nanomed Biotechnol 2019; 47(1): 1295-311. [http://dx.doi.org/10.1080/21691401.2018.1489271] [PMID: 30033768]

[19] Damrongrungruang T, Panpitakkul P, Somudorn J, *et al.* Glutaryl melatonin niosome gel for topical oral mucositis: Anti- inflammatory and anticandidiasis. Curr Drug Deliv 2020; 17(3): 195-206. [http://dx.doi.org/10.2174/1567201817666200122162545] [PMID: 31969103]

[20] Priprem A, Janpim K, Nualkaew S, Mahakunakorn P. Topical niosome gel of zingiber cassumunar roxb. AAPS PharmSciTech 2016; 17(3): 631-9. [http://dx.doi.org/10.1208/s12249-015-0376-z] [PMID: 26292930]

[21] Aggarwal G, Nagpal M, Kaur G. Development and comparison of nanosponge and niosome based gel for the topical delivery of tazarotene. Pharm Nanotechnol 2016; 4(3): 213-28. [http://dx.doi.org/10.2174/2211738504666160804154213] [PMID: 29052500]

[22] Osanloo M, Assadpour S, Mehravaran A, Abastabar M, Akhtari J. Niosome-loaded antifungal drugs as an effective nanocarrier system: A mini review. Curr Med Mycol 2018; 4(4): 31-6. [PMID: 30815615]

[23] Gharbavi M, Amani J, Kheiri-Manjili H, Danafar H, Sharafi A. Niosome: A promising nanocarrier for natural drug delivery through blood-brain barrier. Adv Pharmacol Sci 2018; 2018: 1-15. [http://dx.doi.org/10.1155/2018/6847971] [PMID: 30651728]

[24] Moghassemi S, Hadjizadeh A. Nano-niosomes as nanoscale drug delivery systems: An illustrated review. J Control Release 2014; 185: 22-36. [http://dx.doi.org/10.1016/j.jconrel.2014.04.015] [PMID: 24747765]

[25] Amin ML. P-glycoprotein inhibition for optimal drug delivery. Drug Target Insights 2013; 7: DTI.S12519. [http://dx.doi.org/10.4137/DTI.S12519] [PMID: 24023511]

[26] Chen S, Hanning S, Falconer J, Locke M, Wen J. Recent advances in non-ionic surfactant vesicles (niosomes): Fabrication, characterization, pharmaceutical and cosmetic applications. Eur J Pharm Biopharm 2019; 144: 18-39. [http://dx.doi.org/10.1016/j.ejpb.2019.08.015] [PMID: 31446046]

[27] Abdelkader H, Alani AWG, Alany RG. Recent advances in non-ionic surfactant vesicles (niosomes): Self-assembly, fabrication, characterization, drug delivery applications and limitations. Drug Deliv 2014; 21(2): 87-100.

[http://dx.doi.org/10.3109/10717544.2013.838077] [PMID: 24156390]

[28] Shatalebi MA, Mostafavi SA, Moghaddas A. Niosome as a drug carrier for topical delivery of N-acetyl glucosamine. Res Pharm Sci 2010; 5(2): 107-17.
[PMID: 21589799]

[29] Akbarzadeh I, Shayan M, Bourbour M, *et al.* Preparation, optimization and in-vitro evaluation of curcumin-loaded niosome@calcium alginate nanocarrier as a new approach for breast cancer treatment. Biology (Basel) 2021; 10(3): 173.
[http://dx.doi.org/10.3390/biology10030173] [PMID: 33652630]

[30] Mohamad Saimi NI, Salim N, Ahmad N, Abdulmalek E, Abdul Rahman MB. Aerosolized niosome formulation containing gemcitabine and cisplatin for lung cancer treatment: Optimization, characterization and *in vitro* evaluation. Pharmaceutics 2021; 13(1): 59.
[http://dx.doi.org/10.3390/pharmaceutics13010059] [PMID: 33466428]

[31] Uthaiwat P, Daduang J, Priprem A, *et al.* Topical melatonin niosome gel for the treatment of 5-F--induced oral mucositis in mice. Curr Drug Deliv 2021; 18(2): 199-211.
[http://dx.doi.org/10.2174/1567201817666200525151848] [PMID: 32484102]

[32] Moghtaderi M, Mirzaie A, Zabet N, *et al.* Enhanced antibacterial activity of *Echinacea angustifolia* extract against multidrug-resistant *Klebsiella pneumoniae* through niosome encapsulation. Nanomaterials (Basel) 2021; 11(6): 1573.
[http://dx.doi.org/10.3390/nano11061573] [PMID: 34203811]

[33] Nasseri B. Effect of cholesterol and temperature on the elastic properties of niosomal membranes. Int J Pharm 2005; 300(1-2): 95-101.
[http://dx.doi.org/10.1016/j.ijpharm.2005.05.009] [PMID: 16006080]

[34] Okore VC, Attama AA, Ofokansi KC, Esimone CO, Onuigbo EB. Formulation and evaluation of niosomes. Indian J Pharm Sci 2011; 73(3): 323-8.
[PMID: 22457561]

[35] Bartelds R, Nematollahi MH, Pols T, *et al.* Niosomes, an alternative for liposomal delivery. PLoS One 2018; 13(4): e0194179.
[http://dx.doi.org/10.1371/journal.pone.0194179] [PMID: 29649223]

[36] Abdelbary G, El-gendy N. Niosome-encapsulated gentamicin for ophthalmic controlled delivery. AAPS PharmSciTech 2008; 9(3): 740-7.
[http://dx.doi.org/10.1208/s12249-008-9105-1] [PMID: 18563578]

[37] Vyas SP, Mysore N, Jaitely V, Venkatesan N. Discoidal niosome based controlled ocular delivery of timolol maleate. Pharmazie 1998; 53(7): 466-9.
[PMID: 9742041]

[38] Kara A, Rouillard C, Mathault J, *et al.* Towards a multifunctional electrochemical sensing and niosome generation lab-on-chip platform based on a plug-and-play concept. Sensors (Basel) 2016; 16(6): 778.
[http://dx.doi.org/10.3390/s16060778] [PMID: 27240377]

[39] Barani M, Mirzaei M, Torkzadeh-Mahani M, Nematollahi MH. Lawsone-loaded Niosome and its antitumor activity in MCF-7 breast Cancer cell line: A nano-herbal treatment for Cancer. Daru 2018; 26(1): 11-7.
[http://dx.doi.org/10.1007/s40199-018-0207-3] [PMID: 30159762]

[40] Cetin EO, Salmanoglu DS, Ozden I, Ors-Kumoglu G, Akar S, Demirozer M, *et al.* Preparation of ethanol extract of propolis loaded niosome formulation and evaluation of effects on different cancer cell lines. Nutr Cancer 2021; 1-13.
[PMID: 33590797]

[41] Hedayati Ch M, Abolhassani Targhi A, Shamsi F, *et al.* Niosome□encapsulated tobramycin reduced antibiotic resistance and enhanced antibacterial activity against multidrug□resistant clinical strains of

PSEUDOMONAS AERUGINOSA. J Biomed Mater Res A 2021; 109(6): 966-80.
[http://dx.doi.org/10.1002/jbm.a.37086] [PMID: 32865883]

[42] Pardakhty A, Moazeni E, Varshosaz J, Hajhashemi V, Rouholamini Najafabadi A. Pharmacokinetic study of niosome-loaded insulin in diabetic rats. Daru 2011; 19(6): 404-11.
[PMID: 23008685]

[43] Puras G, Mashal M, Zárate J, *et al.* A novel cationic niosome formulation for gene delivery to the retina. J Control Release 2014; 174: 27-36.
[http://dx.doi.org/10.1016/j.jconrel.2013.11.004] [PMID: 24231407]

[44] Muzzalupo R, Trombino S, Iemma F, Puoci F, La Mesa C, Picci N. Preparation and characterization of bolaform surfactant vesicles. Colloids Surf B Biointerfaces 2005; 46(2): 78-83.
[http://dx.doi.org/10.1016/j.colsurfb.2005.09.003] [PMID: 16257519]

[45] Paolino D, Muzzalupo R, Ricciardi A, Celia C, Picci N, Fresta M. *in vitro* and *in vivo* evaluation of bola-surfactant containing niosomes for transdermal delivery. Biomed Microdevices 2007; 9(4): 421-33.
[http://dx.doi.org/10.1007/s10544-007-9046-6] [PMID: 17252206]

[46] Tareen FK, Shah KU, Ahmad N, Ur Rehman A, Shah SU, Ullah N. Proniosomes as a carrier system for transdermal delivery of clozapine. Drug Dev Ind Pharm 2020; 1-24.
[http://dx.doi.org/10.1080/03639045.2020.1764020] [PMID: 32362194]

[47] Khalil RM, Abdelbary GA, Basha M, Awad GEA, El-Hashemy HA. Design and evaluation of proniosomes as a carrier for ocular delivery of lomefloxacin HCl. J Liposome Res 2017; 27(2): 118-29.
[http://dx.doi.org/10.3109/08982104.2016.1167737] [PMID: 27079800]

[48] Gopinath D, Ravi D, Rao BR, Apte SS, Renuka D, Rambhau D. Ascorbyl palmitate vesicles (Aspasomes): Formation, characterization and applications. Int J Pharm 2004; 271(1-2): 95-113.
[http://dx.doi.org/10.1016/j.ijpharm.2003.10.032] [PMID: 15129977]

[49] Ghosh S, Mukherjee B, Chaudhuri S, Roy T, Mukherjee A, Sengupta S. Methotrexate aspasomes against rheumatoid arthritis: Optimized hydrogel loaded liposomal formulation with *in vivo* evaluation in wistar rats. AAPS PharmSciTech 2018; 19(3): 1320-36.
[http://dx.doi.org/10.1208/s12249-017-0939-2] [PMID: 29340978]

[50] Liu Y, Xia Y, Rad AT, Aresh W, Nieh MP. Stable discoidal bicelles: A platform of lipid nanocarriers for cellular delivery. Methods Mol Biol 2017; 1522: 273-82.
[http://dx.doi.org/10.1007/978-1-4939-6591-5_22] [PMID: 27837547]

[51] Abdelkader H, Ismail S, Kamal A, Alany RG. Design and evaluation of controlled-release niosomes and discomes for naltrexone hydrochloride ocular delivery. J Pharm Sci 2011; 100(5): 1833-46.
[http://dx.doi.org/10.1002/jps.22422] [PMID: 21246556]

[52] Manosroi A, Chankhampan C, Ofoghi H, Manosroi W, Manosroi J. Low cytotoxic elastic niosomes loaded with salmon calcitonin on human skin fibroblasts. Hum Exp Toxicol 2013; 32(1): 31-44.
[http://dx.doi.org/10.1177/0960327112454892] [PMID: 23111885]

[53] Hajizadeh MR, Parvaz N, Barani M, *et al.* Diosgenin-loaded niosome as an effective phytochemical nanocarrier: Physicochemical characterization, loading efficiency, and cytotoxicity assay. Daru 2019; 27(1): 329-39.
[http://dx.doi.org/10.1007/s40199-019-00277-0] [PMID: 31134490]

[54] Obeid MA, Gany SAS, Gray AI, Young L, Igoli JO, Ferro VA. Niosome-encapsulated balanocarpol: Compound isolation, characterisation, and cytotoxicity evaluation against human breast and ovarian cancer cell lines. Nanotechnology 2020; 31(19): 195101.
[http://dx.doi.org/10.1088/1361-6528/ab6d9c] [PMID: 31958777]

[55] Moghassemi S, Hadjizadeh A, Omidfar K. Formulation and characterization of bovine serum albumin-loaded niosome. AAPS PharmSciTech 2017; 18(1): 27-33.

[http://dx.doi.org/10.1208/s12249-016-0487-1] [PMID: 26817764]

[56] Muzzalupo R, Tavano L, La Mesa C. Alkyl glucopyranoside-based niosomes containing methotrexate for pharmaceutical applications: Evaluation of physico-chemical and biological properties. Int J Pharm 2013; 458(1): 224-9.
[http://dx.doi.org/10.1016/j.ijpharm.2013.09.011] [PMID: 24060370]

[57] Shahiwala A, Misra A. Studies in topical application of niosomally entrapped Nimesulide. J Pharm Pharm Sci 2002; 5(3): 220-5.
[PMID: 12553889]

[58] Mali N, Darandale S, Vavia P. Niosomes as a vesicular carrier for topical administration of minoxidil: Formulation and *in vitro* assessment. Drug Deliv Transl Res 2013; 3(6): 587-92.
[http://dx.doi.org/10.1007/s13346-012-0083-1] [PMID: 25786376]

[59] Zarei M, Norouzian D, Honarvar B, Mohammadi M, Shamabadi HE, Akbarzadeh A. Paclitaxel loaded niosome nanoparticle formulation prepared *via* reverse phase evaporation method: An *in vitro* evaluation. Pak J Biol Sci 2013; 16(6): 295-8.
[http://dx.doi.org/10.3923/pjbs.2013.295.298] [PMID: 24498794]

[60] Schlich M, Lai F, Pireddu R, *et al.* Resveratrol proniosomes as a convenient nanoingredient for functional food. Food Chem 2020; 310: 125950.
[http://dx.doi.org/10.1016/j.foodchem.2019.125950] [PMID: 31830712]

[61] Akbarzadeh I, Saremi Poor A, Yaghmaei S, *et al.* Niosomal delivery of simvastatin to MDA-MB-231 cancer cells. Drug Dev Ind Pharm 2020; 46(9): 1535-49.
[http://dx.doi.org/10.1080/03639045.2020.1810269] [PMID: 32808813]

[62] Firozian F, Karami S, Ranjbar A, Azandaryani MT, Nili-Ahmadabadi A. Improvement of therapeutic potential N-acetylcysteine in acetaminophen hepatotoxicity by encapsulation in PEGylated nano-niosomes. Life Sci 2020; 255: 117832.
[http://dx.doi.org/10.1016/j.lfs.2020.117832] [PMID: 32450164]

[63] Laguerre M, Bayrasy C, Panya A, *et al.* What makes good antioxidants in lipid-based systems? The next theories beyond the polar paradox. Crit Rev Food Sci Nutr 2015; 55(2): 183-201.
[http://dx.doi.org/10.1080/10408398.2011.650335] [PMID: 24915410]

[64] Hao YM, Li K. Entrapment and release difference resulting from hydrogen bonding interactions in niosome. Int J Pharm 2011; 403(1-2): 245-53.
[http://dx.doi.org/10.1016/j.ijpharm.2010.10.027] [PMID: 20971171]

[65] Luan LB, Zhu JB, Yu WP, Wei KB. [Studies on the preparation of camptothecin niosomes]. Yao Xue Xue Bao 2002; 37(1): 59-62.
[PMID: 12579902]

[66] Marianecci C, Paolino D, Celia C, Fresta M, Carafa M, Alhaique F. Non-ionic surfactant vesicles in pulmonary glucocorticoid delivery: Characterization and interaction with human lung fibroblasts. J Control Release 2010; 147(1): 127-35.
[http://dx.doi.org/10.1016/j.jconrel.2010.06.022] [PMID: 20603167]

[67] Talsma H, Van Steenbergen MJ, Borchert JCH, Crommelin DJA. A novel technique for the one-step preparation of liposomes and nonionic surfactant vesicles without the use of organic solvents. Liposome formation in a continuous gas stream: The 'bubble' method. J Pharm Sci 1994; 83(3): 276-80.
[http://dx.doi.org/10.1002/jps.2600830303] [PMID: 8207668]

[68] Aliño SF, Garcia-Sanz M, Irruarrizaga A, Alfaro J, Hernandez J. High encapsulation efficiencies in sized liposomes produced by extrusion of dehydration-rehydration vesicles. J Microencapsul 1990; 7(4): 497-503.
[http://dx.doi.org/10.3109/02652049009040472] [PMID: 2266475]

[69] Ali Doosti B, Fjällborg D, Kustanovich K, Jesorka A, Cans AS, Lobovkina T. Generation of

interconnected vesicles in a liposomal cell model. Sci Rep 2020; 10(1): 14040. [http://dx.doi.org/10.1038/s41598-020-70562-5] [PMID: 32820180]

[70] Hope MJ, Cullis PR. The role of nonbilayer lipid structures in the fusion of human erythrocytes induced by lipid fusogens. Biochim Biophys Acta Biomembr 1981; 640(1): 82-90. [http://dx.doi.org/10.1016/0005-2736(81)90533-2] [PMID: 7213694]

[71] Deamer D, Bangham AD. Large volume liposomes by an ether vaporization method. Biochim Biophys Acta 1976; 443(3): 629-34. [PMID: 963074]

[72] Jain CP, Vyas SP. Preparation and characterization of niosomes containing rifampicin for lung targeting. J Microencapsul 1995; 12(4): 401-7. [http://dx.doi.org/10.3109/02652049509087252] [PMID: 8583314]

[73] Waddad AY, Abbad S, Yu F, *et al.* Formulation, characterization and pharmacokinetics of Morin hydrate niosomes prepared from various non-ionic surfactants. Int J Pharm 2013; 456(2): 446-58. [http://dx.doi.org/10.1016/j.ijpharm.2013.08.040] [PMID: 23998955]

[74] Marwa A, Omaima S, Hanaa E-G, Mohammed A-SJI. Jops, research. Preparation and in-vitro evaluation of diclofenac sodium niosomal formulations. 2013; 4(5): 1757.

[75] Zarrabi A, Alipoor Amro Abadi M, Khorasani S, *et al.* Nanoliposomes and tocosomes as multifunctional nanocarriers for the encapsulation of nutraceutical and dietary molecules. Molecules 2020; 25(3): 638. [http://dx.doi.org/10.3390/molecules25030638] [PMID: 32024189]

[76] Hong JS, Stavis SM, DePaoli Lacerda SH, Locascio LE, Raghavan SR, Gaitan M. Microfluidic directed self-assembly of liposome-hydrogel hybrid nanoparticles. Langmuir 2010; 26(13): 11581-8. [http://dx.doi.org/10.1021/la100879p] [PMID: 20429539]

[77] Lo CT, Jahn A, Locascio LE, Vreeland WN. Controlled self-assembly of monodisperse niosomes by microfluidic hydrodynamic focusing. Langmuir 2010; 26(11): 8559-66. [http://dx.doi.org/10.1021/la904616s] [PMID: 20146467]

[78] Yamaguchi S, Tsuchiya K, Sakai K, Abe M, Sakai H. Preparation of nonionic vesicles using the supercritical carbon dioxide reverse phase evaporation method and analysis of their solution properties. J Oleo Sci 2016; 65(1): 21-6. [http://dx.doi.org/10.5650/jos.ess15192] [PMID: 26666274]

[79] Yamaguchi S, Kimura Z, Misono T, *et al.* Preparation and properties of nonionic vesicles prepared with polyglycerol fatty acid esters using the supercritical carbon dioxide reverse phase evaporation method. J Oleo Sci 2016; 65(3): 201-6. [http://dx.doi.org/10.5650/jos.ess15217] [PMID: 26876680]

[80] Uchegbu IF, Vyas SPJIjop. Non-ionic surfactant based vesicles (niosomes) in drug delivery. 1998; 172((1-2)): 33-70.

[81] Chen Q, Schönherr H, Vancso GJ. Block-copolymer vesicles as nanoreactors for enzymatic reactions. Small 2009; 5(12): 1436-45. [http://dx.doi.org/10.1002/smll.200801455] [PMID: 19283796]

[82] Chopineau J, Lesieur S, Ollivon MJJotACS. Vesicle formation by enzymic processes. 1994; 116(25): 11582-3.

[83] Wiggenhorn M, Winter G, Haas H, Drexler K. Liposome preparation by single-pass process. Google Patents 2010.

[84] Mayer LD, Hope MJ, Cullis PR. Vesicles of variable sizes produced by a rapid extrusion procedure. Biochim Biophys Acta Biomembr 1986; 858(1): 161-8. [http://dx.doi.org/10.1016/0005-2736(86)90302-0] [PMID: 3707960]

[85] Nowroozi F, Almasi A, Javidi J, Haeri A, Dadashzadeh S. Effect of surfactant type, cholesterol

content and various downsizing methods on the particle size of Niosomes. Iran J Pharm Res 2018; 17 (Suppl. 2): 1-11.
[PMID: 31011337]

[86] Paecharoenchai O, Niyomtham N, Ngawhirunpat T, Rojanarata T, Yingyongnarongkul B, Opanasopit P. Cationic niosomes composed of spermine-based cationic lipids mediate high gene transfection efficiency. J Drug Target 2012; 20(9): 783-92.
[http://dx.doi.org/10.3109/1061186X.2012.716846] [PMID: 22931523]

[87] Mahale NB, Thakkar PD, Mali RG, Walunj DR, Chaudhari SR. Niosomes: Novel sustained release nonionic stable vesicular systems — An overview. Adv Colloid Interface Sci 2012; 183-184: 46-54.
[http://dx.doi.org/10.1016/j.cis.2012.08.002] [PMID: 22947187]

[88] Fond G, Miot S. Nanopsychiatry. The potential role of nanotechnologies in the future of psychiatry. A systematic review. Encephale 2013; 39(4): 252-7.
[http://dx.doi.org/10.1016/j.encep.2013.02.002] [PMID: 23545476]

[89] Mukherjee B, Patra B, Layek B, Mukherjee A. Sustained release of acyclovir from nano-liposomes and nano-niosomes: An *in vitro* study. Int J Nanomedicine 2007; 2(2): 213-25.
[PMID: 17722549]

[90] Patel P, Barot T, Kulkarni P. Formulation, characterization and *in-vitro* and *in-vivo* evaluation of capecitabine loaded Niosomes. Curr Drug Deliv 2020; 17(3): 257-68.
[http://dx.doi.org/10.2174/1567201817666200214111815] [PMID: 32056523]

[91] Yazdi Rouholamini SE, Moghassemi S, Maharat Z, Hakamivala A, Kashanian S, Omidfar K. Effect of silibinin-loaded nano-niosomal coated with trimethyl chitosan on miRNAs expression in 2D and 3D models of T47D breast cancer cell line. Artif Cells Nanomed Biotechnol 2018; 46(3): 524-35.
[http://dx.doi.org/10.1080/21691401.2017.1326928] [PMID: 28509572]

[92] Tavano L, Aiello R, Ioele G, Picci N, Muzzalupo R. Niosomes from glucuronic acid-based surfactant as new carriers for cancer therapy: Preparation, characterization and biological properties. Colloids Surf B Biointerfaces 2014; 118: 7-13.
[http://dx.doi.org/10.1016/j.colsurfb.2014.03.016] [PMID: 24709252]

[93] Yaghoobian M, Haeri A, Bolourchian N, Shahhosseni S, Dadashzadeh S. The impact of surfactant composition and surface charge of niosomes on the oral absorption of repaglinide as a BCS II model drug. Int J Nanomedicine 2020; 15: 8767-81.
[http://dx.doi.org/10.2147/IJN.S261932] [PMID: 33204087]

[94] Zhang Y, Jing Q, Hu H, *et al.* Sodium dodecyl sulfate improved stability and transdermal delivery of salidroside-encapsulated niosomes *via* effects on zeta potential. Int J Pharm 2020; 580: 119183.
[http://dx.doi.org/10.1016/j.ijpharm.2020.119183] [PMID: 32112930]

[95] Kurmi BD, Kayat J, Gajbhiye V, Tekade RK, Jain NK. Micro- and nanocarrier-mediated lung targeting. Expert Opin Drug Deliv 2010; 7(7): 781-94.
[http://dx.doi.org/10.1517/17425247.2010.492212] [PMID: 20560777]

[96] Li M, Du C, Guo N, *et al.* Composition design and medical application of liposomes. Eur J Med Chem 2019; 164: 640-53.
[http://dx.doi.org/10.1016/j.ejmech.2019.01.007] [PMID: 30640028]

[97] Rezvani M, Hesari J, Peighambardoust SH, Manconi M, Hamishehkar H, Escribano-Ferrer E. Potential application of nanovesicles (niosomes and liposomes) for fortification of functional beverages with Isoleucine-Proline-Proline: A comparative study with central composite design approach. Food Chem 2019; 293: 368-77.
[http://dx.doi.org/10.1016/j.foodchem.2019.05.015] [PMID: 31151624]

[98] Marianecci C, Di Marzio L, Rinaldi F, *et al.* Niosomes from 80s to present: The state of the art. Adv Colloid Interface Sci 2014; 205: 187-206.
[http://dx.doi.org/10.1016/j.cis.2013.11.018] [PMID: 24369107]

[99] Wadhwa S, Garg V, Gulati M, Kapoor B, Singh SK, Mittal N. Nanovesicles for nanomedicine: Theory and practices. Methods Mol Biol 2019; 2000: 1-17. [http://dx.doi.org/10.1007/978-1-4939-9516-5_1] [PMID: 31148004]

[100] Kurmi BD, Paliwal SR. Development and optimization of TPGS-based stealth liposome of doxorubicin using Box-Behnken design: Characterization, hemocompatibility, and cytotoxicity evaluation in breast cancer cells. J Liposome Res 2021; 1-17. [PMID: 33724151]

CHAPTER 13

Resealed Erythrocytes: As A Drug Delivery Tool

Krishna Yadav[1], Monika Kaurav[2], Preeti Patel[3], Ashish K. Parashar[4] and **Balak Das Kurmi[2,*]**

[1] *University Institute of Pharmacy, Pt. Ravishankar Shukla University, Raipur, Chhattisgarh-492010, India*

[2] *KIET School of Pharmacy, Ghaziabad-201206, (U.P.) India*

[3] *ISF College of Pharmacy, Moga-142001, Punjab, India*

[4] *Chameli Devi Institute of Pharmacy, Indore-452020, (M.P.), India*

Abstract: Being the most abundant cell in the human body, resealed erythrocytes have been utilized as a promising natural biological carrier for therapeutic delivery. In various therapeutics, delivery resealed erythrocytes are found to be an alternative delivery approach with overcoming toxic and rapid clearance effects, such as enzyme-loaded bioreactors performing vital reaction along with improving the enzymes circulation time, as drug-loaded carrier affords sustained release of drug and in drug, targeting delivers drugs release in specific target organs without recognition by the immune system. From the research level to clinical development, it has been observed that the drug carrier expedition faces many regulatory and industrial process development challenges. Resealed erythrocytes possess many remarkable properties such as biocompatibility, biodegradability, long circulation and flexibility to encapsulate a wide variety of therapeutic compounds *via* employing different chemical and physical methods. It is possible to obtain resealed RBCs by collecting them from the source of concern (*e.g.*, humans, rats, rabbits, pigs, and so forth) through blood samples following the separation of RBCs. A number of techniques are then used for effective drug loadings, including hypotonic dialysis, hypotonic dilution, hypotonic preswelling, endocytosis, lipid fusion, electric cell fusion, and chemical disturbance. Up to date, resealed erythrocytes have been explored as a carrier for various therapeutic drug substances (antiviral, anti-inflammatory, steroids and anticancer, *etc.*), enzymes, antibiotics, and diagnostic agents. The main objective of this chapter is to emphasize the advantages, limitations, source, isolation, loading methodology, characterization parameters, and finally, to pay attention to *in-vivo* studies, clinical applications, and future potential of resealed erythrocytes.

* **Correspondence author Balak Das Kurmi**: KIET School of Pharmacy, Ghaziabad-201206, (U.P.) India; Tel: +919754275553; E-mail: **bdkurmi@gmail.com**

Keywords: Advantages, Biodegradability, Carrier erythrocyte,RBC, Cellular carrier, Characterization parameters, Clinical applications,drug-loaded carrier, Development challenges, Drug delivery, Drug targeting, Diagnostics, Limitations, Isolation, *in-vivo* studies, Loading methodology, Release of drug, Resealed erythrocyte, Source, Therapeutics delivery.

INTRODUCTION

Currently, the industry is dominated by more than 30 powerful therapeutics formulations, with a gross turnover of about 33 billion US dollars and a steady annual increase of around 15%. The resurgence of the need for safe medications fortified to achieve the goal, and with minimal/trivial side effects is the crucial rationale for such emerging considerations for the conveyance of therapeutics. The biodistribution of medications and APIs in the body is one of the first concerns accompanying the systemic conveyance of therapeutics. An idyllic pharmaceutical should only perform its pharmacological activity on the target location while still employing the lowest feasible dose of medication without any side effects on the non-target areas. The purpose should be to increase therapeutic suitability by reducing dose and its frequency [1].

Researchers are currently focusing on a new effort to design a mechanism for medication conveyance that has the greatest therapeutic benefit. The basic idea is based on the controlled dispersal of pharmacological, bioactive, and biotechnological medicines. Therapeutic targeting is a notion that works to transmit therapeutics to (activity) receptors or bodies or other explicit pieces inside the body to transfer medicines completely. Accordingly, it focuses on a functioning bio-atom from efficacious medication conveyance where pharmacological specialists coordinate explicitly to its objective location. Medication targeting can be accomplished either by chemical transformation or by an apposite conveyance carrier [2]. The fundamental measures accompanied by the determination of the transporter in therapeutic targeting are that transporters utilized in the conveyance of the medication ought to have the option to shield the medication from untimely bio-inactivation and uninterrupted the arrival of the medication to the objective location. The transporter satisfying these standards expands the dose-effect of the medication by diminishing the dose and recurrence of the administration.

Natural transporters, such as antibodies, liposomes, macromolecules, erythrocytes (ERS, Red blood cells, RBCs), and others, achieve these optimal qualities. Unlike synthetic transporters, which must be delivered orally or parenterally, these biological transporters may be introduced unswervingly into the circulatory system, allowing for regulated and sustained pharmaceutical conveyance. The cellular transporters/carriers provide significant prospective benefits in biodegradability, biocompatibility, non-immunogenicity, non-pathogenicity, and self-degradability, combined with excellent therapeutic loading skills for different transporters utilized for therapeutic targeting [1]. The various currently available transport systems of medications are either simple or decomposable, such as microparticles, cells, cell phantoms, lipoproteins, liposomes, leucocytes, platelets, and RBCs dissolvable macromolecules, such as monoclonal antibodies, polysaccharide polymers, and decomposable polymers and unpredictable multi-composing designs.

Every different kinds of transporters utilized RBCs in light of their remarkable conduct and feature in giving an idyllic medication conveyance system. Blood is the main fluid in the body that provides vital nutrients and oxygen to cells while also transporting metabolic waste away from them. The plasma in blood makes up around fifty-five percent of the total, with corpuscles accounting for the other forty-five percent. RBCs, leucocytes (WBC) and platelets constitute forty-five percent of blood corpuscles, suspended in blood plasma, which constitutes fifty-five percent of the body's fluid. The bone marrow is where blood cells are formed. All blood cells, such as stem cells, are made from bone marrow. Stem cells are immortal (*i.e.*, they do not perish). Stem cells are also undifferentiated cells that have not yet been converted into a specific cell kind [1]. As they are pluripotent, they have the command to convert into any kind of blood cell. The RBCs are the most prevalent in the blood, and these endless, undifferentiated pluripotent stem cells grow up to RBCs, Leukocytes(LUE), and platelets of the complete cell. LUE, often known as white platelets, is a collection of closely related cell kinds that participate in immunological responses. Monocytes, basophils, eosinophils, lymphocytes, and neutrophils are all kinds of LUE. The chief function of RBCs is to transfer gases during the respiratory cycle. Erythropoiesis is the process through which RBCs are created. Platelets are responsible for converting fibrinogen into fibrin, which has the important function of clotting the blood [1].

RBCs are the most numerous cells of the human body, with possible transporter capacities for the conveyance of therapeutics. These are biocompatible, decomposable, and have impressively long circulatory ½-lives. They can also be filled with some biologically active substances by a range of physical and chemical methods. RBCs have been thoroughly evaluated based on their drug-carrying capability and loading efficiency. Simply collect blood samples from the organism of interest, remove RBCs from plasma, ensnare the medicine in the ERS, and reseal the resultant cell transporters, and you have drug-loaded transporter ERS [1]. As a result, they are known as resealed erythrocytes(R-ERS). This entire cycle is dependent on how these cells respond under osmotic environments. The R-ERS function as lethargic revolving stores upon reinjection, directing therapeutics to reticuloendothelial systems (RES) [3].

HISTORICAL CONCERN OF R-ERS

RBCs were first discovered in 1658 by a Dutch physician who mistook them for fat globules. On the other hand, RBCs were first depicted by Lee Van Hock in the seventeenth century as particles approximately 25 thousand times smaller than fine particles of sand [1, 4]. Nonetheless, about a century later, Howson discovered that these cells are flat discs rather than globules, and he gave an exact representation of them. By understanding hemoglobin's vital role in oxygen transport to diverse tissues, Hoppe Seyler validated Hunefeld's discovery of hemoglobin in the eighteenth century. Reversible oxygenation (together with CO_2 interchange) was thought to be RBCs' key or even exclusive activity until the late 20^{th}century. In any event, our comprehension of ERS capabilities has now vastly expanded to include O_2, CO_2, H_2S, NOinterchange, immunological clearance, and unquestionably the leeway of several other soluble blood constituents like cytokines.

An inquiry to mount the "ERS ghosts" by ATP was presented by researchers, making the first attempt to catch synthetic chemicals in quite a while [1]. Marsden and Ostling conducted a test on filling dextran in RBCs in 1959, and the results were positive, with efficacious ensnarement of dextran with molecular weights of 10-250 KD in ERS ghosts [5]. Around fourteen years later, the primary outlines entrapping ERS ghosts with pharmacological actives for conveyance purposes [6]. The term "carrier ERS" was originally utilized in 1979 to describe medication-stacked ERS [7].

BIOLOGICAL FEATURES OF RBCS

RBCs are the utmost well-known kind of blood cells in the body. They are the primary mechanism of conveying oxygen to body tissues *via* blood flow *via* the circulatory system of vertebrate living beings. RBCs are formed at over 2 million cells/second in the bone marrow and circulate for roughly 100–120 days throughout the body [1, 8]. During this period, they traverse around 250 kilometers *via* the circulatory system before being recycled by Macrophage (MP). RBCs make up around a fourth of the human body cells during each flow duration of roughly 20 seconds. Erythropoiesis is the interplay of ERS materialization. RBCs are formed in the red bone marrow in adults, under the control of erythropoietin and other hemopoietic hormones. RBCs are the most numerous cells in the body, with 5.4 million cells per mm3 of blood in males and 4.8 million cells per mm3 of blood in females. RBCs have a surface area of roughly 136 μm^2 but can grow to a sphere of approximately 150 fl [8]. RBCs have a typical width of 7.8 µm, a thickness of 2.5 µm at the perimeter, 1 µm in the center, and a capacity of 85–90 µm. A biconcave disc has a significantly larger surface area for gas-particle passage through RBCs than a sphere or a cube. RBCs may pass through narrow channels as small as 3 µm in diameter without bursting because of their biconcave structure and flexible nature. The nuclear-derived human ERS is one of the utmost concentrated cells [8]. RBCs can not manufacture protein, complete oxidative reactions accompanying mitochondria, or go through mitosis since they lack cytoplasmic organelles like mitochondria, ribosomes, and nucleus. As a result, they can not duplicate or carry out extensive metabolic exercises. RBCs are composed of around 35 percent solid matter, the majority of which is hemoglobin, and the residual 65 percent water. Lecithin, cholesterol and cephaeline are all found in the lipid content of RBCs. RBCs have a huge extent of K+ than plasma, while plasma has a huge extent of Na+ [8, 9]. Hemoglobin, a heme-containing protein responsible for O_2–CO_2 binding inside RBCs, is encased in the plasma membrane (MB) of ERS. Each RBC has around 280 million hemoglobin fragments. Hemoglobin molecules are composed of four polypeptide chains of the protein globin, and a ring-like non-protein colored ring is a heme attached to each of the four chains. The heme ring reversibly integrates with one oxygen atom in the center, letting each hemoglobin particle attach to four oxygen atoms [8, 9]. The foremost function of the ERS is to wrap and stabilize hemoglobin so that it may function as an oxygen transporter for a comprehensive length of time. Hemoglobin interacts with small diffusible ligands, including Co_2, O_2, and N_2O, and may influence blood pressure control [10]. RBCs' major occupation is the conveyance of oxygen from the lungs to the tissues and carbon dioxide back to the lungs. RBCs are an extremely specific oxygen transporter mechanism in the body. The deficiency of a core in RBCs means that the entire intracellular space is available for oxygen conveyance. Due to the nonexistence of mitochondria in RBCs, energy is created anaerobically in RBCs, and RBCs do not use any of the oxygen atoms they transport. RBCs, alternatively, extract energy from glucose metabolism *via* direct glycolysis and the hexose monophosphate shunt [1, 8].

The MB skeletal proteins of the RBCs are systematized in an unvarying shell and are bound to the RBCsMB. The RBCstructure can go through various reversible changes. A significant component of RBC's endurance is its deformability. Significant components influencing deformability are inner thickness (mostly contributed by RBCs hemoglobin), natural deformability of the MB, and the surface/volume of the cell [11]. The RBCs additionally have different other extremely interesting features, for example, they act as an osmometer since they squeeze when put into a hypertonic solution or swell when put into a hypotonic solution [1, 8, 12]. The RBCs can magnitude basic hemolytic measurements leading to openings orifices on the MBs ranging from 10 nm to 500 nm. These progressions are typically revocable and following hemolysis, the openings close, and the cell acquires its biconcave structure. RBCs are biocompatible transporters for various bioactive constituents, including proteinous therapeutics, since they highlight some special benefits. As RBCs mature, metabolic pathways gradually become inactive, resulting in the loss of the cell MB's intrinsic integrity and the cells' adaptability and chemical composition [12, 13]. Following entry through most of the spleen trabecular, these changes in cells result in cell obliteration. Peritoneal MP, hepatic Kupffer cells, and alveolar MP of the lung, peripheral blood monocytes, and vascular endothelial cells are the other attractive spots for the decimation of the aberrant RBCs or matured cells in the MP of the RES [14]. It has been widely documented that maturation and the advancement of several factors make RBCs identifiable to phagocytosing MP by transforming the chemical architecture of the endothelial surface, *i.e.*, the phospholipid component [12].

STRUCTURAL FEATURE OF ERYTHROCYTE MEMBRANE

It consists of several indistinguishable lipids and proteins. The surface area of the MB is neatly negative, chiefly due to carboxylic sialic acid groups. This negative surface charge prevents the interaction of RBCs with other RBCs and has sufficient distance between them so that they cannot be aggregated with IgG immediately. The isoelectric point is about pH 2, elevated to pH 4-5 when neuraminidase removes the sialic acid proportionately. There is an increase in N-acetylneuraminic acid per human ERS of around 2.4×10^7. The MB's phosphoglycerides substance accounts for almost half of the final lipid composition and includes phosphatidylcholine and phosphatidylethanolamine as key lipids in animal groups. Sphingomyelin and cholesterol are two additional main lipid components of MBs. RBCs cannot integrate lipids, but they do have the capacity to use plasma lipids for lipid turnover and replacements [15].

SELECTION OF ERS AS A DELIVERY CARRIER

RBCs' ability to maintain their form and morphology when put in isotonic (IST) saline often has a key significance in making them apposite transporters for therapeutics and enzymes. For RBCs to be appropriate for the conveyance of therapeutics, they must have the following characteristics [16]:

1. They ought to be of fitting structure and size to empower their entry through the vessels.

2. They ought to have explicit physicochemical features by which the idyllic objective site could be perceived.
3. They ought to be biocompatible with the least possible harmful results.
4. Their degradation products ought to be biocompatible.
5. There ought to be the most reduced or no spillage or draining of medications from the RBCs before the objective is achieved.
6. They ought to have the capability to convey a comprehensive range of medications with various assets.
7. They ought to be physiochemically viable with therapeutics.
8. The transporter system ought to have significant firmness during storage.
9. The medication release at the spot of activity ought to be in a controlled way.
10. They ought to have high medication stacking productivity for a wide range of medications with various features.
11. There ought to be zero chance of set off immunological response.

PROS AND CONS OF ERYTHROCYTES AS A DELIVERY CARRIER

A broad range of pharmacological targets, mostly based on intravenous leisure discharge along with therapeutic conveyance and various other uses, comprises the therapeutics treatment, controlled medication release, hemoglobin content investigations, enzyme treatment, and RES organ use, which are the potential uses of R-ERS as medication conveying devices. Therefore, it is necessary to consider the pros and cons of the conveyance carrier to determine whether the application is so scalable [17].

Advantages of Erythrocytes as a Delivery Carrier

1. There is no trivial chance of a set-off immune reaction.
2. These are the characteristic result of the form that is decomposable in nature with no formation of unsafe items.
3. They have a substantial-unvarying structure and size of the transporter.
4. They have a reasonably dormant intracellular climate.
5. They empower the filling of proteins and nucleic acids in eukaryotic cells by cell mixture with RBCs.
6. They give an idyllic zero-order therapeutic discharge kinetic.
7. They forestall the decimation of the captured therapeutic from inactivation by endogenous chemicals.
8. A varied assortment of proteins and compounds can be loaded into the cells.
9. The alteration of pharmacokinetics and pharmacodynamics limits of medications or chemical substances should be possible.

10. They aid in accomplishing steady-state plasma concentration, diminishing variations in the therapeutic concentration.
11. They ensure the organic entity against the poisonous impacts of medications.
12. They give effortlessness of circulation and can be targeted to the RES organ.
13. They expand the systemic action of the medication by staying in the body for a drawn-out period.
14. There are conceivable outcomes of a decrease in the side effects of the medication.
15. The encapsulation of medications does not need the chemical alteration of the materials to be stacked.
16. This is intriguing since various systems involve a covalent bonding of the medicine and transporter, which could alter the parent drug's intrinsic mobility.
17. The seclusion of RBCs is an easy procedure, and a lot of medication can be consolidated into a small space of cells.
18. They are non-immunogenic in real life and cable to focus on ailing tissue or organ.
19. They work by securing the untimely debasement, deactivation, and discharge of proteins and chemicals.

Disadvantages of Erythrocytes as a Delivery Carrier

1. The biggest downside is that they are eliminated *in vivo* by the RES due to a change in the loading mechanism in cells.
2. Reliable and firm storage techniques are absent.
3. As transporters, they have a limited perspective on the non-phagocytic objective tissue.
4. They can run over issues, for example, cell amassing or dose dumping.
5. They can experience the spillage of a few of the loaded materials from the encapsulated RBCs.
6. There are possibilities of tainting because of the source of the blood, the apparatus utilized, and the therapeutic entrapping areas.
7. The collection and handling of RBCs require a high degree of fortification.
8. It is not possible to infuse straightforwardly into the cell nucleus.
9. They have a fourteen-day storage lifespan at the very least.
10. It is anything but a monetary procedure.

PROCESS OF ISOLATION OF ERYTHROCYTES

Fresh whole blood is typically utilized for loading the therapeutic or chemical compound. Since the capturing ability of the RBCs obtained from fresh blood is better than that of the matured ones. The fresh whole blood is considered and isolated, followed by promptly chilling to 4°C and keeping it for less than 2 days [1, 3, 17]. For therapeutic conveyance, mammalian RBCs have been utilized like the RBCs of mice, rats, rabbits, chickens, goats, sheep, pigs, monkeys, cows, and humans (Table **13.1**). Blood is removed from the cardiovascular or splenic puncture on account of little animals and by means of veins in the case of huge animals in a syringe holding a drop of the anticoagulant. Blood samples were obtained in tubes containing anticoagulants such as EDTA, heparin, and other anticoagulants to isolate RBCs. In a cooling centrifuge, the obtained whole blood is centrifuged at a speed of 2500 rpm for 5 minutes at a temperature of 4±1°C. After centrifugation, the serum and buffy coatings are cautiously parted, and the encapsulated cells are rinsed many times with 7.4 pH phosphate buffer saline (PBS). The rinsed ERS are then diluted in buffer solution (BFS). The rinsed ERS are then positioned in an acid-citrate-dextrose BFS for up to 48 hours at 40°C before use [1, 3, 17].

Table 13.1. Various processing parameters for the isolation of ERS.

Source of RBCs	Centrifugal Force (g)	Composition of the Buffer Utilized
Mouse	100-500	10 MmMPP /DSP, pH 7.0; 5mm Adenosine; 5mmMagnesium chloride; 10 Mm Glucose
Rabbit	500-1000	10 MmMPP/DSPpH 7.0
Goat	500-1000	10 MmMPP/ DSP, pH 7.0
Sheep	500-1000	10 MmMPP/DSP, pH 7.0; 5 MmMagnesium chloride
Dog	500-1000	15 MmMPP/DSP, pH 7.0; 5 MmMagnesium chloride; 10 Mm Glucose
Pig	500-1000	10 MmMPP/DSP, pH 7.0
Cow	1000	10-15 MmMPP/DSP, pH 7.0; 2MmMagnesium chloride; 10 Mm Glucose
Horse	1000	10 MmMPP/DSP, pH 7.0; 2 MmMagnesium chloride; 10 Mm Glucose
Human	<500	154Mm NaCl Or 10mmMPP/DSP, Ph 7.0; 2mmMagnesium chloride; 10 Mm Glucose
Monopotassium Phosphate: MPP; Disodium phosphate: DSP.		

TECHNIQUES OF DRUG LOADING OR ENCAPSULATION IN ERYTHROCYTES

Different techniques are utilized to encapsulate therapeutics or bioactives in ERS. They involve physical approaches (*e.g.*, electrical pulse), systems based on osmosis, and chemical-basedapproaches (*e.g.*, MBperturbation of the RBCsby chemical agent) (Fig. **13.1**) [18]. Despite the technique utilized, the modelcharacteristics for the effective loading of the medication must have a higher solubilityin water dissolvability, resentment against debasement inside RBCs, absence of any chemical or physical interaction with RBCs, and noticeable pharmacokinetic and pharmacodynamics features [18].

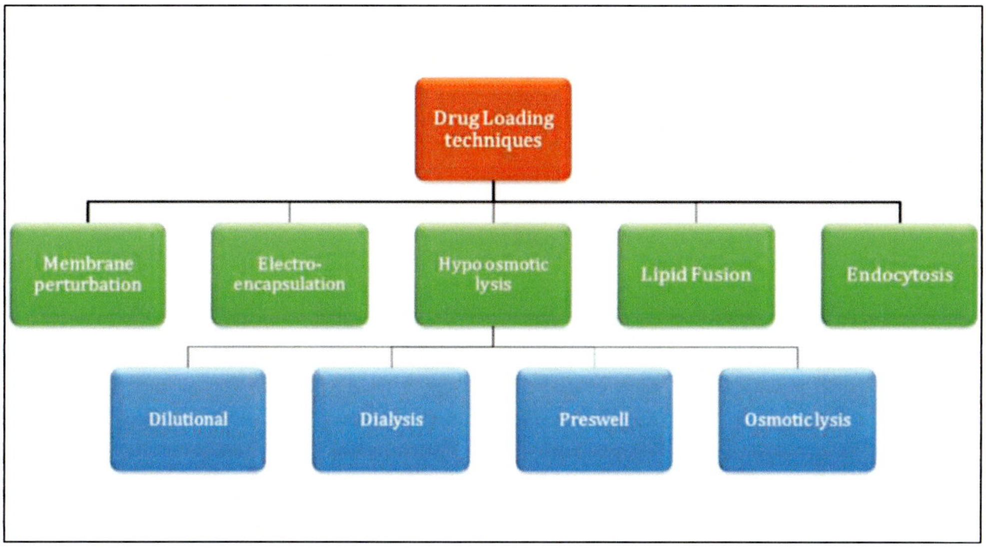

Fig. (13.1). Various techniques of therapeutic loading or encapsulation in ERS.

Hypo-Osmotic Lysis Techniques

This technique relies on the propensity of RBCs to go through reversible swelling when put in the hypotonic solution (Fig. **13.2**). RBCs have a remarkable capacity to go through reversible modifications in structure with or without capacity modification and reversible deform under pressure [19]. The cells embrace a spherical form to contain more capacity while maintaining the same surface area. Nonetheless, the form changes from biconcave to spherical when the volume increases. The absence of the excess MB causes this shift; consequently, the cell's surface area remains constant. The acquisition capacity is approx. 25–50 percent. The cells can sustain their structure till the cellular material reaches ~150 mOsm/kg, over which the MB breaches. Now, on the MB are generated certain temporary holes of 200–500 Å [19]. Cells are emptied following cell lysis. The remains are known as a ghost of an ERS. Heterogeneous and mainly three kinds of ghost populations are found.

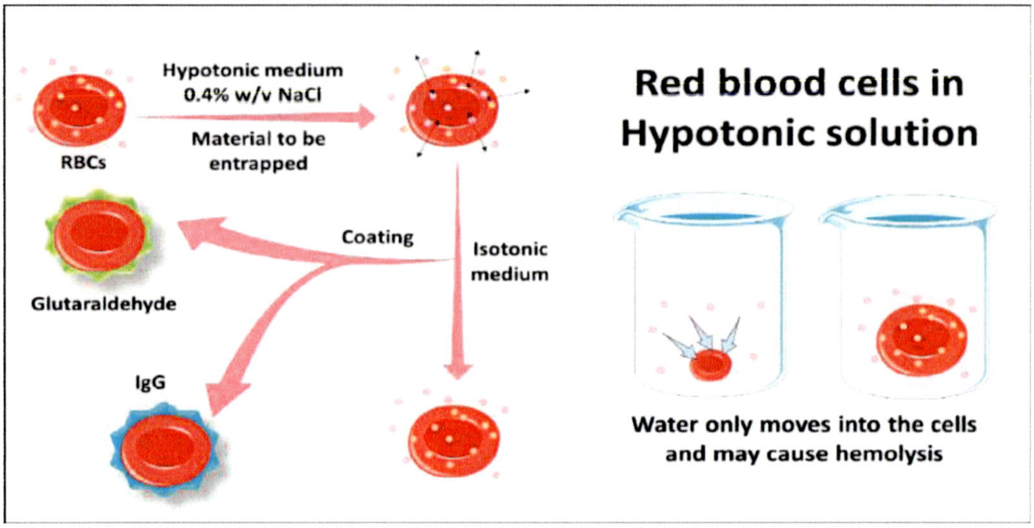

Fig. (13.2). The Hypo-osmotic lysis techniques for therapeutic loading into ERS.

- Kind I ghost is the ones that reseal as soon as the hemolysis stops.
- Kind II ghosts reseal after hemolysis is reversed, *i.e.*, after alkali ions are added.
- Kind III ghosts are the ones that continue to leak under various laboratory conditions.

Depending on how the broken MB may be resealed by reconstruction of IST environments, these RBCs are being utilized as a therapeutic carrier. These cells persist with their peculiar biconcave form after incubating and recover their distinctive impermeable RBCs by introducing enough KCl of 1.54 M, restoring isotonicity [19]. During resealing, 4 mM magnesium salts, 10 mM glucose, and 2 m Madenosine are introduced to the above definitive concentration, where the preservation of cellular energy metabolism is desirable.

The group of experts investigated in this respect for RBC capture of non-diffusible therapeutics and thereby promoted a new methodology for loading pharmaceuticals into RBCs. They developed a tool known as a "red cell loader." Different naturally active substances were embedded in RBCs during blood banking utilizing merely 50 ml of the blood sample within 2 hours at room temperature. During this procedure, the concentration with hemofilter and IST restoration of cells is preceded by 2 hypotonic dilutions for washed ERS [1]. The results have shown that around 30% of therapeutics were loaded with 35-50 percent of cell recuperation. *In vivo*, the treated RBCs displayed conventional durability. It was also shown that by enhancing their detection by tissue MP, identical cells might be utilized to target therapeutics [19].

Hypotonic Dilutional Technique

Hypotonic dilution was the prime technique inspected for the entrapment of chemical substances into RBCs (Fig. **13.3**) and is a unique, least difficult, and quickest strategy. This strategy dilutes a volume of ladenRBCs with 2 to 20 parts of an aqueous solution containing medication [20]. The solution's tonicity is then reconstituted by introducing a hypertonic BFS. The acquired mix is then centrifuged at a predetermined speed, the supernatant fluid is then thrown out, and the pellet is rinsed with IST BFS. The main shortcomings of this technique are low encapsulation and a substantial amount of hemoglobin and other cell fragment depletion. The encapsulated cells' circulatory ½-life is also reduced due to this [21].

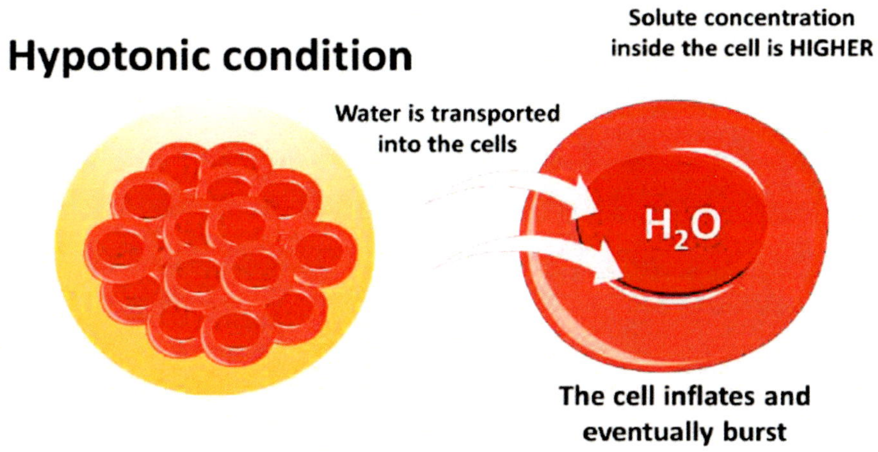

Fig. (13.3). The hypotonic dilutional technique of therapeutic loading.

RES MP quickly phagocytize these cells, allowing them to be utilized to target RES organs in the future. The hypotonic dilutional technique is most frequently utilized to encapsulate catalysts such as B-glycosidase and B-galactosidase, arginase, and asparaginase, just as bronchodilators, for example, salbutamol [20, 21].

Pre-Swell Dilutional Hemolysis

In 1975, Rechsteiner pioneered this approach, later reformed by Jenner and associates for therapeutic loading (Fig. **13.4**) [1]. This strategy includes swelling the ERSprimarily by putting them in a marginally hypotonic solution without going through lysis [22]. The swollen cells are obtained in the subsequent stage by centrifugation at stumpy speed. At that point, comparatively small volumes of watery medication solution are introduced to the lysispoint. The lethargic swelling of cells brings about great preservation of the cytoplasmic elements and subsequently great endurance *in vivo*. The scheme relies on a hypotonic BFS without rupture on the criterion of immediate controlled swelling of RBCs. This fusion is at lower g values at that stage. Therefore, the disposal of the supernatant and thus the introduction of 100-120 ml of an aqueous solution of the therapeutic to the lysis zone is inserted. The mixture is centrifuged between the therapeutic supplement processes [23]. The endpoint of lysis is characterized by the vanishing of a certain barrier between the cell fraction and the supernatant following centrifugation. The formation of a cell combination is reinstated at the lysis stage by introducing a certain hypertonic BFS. The resulting cell suspension is then treated to reseal ERS at 37°C. This strategy is less complicated and faster than many ways and renders cells less detrimental. The therapeutics that are incorporated in ERS utilizing this strategy comprise asparaginase, insulin, propranolol, cortisol-21-phosphate, cyclophosphamide, methotrexate, enalapril levothyroxine, metronidazole, and isoniazid [22, 23].

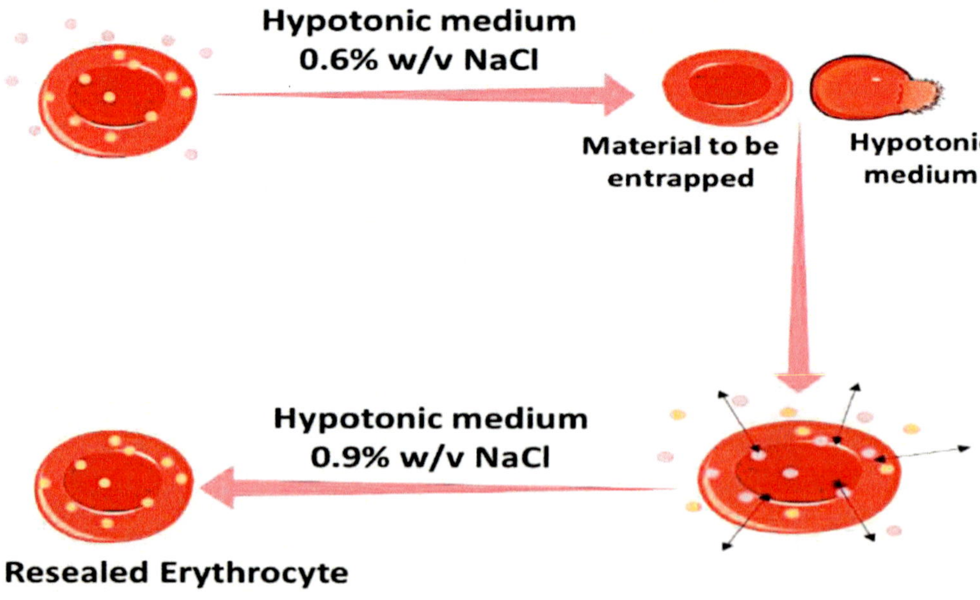

Fig. (13.4). Pre-swell dilutional hemolysis technique of therapeutic loading into ERS.

Hypotonic Dialysis

Klibansky Dale was the first to propose this approach for encapsulating lipids and enzymes (Fig. **13.5**) [1]. Various techniques are based on the idea that a semipermeable dialysis MB increases the intracellular to extracellular volume proportion for biomolecules during lysis and resealing. In this technique, an IST stabilized suspension of RBCs with a hematocrit of 70 to 80 is made and positioned in a standard dialysis tubing flooded with 10 to 20 parts of a hypotonic BFS. The medium is swirled at a slow pace for 2 hours [24]. The tonicity of the dialysis tube can be reestablished by simply introducing a predetermined volume of hypertonic BFS to the nearby medium or by substituting the medium with IST BFS. The medication to be encapsulated can be introduced either at the start of the test by solubilizing the medicine in an IST cell suspending BFS within a dialysis sack or after the shaking is completed by introducing the therapeutic to a dialysis bag. By utilizing,Roper explored a normal hemodialysis device to entrap a therapeutic in RBCs. The erythro-suspension and the drug which is entering the blood chamber arepositioned in this interaction and the hypotonic solution is then positioned in the receptor chamber [1]. This steered to the notion of "continuous flow dialysis" and one of the additional aspects of this methodology was that, with a 70-80 percent recovery, a high entanglement limit, and a significant automation control with interaction variables, the high capture productivity is in the range of 30-50 percent. This incorporates shortcomingslike long handling time and the need for specialized devices. This strategy has been utilized for embodying proteins like inositol, B-galactosidase, glucocerebrosidase, hexaphosphatase, and asparaginase, just as medications, for example, pentamidine, Adriamycin, and gentamicin, interleukin-2, and human recombinant erythropoietin [1, 24].

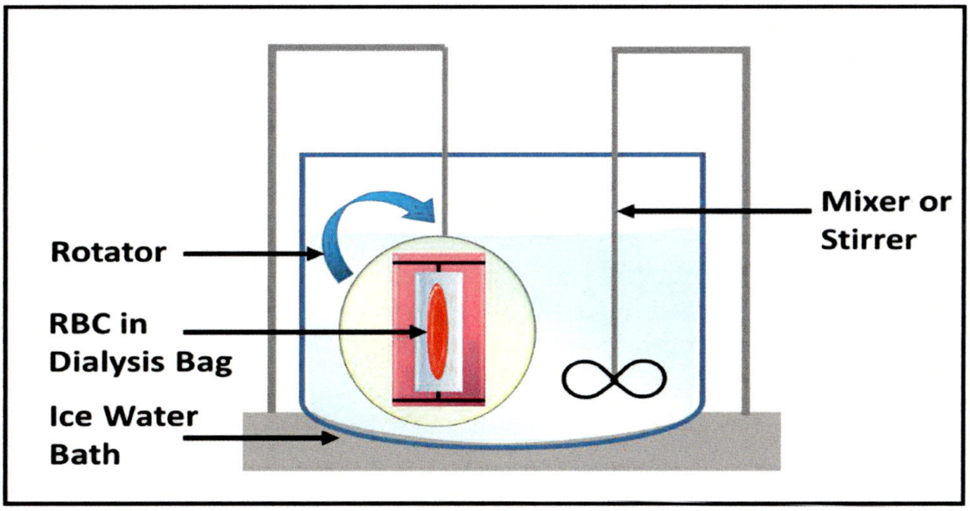

Fig. (13.5). Hypotonic dialysis technique of therapeutic loading into ERS.

Isotonic Osmotic Lysis

Schrier pioneered this method in 1975 [24]. The osmotic pulse method is well-known because it uses chemical or physical techniques to achieve IST hemolysis (Table **13.2**). It might be in the form of IST or non-IST solutions. When ERS are incubated in solutions containing highly permeable fluid to MBs, the solution may diffuse into cells owing to the concentration gradient. Following that, water is added to maintain osmotic balance [25]. Chemicals like urea, ammonium chloride, and polyethylene Glycol have been employed to achieve IST hemolysis. Furthermore, this approach is not resistant to deviations in MB structure.

Table 13.2. The assessment of various kinds of hypo-osmotic lysis techniques.

Technique	Entrapment Efficiency	Pros	Cons
Hypotonic dilution	20-40	The quickest and most simplistic method, particularly for therapeutics with small molecular weights	The effectiveness of entrapment has lowered
Hypotonic dialysis	30-45	ERS with higher structural stability and MB preservation have better *in vivo* survival	It takes a long time. The size variations of R-ERS is heterogeneous
Presswell dilutional hemolysis	30-90	Good cytoplasm retention and *in-vivo* sustainability	-
IST osmotic lysis	-	*in-vivo* stability and good cytoplasm retention	Only giant molecules are impermeable, and the process takes time

Membrane Perturbation

This technique depends on how RBCs, when presented to specific chemical substances like polyene antibiotics, for example, halothane,amphotericin-B, and so on, there is an increment in the layer penetrability of the ERS. The vital drawback of this technique is that it acquires irrevocable alterations in the cell MB; consequently, this strategy is not so renowned. Kitao and Hattori, in 1980, utilized this strategy for productive ensnarement of the antineoplastic medication daunomycin in human and mouse RBCs [26].

Electro Encapsulation or Electro-Insertion

This methodology, also termed electroporation, entails producing electrically induced permeability transformations at large MB potential variances. The methodology is centered on the perception that an electrical jolt causes permanent alterations in the ERSMB, unbolted by a dielectric interruption. By maintaining the orifices in an IST liquid at 37°C, the pores can be resealed. In this interaction, ERS is suspended in IST fluid in an electrical release compartment [27]. To yield a square-wave potential, a capacitor linked to an external circuit is charged to an explicit voltage and then released over a definite period utilizing cell suspension. The idyllic electric field power ranges from 1-10 kW/cm and the optimum release period from 20-160 μ second. There is a reverse link between electrical field power and time of release. The therapeutic to be encapsulated is introduced to the medium in which the cells are dispersed from the commencement of the experimentation [15]. Either inter and intracellular electrodes directly or by magnitude, supplying an inner electrical field to the cells produces possible MB-wide disparities. The pore generation level is determined by pulse resistance, electric field strength, and ionic strength of the suspension media [27].

In addition, the MB, when breached, is impermeable to its cytoplasmic macromolecules, regardless of the size of the holes, instantly spreads between the additional space and the intracellular space. Due to its macromolecular substance's colloidal osmotic pressure factors, the cell layer finally denatures. The colloidal osmotic hemoglobin pressure factor is approximately 30 mOsm attributable to ERS. This pressing element promotes water and particulate flooding, which causes cell expansion. However, when the cell capacity reaches 155 percent of its characteristic volume, the MB bursts [27].

As a result, cell lysis might be viewed as a secondary impact of electrical MB alteration. Because cell lysis is induced by colloidal osmotic swelling, avoiding lysis is to transform the colloidal osmotic pressure factor of the cell macromolecules. This is thought to be possible due to the formation of massive particles such as serum bovine or tetrasaccharide stachyose, and ribonucleases. It aids in the neutralization of colloidal osmotic swelling caused by electrically punctured ERS. Under osmotically controlled conditions, pores stay open for a few days at 40°C. As a result, therapeutics may be loaded into RBCs. If medication expansion is completed at this time, medications will overflow into RBCs. To gradually reseal these pores, an appropriate technique might be applied [1].

One benefit of this process is that it enables for more even transport of entrapped cells utilizing osmotic techniques. The necessity for specialized equipment and the operation's intricacy is this technique's key restrictions. Nonetheless, the approach's entrapment capability is up to nearly 35 percent. Its average lifespan of resealed cells is virtually the same as that of conventional cells made by this current method. This method may encapsulate various substances in the core of ERS, including urease, sucrose, methotrexate, human glycophorin, isoniazid,

DNA strands, and latex particles ranging in diameter from 0.2 μm to 5 μm [28, 29].

Encapsulation by Endocytosis

Schrier and his colleagues were the first to explain this methodology in 1975. This includes mixing 1part of washed compressed RBCs with 9parts of BFS solution comprising 2.5 mM ATP, 2.5 mM $MgCl_2$, and 1 mM $CaCl_2$ for two minutes at room temperature. The holes generated by this technique are resealed by utilizing 154 mM of NaCl and incubating at 37°C for 2 min. The capture of medication content ensues by endocytosis. The vesicle layer isolates endocytosed content from the cytoplasm, shielding it from the ERS and the other way around [3, 15]. The different medications captured by this technique are primaquine and vinblastine, amino-quinolones, chlorpromazine, and hydrocortisone, phenothiazines, propranolol, Vitamin A, and tetracaine.

Loading of the Drug by an Electric Cell Fusion Technique

The drugs are entrapped in the ERS ghost, which is also trailed by the adherence of these cells to the desired cells in this procedure. The utilization of an electric pulse, which induces the release of a captured agent, emphasizes the combination even more. This approach infuses a cell-explicit monoclonal antibody into a ghost ERS. Chemical cross-linking of a particular surface protein of intended cells may be utilized to induce a reaction in the immune system to manage loaded cells and guide them to the targeted cells [30].

Lipid Fusion Method

The exchange of lipid-encased therapeutic vesicles occurs in this mechanism, which involves fusing lipid vesicles carrying bioactives with human ERS. The encapsulation efficacy of this approach is modest. The researchers fused human ERS with lipid vesicles containing inositol hexaphosphate and discovered that inositol hexaphosphate loading in RBCs might diminish hemoglobin's oxygen proclivity in intact ERS. Another set of researchers attempted to reseal tyrosine kinase into human RBCs by rapidly freezing and defrosting them in fluid, encouraging results [1, 15].

CHARACTERIZATION OF R-ERS

ERS act as a transporter to convey therapeutics to the desired cells when they are filled with the right therapeutic candidate and sealed. Therefore, the characterization of formulated carriers for the conveyance of therapeutics is important. The R-ERS are tested for the conveyance of therapeutics suitability utilizing different *in vitro* and *in vivo* characterization parameters.

In Vitro Characterization

The Structure and Surface Morphology

The morphology of ERS determines how long they will survive once they have been administered. R-ERS are morphologically represented by comparing them with untreated RBCs by utilizing transmission electron microscopy (TEM) or Scanning electron microscopy (SEM). Different methods, such as stage contrast microscopy, can similarly be utilized. In a few cases when spherical ERS (spherocytes) is detected, light microscopy reveals no discernible alteration in R-ERS. The SEM examinations have uncovered that a greater part of the cells keeps up their biconcave discoid structures after the drug encapsulation step, and few stomatocytes are spherocytes with introversion in one point framed. Sometimes, cells of more modest size (microcyte) are likewise noticed [31]. Electron microscopy perception might be made of the morphological modifications in the ERS incited as a natural osmosis-based entrapment strategy when they are exposed to solutions of various osmolality. In an examination of rats, it was seen that when rat's ERS are presented to IST solutions (300 mosM/kg), they show the typical structure of discocyte (biconcave). This advances the surface structure of stomatocytes (uniconcave) when they are presented with solutions of 200 mosM/kg, accomplishing the spherocytic structure (the utmost delicate of the three) when the solution is 150 mosM/kg [32, 33].

Drug Content

Determining encapsulation efficiency has mainly been utilized to detect therapeutic content within cells. The procedure involves deproteinizing sealed, loaded RBCs (0.5 mL) with acetonitrile (2.0 mL), then centrifuging for 10 minutes at 2500-3000 rpm. After that, the composition of the distinct supernatant is determined by utilizing spectrophotometry [3, 15].

In Vitro Release of Drug and Content Hemoglobin Study

The drug loading may result in prolonged drug release, affecting the pharmacokinetic profile of the encapsulated ERS *in vivo*. The drug spillage from loaded ERS is investigated *in vitro* by utilizing autologous plasma or an isosmoticBFS at 37°C with the hematocrit level maintained between 0.5-50 percent. At predetermined adjusted time intervals, the supernatant is examined and substituted with an equivalent measurement of autologous plasma or BFS.

Several inventors proposed utilizing a dialysis bag to investigate *in vitro* release from encapsulated ERS [32].

Modifications in the permeability of the RBCs MB during the entrapment process may reduce the amount of hemoglobin in ERS. Furthermore, the relationship between hemoglobin and therapeutic release aids in identifying the components involved in the release of drugs lodged in ERS [34]. The RBCs suspension is utilized to evaluate hemoglobin leakage, and the absorbance of the supernatant at 540 nm is measured by utilizing a spectrophotometer. Drug/hemoglobin releases are directed simultaneously from drug-loaded cells. The cell suspension (5 percent hematocrit in PBS) is kept at 40 degrees Celsius in amber-colored glass vessels [21, 33]. The supernatant is removed at a pre-decided interval span utilizing a hypodermic needle outfitted with a 0.45 m filter and afterward deproteinized utilizing methanol and therefore are, assessed for drug content. After centrifugation, the supernatant from each sample is extracted and analyzed, and the percent hemoglobin release can be determined by utilizing the formula:

$$Percent\ hemoglobin\ release = \frac{A_{540}\ of\ sample\ - A_{540\ of\ blank}}{A_{540}\ of\ 100\%\ hemoglobin}$$

Or

$$Mean\ copuscular\ hemoglobin\ [MCH(PG)] = \frac{\text{Hemoglobin}\ \left(\frac{\text{gm}}{\text{100 ml}}\right) \text{X 10}}{\text{Erythrocyte counts}\ \left(\frac{\text{Millions}}{Cu\ mm}\right)}$$

Cell Counting and Recovery Study

This entails calculating the total number of RBCs per unit volume of whole blood, mainly by utilizing mechanical counting equipment. The volume of the ERS suspension when entrapped and the hematocrit might be utilized to assess how many red cells were recovered. The key goal is to reduce cell loss and improve cell recovery during the entrapment process [32].

Osmotic Shock and Fragility Study

The unusual fragility of red cells is ascertained by osmotic fragility. By exposing untreated or encapsulated ERS to hypotonic solutions and causing them to swell, the overall fragility of the red cells can be examined. When RBCs are presented with solutions of various constitutions, their structure transforms because of osmotic irregularity [30]. In order to take into account the effects of shifting constitutions, drug-encapsulated RBCs are incubated separately for 10 minutes at 37 ± 2 °C, followed by centrifugation for 10 minutes at 2000 rpm. The R-ERS solution in deionized water is dispersed and centrifuged at 300 rpm over 15 min to determine the osmotic shock. The supernatant is spectrometrically evaluated for a percentage of hemoglobin release [30].

Turbulence Fragility (TF)

The TF is one more feature that hinges upon alterations in the veracity of the cell layer and mirrors the opposition of encapsulated cells counter to hemolysis coming about because of the turbulence stream inside the flow. Turbulence stun assists in determining the stability of stacked ERS in the face of turbulence pressure exerted by the cells in the presence of *in vivo* circulation turbulence. It is the level of reproducing the obliteration of encapsulated cells in infusion [21]. The TF is assessed by passing the cell suspension *via* needles with a smaller inner diameter, such as 30 gauges, at a flow velocity of 10 ml/min, equivalent to blood flow, or by rapidly quivering the cell suspension. It is accompanied by the collection of an aliquot, after which the centrifuged sample is evaluated. Medication encapsulated ERS seem to be less impervious to disturbance, most likely showing obliteration of cells after shaking. In this way, hemoglobin and medication delivered after the method are resolved in the two cases. The findings show that resealed cells are more vulnerable to turbulence than previously reported [21, 32].

Erythrocyte Sedimentation Rate (ESR)

It is a measurement of the stability of RBCs suspension in plasma that is linked to the quantity and size of red cells and the general grouping of plasma protein, particularly fibrinogen and globulins. The rate of RBCs sedimentation in a typical tube is determined to complete this measure. A typical blood ESR ranges from 0 to 15 mm/hour, implying dynamic and nonsensical sickness measures exist [16].

Determination of Entrapped Magnetite

To confirm the quantity of a given metal in a sample, the atomic absorption spectroscopic technique is utilized. The HCl is introduced to a static measure of magnetite-bearing ERS, and the substance is warmed for 2 hours at 60°C, at that point 20 percent w/v trichloroacetic acid is added; consequently, the supernatant acquired afterward centrifugation is utilized to decide magnetite quantity utilizing atomic absorption spectroscopy [16].

In Vitro Stability

The R-ERS' stability is assessed by seeding the cells in an iso-osmotic BFS or autologous plasma with a 0.5 to 5% hematocrit at temperatures ranging from 4-37°C [3, 15].

Storage

In vitro storage has an indisputable effect on the therapeutic attainment of R-ERS as a conveyance of the therapeutics method. By utilizing fair storage strategies, drug-loaded ERS may be developed on a wide scale while upholding their endurance and therapeutic material. However, consistent and feasible storage options have become a stumbling block to the ERS carrier for clinical use [25].

Hank's balanced salt solution and acid citrate-dextrose at 4°C are the most popularly known storage media [25]. Cells retain their physiologic and transporter features at this temperature for at least fourteen days. The adding of calcium-chelating agents or purine nucleosides extends the duration that cells last in the bloodstream after being reinjected. Similarly, to achieve stabilization, R-ERS are exposed to MB stabilizing agents such as dimethyl 3, 3-dithio-bis propionamide, dimethyl sulfoxide, toluene-2-4-diisocyanate, glutaraldehyde, and toluene-2-4-diisocyanate, preceded by lyophilization or sintered glass filtration [25]. The resulting powder remained stable for at least a month, with no visible alterations. The other storage strategies observed are entrapment of a prodrug that transforms to the parent therapeuticmerely at internal heat levels, more glycerol freezing, and rescindable immobilization in alginate or gelatin gels.

In Vivo Characterization

The survival time available for use after resealing ERS is utilized to determine their adequacy. Labeling cells with ^{51}Cr or fluorescent markers, including fluorescein isothiocyanate and capturing 14C sucrose or gentamicin, are some of the approaches utilized to detect *in vivo* survival time. The flow survivability energy of R-ERS has a bimodal manner, with a quick islay of cells in the initial twenty-four hours after injection, trailed by a leisurely decay stage with a half-life of days or weeks. Biological characteristics affect R-ERS' *in vivo* ability in general [15].

ADMINISTRATION OF R-ERS

Intravenous is the foremost typical route of administration, preceded by subcutaneous, intraperitoneal, intranasal, and then oral. Intraperitoneal injection demonstrated that the longevity of cells accessible for use was comparable to intravenous injection [35]. An ERS-based bioadhesive system for the nasal conveyance of propranolol. They discovered that twenty-five percent of resealed cells stayed usable for fourteen days, and they suggested this injection approach as a technique for extravascular steering of RBCs to peritoneal MP. The primed cell delivered entrapped therapeutics at the injection site after subcutaneous administration for modest release of captured therapeutics [35].

DRUG RELEASE MECHANISM FROM R-ERS

Since these transporters are proteins with certain features similar to catalysts, comprising particularity, a variety of substances penetrate cells through a specific MB protein system. A drug can efflux out of ERS transporters in one of three different ways: 1. Diffusion across the cell's MB. 2. Phagocytosis of resealed cells by RES MP, resulting in therapeutic aggregation within the macrophage, followed by stagnant conveyance, and 3. Making use of a specific mode of transportation. The other method involves the subcutaneous conveyance of ERS to lymph nodes, preceded by hemolysis to administer the therapeutic [1, 3].

The process of phagocytosis is widely utilized to remove RBCs from circulation. Cross-linking determines when the cells will be eliminated, mostly by the liver or the spleen. Following antibody cross-linking or heat therapy, R-ERS are swiftly eliminated from circulation by phagocytic cells situated mostly in the liver and spleen. The pace at which a single molecule infiltrates into a lipid bilayer determines the diffusion rate. It is most noticeable in a molecule with maximum lipid solvency [1, 3].

APPLICATIONS OF R-ERS

The impending therapeutic use of R-ERS as a medication conveyance system encompasses an extensive range of pharmacological and therapeutic goals, the majority of which are based on intravenous gradual medication discharge and targeted conveyance of therapeutics. The R-ERS have a wide range of possible uses in veterinary and human medication [1, 3]. These cells could be utilized as free-flowing transporters to distribute (convey) drugs over a significant time or to a particular body part, such as the spleen, liver, and lymph nodes. The drug-loaded R-ERS are also in the preclinical stage for a significant proportion of the medication conveyance.

Drug Targeting

The conveyance of therapeutics should be transported to a designated destination with a specific goal in mind, showing the highest therapeutic index and the fewest side effects. R-ERS can go about as medication transporters just as targeting nanobots. Since the alteration of the MB is experienced by MP, ERS with surface reform is often utilized to target organs of mononuclear phagocytic systems/RES [20].

Targeting RES Organs

Since the modifications in the MB are identifiable by MP, ERS with surface functionalization is utilized to target organs in mononuclear phagocytic systems/ RES. Surface modulation of glutaraldehyde, carbohydrates including sialic acid, sulfhydryl, and chemical cross-linking are some of the approaches utilized. Antibodies such as ant-Rh or other kinds of antibodies can also be utilized to cover the surface of ERS [1, 3].

TargetingNon-RES

Other organs have also been targeted with R-ERS. The use of ultrasound waves, loading of photosensitive material, paramagnetic particles alongside the therapeutic, and antibody linkage to the ERS layer to obtain the specificity of action are all examples of various methodologies for targeting non-RES organs [15].

Targeting the Liver

A massive amount of metabolic abnormalities which reflect the extent of insufficiency or lacking enzymes can be controlled by introducing these enzymes. The reduced distribution 1/2-life of enzymes, adverse reactions, and toxic symptoms are the most common side effects accompanied by exogenous enzyme therapy. However, these complications can be effectively addressed by administering these enzymes as R-ERS. P-galactosidase, P-glucosidase, and P-glucuronidase are some of the enzymes employed. Glucocerebrosidase-loaded ERS can treat the symptoms caused by glucocerebrosidase accumulation in the liver and spleen [20].

Delayed Drug Release

Delayed-release conveyance methods are specifically designed to achieve a long-term pharmacological effect of the therapeutic by continuously administering the medication over a long period after the administration of a single dose. Since R-ERS in the bloodstream has a long life span, they can be utilized as circulating storehouses for antitumor, anti-parasitic, and antibiotic therapeutics, much like cardiovascular therapeutics [36]. This is only possible if the therapeutic and the medication loading technique is chosen and do not alter the biochemical and anatomical features of ERS. Various bioactives are entrapped in ERS to provide prolonged therapeutic release in the systemic circulation to effectively treat ailments. Antimicrobials, antineoplastic, supplements, and steroids are all transported efficiently by R-ERS. Thus, they have been utilized as a depot device for the regulated and delayed release of anti-parasitic, anti-amoebic, antineoplastic, vitamins, veterinary, steroids, anti-biotic, and cardiovascular therapeutics [36].

Elimination of Toxic Agents

The researchers utilized R-ERS to investigate cyanide inebriation and discovered that cyanide inebriation was hampered by a murine ERS carrier holding bovine rhodanese and $Na_2S_2O_3$. Antagonizing organophosphorus intoxication by a delivered ERS carrying a recombinant phosphodiesterase has also been taken into consideration [37].

Enzyme Therapy

Enzyme therapy has a significant capacity for the long-term treatment of a metabolic condition. The transporter preferred for enzyme treatment should have a long circulatory life, though extreme take-up would also be advantageous. For both of these causes and an overall carrier of other therapeutic agents, ERS provides the strongest prospects [36]. They are a stereotypical transporter of endogenous substrates, non-immunogenic, non-harmful, decomposable, and easy to obtain. By steering these, *i.e.*, enzymes β-Glucoside, β-galactosidase, and β-glucuronidase as R-ERS, metabolic diseases caused by deficient or absent enzymes may be treated [36, 38].

Targetingof Parasitic Disease

The exceptional capacity of R-ERS to specifically amass inside RES organs makes them helpful in the conveyance of parasitic medications. Parasitic illnesses include holding parasites in the RES structures that can be effectively constrained by using R-ERS by this strategy. The investigations carried out on animal model outcomes were positive for encapsulated ERS against malarial, leishmanial, and amoebic disorders [33, 39].

Delivery of Therapeutic Agents

Antiviral therapeutics encapsulated and other therapeutic agents in R-ERS for effective conveyance and targeting have been the subject of several studies (Table **13.3**). Since nucleotides and nucleotide analogs make up a considerable portion of antiviral therapeutics, their encapsulation in ERS and passage across the MB must be carefully considered [40]. The ability of ERS to deliver anticancer therapeutics, including methotrexate, asparaginase, bleomycin, and Adriamycin, has been reported [15]. A preferential treatment affecting the liver, accompanied by the lungs, kidneys, and spleen, was also reported during a methotrexate investigation in ERS. Desferrioxamine-loaded ERS were utilized to treat excess iron deposition caused by repeated transfusions in thalassemic patients. Since mature ERS are killed in RES organs, which contributes to an aggregation of iron in these body parts, targeting this agent to the RES is hugely advantageous [1].

Table 13.3. Application of R-ERS in different therapeutic approaches.

Approaches	Therapeutic or Targeting Agents	Application
Application of R-ERS in the targeting of RES organs		
Diseases in lysosomal storage	C-glucuronidase; Lysosomal enzymes; 13-galactosidase and 6-glucosidase	To carry lysosomal enzymes and medicines to erythrophagocytic cell lysosomes
Gaucher's disease	Glucocerebrosidase	The loaded cells stayed in the treated patient for ten days without causing any side effects. Atypical blood counts, blood pressure, and kidney functions were also reported.
Liver cancer	Adriamycin, Bleomycin, Carboplatin, Gentamycin, and other anticancer therapeutics	Hepatic carcinomas are being targeted.
Parasitic condition	ERS loaded with pentamidine and immunoglobulin G, and ERS treated with glutaraldehyde	Therapeutics that target parasitic infections in which the parasite is found in the organs of RES, such as macrophage-enclosed leishmaniasis.
RES Iron Overload Removal	Deferoxamine, an iron-chelating therapeutic, is utilized.	An antimalarial medication, primaquine phosphate, and an antiamoebic therapeutic, metronidazole, are also targeted at the liver.

(Table 13.3) cont.....

Approaches	Therapeutic or Targeting Agents	Application
Toxic Agent Elimination	Bovine rhodanese and sodium thiosulphate-containing murine carrier ERS	Antagonize the fatal impacts of potassium cyanide in mice by antagonizing cyanide toxicity
Application of R-ERS in the targeting of non-RES organs		
ERS that react to magnets	Small paramagnetic elements are encapsulated in ERS	Due to the impact of an outward magnetic arena, localization to a specific area
Photosensitized ERS	Methotrexate was utilized to photosensitize the mice, which were then exposed to a haematoporphyrin derivative	The use of a combination of chemotherapy and photodynamic therapy in the treatment of cancers in the body that are not found in the RES dominant organs may be beneficial. OR as a photo-activated methotrexate carrier/conveyance device in tumor therapy
Antibody attached ERS	Antibody decoration of therapeutic carrier ERS that have been resealed	The targeting of therapeutic to the RES
Ultrasound-guided ERSconveyance	RBCs and colloidal particles	Targeted micro particle disruption with ultrasound causes microvessel ruptures, allowing conveyance to tissue.
Application of R-ERS in therapeutic conveyance		
Antiviral agents	ERS loaded with azidothymidine homodinucleotide	Azidothymidine, antiretroviral therapy, is delivered gradually.
	Analogue of an antiviral nucleotide	Encapsulated in ERS for macrophage targeting
	Azidothymidine heterodinucleotide and Acyclovir	Defense against the Human Immunodeficiency Virus or the Herpes Simplex Virus *via* selective conveyance to MP.
Enzymes	Asparaginase (L-asparaginase) Dehydratase of aminolevulinate	It's utilized to cure leukemia. To help an adolescent who has been poisoned by lead.

CONCLUSION

This chapter centers on the aptness of ERS as natural carriers. It displays the different idle biomedical utilization of RBCs-centered medication conveyance systems that open new points of view to the idea of utilizing own cells for health benefits. Subsequently, the R-ERS is the proficient transporter for different biological proteins and medications for conveyance and targeting. Nonetheless, the idea desires more rationalization to turn into a customized medication conveyance system. The vast majority of the investigations in this space are in the *in vitro* stage. The continuous activities overall stay behind to venture into preclinical and, at that point, clinical examinations to demonstrate the capacities of these capable conveyance carriers.

FUTURE PROSPECTS

Aside from the broad-spectrum aids of utilizing ERS as a conveyance of therapeutics carrier, they may also be utilized for vaccine conveyance to achieve controlled release of immunizing agents to lessen the recurrence of doses for prime immunization or foster single-dose antibodies. They work as a vehicle for the antigen to be delivered to antigen-presenting cells, MP, and dendritic cells. Based on the magnitude of alterations in functioning and structure that occurred in the antigen capture process, ERS loaded with antigens may be configured to serve as regulated antigen release (due to minor cell alterations) or antigen targeting (due to major cell alterations) vehicles. The loading technique is responsible for the inborn adjuvant of encapsulated ERS.

CONSENT FOR PUBLICATION

Not applicable.

CONFLICT OF INTEREST

The authors declare no conflict of interest, financial or otherwise.

ACKNOWLEDGEMENT

Declared none.

REFERENCES

[1] Bellad K, Nanjwade B, Kamble M, *et al.* Resealed erythrocyte based drug delivery system. World J Pharm Pharm Sci 2017; 6: 446-82.

[2] Sawant K, Soni H, Rayasa M. Investigation on resealed erythrocytes as carriers for 5-fluorouracil. 2001; 63: 105-9.

[3] Begum GS, D M. An advanced review on resealed erythrocytes. Asian Journal of Pharmaceutical Research and Development 2019; 7(6): 55-61. [http://dx.doi.org/10.22270/ajprd.v7i6.606]

[4] Moras M, Lefevre SD, Ostuni MA. From erythroblasts to mature red blood cells: Organelle clearance in mammals. Front Physiol 2017; 8: 1076. [http://dx.doi.org/10.3389/fphys.2017.01076] [PMID: 29311991]

[5] Marsden NV, Ostling SG. Accumulation of dextran in human red cells after haemolysis. Nature1959; 184(723–724)

[6] Ihler GM, Glew RH, Schnure FW. Enzyme loading of erythrocytes. Proc Natl Acad Sci USA 1973; 70(9): 2663-6. [http://dx.doi.org/10.1073/pnas.70.9.2663] [PMID: 4354859]

[7] Magnani M, Rossi L, D'ascenzo M, Panzani I, Bigi L, Zanella A. Erythrocyte engineering for drug delivery and targeting. Biotechnol Appl Biochem 1998; 28(1): 1-6. [PMID: 9693082]

[8] Tortora GJ, Sandra RG. Principles of Anatomy and Physiology. 7th ed., New York: Harper Collins College Publishers 1993.

[9] Allen TM, Williamson P, Schlegel RA. Phosphatidylserine as a determinant of reticuloendothelial recognition of liposome models of the erythrocyte surface. Proc Natl Acad Sci USA 1988; 85(21): 8067-71.
[http://dx.doi.org/10.1073/pnas.85.21.8067] [PMID: 3186707]

[10] Jia L, Bonaventura C, Bonaventura J, Stamler JS. S-nitrosohaemoglobin: A dynamic activity of blood involved in vascular control. Nature 1996; 380(6571): 221-6.
[http://dx.doi.org/10.1038/380221a0] [PMID: 8637569]

[11] Millán CG, Marinero MLS, Castañeda AZ, Lanao JM. Drug, enzyme and peptide delivery using erythrocytes as carriers. J Control Release 2004; 95(1): 27-49.
[http://dx.doi.org/10.1016/j.jconrel.2003.11.018] [PMID: 15013230]

[12] Serafini S, Rossi L, Antonelli A, *et al.* Drug delivery through phagocytosis of red blood cells. Transfus Med Hemother 2004; 31(2): 92-101.
[http://dx.doi.org/10.1159/000078042]

[13] Rossi L, Serafini S, Pierigé F, *et al.* Erythrocyte-based drug delivery. Expert Opin Drug Deliv 2005; 2(2): 311-22.
[http://dx.doi.org/10.1517/17425247.2.2.311] [PMID: 16296756]

[14] Loegering DJ, Grover GJ, Schneidkraut MJ. Effect of red blood cells and red blood cell ghosts on reticuloendothelial system function. Exp Mol Pathol 1984; 41(1): 67-73.
[http://dx.doi.org/10.1016/0014-4800(84)90008-X] [PMID: 6468637]

[15] Jain S, Jain NK. Resealed erythrocytes as drug carriers. In: Jain N, Ed. Controlled and Novel Drug Delivery. New Delhi: CBS Publishers and Distributors Pvt Ltd 2004; pp. 256-81.

[16] Hirlekar R, Patel P, Dand N, Kadam V. Drug loaded erythrocytes: As novel drug delivery system. Curr Pharm Des 2008; 14(1): 63-70.
[http://dx.doi.org/10.2174/138161208783330772] [PMID: 18220819]

[17] Gill R. Resealed erythrocytes as a potential drug carrier system. Int J Pharm Sci Res 3.

[18] Hamidi M, Tajerzadeh H. Carrier erythrocytes: An overview. Drug Deliv 2003; 10(1): 9-20.
[http://dx.doi.org/10.1080/713840329] [PMID: 12554359]

[19] DeLoach JR, Harris RL, Ihler GM. An erythrocyte encapsulator dialyzer used in preparing large quantities of erythrocyte ghosts and encapsulation of a pesticide in erythrocyte ghosts. Anal Biochem 1980; 102(1): 220-7.
[http://dx.doi.org/10.1016/0003-2697(80)90342-5] [PMID: 6766688]

[20] Deloach J, Ihler G. A dialysis procedure for loading erythrocytes with enzymes and lipids. Biochim Biophys Acta, Gen Subj 1977; 496(1): 136-45.
[http://dx.doi.org/10.1016/0304-4165(77)90121-0] [PMID: 836891]

[21] Talwar N, Jain NK. Erythrocytes as carriers of metronidazole: In-vitro characterization. Drug Dev Ind Pharm 1992; 18(16): 1799-812.
[http://dx.doi.org/10.3109/03639049209040903]

[22] Alpar HO, Lewis DA. Therapeutic efficacy of asparaginase encapsulated in intact erythrocytes. Biochem Pharmacol 1985; 34(2): 257-61.
[http://dx.doi.org/10.1016/0006-2952(85)90133-9] [PMID: 3966927]

[23] Rechsteiner MC. Uptake of proteins by red blood cells. Exp Cell Res 1975; 93(2): 487-92.
[http://dx.doi.org/10.1016/0014-4827(75)90478-4] [PMID: 1098917]

[24] Dale GL, Villacorte DG, Beutler E. High-yield entrapment of proteins into erythrocytes. Biochem Med 1977; 18(2): 220-5.
[http://dx.doi.org/10.1016/0006-2944(77)90093-X] [PMID: 410409]

[25] Muzykantov VR. Drug delivery by red blood cells: Vascular carriers designed by mother nature. Expert Opin Drug Deliv 2010; 7(4): 403-27.
[http://dx.doi.org/10.1517/17425241003610633] [PMID: 20192900]

[26] Kitao T, Hattori K, Takeshita M. Agglutination of leukemic cells and daunomycin entrapped erythrocytes with lectin *in vitro* and *in vivo*. Experientia 1978; 34(1): 94-5.
[http://dx.doi.org/10.1007/BF01921924] [PMID: 620752]

[27] Kinosita K Jr, Tsong TT. Hemolysis of human erythrocytes by transient electric field. Proc Natl Acad Sci USA 1977; 74(5): 1923-7.
[http://dx.doi.org/10.1073/pnas.74.5.1923] [PMID: 266714]

[28] Tsong TY, Kinosita K Jr. Use of voltage pulses for the pore opening and drug loading, and the subsequent resealing of red blood cells. Curr Stud Hematol Blood Transfus 1985; 51(51): 108-14.
[http://dx.doi.org/10.1159/000410233] [PMID: 4004753]

[29] Mitchell DH, James GT, Kruse CA. Bioactivity of electric field-pulsed human recombinant interleukin-2 and its encapsulation into erythrocyte carriers. Biotechnol Appl Biochem 1990; 12(3): 264-75.
[PMID: 2360992]

[30] Li LH, Hensen ML, Zhao YL, Hui SW. Electrofusion between heterogeneous-sized mammalian cells in a pellet: Potential applications in drug delivery and hybridoma formation. Biophys J 1996; 71(1): 479-86.
[http://dx.doi.org/10.1016/S0006-3495(96)79249-4] [PMID: 8804630]

[31] Pierigè F, Serafini S, Rossi L, Magnani M. Cell-based drug delivery. Adv Drug Deliv Rev 2008; 60(2): 286-95.
[http://dx.doi.org/10.1016/j.addr.2007.08.029] [PMID: 17997501]

[32] Luque J, Garı'n M, Sanz S, *et al.* The use of resealed erythrocytes as carriers and bioreactors. In: Magnani M, DeLoach JR, Eds. Advances in Experimental Medicine and Biology. Springer Nature Switzerland AG 1992; pp. 81-9.

[33] Hamidi M, Tajerzadeh H, Dehpour AR, Rouini MR, Ejtemaee-Mehr S. *in vitro* characterization of human intact erythrocytes loaded by enalaprilat. Drug Deliv 2001; 8(4): 223-30.
[http://dx.doi.org/10.1080/107175401317245903] [PMID: 11757780]

[34] Garín MI, López RM, Sanz S, Pinilla M, Luque J. Erythrocytes as carriers for recombinant human erythropoietin. Pharm Res 1996; 13(6): 869-74.
[http://dx.doi.org/10.1023/A:1016049027661] [PMID: 8792424]

[35] Vyas SP, Talwar N, Karajgi JS, Jain NK. An erythrocyte based bioadhesive system for nasal delivery of propranolol. J Control Release 1993; 23(3): 231-7.
[http://dx.doi.org/10.1016/0168-3659(93)90004-O]

[36] Gupta A, Mishra A, Bansal P, *et al.* Cell based drug delivery system through resealed erythrocyte - A review. Int J Pharm Sci Drug Res 2010; 02: 23-30.

[37] Pei L, Omburo G, Mcguinn WD, *et al.* Encapsulation of phosphotriesterase within murine erythrocytes. Toxicol Appl Pharmacol 1994; 124(2): 296-301.
[http://dx.doi.org/10.1006/taap.1994.1035] [PMID: 8122276]

[38] Ropars C, Avenard G, Chassaigne MBT-M. Large-scale entrapment of drugs into resealed red blood cells using a continuous-flow dialysis system. Drug and Enzyme Targeting Part B. 242-8.

[39] Talwar N, Jain NK. Erythrocytes as carriers of primaquine-preparation: Characterization and evaluation. J Control Release 1992; 20(2): 133-41.
[http://dx.doi.org/10.1016/0168-3659(92)90159-O]

[40] Fraternale A, Rossi L, Magnani M. Encapsulation, metabolism and release of 2-fluoro-ara-AMP from human erythrocytes. Biochim Biophys Acta, Gen Subj 1996; 1291(2): 149-54. [http://dx.doi.org/10.1016/0304-4165(96)00059-1] [PMID: 8898876]

CHAPTER 14

Gene Therapy: A New Avenue for the Management of Ophthalmic Diseases

Kesavan Karthikeyan[1,*], Nivedita Gautam[1], Olivia Parra-Marín[2] and Selvasankar Murugesan[3]

[1] *Department of Pharmacy, Guru Ghasidas Vishwavidyalaya (A Central University), Bilaspur, Chhattisgarh, India*

[2] *Departamento de Biología Molecular y Biotecnología, Instituto de Investigaciones Biomédicas, Universidad Nacional Autónoma de México, Ciudad Universitaria, 04510, Ciudad de México, Mexico*

[3] *Mother and Child Health Department, Sidra Medicine, Doha, Qatar*

Abstract: Gene therapy aims at intercellular delivery of functional genetic material to the affected area to restore its function or block a dysfunctional gene using viral vectors (Adeno-associated virus) or non-viral vectors (liposomes, SLNs). Gene therapy for the management of ocular diseases is emerging with improved and encouraging results. The Eye has well-defined anatomy, tight ocular barriers, and immune-privileged. It is a perfect target for gene therapy. Recently, many clinical trials are underway or have been completed. The success of these clinical trials promotes the treatment of several ocular diseases (Age-related macular degeneration, glaucoma, retinitis pigmentosa, and choroideremia). Gene therapy should possess an efficient targeting capacity and longstanding gene expression. Viral vectors are mainly used for gene therapy, but due to the risk associated with immunogenicity and mutagenesis, non-viral vectors are widely utilized. This chapter summarizes the recent development of therapeutic gene delivery approaches for the effective management of ocular diseases and their use in ophthalmology.

Keywords: Gene therapy, Non-viral, Ocular delivery, Ocular gene therapy, Viral.

INTRODUCTION

The human eye is an inaccessible, unique, and highly complex organ specified for photoreception. Its complex anatomy and physiology make it a vastly protected organ [1]. The eye ball consists of three primary layers, i) sclera and cornea (on the outside), ii) the retina (on the inside), and iii) in between is the uvea layer.

* **Corresponding author Kesavan Karthikeyan:** Department of Pharmacy, Guru Ghasidas Vishwavidyalaya (A Central University), Bilaspur, Chhattisgarh, India; Tel: +917587483123; E-mails: **kesavanmpharm@gmail.com** and **k7_76@rediffmail.com**

Akhlesh K. Jain & Keerti Mishra (Eds.)

Generally, the whole human eye is partitioned into two chambers: the anterior (at the front lobe) and the posterior (at the back lobe) [2]. The eye chambers (anterior and posterior) function individually after the ocular administration of any drug [3]. The most popular and accepted administration route for ocular disorders, especially for the eye's anterior segments, is the topical route, as it offers easy administration, low cost, and patient compliance [4]. But the topical route is associated with problems like attaining the optimum amount of drug at the target action. Moreover, conventional ocular dosage forms have poor or low bioavailability because of precorneal loss aspects: tear drainage, brief residence time in the cul-de-sac, non-productive absorption, and relatively low permeability feature of the corneal epithelial membrane [5]. Consequently, of these factors, not more than only 5% of administered drugs penetrate the eye [6].

Ocular disorders like diabetic retinopathy, glaucoma, age-related macular degeneration (AMD), and different types of retinitis pigmentosa cause damage to the eye's posterior segment, leading to impaired vision and blindness [7]. Approaches like topical (local), systemic, intravitreal, and periocular (comprising subconjunctival, sub-Tenon's, and retrobulbar) routes are the different administration routes for the treatment of posterior eye segment diseases. But the delivery of drugs to the rear section of the eye is the most challenging task due to protecting biological barriers. In contrast, the current approaches for managing ocular diseases have had limited achievements [8, 9]. Due to instant drainage *via* nasolacrimal ducts, impermeability of the corneal epithelium, absorption in the systemic circulation, and the blood-aqueous barrier restrict the topical route of administration.

On the contrary, the systemic route of administration to the posterior segment gets obstructed by the blood-retinal barriers and toxicities caused due to repeated systemic administration of drugs which are liable to aggravate because of nonspecific absorption [10, 11]. Therefore, intravitreal injections are the most preferred to deliver the drug to the tissues of the posterior section, and effective drug concentration can be achieved. Still, retinal detachment, hemorrhage, endophthalmitis, and cataract are some of the inbuilt side effects associated with this route of administration. Recently, intravitreal sustained-release devices, including implant devices, liposomes, and microspheres, offer effective treatment of posterior segment diseases. However, they necessitate intraocular surgery, and periodical substitution and are liable to side effects like intravitreal injections [12]. Different approaches such as permeation enhancers/cyclodextrins addition and viscosity enhancers were less significant to improve bioavailability. In recent times, enhanced ocular drug absorption was achieved by evasion/inhibition of drug efflux pumps. However, unwanted effects are evident due to their long-term use [13].

Many vivid changes have been observed in ocular drug delivery areas over a period. Understanding various approaches to gene delivery on the eye is a new opening of opportunities. The human eye is a highly immune-privileged spot with unique characteristics for designing successful ocular gene therapy. The anterior segment of the eye is protected from total immunological responses. Transportation of exogenous genes (*in vivo*) to the eye possesses high potential for ocular disease prevention and cure, employing genes as drugs. Genes are advantageous compared to conventional drugs as when the genes are inserted into the cells, they can release products for a longer period, which will enhance the duration of action of the commercial drugs available. The potential use of specific promoters targets the desired transgene expression. Restricting the gene expression to the particular cell type would prevent the adjacent tissues and reduce the subsidiary effects. In addition to this, gene expression can be easily regulated [14].

Ongoing studies in developing an improved gene-drug delivery system for ocular diseases will enhance drug delivery to the cell-specific targeting to minimize the immune responses. Therefore, this chapter is formed to summarize the latest development in the field of gene-drug delivery, surveyed in relevance to their application in ophthalmology.

Anatomy and Physiology of Eye

The human eye has distinctive anatomy and is a complex organ. Structurally, the whole eye is categorized into two major parts: the anterior and posterior segments (Fig. **14.1**). Approximately 1/3rd of the eye covering the conjunctiva, cornea, aqueous humor, ciliary body, iris, and lens make up the anterior segment. On the other hand, the remaining back portion of the eye, *i.e.*, choroid, sclera, retinal pigment epithelium, optic nerve, neural retina, and vitreous humor, frame the posterior segment. Some diseases cause significant risk to the eye's vision, such as the anterior segment suffering from allergic conjunctivitis, glaucoma, anterior uveitis, and cataract. In contrast, diabetic retinopathy and age-related macular degeneration (AMD) affect the posterior segment of the eye [15].

In contrast with the other drug delivery systems of the body, more significant challenges are being faced by the ocular drug delivery system, due to the manifestation of various ocular barriers. Usually, these innate and unique ocular barriers are anatomically and physiologically meant to protect the eye from foreign materials [16] and maintain vital ocular functions [17]. These barriers are particular, *viz.* topical, systemic, and injectable, based on the route of administration [16].

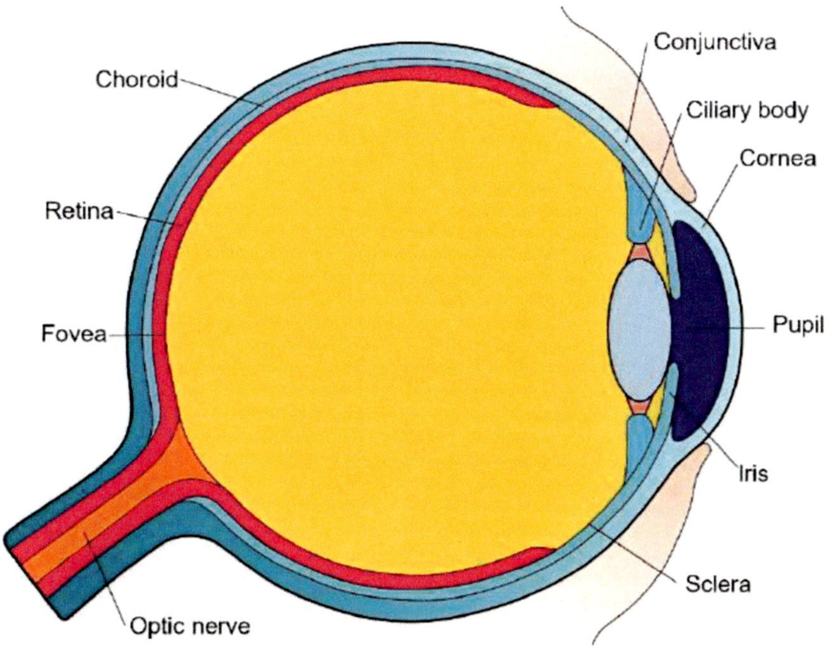

Fig. (14.1). Structure of the eye.

Barriers to Ocular Drug Delivery

The eye is a unique and complex organ, and the ocular barriers pose a difficult challenge for framing a drug delivery system. In order to alter and improve ocular absorption, it is essential to conquer these ocular barriers as they hinder the permeation of drugs to both the segments of the eye (anterior and posterior), making the delivery system a complicated and challenging job. Barriers to the anterior segment permeation are static barriers, including stroma, corneal epithelium, and blood-aqueous barrier (Fig. **14.2**) Dynamic barriers include lymph flow, conjunctival blood flow, and tear drainage [18]. At the same time, posterior segment barriers are most challenging for drug delivery in the back of the eye, like the retina and choroid.

Ocular Barriers

The topical route for treating the diseases of the anterior eye segment is extensively adopted as a non-invasive route. About 90% of the commercial formulations are in convectional dosage form (eye drops) due to effortless administration and patient comfort [19, 20]. After administration, only a tiny amount of eye drops (approx 1-5%) reaches the intraocular tissues, whereas 90-95% gets eliminated frequently within 5-6 minutes, irrespective of the volume administered [21].

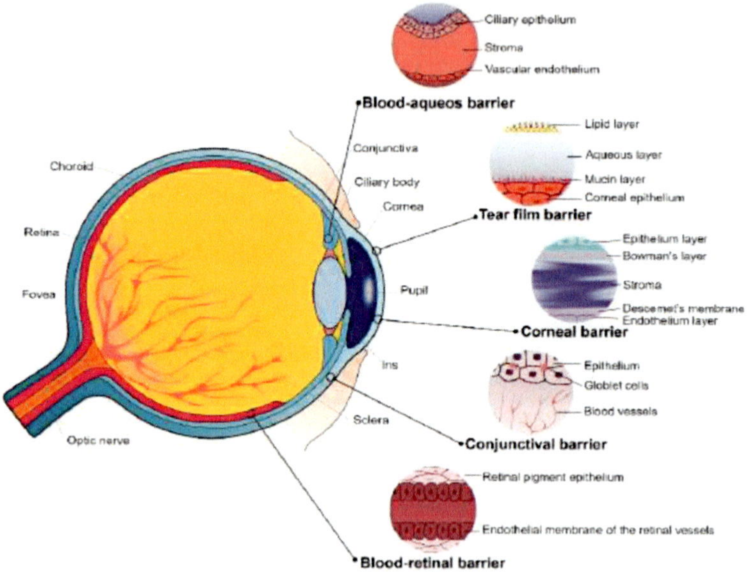

Fig. (14.2). Barriers to ocular drug delivery.

Tear

Tear film prevents dehydration and furnishes protection to the corneal epithelial layer in the eye. The tear film consists of three distinct layers: an inside mucin layer (secreted by goblet cells in the conjunctiva), an aqueous middle layer, and an outer layer of lipid [22]. It is the first precorneal barrier that decreases the effective concentration of the instilled drug. Significantly less dose (less than 5%) reaches aqueous humor after topical administration. A large fraction vanished due to lacrimation, dilution with tear fluid, nasolacrimal drainage, and tear turnover, resulting in reduced bioavailability [11]. Additionally, accelerated clearance and drug binding to teat proteins cause a reduction in the effective concentration of the drug [21].

Cornea

The cornea, the anterior-most layer, a clear and avascular structure of the eye having 12 mm diameter and 520 mm thickness, acts as a mechanical barrier by limiting the passage of exogenic substances inside the eye and protecting ocular tissues [23]. The human corneal layers are: i) corneal epithelium layer, ii) basement membrane layer, iii) Bowman's layer, iv) stroma, v) Descemet's membrane, and vi) endothelium layer [24].

The epithelium layer: Layers of columnar cells originated from the epidermal ectoderm form the epithelium layer. Tear film covers it from the outer region, and internally it comes in connection to the aqueous humor. The lipophilic nature and tight junction in the mature epithelial cells confine access to hydrophilic drugs and macromolecules [25, 26].

The stroma: The stroma structurally is formed by a lamellar arrangement of collagen fibrils and is composed of an extracellular matrix. About 85-90% of corneal thickness comprises stroma. They are extremely hydrated composition (collagen) exerting a significant diffusional permeation barrier of highly lipophilic drug moiety as it is hydrophilic [27].

The endothelial layer: A monolayered endothelium is packed between stroma (aqueous compartment) and aqueous humor has permeable tight junctions (also known as desmosomes) that permit the free flow of molecules in between the aqueous compartments [28].

Factors like lipophilicity, charge, molecular weight and degree of ionization affect the passage of topically administered drugs *via* the corneal route [27]. Small-sized lipophilic drugs can easily permeate through the cornea. After passing it, they reach aqueous humor and the anterior uvea [25]. Another major significant barrier is the efflux transporter (active on the plasma membrane of corneal cells) that bounds the permeation of active constituents from reaching targeted ocular sites. Various researchers have identified and revealed the expression of drug discharge pumps such as multidrug-resistant proteins (MRPs), P-glycoprotein (P-gp), breast cancer resistant protein (BCRP), and their contribution to drug discharge at cell surface using human and rabbit cornea [29 - 31].

Conjunctiva

Conjunctiva is a thin, transparent, and highly vascularized membrane subsisting of an epithelium (2-3 cell thick layers). The former surface of the sclera is covered by the bulbar conjunctiva and is folded to form the Palpebral conjunctiva at the fornix (fornix conjunctiva). The first barrier is the bulbar conjunctiva, which strictly permeates the topically administered therapeutic agent into the eye. Compared to the corneal route, this way of permeation is appropriate for large and water-soluble drugs [32, 33]. Conjunctiva possesses rich vasculature different from the cornea, and after crossing the conjunctiva, a large volume of applied drug is eliminated by the systemic circulation. Whereas the residual drugs get penetrated *via* sclera, which (its permeability lies between conjunctiva and cornea) is higher permeable than the cornea but less permeable than the conjunctiva [34].

Blood Ocular Barriers

The aqueous lens and vitreous constitute the interior portion of the eye. A clear liquid filled in the anterior and posterior chambers of the eye is aqueous. In contrast, transparent and avascular connective tissues of the vitreous are filled in the space between the lens and the retina. This inert gel, like vitreous, consists of water (99%), collagen, hyaluronic acid, and ions [35]. Systemic application through oral or intravenous administration is the main route for attaining and maintaining significant drug concentrations at the retina and the vitreous in various posterior segment disorders. However, this route has several disadvantages with high doses, and due to blood-ocular barriers, a tiny proportion of the drug reaches ocular tissues [36]. Blood-ocular barrier (BOB), blood-aqueous barrier (BAB), and blood-retinal barrier (BRB) systems, split the interior portion of the eye and functionally control the traverse of blood between the posterior and anterior chambers, thus maintaining the clarity and transparency of ocular fluids [35]. Despite various biological obstructions, an intravitreal injection can overcome the BOB. Still, the threats of lens impairment, endophthalmitis, retinal detachment, and low compliance are the drawbacks of this route [36].

The Blood–Aqueous Barrier

The ciliary body and iris are the main structures that form the BAB at the anterior segment of the eye and are situated at the anterior part of the eye. The ciliary epithelium (non-pigmented cell layer) and endothelial cells of iris blood vessels form tight junctional complexes responsible for preventing the nonspecific transfer of solutes into the internal ocular milieu, thus influencing chemical equilibrium and transparency of the ocular fluids [37]. Tight junctions between the non-pigmented ciliary epithelial cells are the type of epithelial barrier. In contrast, tight junctions between the vascular endothelial cells, which contain proteins similar to the tight epithelial junctions, are the type of endothelial barrier [38]. BAB is a structurally integral part, but its barrier function is incomplete. For example, it has been reported that horseradish peroxidase (HRP, molecular mass 40 kDa), when injected, is impermeable over the iris blood vessels but can infuse over the fine capillaries of the ciliary processes and reaches the aqueous humor [39, 40]. As a result, there is less restriction for the external motion of the substances from the aqueous humor athwart the iris blood vessels toward systemic circulation [41].

BAB has such structural and functional arrangements that allow small and lipophilic drugs to enter the uveal blood circulation and remove them from the anterior chamber more rapidly than water-soluble drugs, which are exterminated by aqueous humor turnover only [42, 43]. For example, the pilocarpine clearance rate was 13.0 μl/min, whereas the inulin clearance is similar to the rate of aqueous humor turnover [44, 45], which is 3.0-4.7 ml/min in rabbits and 2.0-3.0 ml/min in humans.

The Blood Retinal Barrier

The posterior part of the eye consists of BRB between the bloodstream, and the eye is formed by the junctions between the tight walls of retinal capillaries (inner BRB) and retinal pigment epithelium (RPE) (outer BRB) [46]. RCE cells consist of tight intercellular junctions made up of intercellular communications of RCE and glial cells [47]. Due to their functional expression and biological characteristics, the blood-retinal barriers possess barrier properties similar to the blood-brain barrier formed by brain capillary endothelial cells, pericytes, and astrocytes with transepithelial electrical resistance (TEER) value of approximately 15002000 (Ω.cm) [48 - 51]. The retinal vessels become impermeable to larger molecules (more than 20-30kDa) due to inner BRB [52]. Small protein tracers like microperoxidase (19 kDa) can be transported to perioxonal space, but zonulae occludens present at the intercellular junction of the retinal endothelium obstruct them from penetrating the retina [53]. This barrier is permeable for lipophilic substances across RCE cells, but they possess poor permeability for small hydrophilic compounds and proteins [54, 55]. A higher loading dose of the drug is required, either administrated by the oral or intravenous route, as the blood flow and restrictions of BRB allow passage of a tiny fraction of the drug to permeate the posterior chamber, usually only 12% of plasma concentration. Hence, the large remaining proportion of the drug is distributed within the other body parts leading to unwanted consequences.

GENE THERAPY

Gene therapy is a treatment approach for different medication conditions based on transferring genetic material into cells, tissues, or organs for treating a disease or improving a patient's clinical status. The prime objective of gene therapy is to substitute nonfunctional or defective genes with new functional genes to attain a normal level of genetic expression [56, 57]. Various gene delivery methods are developed for different types of cells and tissues, from bacteria to mammalian. Viral and non-viral are the two categories of gene delivery systems.

• In virus-mediated gene delivery, viruses insert their DNA into the host cell, and therapeutic genes meant for delivery are encapsulated inside a viral particle.

• Non-viral gene delivery systems consist of physical methods such as Fhydrostatic pressure, continuous infusion, microinjection, impalefection, gene gun, electroporation, sonication, and chemical (lipofection), including the use of polymeric gene carriers (polyplexes).

Among the latest innovations in gene therapy, many of them have achieved great possibilities in treating various ocular disorders. The eye is suitable for gene therapy targeting because it is readily accessible, small size, and compact structure allows access to small vectors dose to produce the desired effect. The tight junctions in RPE cells and BOB restrict the loss of vector/gene into the systemic circulation, thus preventing any immune response production. Various *in vivo* with non-invasive techniques are available to monitor the external layers of the eye and the retina, such as optical coherence tomography (OCT) for retinal structure and electroretinography (ERG), visual evoked potentials (VEPs), and measurement of afferent pupillary light responses (PLRs) for retinal functions) [58, 59].

Ocular Gene Therapy

A successful gene therapy depends on designing effective, non-toxic gene vectors that can envelop and transport foreign genetic matters into targeted cell types [60]. Ocular gene therapy vectors are categorized into two groups, viral and non-viral gene delivery systems. Viral vectors, for example, adeno-associated virus (AAV), have attractive properties of high gene transduction capability, encounter biosafety problems, specifically innate and immune barriers [60], toxicity [61], and potential recombination of or complementation [62] to vector delivery. The size of viral vectors is another limitation that restricts the insertion of genes <5 kb [63]. Viral vectors target only functional genes to the retina. Still, non-viral vectors can transport genes (LPD/lipoplexes and CK30-PEG) and drugs (nanoparticles/solid lipid nanoparticles and liposomes) to the retina. A brief discussion on gene delivery systems is presented below.

Viral-mediated Gene Delivery

Viral gene delivery is an approach in which viruses are modified into genetic carriers to achieve gene delivery to the targeted site. Advanced gene delivery and therapy have been made possible with viral vectors because of their high transduction efficiency into the targeted cells. Presently, viral vector systems, including lentiviruses, retroviruses, adenoviruses, and adeno-associated viruses, tend to be the best alternative for effective gene delivery [64 - 66]. Adenoviruses (Ad) and adeno-associated viruses (AAV) are the most commonly used DNA viral vectors. The viral gene delivery system is schematically presented in Fig. (**14.3**). Recent developments in viral-mediated gene delivery systems are summarized in Table **14.1**.

Table 14.1. Recent studies on Virus mediated gene delivery systems.

Gene	Vector	Results	Ref.
p21transgene	Adenovirus	Effective anti-proliferative for the inhibition of wound healing following glaucoma surgery.	[70]
Human von hippel-lindau (VHL) protein	Adenovirus	Effectively inhibited angiogenesis in retina and iris in laser-induced multiple BRVO in monkey eyes.	[71]
sFlt-1	Adeno-associated virus	Long-term suppression of ocular neovascularisation by secretion gene therapy.	[79]
siRNA	Adeno-associated virus type 8 vector	Reduction in VEGF was found when siRNA was targeted using an AAV type 8 vector, and inhibition of CNV was observed.	[80]
Bevacizumab	Adeno-associated virus	Suppression of ocular neovascularization in murine mode was found.	[81]
sFLT01	Adeno-associated virus	Effective and local expression of sFLT01 and reduction in VEGF protein level	[83]
Flt23k	Adeno-associated virus	Significant reduction in VEGF levels in RPE/choroid complex and inhibition of the laser-induced murine choroidal neovascularization.	[84]
rAAV.sFLT-1	Adeno-associated virus	The first-in-human study revealed a safe and highly reproducible single subretinal injection of rAAV.sFLT-1 with no toxicity.	[85]
Human RS1 Protein	Adeno-associated virus	Safe and well-tolerated novel therapeutic approach for the treatment of X-linked retinoschisis (XLRS).	[86]
Cartilage oligomeric matrix protein angiopoietin-1 (COMP-Ang1)	Adeno-associated virus	Significant reduction in VEGF levels and choroid neovascularization volume (CNV).	[87]
Anti-human VEGF antibody fragment (antiVEGFfab)	Adeno-associated virus	Dose-dependent response and a significant reduction in the area of neovascularization.	[88]
Retinitis pigmentosa GTPase regulator	Adeno-associated virus	Successful rescue of the disease phenotype in an animal model of X-linked retinitis pigmentosa.	[89]

(Table 14.1) cont.....

Gene	Vector	Results	Ref.
RPE65-*RPE65*	Adeno-associated virus	Safe and efficient subretinal injection of AAV/ RPE65-*RPE65* vector in Leber Congenital Amaurosis (LCA) patients.	[90]
Recombinant Alstrom syndrome type I (ALMS1)	Adeno-associated virus	Showed exact localization of recombinant Alstrom syndrome type I (ALMS1).	[91]
Green fluorescent protein (GFP) gene	Lentiviral	High transduction efficiency of TM and corneal endothelial cells can be effectively obtained after a single dose of recombinant lentivirus with elongation factor 1 alpha (EF-1α) as a promoter.	[98]
Netrin-1 shRNA	Lentiviral	Retinal neovascularization and nonperfused areas are reduced in the oxygen-induced retinopathy (OIR) model.	[99]
RPE65	Lentiviral	Prolonged reattachment times in LV-RPE65 treated mice in comparison to vehicle-treated mice.	[100]

Adenovirus

Adenovirus (Ad), one of the most essential systems developed, is widely employed as they are easily accessible compared to remaining vectors and can be designed at very high titers. They can transduce an extensive range of dividing and postmitotic or terminally differentiated cells and express foreign genes to a detectable or abundant level. Some studies have revealed complications like harsh inflammatory reactions and high-neutralizing antibody titers associated with applicant ion of adenovirus vectors [67, 68]. A significant disruption of focal adhesions, cytoskeleton, and cell-cell adhesions of human TM cells in culture was achieved by adenovirus-mediated delivery of exoenzyme C3 transferase Liu X and their co-workers and enhanced drainage facility 90% in organ-cultured monkey former segment was also observed [69].

Ocular gene therapy with rAd-p21 employing an adenovirus vector was developed by Wen *et al.* Quantitative PCR, and RTPCR assays were following a single subconjunctival injection to evaluate rAd-p21 dissemination and gene transfer. Targeted delivery of rAd-p21 was achieved for filtration surgery with minimal systemic exposure after local administration. Neither delivery of vector nor transgene expression was affected by the production of serum neutralizing anti-adenovirus antibodies in a subsequent administration to the contralateral eye [70]. Akiyama *et al.* studied the effect of the human von Hippel-Lindau (VHL) protein-loaded adenovirus vector on the inhibition of ocular angiogenesis in a monkey model of multiple branch retinal vein occlusion (BRVO). Finding revealed successful transfer of VHL into intraocular tissues and significant reduction in Vascular Endothelial Growth Factor (VEGF) expression [71].

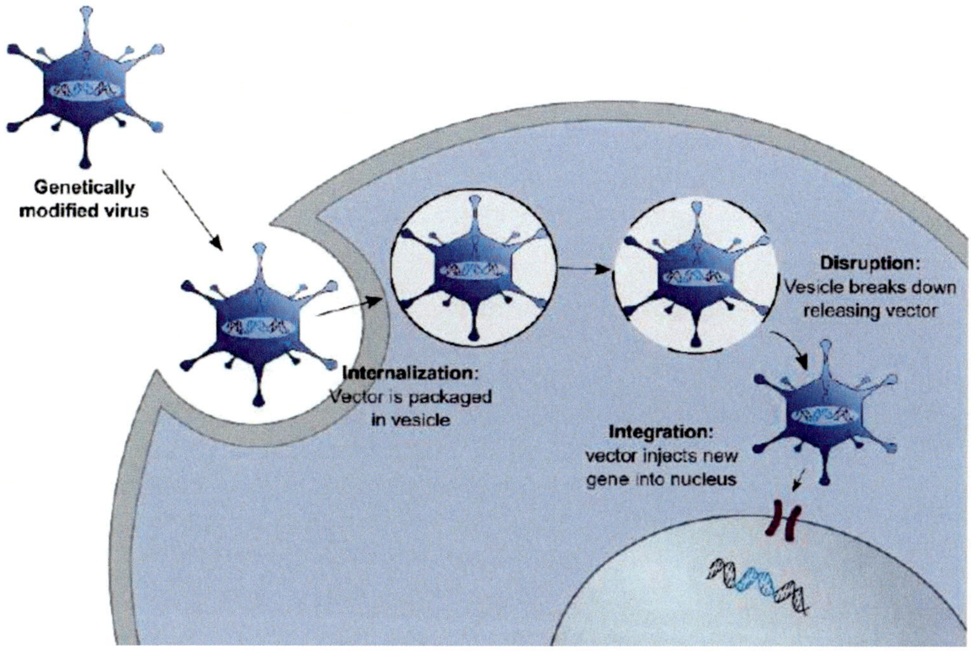

Fig. (14.3). Schematic representation of Viral based gene therapy.

Adeno-associated Virus

Adeno-associated vectors (AAV) have similar features as adenoviral vectors but are invulnerable due to some deficiency in their replication and pathogenicity [72]. It was reported that AAV-based vectors possess long-term gene transferring potential devoid of any observable side effects in several animal models. After injecting AAV, subretinally competent gene delivery to pigmented epithelial cells and photoreceptors was achieved in various models [73 - 76]. In the case of primary photoreceptor diseases in rodent models and a natural disease in dogs analogous to human Leber congenital amaurosis, AAV-mediated gene therapy delayed the loss of photoreceptors. Generally, AAV vectors develop a neutralizing antibody response, despite producing any severe inflammation [77]. Examinations on biodistribution and toxicity linked with vectors were performed in non-human primates, and very soon, Human clinical trials for RPE65 gene therapy were programmed [78].

Patients of neovascular age-related macular degeneration (NVAMD) necessitate sustained suppression of VEGF, which could be achieved by the transfer of VEGF neutralizing protein (gene transfer). Lai *et al.* studied the recombinant AAV vector encoding soluble VEGF receptor 1, sFlt-1 (AAV-CMV.sFLT) for the inhibition of cautery-induced corneal neovascularisation and laser-induced choroidal neovascularisation [79]. Transgene expression in the iris pigment epithelium and corneal endothelium was observed following AAV-CMV.sFLT delivery into the anterior chamber minimized the development of corneal neovascularization in the stroma of cauterized rats by 36% compared with cauterized control groups. Subretinal delivery of AAV-CMV.sFLT on the eye leads to suppressed choroidal neovascularization at the laser lesions around the optic nerve by 19%, which indicated diffusion of the secreted anti-angiogenic protein across the retina.

Igarashi and co-workers have already proved that type 8 adeno-associated viral (AAV) vectors mediating the expression of FLT-1 are effective in inhibiting neovascularization in a CNV mouse model [80]. Mao *et al.* assumed that long-term suppression of ocular neovascularization could be achieved using an AAV vector expressing bevacizumab [81]. Bevacizumab independently is effective for only 14 days. Still, when an AAV vector expressing bevacizumab is administered intravitreally (single dose), it suppresses ocular neovascularization for at least 168 days in a murine model, the highest time point calculated [82].

Another study performed by Tuo *et al.* was on the retinal lesions in $Ccl2^{-/-}/Cx3cr1^{-/-}$ mice for age-related macular degeneration (AMD). They evaluated the effects of adeno-associated virus encoding sFLT01 (AAV5.sFLT01). After subretinal injection into the right eye, they observed a proficient and local expression of sFLT01 and a decrease in the level of VEGF protein in the retina, which can either stabilizes or arrests the progression of retinal lesions in $Ccl2^{-/-}/Cx3cr1^{-/-}$ mice. Furthermore, alteration of VEGFA, ERK phosphorylation, and iNOS within the retinal tissues urged the participation of reactive nitrogen species within the retinal lesions. These findings signify the possible beneficial effects of sFLt01 gene therapy in oxidative stress management and angiogenesis for AMD patients [83].

A novel intracellular approach was developed to inhibit retinal pigment epithelium (RPE)-derived VEGF for age-related macular degeneration treatment. Previously many studies have investigated employing AAV vectors for effective inhibition of VEGF (AAV2.PlGF1-DE, type 8 AAV-sFLT-1, AAV2 conjugated with anti-VEGF shRNA, AAV5.sFLT-1, and AAV2-sFLT-1). Zhang *et al.*, found that AAV2-mediated expression of Flt23k was sustained till six months, followed by post-subretinal injection in mice. Elisa and Western blot analysis of AAV2.FLT-23k showed a significantly reduced VEGF level in RPE/choroid complex and inhibited the laser-induced murine choroidal neovascularization. Other findings of this study; AAV2.FLT-23k had no adverse effects on the structure and function of the retina, and it does not induce apoptosis in the RPE or choroid [84]. Rakoczy *et al.* studied the safety of rAAV.sFLT-1 for wet age-related macular degeneration treatment in their single-center, phase 1, randomized controlled clinical trial.. They have previously reported that rAAV.sFLT-1 facilitated long-term secretion of sFLT-1 and was found to be safe and efficient in different animal models of retinal and choroid neovascularization (CNV). This first-in-human study revealed that a single subretinal injection of rAAV.sFLT-1 was found to be highly reproducible. After surgery, temporary and mild intraocular inflammation was observed with no dose-limiting toxicity. Results depicted that rAAV.sFLT-1 was well tolerated and safe and could be an enduring treatment option for wet age-related macular degeneration [85].

Mutation in the retinoschisis gene results in X-linked retinoschisis, a rare type of ocular disorder. Lack of retinoschisis protein interrupts the retinal structure, retinal layers splitting, intraretinal cavities formation, and progressive decline of visual function. To date, no approved therapy is available for XLRS patients. Marangoni *et al.* studied a novel therapeutic approach based on the intravitreal delivery of an adeno-associated viral vector coding the human RS1 Protein (AAV8-scRS/IRBPhRS) X-linked retinoschisis (XLRS) treatment. Studies performed under Good Laboratory Practices showed that intravitreal administration of AAV8-scRS/IRBPhRS is safe and well-tolerated in normal rabbits and mice of XLRS. Self-resolving and dose-dependent vitreal inflammation was the main ocular finding, and no other ocular adverse effects were reported with no systemic toxicity. Biodistribution study stated the spread of vector genome in the extraocular tissues; however, no organ or tissue damage was found [86].

Anti-VEGF agents are associated with certain risks and need advancement in safety, efficacy, applicability, and easy usage. Previously, Lee and his group reported that the cartilage oligomeric matrix protein angiopoietin-1 (COMP-Ang1) and VEGF inhibitor fusion protein aflibercept are similar in the AMD model in suppressing CNV formation and more advanced in vascular leakage suppression. To build on this work, Lambert *et al.* studied the suppression of choroid neovascularization and vascular endothelial growth factor *via* subretinal administration of adeno-associated virus with COM-Ang1 (AAV2.COM-Ang1). When mice were treated with subretinal AAV2.COM-Ang1, localization AAV2 and plasmid protein expression were confirmed in the RPE/choroid of mice. In the laser-induced neovascular AMD, author found a significant decrease in VEGF levels (29-33%, $p<0.01$) and CNV volume (60-70%, $p<0.01$), but no associated reduction was observed in hypoxia-inducible factor (HIF1-α) in comparison to the control [87]. Another researcher has studied a new approach for the neovascular age-related macular degeneration (NVAMD) treatment. They demonstrated the expression of anti-human VEGF antibody fragment (antiVEGFfab) following subretinal administration of AAV8-antiVEGFfab in mice models. $\geq 1x10^7$ gene copies (GC) of AAV8-antiVEGFfab were injected into the retina of *rho/VEGF mice*. A dose-dependent response and a significant reduction in the area of neovascularization were found in comparison to placebo-vector injected eye. The author found 70-80% sustained reduction with $3x10^9$ or $1x10^9$ GC in retinal detachment caused by doxycycline-induced high expression of VEGF in Tet/opsin/VEGF mice [88].

X-linked retinitis pigmentosa (a blinding disorder of the retina) causes a mutation in the retinitis pigmentosa GTPase regulator ($RPGR^{ORF15}$). Many studies have been successfully established with gene therapy employing AAV vectors in numerous animal models. But few unpredictable recombination errors are evident due to intrinsic sequence instability at the purine region of $RPGR^{ORF15}$. For the improvement of stability and efficacy of the AAV8 gene therapy for the treatment of XLRP, Fischer *et al*. described a codon-optimized gene therapy. The developed codon-optimized sequence does not significantly change the post-translation modification and shows better stability and expression levels *in vitro*. The codon-optimized RPGR with AAV8 successfully rescues the disease phenotype in two animal models ($Rpgr^{-/y}$ and C57BL/$6J^{Rd9/Boc}$) [89].

Increased AMD risk is associated with polymorphisms hindering factor H (fH) function, and complement activation plays a significant role in AMD pathogenesis. Previously a fusion protein having complement receptor-2 fragments linked with the inhibitory domain of fH (CR2-fH), an alternative pathway inhibitor, has been validated to treat choroid neovascularization (CNV) intravenously. The safety and efficacy of subretinal injection of the AAV2/4 RPE65-RPE65 vector were evaluated by Meur *et al*. in a group of 9 patients with Leber Congenital Amaurosis (LCA). LCA is a severe and initial type of retinal degeneration that accounts for 5% of retinal dystrophy cases. Either low (1.22×10^{10} vg to 2×10^{10} vg) or high (3.27×10^{10} to $4.8x10^{10}$ vg) vector doses were administered to the patients. Results revealed good ocular and general tolerance to the rAAV2/4-RPE65-*RPE65* vector. Nystagmus patients showed better visual acuity. MRI analysis reported stabilization and visible improvement and cortical activation beside visual pathways. OCT analysis showed no retinal thinning after vector administration, excluding macular detachment [90].

Single AAV vectors have a gene transferring capacity of only 5 kb, limiting their applicability for inherited retinal degenerations (IRDs) treatment. IRDs are caused due to mutation in genes more expressed in retinal photoreceptors than in retinal pigmented epithelium (RPE). To extend the transfer capacity of AAV, Maddalena and coworkers generated triple AAV, with a maximum transfer capacity of about

14kb. The transcriptomic analysis reported total-length products along with numerous aberrant transcripts after transduction of triple AAV. Further results showed that 4% (approx) of mouse photoreceptors were transduced by a triple AAV vector and showed exact localization of recombinant Alstrom syndrome type I (ALMS1). In the mouse model of ALMS, the low photoreceptor transduction levels may validate the modest and transitory retinal improvement. While in the case of pig retina, transduction levels were 40% of those found with single vectors [91].

Lentiviral Vectors

Lentiviral (LV) vectors are a type of vectors that are single-stranded RNA. They hold properties like the ability to infect both dividing and non-dividing cells and primary cells, high and stable expression, and a deficit of associated intraocular inflammation, making them promising for gene delivery in ocular disorders [92]. Integration of lentivirus vectors is inserted into the host genome. Lentiviral vectors have been reported to obtain stable transgene expression in the animal model and human *in-vitro* [93]. They are capable of transducing retinal cells [94 - 96], and they were also used to treat the wet form of age-related macular degeneration [(RetinoStat®] *via* subretinal routes [97].

Challa *et al.* studied the *in vivo* efficiency of lentiviral vectors for gene delivery to the trabecular meshwork (TM) of rodent eyes. Elongation factor 1 alpha (EF-1α) promoter stimulates high expression of the reporter gene and to attain a stable and long-term expression. It is a consistent substitute for the cytomegalovirus (CMV) promoter. The work suggested that targeting gene expression to the trabecular meshwork cells, necessitates the effective use of such specific promoters. Additionally, *in vivo* lentiviral mediated gene transfer might be a potential means to study the normal and pathologic physiology of the corneal endothelium [98]. Mutation in the *ABCA4* gene causes impaired vision and blindness in Stargardt disease (STGD1), a most common type of inherited juvenile macular degeneration. Till now, there has been no approved therapy for STGD1 disease. Introducing the normal ABCA1 gene to PR cells in STGD patients would lead to sustained levels of active protein at the disease site. Binley *et al.* selected a lentiviral vector (StarGen) due to the large size of *ABCA1* cDNA (6.8 kb) to deliver long-term gene expression for STGD1 treatment. The results showed that the developed EIAV-CMV-GFP receptor vector could transduce both rod and cones photoreceptors (PRs) and RPE with high efficiency in macaque after subretinal administration. Initially, a slightly elevated level of inflammation was noticed, which was momentary, and no toxicity was monitored. Biodistribution studies reveal that StarGen vectors are localized to the ocular compartment following the subretinal administration. Furthermore, it was concluded that

StarGen is a safe and well-tolerated gene therapy with no detrimental changes after subretinal administration [96].

Pathological retinal neovascularization is a sight-threatening ocular disease that includes a sequence of events like extracellular matrix components degradation, expansion, and migration of endothelial cells and tube formation. Various proangiogenic molecules, including VEGF, play a vital role in retinal neovascularization. However, anti-VEGF alone cannot entirely eradicate pathological angiogenesis. It necessitates utilizing other angiogenic factors like hypoxia-inducible factors (HIF) 1α, erythropoietin, and netrin-1. Xu *et al.*, investigated the function of lentivirus-mediated netrin-1 in pathological angiogenesis and retinal neovascularization in the retinas of oxygen-induced retinopathy (OIR) mice. Results showed that expression of both netrin-1 mRNA and protein was up-regulated in the retinas of OIR mice in comparison to control, signifying its vital role in pathological retinal neovascularization. Transfection *via* lentivirus-mediated netrin-1 shRNA reduced the retinal neovascularization and nonperfused areas in the OIR model [99].

Various gene therapy strategies have been investigated for RPE65-related Leber congenital amaurosis (LCA), which mainly rely on AAV vectors; however, they are associated with limited long-term effects. Therefore, Matet *et al.* evaluated the ocular and systemic tolerance of lentiviral mediated gene therapy vector (LV-RPE65) *via* subretinal route in context with structure and function of the retina and systemic biodistribution on healthy non-human primates (NHPs). In this study, the early kinetics of retinal detachment was described for the first time at 2, 4, and 7 days following subretinal administration using multimodal imaging in 5 NHPs. Results revealed extended reattachment times in LV-RPE65 treated mice compared to the control group. Despite initial perivascular reaction and foveal structure changes, the whole of the retinal function was preserved ultimately. Immunohistochemistry results revealed no difference in glial, microglial, or leucocyte ocular activation, varying from low to high dose and control group. No signs of vector shedding or extraocular targeting were observed, indicating the safety of the LV-RPE65 vector [100].

Non-Viral Mediated Gene Delivery

Irrespective of the benefits of viral vectors in ocular gene therapy, there reside significant possibilities for further advancements. For developing a potential gene substitution therapy and to overcome the limitations of viral vectors, non-viral vectors have been created. A variety of non-viral vectors is available, allowing for a wide range of products, accessibility, applicability, low cost of production, and enhanced "genomic" safety [101].

Non-viral vectors have several advantages. They are mostly found to be safe and non-toxic to ophthalmic tissues. Low transfection rate and short lifespan are the two major drawbacks of non-viral vectors being overcome *via* slow-release devices and requiring repeated treatments. While the latest viral vectors, lentiviral, non-integrating, and self-inhibiting, offer promising strategies to improve a few of these concerns, there is a constant prerequisite for enhancing and developing gene therapy vectors for the eye. Consequently, in recent times various significant research efforts have been made to develop non-viral DNA delivery systems. Recent developments of non-viral mediated gene delivery systems are summarized in Table **14.2**.

Table 14.2. Recent studies on Non-viral mediated gene delivery systems.

Gene	Carrier	Results	Ref.
Oligonucleotides (ODNs)	Liposomes	Protection of ODNs against degradation by nuclease and enhanced DNA properties were observed.	[111]
Phosphodiester oligonucleotide (ONDs)	Liposomes	Reduction in the rate of degradation of native oligonucleotide and enhanced half-life. Sustained release of the OND and reduced distribution in non-target regions.	[112]
Brain-specific angiogenesis inhibitor 1 (BAI1-ECR) gene	Liposomes	Significant inhibition of corneal neovascularization.	[113]
Plasmid DNA	Liposomes	Showed better and safe transfection efficiency and gene expression.	[114]
Plasmid DNA complexed with Gemini surfactant	Nanoparticle (Gemini NPs)	The better alternative for targeting glaucoma-relevant tissues *via* both intravitreal and topical route of administration	[133]
PRPF31	Span poly-- -arginin (SP-OA) nanoparticles	Significant visual acuity improvement and retinal thickness were found in Prpf31$^{A216P/+}$ mice treated with SP-PAPRPF31 nanoparticles.	[134]
Plasmid DNA	Polymeric nanoparticles	Capable for the pDNA protection from premature release and degradation in the extracellular media. Additionally, the cellular uptake and transfection efficacy were also altered.	[135]
Human FLT1	Polyethylene glycol (PEG)-POD nanoparticles	A 50% reduction in choroid neovascularization in a murine model of age-related macular degeneration was observed.	[136]

(Table 14.2) cont.....

Gene	Carrier	Results	Ref.
Plasmid DNA	Nanoparticles	Significantly improved electroretinography (ERG) activity indicating good transfection efficiency	[137]
pCMSEGPE plasmid	Noisome	Protected the incorporated DNA from enzymatic digestion with successful transfection in both HEK-293 and ARPE-19 cells with no cell viability.	[138]
pCMS-EGFP plasmid	Noisome	Enhanced transfection efficacy was observed with no cell viability.	[139]
Plasmid DNA with lacZ gene	PEO-PPO-PEO non-ionic copolymeric Micelles	Efficient and stable transfer of the functional gene through topical delivery in mice and rabbits.	[142]
Lutein and Zeaxanthin	Micelles	Formulations prepared with ethanol/ Tween40 resulted in the lowest lactate dehydrogenase (LDH) release, the highest carotenoid uptake, and the most inadequate stress response.	[143]
Anti-apoptotic gene (bcl-x_L)	Micelles	Efficient reduction apoptosis in the wounded cornea was found after administration of plasmid encoding anti-apoptotic gene bcl- x_L *via* eye drop.	[144]
Plasmid DNA	Polyplexes	Therapeutic DNA material diffused in the vitreous cavity then reached all areas of the retina.	[147]
Plasmid DNA	Polyplexes	Protected the plasmid against enzymatic digestion with a significant increase in transfection efficiency.	[148]
Plasmid DNA (pDNA)/polyethylenimine (PEI)	Polyplexes	Showed high gene expression on ARPE-19 cells without cytotoxicity and aggregation in the vitreous body when compared with cationic ternary complexes.	[152]
Plasmid DNA	Polyplexes	Successful induction of GFP expression in a cell line (*in vitro*) with no apparent cytotoxicity.	[153]
Plasmid DNA	Polyplexes	Co-transfection with integrase showed sustained expression.	[154]

Naked DNA Injection

One of the most effortless and common types of non–viral gene therapy is the Naked DNA injection, which involves the injection into the local tissues. Research revealed the possible approach for transferring exogenous genes to photoreceptor cells present in the primate retina by employing a vascular route and an ocular-specific promoter (opsin promoter). Plasmid DNA does not get incorporated into the host chromosome; thus, plasmid-based gene expression is temporary and frequently needs repeatable administrations [102]. In light of further advancement, a non-viral method incorporating mannitol in plasmid solution showed enhanced efficiency *in vivo* for gene transfer into RGCs of an adult C57Bl6 mouse [103].

Physical Methods

The cellular uptake of Naked DNA is minor, therefore making them more feasible for ocular gene therapy. Various researches have been done using electroporation or iontophoresis to improve the uptake and expression of naked DNA [104 - 107]. These methods use electric currents to facilitate DNA uptake and its movement into the cells. Electroporation in animal models is one of the best methods for testing DNA vectors in proof-of-principle studies. However, they are not considered a feasible delivery catalyst for clinical therapies due to their side effects. On the other hand, Iontophoresis is not associated with severe side effects and can effectively increase the retinal uptake of oligonucleotides [108]. Still, some reports disagree with the effectiveness of these methods in improving the uptake of complete genes or expression vectors [107]. Further examples of physical methods for gene transfer are ultrasound, pressure-perfusion, magnetic fields, focused laser, and ballistic (gene gun) approaches and these methods can improve plasmid delivery [109] but have not been utilized in experimental gene therapy for glaucoma.

Chemical Approaches

Chemical approaches have matured to guard the therapeutic genetic components and allow a more capable delivery. Amongst, positively charged lipid- and polymer-based nanocarriers have been primarily studied (Fig. **14.4**). Lipids and polymer-based nanocarriers can connect with genetic materials and form nanosized complexes that can go over the cell membrane.

Liposomes

Liposomes have one or more concentric lipid bilayer membranes that enclose their hydrophilic spaces. They possess various benefits as drug, antigen, and gene delivery carriers, and their size can be easily modified. Additionally, they can be altered to attach a targeting function. Liposomes are biodegradable, sustain the drug release, and remain localized at the targeted site offering an attractive ocular drug delivery [110]. Naked genetic materials can be degraded upon administration and necessitate intraocular tissue protection Bochot *et al.* employed liposomes for intravitreal administration of oligonucleotides (ODNs) to treat ocular viral infections. The authors found that using liposomes after intravitreal administration can protect ODNs against degradation by nuclease. In addition, the DNA properties can be improved by using the haemagglutinating virus of Japan (HVJ), having viral high-mobility group 1 protein (a non-histone nuclear protein) which facilitates the intracellular trafficking of the plasmid DNA into the nuclei. It also assists in arbitrating the binding of liposomes with the cell membrane [111].

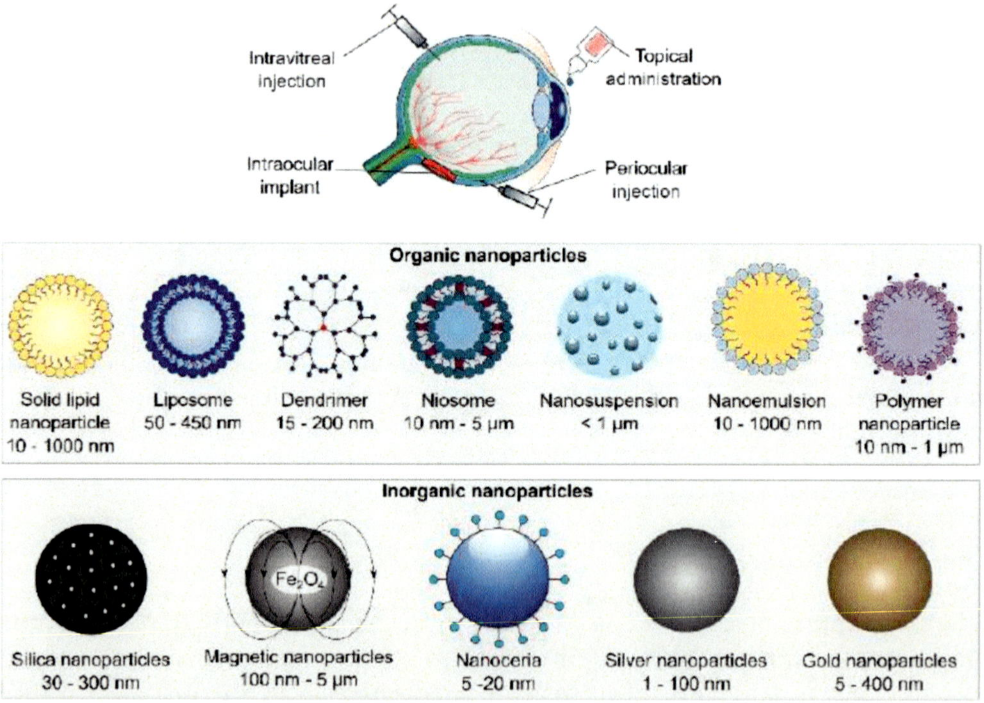

Fig. (14.4). Nanocarrier-based non-viral gene therapy.

Moreover, Bochot *et al.*, investigated intravitreal injection of a model phosphodiester oligonucleotide (OND) delivered through pegylated liposomes in a rabbit model. The developed liposomes decreased the rate of degradation of native oligonucleotide and enhanced the half-life in the vitreous humor resulting in sustained release of the OND compared to solution into the vitreous. Additionally, the distribution of non-target tissues (Sclera and lens) was significantly reduced [112].

Yoon *et al.* investigated the effect of lipid-mediated subconjunctival injection of the brain-specific angiogenesis inhibitor 1 (BAI1-ECR) gene on an *in-vivo* rabbit model of corneal angiogenesis. The author reported significant inhibition of corneal neovascularization after twice or thrice weekly subconjunctival injection of plasmid enclosing the extracellular region of BAI1-ECR gene complexed with fluorescent protein vector in liposomes [113].

Non-viral DNA carriers (cationic liposomes) are safe, non-immunogenic, and less toxic than viral vectors but have low transfection efficiency. Peters *et al.* investigated strategies for improving DNA transfer by cationic lipid-based carriers to RPE cells. They evaluated whether the development of pegylated lipoplexes will result in efficient transfection of RPE cells. Further, they designed post-pegylated lipoplexes and studied their transfection capacity into RPE cells and their behavior in the vitreous. Results of transfection efficiency and gene expression revealed that lipoplexes post-pegylated with PEG-ceramides were better and less toxic than pre-pegylated lipoplexes. Confocal images show no aggregation of post-pegylated lipoplexes in the vitreous, leading to more efficient transport through the neural retina. Upon contact with RPE membranes, the post-pegylated lipoplexes undergo de-pegylation and successfully deliver DNA [114].

Nanoparticles

DNA nanoparticle technology can overcome numerous barrier systems of the eye to achieve a successful gene therapy for the ocular drug delivery system. For more than 25 years, studies have explored the various forces (structural and energetic) involved in DNA condensation. Still, recently because of its application in gene therapy, this technology has gained the interest of researchers. Nanoparticle vectors have massive payloads (examined up to 20 kb), no significant harmful responses, and their nano size presents extensive cellular uptake [115]. The DNA nanoparticles' size ranges between 10 to 400 nm in diameter. Results revealed that Compacted-DNA nanoparticles could be a potential candidate for targeting genes in the retina and RPE cells [116].

Retinal pigment epithelium (RPE) is crucial in ocular disorders (correlated with senescence and dystrophies of the photoreceptors). Its reliability and function are vital for neural retina homeostasis. To detain the processes leading to these diseases, RPE cells offer potential goals for drug delivery and gene transfer. Therefore, microparticles of PLA or PLGA were previously studied for biodegradation and ocular tissue reactions both *in-vitro* [117, 118] and *in-vivo* [119 - 121]. PLA microspheres were phagocytosed by RPE and debased in their cytoplasm when administered in subretinal space [115]. Bejjani *et al.* evaluated the potential benefits of poly(lactic) acid (PLA) and poly(lactide-co-glycolide)

(PLGA) nanoparticles (NPs) as vectors for transferring a gene to retinal pigment epithelium (RPE) cells. They found about 10%-35% of cells expressed the transfected gene, with the absence of cell toxicity even when at higher PLGA NPs concentrations (up to 4 mg/ml). PLGA polyplex NPs were non-toxic and can be a valuable mode of gene transfer into RPE cells *in vitro* and *in vivo* [116].

Non-viral vectors are regarded as beneficial for gene therapy owing to their capability to diminish the host's immune response, which is a major apprehension for viral vectors. Protection of plasmid biodegradation, facilitating cell entry and nuclear targeting, lack cytotoxicity, and escape endo/lysosome entrapment define an ideal non-viral vector [122].

Mo *et al.* investigated the probability of human serum albumin nanoparticles (HSA NP) containing a plasmid encoding the genes for SOD1 as a non-viral vector for ocular delivery. Various studies have been previously reported, but for the first time, the authors have used HSA as a single carrier material for gene delivery [123]. Superoxide dismutase 1 (SOD1) or Cu, Zn SOD, is the most abundant SOD present in the cell cytosol in the eye [124]. SOD1 cuts down oxidative stress in the retina (Cellular damage due to reactive species) as they convert free oxygen radicals into hydrogen peroxide, and enzymes such as glutathione peroxidase or catalase break down the peroxides into water [125]. Human serum albumin (HSA) possesses a unique feature of reversibly/covalently binding to different types of endogenous or exogenous ligands with significant affinity; this makes HSA a protein transporter and depot for many compounds [126]. HAS Nanoparticles were prepared by the modified desolvation-crosslinking method. No cytotoxicity was found in ARPE 19 cells, and protection of the plasmid DNA against the DNase I (biodegradation) was observed, indicating their stability. *In vitro* studies of the HAS nanoparticles showed sustained plasmid release for six days. Uptake of HSA NP *via* cells is an energy-dependent mechanism arbitrated by caveolae and clathrin-dependent endocytosis.

Additionally, its endogenous nature might turn it into a highly proficient and safe carrier for gene delivery [127 - 129]. Efficient gene expression and transfection were observed under *in vitro* and *in vivo* conditions. The swift uptake, less toxicity, and sluggish clearance of PEI2-GNPs in the rabbit cornea consider it a gorgeous approach for gene therapy to the cornea. Additionally, after delivering the genetic material to its target, the empty vector diffuses out of the tissues. Whereas, Jiang *et al.*, found that the formed nanoparticles have a dual cationic-shell structure and consist of various advantageous features like good cellular uptake efficiency, DNA protecting effect, use of multiple endocytic pathways, and endo-lysosome escaping ability resulting in better transfection efficiency and concluding DLCS-NP as a promising non-viral vector for effectual ocular gene therapy [130].

Solid lipid nanoparticles (SLNs) are colloidal nanostructured systems consisting of oil-in-water microemulsions, wherein dispersed phases are formed by one or more lipids and usually remain solid at room temperature. The quality and quantity of the components employed in the production of SLNs can lead to toxicity and cell death by causing the breakdown of the membranes. Fabregas *et al.* aimed at optimizing a formula for SLN production to get efficient DNA binding and minimum cell toxicity. The developed SLNs were of approx 120nm size and had a positive surface charge of 42 mV. DNA binding efficiency of the optimized SLN was found suitable after evaluation in the TCERG1 gene. *In vivo* studies revealed that the SLNs have high DNA binding efficiency with no toxicity [131]. Apaolaza *et al.* prepared solid lipid nanoparticles (SLN) using hyaluronic acid (HA) and protamine (P) as non-viral carriers for gene therapy. SLN with Gene complexes were obtained with a particle size of 240 nm to 340 nm and positively surfaced charged. In ARPE 19cells, the addition of P and HA encouraged approximately a 7-fold increase in the transfection ability of SLNs. The intracellular complexion of DNA exhibited that the HA can adapt to the high level of condensation of DNA owing to the protamine within the cells; an interesting fact if the vector is uptaken *via* non-degradative endocytosis. In addition, the therapeutic genetic material which encodes the protein retinoschisin attained a positive transfection in ARPE-19 cells, proving a potential use of this novel non-viral system for the management of X-linked juvenile retinoschisis by gene therapy [132].

Alqawlaq *et al.* aimed to develop a nanoparticle system consisting of plasmid DNA compiled with Gemini surfactant with the subsequent inclusion of helper lipid vesicles to effectively treat glaucoma. The optimized GL-NPs were found to be biocompatible with rat retinal ganglion cells (RGC-5) with > 95% viability and were in the nano-size range (150-180nm). GL-NPs were confined within the nerve fiber retinal layer and in several anterior chamber tissues after intravitreal and topical administration, respectively. After intravitreal and topical injection, the GL-NPs were found to be thermodynamically stable in the vitreous and tear film and exchanged as a unit, non-aggregated particles [133]. The author concluded that Gemini NPs' capability to deliver pDNA to the former chamber and retina could be a better alternative for targeting glaucoma-relevant tissues *via* both intravitreal and topical routes of administration. Mutations in the PRPF31 gene lead to autosomal dominant retinitis pigmentosa (adRP). Previously viral gene therapies have been explored for the treatment of adRP but are associated with certain major drawbacks. Pensado *et al.* evaluated Span poly-L-arginine (SP-OA) nanoparticles to mediate gene transfer carrying a point mutation (A216P) in the *Prpf31*. The developed nanoparticles were of size range from 182nm -228nm with positive surface charge (+42mV to +33mV) that become negative after incubation with GFP plasmid or PRPF31. The Western blot analysis showed a higher transfection efficacy of the developed SP-PA nanoparticles non-viral vectors compared to viral vectors. Significant visual acuity improvement and retinal thickness were found in $Prpf31^{A216P/+}$ mice treated with SP-PAPRPF31 nanoparticles [134].

It is well known that dysfunction of RPE cells leads to many hereditary and acquired ocular diseases, and gene imbalance occurs due to such pathological conditions. Gene therapy is considered a therapeutic strategy to restore gene expression in such conditions. The vectors intended for gene delivery have their physicochemical properties that interact with the constituents present in the surrounding environment. Such interactions can result in irregular/unexpected release of the genetic material or undergo degradation, and even the transfection efficiency can be affected. Tasharrofi *et al.* studied the importance of interaction between gene delivery vectors and the surrounding environment. Polymeric nanoparticles with different vectors and mixing orders were formulated (pDNA, PLGA/PEI, and PEI polymer or PLGA nanoparticles). Characterization and efficacy of the developed nanoparticles for delivering a gene to RPE cells were evaluated in the existence of vitreous or fetal bovine serum (FBS). All the developed formulations exhibited no cytotoxicity in hRPE cells and were capable of pDNA protection from immature release and deterioration in the extracellular media. Furthermore, the cellular uptake and transfection efficacy was also altered due to the adsorption of vitreous or serum proteins onto the vector surface [135].

Dasari *et al.* have described a 3.5 kDa peptide for ocular delivery (POD); in their study, they targeted cell surface sialic acid. The developed plasmid DNA containing polyethylene glycol (PEG)-POD nanoparticles facilitated moderate gene transfer and rescue of retinal degeneration. *In vitro* analysis showed that gene transfer by PEG-POD nanoparticles was hindered at different stages in systemic investigation. Therefore, they functionalized POD with PEG using a reducible orthopyridyl disulfide bond. The author found that these reduced nanoparticles had the capability of gene transfer *in vitro* while holding their *in vivo* gene transfer properties. They consumed this strategy for delivering human FLT1 to the retina and gained a 50% reduction in choroid neovascularization in a murine model of age-related macular degeneration [136]. Sun *et al.*, in their research, utilized a multifunctional lipid (1-aminoethyl)iminobis [N-9oleicylcysteinyl-1-amino-ethyl0propionamide] (ECO) for designing a gene delivery carrier for the treatment of LCA. ECO consists of a protonatable ethylenediamine (E) head group, two cysteine (C) functional linkers, and two oleoyls (O) lipophilic tails. The designed gene system is based on the ECO's pH-sensitive amphiphilic endosomal escape and reductive cytosolic release of nucleic acids. Previously ECO has been reported for its excellent transfection efficiency for RNA cancer therapy. The ECO/dendrimer system has also been successfully utilized to transfect the retinal tissue with GFP. Here in this study author has prepared all-trans-retinylamine modified ECO plasmid DNA (pDNA) nanoparticles with PEG spacer (Ret-PEG-ECO/pRPE65 nanoparticles) intending to target interphotoreceptor retinoid-binding protein (IRBP) for improved gene delivery into the retina. *In vivo* results showed that nanoparticles have significantly enhanced the electroretinography (ERG) activity, indicating good transfection efficiency and vision of Rpe65$^{-/-}$ mice. This effect was sustained for at least 120 days after gene therapy., A safety assessment study conducted in BALB/c mice showed that the developed nanoparticles could be safely administered through the subretinal route in gene replacement therapy [137].

Niosomes

Niosomes are bilayer structures consisting of non-ionic surfactant vesicles and represent an alternative to liposomes. Few studies have been reported on the applicability of niosomes for gene delivery purposes. Puras *et al.* studied a novel cationic noisome for delivering a gene to the retina. Author detailed and characterized method of preparing niosome based on cationic lipids 2,3-di (tetradecyloxy)propane-1-amine, blended with squalene and polysorbate 80 consisting of pCMSEGPE plasmid. The prepared lipoplexes at ratio 15/1 were in the size range of 200nm with a zeta potential of 25mV and spherical. In this ratio, niosomes effectively condensed and protected the incorporated DNA from enzymatic digestion. Successful transfection was observed in HEK-293 and ARPE-19 cells with no cell viability. HEK-293 showed caveolae-dependent entry, and lipoplexes entered with clathrin-mediated endocytosis into the retinal cells. The expression of EGFP was identified in different retinal cells; subretinal injections transfected the RPE layers, whereas a broad surface in the inner retinal layer was transfected through intravitreal administration [138].

Mashal *et al.* formulated niosomes incorporating lycopene (natural lipid) using cationic lipid DOTMA and polysorbate 60 for targeting genetic material in the rat retina. Niosomes with and without lycopene were formulated and evaluated for size and morphology. The capacity to condense, release, and protection of DNA against enzymatic digestion was also studied. Niosomes containing lycopene complexed with pCMS-EGFP plasmid at an 18/1 mass ratio of cationic lipid/DNA were found to be of nano-size range with positive zeta potential and low PDI. Moreover, the *in vitro* study in ARPE 19 cells revealed that the developed niosomes were effectively capable of condensing, releasing, and protecting DNA.

Around 35% transfection efficacy was observed with no cell viability. The author found a caveolae caveolae-mediated endocytosis and macropinocytosis with the internalization pathway study. Nioploxex showed efficient transfection in the outer segment of the retina *via* both the subretinal and intravitreal routes [139].

Micelles

Further study was conducted taking non-ionic PEO-PPO-PEO copolymer in concern. A non-ionic PEO-PPO-PEO copolymer derived from ethylene oxide (80%) and propylene oxide (20%) has previously been reported to show up to 5 times prolonged half-life ($t_{1/2}$) of fentanyl in the bloodstream *via* pharmacokinetic data analysis of patch formulation [140, 141]. Thus, the author found copolymer micelle carrier a potential topical drug delivery approach to prevent interaction of serum/protein, and the micelle carrier has excellent stability properties. Liaw *et al.* investigated the practicability of using PEO-PPO-PEO non-ionic copolymeric micelles to deliver plasmid DNA with the lacZ gene into ocular tissues. Results revealed that the formed micelles were above 0.1% (w/v) of a block copolymer with a size and a surface charge of 160 nm of -4.4 mV, respectively. EDTA and cytochalasin B were incorporated to augment the transfection properties of developed micelles. The augmented mechanism seems to comprise the plasmid/PEO-PPO-PEO micelles for the tight junction opening of ocular tissues and elevating the paracellular pathway for other distribution (endocytosis) [142].

In addition to the previous studies related to vectors for gene transfer, another set of researchers, Schafer *et al.*, studied the micelles as a carrier for delivery of dietary carotenoids, lutein, and zeaxanthin to protect against damages due to free radicals, which can cause disorders like cataract and age-related macular degeneration (AMD). The micelles' solubility, uptake, and biocompatibility were evaluated in the human retinal pigment epithelial cells. After various experiments, ethanol/Tween40 vehicles were effective as delivery vehicles for lutein and zeaxanthin to supply these carotenoids to differentiated ARPE-19 cells when the vehicle concentration does not exceed 0.01% [143]. Further carrying on the concept of micelles as a non-viral gene delivery system, Tong *et al.* delivered plasmid (pCMV–bcl-x_L–eGFP) encoding an anti-apoptotic gene, the bcl-x_L with a nano-carrier, polymeric micelles (PM) to reduce the apoptosis activated by corneal epithelial debridement *via* eye drop. Results showed a significant reduction in apoptosis of wounded cornea. Thus, delivery of pCMV–bcl-x_L–eGFP/ PM *via* eye drop may be therapeutically effective and beneficial in diminishing apoptosis in the cornea [144].

Polyplexes

Cationic polymers complex with nucleic acids such as plasmid DNA are polyplexes (Fig. **14.5**). Nanosized complexes contain vector capacity, stability in nuclease-abundant environments, and relatively high transfection efficiency for dividing and non-dividing cells [145]. The use of these polyplexes in gene therapy is based on the theory that they adsorb more efficiently with mammalian cells' negatively charged plasma membrane *via* electrostatic interactions.

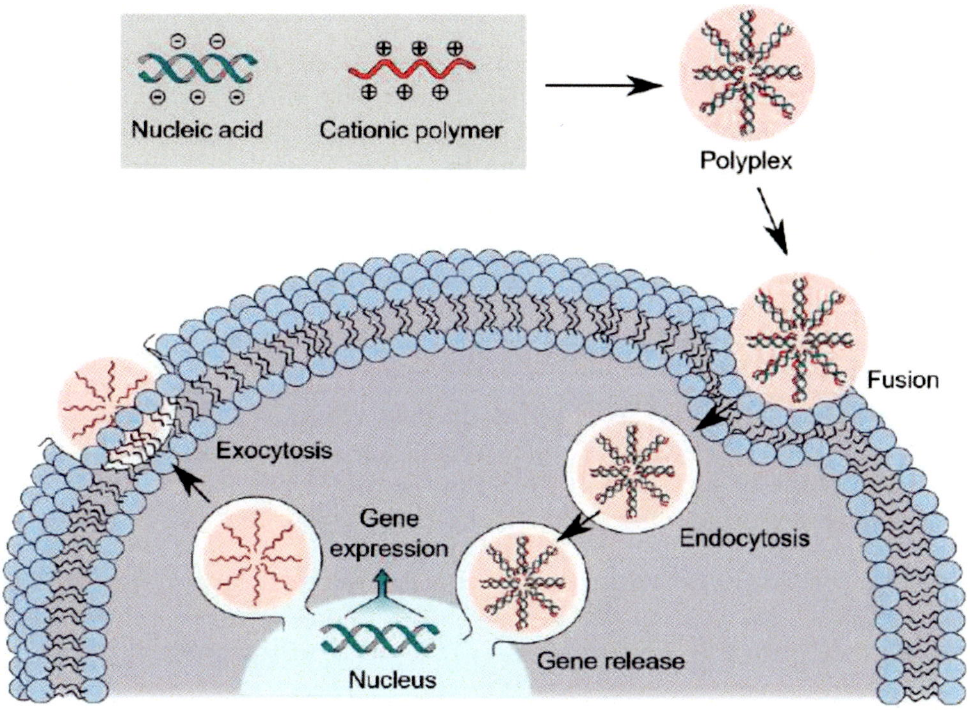

Fig. (14.5). Schematic representation of polyplexes-based gene therapy.

A group of researchers investigated a non- invasive and non-viral delivery system that could be used to treat retinal degenerations, which would be safe and efficient. Different researchers in the past have conducted various gene therapy trials, and the majority of those studies concluded winning recovery of photoreceptor cells, but direct administration of a needle into the eye is associated with an inherent risk of vision trauma like intraocular infection and retinal detachment or bleeding. Souied *et al.*, investigated the transfer of 'naked' plasmid DNA into the mouse retina using transscleral iontophoresis holding gene therapy material to avoid the risk associated with injections. The dazzling GFP fluorescence and photoreceptor recovery found in the retina area revealed the successful direct transfer of DNA through the sclera. Proof of gene transfer to the posterior part of the retina suggested DNA transfer into the retina could be *via* the vitreous cavity. Findings indicated that transscleral iontophoresis can be employed as the method of choice to treat various inherited retinal disorders [146].

Puras *et al.* incorporated ultra-pure oligochitosans (NOVAFECT O15) for designing polyplexes (EGFP plasmid) as they easily get attached to the DNA through electrostatic interactions [147]. Corneal gene delivery studies of NOVAFECT O15 after intrastromal injection have been done [148, 149]. Accordingly, the author administered low molecular weight ultrapure oligochitosan and EGFP plasmid polyplexes *via* subretinal and intravitreal injections to explore the potential use of ultrapure oligochitoan as DNA (EGFP plasmid) carries in other ocular tissues such as retinal [150]. They also evaluated the expression of the EGFP (plasmid) (after 72h) in different cells (Human Embryonic Kidney (HEK-293) and Human Retinal Pigmented Epithelial Cells (ARPE-19)) and retinal layers by confocal microscopy. The resulting polyplexes protect the plasmid against enzymatic digestion. A significant increase in transfection efficiency in HEK-293 cultured cells and no significant transfection in ARPE-19 cultured cells were observed. The light-sensitive photoreceptor cells and pigmented cells of the retinal pigment epithelium were transfected by subretinal administration. In contrast, cells in the ganglion cell layer and blood vessels (inner retinal layer and photoreceptors) were transfected by intravitreal injections. These results support the potential use of oligochitosans for delivering genetic material into retinal cells *in vivo*.

In recent years many researchers have been going forward to achieve a suitable and safe non-viral system for gene therapy. Anionic ternary complexes were developed by coating plasmid DNA (pDNA)/polyethyleneimine (PEI) complex with anionic polymers such as γ-polyglutamic acid (γ-PGA) and chondroitin sulfate (CS). More gene expression on ARPE-19 cells was observed by anionic complexes without cytotoxicity and aggregation in the vitreous body compared with cationic ternary complexes [151].

Martens *et al.* investigated the applicability of hyaluronic acid (HA) for improving intravitreal mobility of non-viral polymeric nanocarrier (p(CBA-ABOL)/pDNA complexes). Uncoated polyplexes were 108nm in size, followed by a zeta potential of +29mV. The zeta potential of HA-coated polyplexes became anionic at 4-fold molar excess of HA-monomers compared to cationic monomers. HA-coated polyplexes showed good mobility in vitreous humor when evaluated in an *ex-vivo* model by fluorescence single particle tracking microscopy except for coating with high molecular weight HA (2700 kDa). The HA-coated polyplexes had negative charges and were efficiently taken up by ARPE-19 cells *in vitro* study; it indicates uptake through CD44receptor-mediated endocytosis. Findings revealed that the HA polyplexes could induce GFP expression in a cell line (*in vitro*) with no apparent cytotoxicity. In contrast, the highest expression was observed with low molecular weight HA (22 kDa) coated polyplexes [152].

Oliveira *et al.*, aimed at enhancing the gene transfer efficiency and sustained gene expression by developing a chitosan polyplexes-mediated gene delivery combined with phiC311-integrase. Different polyplexes were developed by incorporating GFP (small transgene 1 Kb) plasmid and CEP290 (large transgene >8 Kb) with or without integrase plasmid in varying sizes of chitosan polymer. Developed polyplexes were characterized, and co-transfection with integrase was performed. DNA complexation efficiency, particle size, and surface morphology were the same for all the formulations; however, the transfection efficiency and transgene expression varied with varying polymer and polymer sizes. Co-transfection with integrase showed sustained expression for over 16 weeks and at least six weeks for GFP and CEP290, respectively. Results showed that this combined approach could overcome the size limitation usually observed with AAV vectors, and a safe, prolonged gene expression can be achieved [153].

CONCLUSION

Progress in developing pre-clinical efficacy and safety profiles of the vectors have made gene therapy a promising alternative to the conventional treatment approaches for several ocular diseases. Ocular gene therapy is the best approach for Leber Congenital Amaurosis, which has urged more research for treating other ocular diseases (glaucoma, age-related macular degeneration, retinitis pigmentosa, or choroideremia). Effective, non-toxic gene carrier development, targeted delivery of therapeutic genes to the tissues, and long-term gene expression are the desired features of successful ocular gene therapy. Both the viral and non-viral gene therapies are showing encouraging results. Still, viral gene therapy has immunogenicity and mutagenesis-associated risks, which urged the development of non-viral gene therapy. Interaction between cationic lipids/ polymers and negatively charged nucleic acids leads to material condensation into nanosized particles, protection of nucleic acids from enzymes, and mediation of cellular entry. Recent approaches in the literature illustrated the benefits of viral and non-viral vectors for the ocular delivery of therapeutic agents. A significant analysis of the mechanism and variations behind ocular diseases and the development of effective gene carriers would lead to improved treatment approaches.

CONSENT FOR PUBLICATION

Not applicable.

CONFLICT OF INTEREST

The authors declare no conflict of interest, financial or otherwise.

ACKNOWLEDGEMENT

Declared none.

REFERENCES

[1] Vadlapudi AD, Cholkar K, Dasari SR, Mitra AK. Ocular drug delivery.Drug Delivery. Burlington, MA, USA: Jones & Bartlett Learning 2015; pp. 219-63.

[2] Chen H. Recent developments in ocular drug delivery. J Drug Target 2015; 23(7-8): 597-604. [http://dx.doi.org/10.3109/1061186X.2015.1052073] [PMID: 26453157]

[3] Nagarwal RC, Kant S, Singh PN, Maiti P, Pandit JK. Polymeric nanoparticulate system: A potential approach for ocular drug delivery. J Control Release 2009; 136(1): 2-13. [http://dx.doi.org/10.1016/j.jconrel.2008.12.018] [PMID: 19331856]

[4] Cholkar K, Patel SP, Vadlapudi AD, Mitra AK. Novel strategies for anterior segment ocular drug delivery. J Ocul Pharmacol Ther 2013; 29(2): 106-23. [http://dx.doi.org/10.1089/jop.2012.0200] [PMID: 23215539]

[5] Souza JG, Dias K, Pereira TA, Bernardi DS, Lopez RFV. Topical delivery of ocular therapeutics: Carrier systems and physical methods. J Pharm Pharmacol 2014; 66(4): 507-30. [http://dx.doi.org/10.1111/jphp.12132] [PMID: 24635555]

[6] Liu S, Jones L, Gu FX. Nanomaterials for ocular drug delivery. Macromol Biosci 2012; 12(5): 608-20. [http://dx.doi.org/10.1002/mabi.201100419] [PMID: 22508445]

[7] Yavuz B, Kompella UB. Ocular drug delivery.Pharmacologic Therapy of Ocular Disease. Cham: Springer 2016; pp. 57-93. [http://dx.doi.org/10.1007/164_2016_84]

[8] Mitra AK, Anand BS, Duvvuri S. Drug delivery to the eye.The biology of eye. New York: Academic Press 2006; pp. 307-51.

[9] Ruponen M, Urtti A. Undefined role of mucus as a barrier in ocular drug delivery. Eur J Pharm Biopharm 2015; 96: 442-6. [http://dx.doi.org/10.1016/j.ejpb.2015.02.032] [PMID: 25770770]

[10] Kang-Mieler JJ, Osswald CR, Mieler WF. Advances in ocular drug delivery: Emphasis on the posterior segment. Expert Opin Drug Deliv 2014; 11(10): 1647-60. [http://dx.doi.org/10.1517/17425247.2014.935338] [PMID: 24975820]

[11] Kaur IP, Kakkar S. Nanotherapy for posterior eye diseases. J Control Release 2014; 193: 100-12. [http://dx.doi.org/10.1016/j.jconrel.2014.05.031] [PMID: 24862316]

[12] Koo H, Moon H, Han H, *et al.* The movement of self-assembled amphiphilic polymeric nanoparticles in the vitreous and retina after intravitreal injection. Biomaterials 2012; 33(12): 3485-93. [http://dx.doi.org/10.1016/j.biomaterials.2012.01.030] [PMID: 22322197]

[13] Bansal P, Garg S, Sharma Y, Venkatesh P. Posterior segment drug delivery devices: Current and novel therapies in development. J Ocul Pharmacol Ther 2016; 32(3): 135-44. [http://dx.doi.org/10.1089/jop.2015.0133] [PMID: 26811883]

[14] Vicentini FTMC, Borgheti-Cardoso LN, Depieri LV, *et al.* Delivery systems and local administration routes for therapeutic siRNA. Pharm Res 2013; 30(4): 915-31. [http://dx.doi.org/10.1007/s11095-013-0971-1] [PMID: 23344907]

[15] Patel A, Cholkar K, Agrahari V, Mitra AK. Ocular drug delivery systems: An overview. World J Pharmacol 2013; 2(2): 47-64.
[http://dx.doi.org/10.5497/wjp.v2.i2.47] [PMID: 25590022]

[16] Gaudana R, Ananthula HK, Parenky A, Mitra AK. Ocular drug delivery. AAPS J 2010; 12(3): 348-60.
[http://dx.doi.org/10.1208/s12248-010-9183-3] [PMID: 20437123]

[17] Toropainen E, Hornof M, Kaarniranta K, Johansson P, Urtti A. Corneal epithelium as a platform for secretion of transgene products after transfection with liposomal gene eyedrops. J Gene Med 2007; 9(3): 208-16.
[http://dx.doi.org/10.1002/jgm.1011] [PMID: 17351984]

[18] Gautam N, Kesavan K. Development of microemulsions for ocular delivery. Ther Deliv 2017; 8(5): 313-30.
[http://dx.doi.org/10.4155/tde-2016-0076] [PMID: 28361605]

[19] Almeida H, Amaral MH, Lobão P, Lobo JMS. *in situ* gelling systems: A strategy to improve the bioavailability of ophthalmic pharmaceutical formulations. Drug Discov Today 2014; 19(4): 400-12.
[http://dx.doi.org/10.1016/j.drudis.2013.10.001] [PMID: 24120893]

[20] Bucolo C, Drago F, Salomone S. Ocular drug delivery: A clue from nanotechnology. Front Pharmacol 2012; 3: 188-90.
[http://dx.doi.org/10.3389/fphar.2012.00188] [PMID: 23125835]

[21] Kuno N, Fujii S. Recent advances in ocular drug delivery systems. Polymers (Basel) 2011; 3(1): 193-221.
[http://dx.doi.org/10.3390/polym3010193]

[22] Stahl U, Willcox M, Stapleton F. Osmolality and tear film dynamics. Clin Exp Optom 2012; 95(1): 3-11.
[http://dx.doi.org/10.1111/j.1444-0938.2011.00634.x] [PMID: 22022802]

[23] Başaran E, Yazan Y. Ocular application of chitosan. Expert Opin Drug Deliv 2012; 9(6): 701-12.
[http://dx.doi.org/10.1517/17425247.2012.681775] [PMID: 22530690]

[24] Tan DTH, Dart JKG, Holland EJ, Kinoshita S. Corneal transplantation. Lancet 2012; 379(9827): 1749-61.
[http://dx.doi.org/10.1016/S0140-6736(12)60437-1] [PMID: 22559901]

[25] Hornof M, Toropainen E, Urtti A. Cell culture models of the ocular barriers. Eur J Pharm Biopharm 2005; 60(2): 207-25.
[http://dx.doi.org/10.1016/j.ejpb.2005.01.009] [PMID: 15939234]

[26] Yang Y, Hong J, Deng SX, Xu J. Age-related changes in human corneal epithelial thickness measured with anterior segment optical coherence tomography. Invest Ophthalmol Vis Sci 2014; 55(8): 5032-8.
[http://dx.doi.org/10.1167/iovs.13-13831] [PMID: 25052994]

[27] Pahuja P, Arora S, Pawar P. Ocular drug delivery system: A reference to natural polymers. Expert Opin Drug Deliv 2012; 9(7): 837-61.
[http://dx.doi.org/10.1517/17425247.2012.690733] [PMID: 22703523]

[28] Fischbarg J, Diecke FPJ. A mathematical model of electrolyte and fluid transport across corneal endothelium. J Membr Biol 2005; 203(1): 41-56.
[http://dx.doi.org/10.1007/s00232-004-0730-7] [PMID: 15834688]

[29] Karla PK, Pal D, Quinn T, Mitra AK. Molecular evidence and functional expression of a novel drug efflux pump (ABCC2) in human corneal epithelium and rabbit cornea and its role in ocular drug efflux. Int J Pharm 2007; 336(1): 12-21.
[http://dx.doi.org/10.1016/j.ijpharm.2006.11.031] [PMID: 17156953]

[30] Karla PK, Earla R, Boddu SH, Johnston TP, Pal D, Mitra A. Molecular expression and functional evidence of a drug efflux pump (BCRP) in human corneal epithelial cells. Curr Eye Res 2009; 34(1):

1-9.
[http://dx.doi.org/10.1080/02713680802518251] [PMID: 19172464]

[31] Dey S, Patel J, Anand BS, *et al.* Molecular evidence and functional expression of P-glycoprotein (MDR1) in human and rabbit cornea and corneal epithelial cell lines. Invest Ophthalmol Vis Sci 2003; 44(7): 2909-18.
[http://dx.doi.org/10.1167/iovs.02-1142] [PMID: 12824231]

[32] del Amo EM, Rimpelä AK, Heikkinen E, *et al.* Pharmacokinetic aspects of retinal drug delivery. Prog Retin Eye Res 2017; 57: 134-85.
[http://dx.doi.org/10.1016/j.preteyeres.2016.12.001] [PMID: 28028001]

[33] Ahmed I. The noncorneal route in ocular drug delivery.Ophthalmic drug delivery systems. New York: Marcel Dekker 2003; pp. 335-63.
[http://dx.doi.org/10.1201/9780203912072.ch11]

[34] Willoughby CE, Ponzin D, Ferrari S, Lobo A, Landau K, Omidi Y. Anatomy and physiology of the human eye: Effects of mucopolysaccharidoses disease on structure and function - a review. Clin Exp Ophthalmol 2010; 38: 2-11.
[http://dx.doi.org/10.1111/j.1442-9071.2010.02363.x]

[35] Dubald M, Bourgeois S, Andrieu V, Fessi H. Ophthalmic drug delivery systems for antibiotherapy—a review. Pharmaceutics 2018; 10(1): 10.
[http://dx.doi.org/10.3390/pharmaceutics10010010] [PMID: 29342879]

[36] Barar J, Asadi M, Mortazavi-Tabatabaei SA, Omidi Y. Ocular drug delivery; impact of *in vitro* cell culture models. J Ophthalmic Vis Res 2009; 4(4): 238-52.
[PMID: 23198080]

[37] Klaassen I, Van Noorden CJF, Schlingemann RO. Molecular basis of the inner blood-retinal barrier and its breakdown in diabetic macular edema and other pathological conditions. Prog Retin Eye Res 2013; 34: 19-48.
[http://dx.doi.org/10.1016/j.preteyeres.2013.02.001] [PMID: 23416119]

[38] Hayreh SS. Blood supply of the anterior segment.Ocular Vascular Occlusive Disorders. Cham: Springer 2015; pp. 111-41.

[39] Freddo TF. A contemporary concept of the blood–aqueous barrier. Prog Retin Eye Res 2013; 32: 181-95.
[http://dx.doi.org/10.1016/j.preteyeres.2012.10.004] [PMID: 23128417]

[40] Barar J, Aghanejad A, Fathi M, Omidi Y. Advanced drug delivery and targeting technologies for the ocular diseases. Bioimpacts 2016; 6(1): 49-67.
[http://dx.doi.org/10.15171/bi.2016.07] [PMID: 27340624]

[41] Jumbe NL, Miller MH. Ocular drug transfer following systemic drug administration.Ophthalmic Drug Delivery Systems. CRC Press 2003; pp. 130-55.
[http://dx.doi.org/10.1201/9780203912072.ch4]

[42] Freddo TF. Shifting the paradigm of the blood-aqueous barrier. Exp Eye Res 2001; 73(5): 581-92.
[http://dx.doi.org/10.1006/exer.2001.1056] [PMID: 11747359]

[43] Pathak Y, Sutariya V, Hirani AA, Eds. Nano-biomaterials for ophthalmic drug delivery. Switzerland: Springer International Publishing 2016.
[http://dx.doi.org/10.1007/978-3-319-29346-2]

[44] Conrad JM, Robinson JR. Aqueous chamber drug distribution volume measurement in rabbits. J Pharm Sci 1977; 66(2): 219-24.
[http://dx.doi.org/10.1002/jps.2600660222] [PMID: 839419]

[45] Schoenwald RD. Ocular pharmacokinetics and pharmacodynamics.Ophthalmic drug delivery systems. CRC Press 2003; pp. 156-201.
[http://dx.doi.org/10.1201/9780203912072.ch5]

[46] Urtti A. Challenges and obstacles of ocular pharmacokinetics and drug delivery. Adv Drug Deliv Rev 2006; 58(11): 1131-5.
[http://dx.doi.org/10.1016/j.addr.2006.07.027] [PMID: 17097758]

[47] Strotmann F, Wolf I, Galla HJ. The biocompatibility of a polyelectrolyte vitreous body substitute on a high resistance *in vitro* model of the blood-retinal barrier. J Biomater Appl 2013; 28(3): 334-42.
[http://dx.doi.org/10.1177/0885328212450597] [PMID: 22693043]

[48] Barar J, Omidi Y. Bioelectrical and permeability properties of brain microvasculature endothelial cells: Effects of tight junction modulators. Res J Biol Sci 2008; 8(3): 556-62.

[49] Omidi Y, Barar J, Ahmadian S, Heidari HR, Gumbleton M. Characterization and astrocytic modulation of system L transporters in brain microvasculature endothelial cells. Cell Biochem Funct 2008; 26(3): 381-91.
[http://dx.doi.org/10.1002/cbf.1455] [PMID: 18210381]

[50] Omidi Y, Campbell L, Barar J, Connell D, Akhtar S, Gumbleton M. Evaluation of the immortalised mouse brain capillary endothelial cell line, b.End3, as an *in vitro* blood–brain barrier model for drug uptake and transport studies. Brain Res 2003; 990(1-2): 95-112.
[http://dx.doi.org/10.1016/S0006-8993(03)03443-7] [PMID: 14568334]

[51] Smith M, Omidi Y, Gumbleton M. Primary porcine brain microvascular endothelial cells: Biochemical and functional characterisation as a model for drug transport and targeting. J Drug Target 2007; 15(4): 253-68.
[http://dx.doi.org/10.1080/10611860701288539] [PMID: 17487694]

[52] Haghjou N, Abdekhodaie MJ, Cheng YL. Retina-choroid-sclera permeability for ophthalmic drugs in the vitreous to blood direction: Quantitative assessment. Pharm Res 2013; 30(1): 41-59.
[http://dx.doi.org/10.1007/s11095-012-0847-9] [PMID: 23054085]

[53] Murata M, Sanbe A, Lee JW, Nishigori H. Laser-induced intrachoroidal dexamethasone drug delivery system to posterior eye segment. Invest Ophthalmol Vis Sci 2013; 54(13): 8317-24.
[http://dx.doi.org/10.1167/iovs.13-13078] [PMID: 24265021]

[54] Hornof M, Weyenberg W, Ludwig A, Bernkop-Schnürch A. Mucoadhesive ocular insert based on thiolated poly(acrylic acid): Development and *in vivo* evaluation in humans. J Control Release 2003; 89(3): 419-28.
[http://dx.doi.org/10.1016/S0168-3659(03)00135-4] [PMID: 12737844]

[55] Mitra AK. Ophthalmic drug delivery systems. New York: Marcel Dekker 2003.
[http://dx.doi.org/10.1201/9780203912072]

[56] Al-Saikhan FI. The gene therapy revolution in ophthalmology. Saudi J Ophthalmol 2013; 27(2): 107-11.
[http://dx.doi.org/10.1016/j.sjopt.2013.02.001] [PMID: 24227970]

[57] Mulligan RC. The basic science of gene therapy. Science 1993; 260(5110): 926-32.
[http://dx.doi.org/10.1126/science.8493530] [PMID: 8493530]

[58] Borrás T. Recent developments in ocular gene therapy. Exp Eye Res 2003; 76(6): 643-52.
[http://dx.doi.org/10.1016/S0014-4835(03)00030-7] [PMID: 12742346]

[59] Colella P, Cotugno G, Auricchio A. Ocular gene therapy: Current progress and future prospects. Trends Mol Med 2009; 15(1): 23-31.
[http://dx.doi.org/10.1016/j.molmed.2008.11.003] [PMID: 19097940]

[60] Rajala A, Wang Y, Zhu Y, *et al.* Nanoparticle-assisted targeted delivery of eye-specific genes to eyes significantly improves the vision of blind mice *in vivo*. Nano Lett 2014; 14(9): 5257-63.
[http://dx.doi.org/10.1021/nl502275s] [PMID: 25115433]

[61] Wang Y, Rajala A, Rajala R. Lipid nanoparticles for ocular gene delivery. J Funct Biomater 2015; 6(2): 379-94.

[http://dx.doi.org/10.3390/jfb6020379] [PMID: 26062170]

[62] Ali M, Lemoine NR, Ring CJ. The use of DNA viruses as vectors for gene therapy. Gene Ther 1994; 1(6): 367-84.
[PMID: 7584103]

[63] Wu Z, Yang H, Colosi P. Effect of genome size on AAV vector packaging. Mol Ther 2010; 18(1): 80-6.
[http://dx.doi.org/10.1038/mt.2009.255] [PMID: 19904234]

[64] Wirth T, Parker N, Ylä-Herttuala S. History of gene therapy. Gene 2013; 525(2): 162-9.
[http://dx.doi.org/10.1016/j.gene.2013.03.137] [PMID: 23618815]

[65] Cevher E, Sezer AD, Çağlar E. Gene delivery systems: Recent progress in viral and non-viral therapy. Recent advances in novel drug carrier systems. 2012; pp. 437-70.

[66] Verma IM, Weitzman MD. Gene therapy: Twenty-first century medicine. Annu Rev Biochem 2005; 74(1): 711-38.
[http://dx.doi.org/10.1146/annurev.biochem.74.050304.091637] [PMID: 15952901]

[67] Crystal RG. Adenovirus: The first effective *in vivo* gene delivery vector. Hum Gene Ther 2014; 25(1): 3-11.
[http://dx.doi.org/10.1089/hum.2013.2527] [PMID: 24444179]

[68] Ginsberg HS. The ups and downs of adenovirus vectors. Bull N Y Acad Med 1996; 73(1): 53-8.
[PMID: 8804738]

[69] Liu X, Hu Y, Filla MS, *et al.* The effect of C3 transgene expression on actin and cellular adhesions in cultured human trabecular meshwork cells and on outflow facility in organ cultured monkey eyes. Mol Vis 2005; 11: 1112-21.
[PMID: 16379023]

[70] Wen SF, Chen Z, Nery J, Faha B. Characterization of adenovirus p21 gene transfer, biodistribution, and immune response after local ocular delivery in New Zealand white rabbits. Exp Eye Res 2003; 77(3): 355-65.
[http://dx.doi.org/10.1016/S0014-4835(03)00122-2] [PMID: 12907168]

[71] Akiyama H, Tanaka T, Itakura H, *et al.* Inhibition of ocular angiogenesis by an adenovirus carrying the human von Hippel-Lindau tumor-suppressor gene *in vivo*. Invest Ophthalmol Vis Sci 2004; 45(5): 1289-96.
[http://dx.doi.org/10.1167/iovs.03-0282] [PMID: 15111579]

[72] Vandenberghe LH, Auricchio A. Novel adeno-associated viral vectors for retinal gene therapy. Gene Ther 2012; 19(2): 162-8.
[http://dx.doi.org/10.1038/gt.2011.151] [PMID: 21993172]

[73] Hauswirth WW, Lewin AS, Zolotukhin S, Muzyczka N. Production and purification of recombinant adeno-associated virus. Methods Enzymol 2000; 316: 743-61.
[http://dx.doi.org/10.1016/S0076-6879(00)16760-6] [PMID: 10800712]

[74] Peel AL, Klein RL. Adeno-associated virus vectors: Activity and applications in the CNS. J Neurosci Methods 2000; 98(2): 95-104.
[http://dx.doi.org/10.1016/S0165-0270(00)00183-7] [PMID: 10880823]

[75] Kiyota T, Ingraham KL, Swan RJ, Jacobsen MT, Andrews SJ, Ikezu T. AAV serotype 2/1-mediated gene delivery of anti-inflammatory interleukin-10 enhances neurogenesis and cognitive function in APP+PS1 mice. Gene Ther 2012; 19(7): 724-33.
[http://dx.doi.org/10.1038/gt.2011.126] [PMID: 21918553]

[76] Han Z, Conley SM, Makkia R, Guo J, Cooper MJ, Naash MI. Comparative analysis of DNA nanoparticles and AAVs for ocular gene delivery. PLoS One 2012; 7(12): e52189.
[http://dx.doi.org/10.1371/journal.pone.0052189] [PMID: 23272225]

[77] Dismuke D, Tenenbaum L, Samulski R. Biosafety of recombinant adeno-associated virus vectors. Curr Gene Ther 2014; 13(6): 434-52.
[http://dx.doi.org/10.2174/1566523211313666007] [PMID: 24195602]

[78] Jacobson SG, Boye SL, Aleman TS, *et al.* Safety in nonhuman primates of ocular AAV2-RPE65, a candidate treatment for blindness in Leber congenital amaurosis. Hum Gene Ther 2006; 17(8): 845-58.
[http://dx.doi.org/10.1089/hum.2006.17.845] [PMID: 16942444]

[79] Lai YKY, Shen WY, Brankov M, Lai CM, Constable IJ, Rakoczy PE. Potential long-term inhibition of ocular neovascularisation by recombinant adeno-associated virus-mediated secretion gene therapy. Gene Ther 2002; 9(12): 804-13.
[http://dx.doi.org/10.1038/sj.gt.3301695] [PMID: 12040462]

[80] Igarashi T, Miyake K, Masuda I, Takahashi H, Shimada T. Adeno-associated vector (type 8)-mediated expression of soluble Flt-1 efficiently inhibits neovascularization in a murine choroidal neovascularization model. Hum Gene Ther 2010; 21(5): 631-7.
[http://dx.doi.org/10.1089/hum.2009.153] [PMID: 20053138]

[81] Mao Y, Kiss S, Boyer JL, *et al.* Persistent suppression of ocular neovascularization with intravitreal administration of AAVrh.10 coding for bevacizumab. Hum Gene Ther 2011; 22(12): 1525-35.
[http://dx.doi.org/10.1089/hum.2011.090] [PMID: 21801028]

[82] Miki K, Miki A, Matsuoka M, Muramatsu D, Hackett SF, Campochiaro PA. Effects of intraocular ranibizumab and bevacizumab in transgenic mice expressing human vascular endothelial growth factor. Ophthalmology 2009; 116(9): 1748-54.
[http://dx.doi.org/10.1016/j.ophtha.2009.05.020] [PMID: 19643496]

[83] Tuo J, Pang JJ, Cao X, *et al.* AAV5-mediated sFLT01 gene therapy arrests retinal lesions in Ccl2−/−/Cx3cr1−/− mice. Neurobiol Aging 2012; 33(2): 433-e1-10.

[84] Zhang X, Das SK, Passi SF, *et al.* AAV2 delivery of Flt23k intraceptors inhibits murine choroidal neovascularization. Mol Ther 2015; 23(2): 226-34.
[http://dx.doi.org/10.1038/mt.2014.199] [PMID: 25306972]

[85] Rakoczy EP, Lai CM, Magno AL, *et al.* Gene therapy with recombinant adeno-associated vectors for neovascular age-related macular degeneration: 1 year follow-up of a phase 1 randomised clinical trial. Lancet 2015; 386(10011): 2395-403.
[http://dx.doi.org/10.1016/S0140-6736(15)00345-1] [PMID: 26431823]

[86] Marangoni D, Bush RA, Zeng Y, *et al.* Ocular and systemic safety of a recombinant AAV8 vector for X-linked retinoschisis gene therapy: GLP studies in rabbits and Rs1-KO mice. Mol Ther Methods Clin Dev 2016; 3: 16011.
[http://dx.doi.org/10.1038/mtm.2016.11] [PMID: 27626041]

[87] Lambert NG, Zhang X, Rai RR, *et al.* Subretinal AAV2.COMP-Ang1 suppresses choroidal neovascularization and vascular endothelial growth factor in a murine model of age-related macular degeneration. Exp Eye Res 2016; 145: 248-57.
[http://dx.doi.org/10.1016/j.exer.2016.01.009] [PMID: 26775053]

[88] Liu Y, Fortmann SD, Shen J, *et al.* AAV8-antiVEGFfab ocular gene transfer for neovascular age-related macular degeneration. Mol Ther 2018; 26(2): 542-9.
[http://dx.doi.org/10.1016/j.ymthe.2017.12.002] [PMID: 29292162]

[89] Fischer MD, McClements ME, Martinez-Fernandez de la Camara C, *et al.* Codon-optimized RPGR improves stability and efficacy of AAV8 gene therapy in two mouse models of X-linked retinitis pigmentosa. Mol Ther 2017; 25(8): 1854-65.
[http://dx.doi.org/10.1016/j.ymthe.2017.05.005] [PMID: 28549772]

[90] Le Meur G, Lebranchu P, Billaud F, *et al.* Safety and long-term efficacy of AAV4 gene therapy in patients with RPE65 Leber congenital amaurosis. Mol Ther 2018; 26(1): 256-68.
[http://dx.doi.org/10.1016/j.ymthe.2017.09.014] [PMID: 29033008]

[91] Maddalena A, Tornabene P, Tiberi P, *et al.* Triple vectors expand AAV transfer capacity in the retina. Mol Ther 2018; 26(2): 524-41.
[http://dx.doi.org/10.1016/j.ymthe.2017.11.019] [PMID: 29292161]

[92] Balaggan KS, Ali RR. Ocular gene delivery using lentiviral vectors. Gene Ther 2012; 19(2): 145-53.
[http://dx.doi.org/10.1038/gt.2011.153] [PMID: 22052240]

[93] Parker DGA, Kaufmann C, Brereton HM, *et al.* Lentivirus-mediated gene transfer to the rat, ovine and human cornea. Gene Ther 2007; 14(9): 760-7.
[http://dx.doi.org/10.1038/sj.gt.3302921] [PMID: 17301843]

[94] Bemelmans AP, Kostic C, Crippa SV, *et al.* Lentiviral gene transfer of RPE65 rescues survival and function of cones in a mouse model of Leber congenital amaurosis. PLoS Med 2006; 3(10): e347.
[http://dx.doi.org/10.1371/journal.pmed.0030347] [PMID: 17032058]

[95] Kong J, Kim S-R, Binley K, *et al.* Correction of the disease phenotype in the mouse model of Stargardt disease by lentiviral gene therapy. Gene Ther 2008; 15(19): 1311-20.
[http://dx.doi.org/10.1038/gt.2008.78] [PMID: 18463687]

[96] Binley K, Widdowson P, Loader J, *et al.* Transduction of photoreceptors with equine infectious anemia virus lentiviral vectors: Safety and biodistribution of StarGen for Stargardt disease. Invest Ophthalmol Vis Sci 2013; 54(6): 4061-71.
[http://dx.doi.org/10.1167/iovs.13-11871] [PMID: 23620430]

[97] Binley K, Widdowson PS, Kelleher M, *et al.* Safety and biodistribution of an equine infectious anemia virus-based gene therapy, RetinoStat(®), for age-related macular degeneration. Hum Gene Ther 2012; 23(9): 980-91.
[http://dx.doi.org/10.1089/hum.2012.008] [PMID: 22716662]

[98] Challa P, Luna C, Liton PB, *et al.* Lentiviral mediated gene delivery to the anterior chamber of rodent eyes. Mol Vis 2005; 11: 425-30.
[PMID: 15988411]

[99] Xu H, Liu J, Xiong S, Le Y, Xia X. Suppression of retinal neovascularization by lentivirus-mediated netrin-1 small hairpin RNA. Ophthalmic Res 2012; 47(3): 163-9.
[http://dx.doi.org/10.1159/000331428] [PMID: 22122983]

[100] Matet A, Kostic C, Bemelmans AP, *et al.* Evaluation of tolerance to lentiviral LV-RPE65 gene therapy vector after subretinal delivery in non-human primates. Transl Res 2017; 188: 40-57.e4.
[http://dx.doi.org/10.1016/j.trsl.2017.06.012] [PMID: 28754419]

[101] Harvey AR. Combined therapies in the treatment of neurotrauma: Polymers, bridges and gene therapy in visual system repair. Neurodegener Dis 2007; 4(4): 300-5.
[http://dx.doi.org/10.1159/000101886] [PMID: 17627133]

[102] Zhang Y, Schlachetzki F, Li JY, Boado RJ, Pardridge WM. Organ-specific gene expression in the rhesus monkey eye following intravenous non-viral gene transfer. Mol Vis 2003; 9: 465-72.
[PMID: 14551536]

[103] Chung DC, Wei Z, Bennett J. *in vivo* non–viral gene transfer to retinal ganglion cells. Invest Ophthalmol Vis Sci 2006; 47(13): 836.

[104] Mamiya K, Ohguro H, Ohguro I, *et al.* Effects of matrix metalloproteinase-3 gene transfer by electroporation in glaucoma filter surgery. Exp Eye Res 2004; 79(3): 405-10.
[http://dx.doi.org/10.1016/j.exer.2004.06.017] [PMID: 15336503]

[105] Chalberg TW, Genise HL, Vollrath D, Calos MP. phiC31 integrase confers genomic integration and long-term transgene expression in rat retina. Invest Ophthalmol Vis Sci 2005; 46(6): 2140-6.
[http://dx.doi.org/10.1167/iovs.04-1252] [PMID: 15914635]

[106] Davies JB, Ciavatta VT, Boatright JH, Nickerson JM. Delivery of several forms of DNA, DNA-RNA hybrids, and dyes across human sclera by electrical fields. Mol Vis 2003; 9(68-69): 569-78.

[PMID: 14566222]

[107] Asahara T, Shinomiya K, Naito T, Shiota H. Induction of gene into the rabbit eye by iontophoresis: Preliminary report. Jpn J Ophthalmol 2001; 45(1): 31-9.
[http://dx.doi.org/10.1016/S0021-5155(00)00291-4] [PMID: 11163043]

[108] Shuler RK Jr, Dioguardi PK, Henjy C, Nickerson JM, Cruysberg LPJ, Edelhauser HF. Scleral permeability of a small, single-stranded oligonucleotide. J Ocul Pharmacol Ther 2004; 20(2): 159-68.
[http://dx.doi.org/10.1089/108076804773710830] [PMID: 15117572]

[109] Wells DJ. Gene therapy progress and prospects: Electroporation and other physical methods. Gene Ther 2004; 11(18): 1363-9.
[http://dx.doi.org/10.1038/sj.gt.3302337] [PMID: 15295618]

[110] Singh K, Mezei M. Liposomal ophthalmic drug delivery system I. Triamcinolone acetonide. Int J Pharm 1983; 16(3): 339-44.
[http://dx.doi.org/10.1016/0378-5173(83)90152-7]

[111] Bochot A, Couvreur P, Fattal E. Intravitreal administration of antisense oligonucleotides: Potential of liposomal delivery. Prog Retin Eye Res 2000; 19(2): 131-47.
[http://dx.doi.org/10.1016/S1350-9462(99)00014-2] [PMID: 10674705]

[112] Bochot A, Fattal E, Boutet V, *et al.* Intravitreal delivery of oligonucleotides by sterically stabilized liposomes. Invest Ophthalmol Vis Sci 2002; 43(1): 253-9.
[PMID: 11773039]

[113] Yoon KC, Ahn KY, Lee JH, *et al.* Lipid-mediated delivery of brain-specific angiogenesis inhibitor 1 gene reduces corneal neovascularization in an *in vivo* rabbit model. Gene Ther 2005; 12(7): 617-24.
[http://dx.doi.org/10.1038/sj.gt.3302442] [PMID: 15703766]

[114] Peeters L, Sanders NN, Jones A, Demeester J, De Smedt SC. Post-pegylated lipoplexes are promising vehicles for gene delivery in RPE cells. J Control Release 2007; 121(3): 208-17.
[http://dx.doi.org/10.1016/j.jconrel.2007.05.033] [PMID: 17630013]

[115] Farjo R, Skaggs J, Quiambao AB, Cooper MJ, Naash MI. Efficient non-viral ocular gene transfer with compacted DNA nanoparticles. PloS one 2006; 1(1): e38:1-8.
[http://dx.doi.org/10.1371/journal.pone.0000038]

[116] Bejjani RA, BenEzra D, Cohen H, *et al.* Nanoparticles for gene delivery to retinal pigment epithelial cells. Mol Vis 2005; 11(2): 124-32.
[PMID: 15735602]

[117] Giordano GG, Chevez-Barrios P, Refojo MF, Garcia CA. Biodegradation and tissue reaction to intravitreous biodegradable poly(D,L-lactic-co-glycolic)acid microspheres. Curr Eye Res 1995; 14(9): 761-8.
[http://dx.doi.org/10.3109/02713689508995797] [PMID: 8529414]

[118] Kimura H, Ogura Y, Moritera T, Honda Y, Tabata Y, Ikada Y. *in vitro* phagocytosis of polylactide microspheres by retinal pigment epithelial cells and intracellular drug release. Curr Eye Res 1994; 13(5): 353-60.
[http://dx.doi.org/10.3109/02713689409167299] [PMID: 8055699]

[119] Zimmer A, Kreuter J, Robinson JR. Studies on the transport pathway of PBCA nanoparticles in ocular tissues. J Microencapsul 1991; 8(4): 497-504.
[http://dx.doi.org/10.3109/02652049109021873] [PMID: 1798020]

[120] Ogura Y, Kimura H. Biodegradable polymer microspheres for targeted drug delivery to the retinal pigment epithelium. Surv Ophthalmol 1995; 39 (Suppl. 1): S17-24.
[http://dx.doi.org/10.1016/S0039-6257(05)80069-4] [PMID: 7660308]

[121] Giordano GG, Thomson RC, Ishaug SL, *et al.* Retinal pigment epithelium cells cultured on synthetic biodegradable polymers. J Biomed Mater Res 1997; 34(1): 87-93.
[http://dx.doi.org/10.1002/(SICI)1097-4636(199701)34:1<87::AID-JBM12>3.0.CO;2-M] [PMID:

8978657]

[122] Luo D, Saltzman WM. Synthetic DNA delivery systems. Nat Biotechnol 2000; 18(1): 33-7. [http://dx.doi.org/10.1038/71889] [PMID: 10625387]

[123] Mo Y, Barnett ME, Takemoto D, Davidson H, Kompella UB. Human serum albumin nanoparticles for efficient delivery of Cu, Zn superoxide dismutase gene. Mol Vis 2007; 13: 746-57. [PMID: 17563725]

[124] Lin D, Barnett M, Grauer L, *et al.* Expression of superoxide dismutase in whole lens prevents cataract formation. Mol Vis 2005; 11(11): 853-8. [PMID: 16254550]

[125] Imamura Y, Noda S, Hashizume K, *et al.* Drusen, choroidal neovascularization, and retinal pigment epithelium dysfunction in SOD1-deficient mice: A model of age-related macular degeneration. Proc Natl Acad Sci USA 2006; 103(30): 11282-7. [http://dx.doi.org/10.1073/pnas.0602131103] [PMID: 16844785]

[126] Kragh-Hansen U. Structure and ligand binding properties of human serum albumin. Dan Med Bull 1990; 37(1): 57-84. [PMID: 2155760]

[127] Syga MI, Nicolì E, Kohler E, Shastri VP. Albumin incorporation in polyethylenimine–DNA polyplexes influences transfection efficiency. Biomacromolecules 2016; 17(1): 200-7. [http://dx.doi.org/10.1021/acs.biomac.5b01308] [PMID: 26652656]

[128] Kompella UB, Amrite AC, Pacha Ravi R, Durazo SA. Nanomedicines for back of the eye drug delivery, gene delivery, and imaging. Prog Retin Eye Res 2013; 36: 172-98. [http://dx.doi.org/10.1016/j.preteyeres.2013.04.001] [PMID: 23603534]

[129] Tschopp M, Stary J, Frueh BE, *et al.* Impact of corneal cross-linking on drug penetration in an ex vivo porcine eye model. Cornea 2012; 31(3): 222-6. [http://dx.doi.org/10.1097/ICO.0B013E31823E29D5] [PMID: 22316648]

[130] Jiang M, Gan L, Zhu C, Dong Y, Liu J, Gan Y. Cationic core–shell liponanoparticles for ocular gene delivery. Biomaterials 2012; 33(30): 7621-30. [http://dx.doi.org/10.1016/j.biomaterials.2012.06.079] [PMID: 22789720]

[131] Fàbregas A, Sánchez-Hernández N, Ticó JR, *et al.* A new optimized formulation of cationic solid lipid nanoparticles intended for gene delivery: Development, characterization and DNA binding efficiency of TCERG1 expression plasmid. Int J Pharm 2014; 473(1-2): 270-9. [http://dx.doi.org/10.1016/j.ijpharm.2014.06.022] [PMID: 24999055]

[132] Apaolaza PS, Delgado D, Pozo-Rodríguez A, Gascón AR, Solinís MÁ. A novel gene therapy vector based on hyaluronic acid and solid lipid nanoparticles for ocular diseases. Int J Pharm 2014; 465(1-2): 413-26. [http://dx.doi.org/10.1016/j.ijpharm.2014.02.038] [PMID: 24576595]

[133] Alqawlaq S, Sivak JM, Huzil JT, *et al.* Preclinical development and ocular biodistribution of gemini-DNA nanoparticles after intravitreal and topical administration: Towards non-invasive glaucoma gene therapy. Nanomedicine 2014; 10(8): 1637-47. [http://dx.doi.org/10.1016/j.nano.2014.05.010] [PMID: 24905400]

[134] Pensado A, Diaz-Corrales FJ, De la Cerda B, *et al.* Span poly-L-arginine nanoparticles are efficient non-viral vectors for PRPF31 gene delivery: An approach of gene therapy to treat retinitis pigmentosa. Nanomedicine 2016; 12(8): 2251-60. [http://dx.doi.org/10.1016/j.nano.2016.06.007] [PMID: 27381066]

[135] Tasharrofi N, Kouhkan F, Soleimani M, *et al.* Efficient gene delivery to primary human retinal pigment epithelial cells: The innate and acquired properties of vectors. Int J Pharm 2017; 518(1-2): 66-79. [http://dx.doi.org/10.1016/j.ijpharm.2016.12.048] [PMID: 28017770]

[136] Dasari BC, Cashman SM, Kumar-Singh R. Reducible PEG-POD/DNA nanoparticles for gene transfer *in vitro* and *in vivo*: Application in a mouse model of age-related macular degeneration. Mol Ther Nucleic Acids 2017; 8: 77-89.
[http://dx.doi.org/10.1016/j.omtn.2017.06.004] [PMID: 28918058]

[137] Sun D, Sahu B, Gao S, *et al.* Targeted multifunctional lipid ECO plasmid DNA nanoparticles as efficient non-viral gene therapy for Leber's congenital amaurosis. Mol Ther Nucleic Acids 2017; 7: 42-52.
[http://dx.doi.org/10.1016/j.omtn.2017.02.005] [PMID: 28624218]

[138] Puras G, Mashal M, Zárate J, *et al.* A novel cationic niosome formulation for gene delivery to the retina. J Control Release 2014; 174: 27-36.
[http://dx.doi.org/10.1016/j.jconrel.2013.11.004] [PMID: 24231407]

[139] Mashal M, Attia N, Puras G, Martínez-Navarrete G, Fernández E, Pedraz JL. Retinal gene delivery enhancement by lycopene incorporation into cationic niosomes based on DOTMA and polysorbate 60. J Control Release 2017; 254: 55-64.
[http://dx.doi.org/10.1016/j.jconrel.2017.03.386] [PMID: 28347807]

[140] Kwon GS, Kataoka K. Block copolymer micelles as long-circulating drug vehicles. Adv Drug Deliv Rev 1995; 16(2-3): 295-309.
[http://dx.doi.org/10.1016/0169-409X(95)00031-2]

[141] Liaw J, Lin YC. Evaluation of poly(ethylene oxide)–poly(propylene oxide)–poly(ethylene oxide) (PEO–PPO–PEO) gels as a release vehicle for percutaneous fentanyl. J Control Release 2000; 68(2): 273-82.
[http://dx.doi.org/10.1016/S0168-3659(00)00268-6] [PMID: 10925135]

[142] Liaw J, Chang S-F, Hsiao F-C. *in vivo* gene delivery into ocular tissues by eye drops of poly(ethylene oxide)-poly(propylene oxide)-poly(ethylene oxide) (PEO-PPO-PEO) polymeric micelles. Gene Ther 2001; 8(13): 999-1004.
[http://dx.doi.org/10.1038/sj.gt.3301485] [PMID: 11438834]

[143] Lornejad-Schäfer MR, Lambert C, Breithaupt DE, Biesalski HK, Frank J. Solubility, uptake and biocompatibility of lutein and zeaxanthin delivered to cultured human retinal pigment epithelial cells in tween40 micelles. Eur J Nutr 2007; 46(2): 79-86.
[http://dx.doi.org/10.1007/s00394-006-0635-6] [PMID: 17225922]

[144] Tong YC, Chang SF, Kao WWY, Liu CY, Liaw J. Polymeric micelle gene delivery of bcl-xL *via* eye drop reduced corneal apoptosis following epithelial debridement. J Control Release 2010; 147(1): 76-83.
[http://dx.doi.org/10.1016/j.jconrel.2010.06.006] [PMID: 20600407]

[145] Li Z, Yin H, Zhang Z, Liu KL, Li J. Supramolecular anchoring of DNA polyplexes in cyclodextrin-based polypseudorotaxane hydrogels for sustained gene delivery. Biomacromolecules 2012; 13(10): 3162-72.
[http://dx.doi.org/10.1021/bm300936x] [PMID: 23016966]

[146] Souied EH, Reid SNM, Piri NI, Lerner LE, Nusinowitz S, Farber DB. Non-invasive gene transfer by iontophoresis for therapy of an inherited retinal degeneration. Exp Eye Res 2008; 87(3): 168-75.
[http://dx.doi.org/10.1016/j.exer.2008.04.009] [PMID: 18653181]

[147] Puras G, Zarate J, Aceves M, *et al.* Low molecular weight oligochitosans for non-viral retinal gene therapy. Eur J Pharm Biopharm 2013; 83(2): 131-40.
[http://dx.doi.org/10.1016/j.ejpb.2012.09.010] [PMID: 23059418]

[148] Klausner EA, Zhang Z, Chapman RL, Multack RF, Volin MV. Ultrapure chitosan oligomers as carriers for corneal gene transfer. Biomaterials 2010; 31(7): 1814-20.
[http://dx.doi.org/10.1016/j.biomaterials.2009.10.031] [PMID: 19879644]

[149] Klausner EA, Zhang Z, Wong SP, Chapman RL, Volin MV, Harbottle RP. Corneal gene delivery:

Chitosan oligomer as a carrier of CpG rich, CpG free or S/MAR plasmid DNA. J Gene Med 2012; 14(2): 100-8.
[http://dx.doi.org/10.1002/jgm.1634] [PMID: 22106057]

[150] Bassnett S, Duncan G. Direct measurement of pH in the rat lens by ion-sensitive microelectrodes. Exp Eye Res 1985; 40(4): 585-90.
[http://dx.doi.org/10.1016/0014-4835(85)90080-6] [PMID: 4007073]

[151] Kurosaki T, Uematsu M, Shimoda K, *et al.* Ocular gene delivery systems using ternary complexes of plasmid DNA, polyethylenimine, and anionic polymers. Biol Pharm Bull 2013; 36(1): 96-101.
[http://dx.doi.org/10.1248/bpb.b12-00728] [PMID: 23302641]

[152] Martens TF, Remaut K, Deschout H, *et al.* Coating nanocarriers with hyaluronic acid facilitates intravitreal drug delivery for retinal gene therapy. J Control Release 2015; 202: 83-92.
[http://dx.doi.org/10.1016/j.jconrel.2015.01.030] [PMID: 25634806]

[153] Oliveira AVV, Silva GA, Chung DC. Enhancement of chitosan-mediated gene delivery through combination with phiC31 integrase. Acta Biomater 2015; 17: 89-97.
[http://dx.doi.org/10.1016/j.actbio.2015.01.013] [PMID: 25600399]

CHAPTER 15

Biological Approaches to Nanoparticles Synthesis and their Applications in the Development Of Herbal Formulations

Vivek Shrivastava[1], **Bhavisha Patel**[1] and **Akhlesh K. Jain**[2,*]

[1] *School of Pharmacy, Parul University, Vadodara, Gujarat, India*

[2] *School of Pharmaceutical Sciences, Guru Ghasidas Central University, Bilaspur- 495 009 (C.G.), India*

Abstract: This chapter focuses on the sustainable environment for the synthesis of nanoparticles using microorganisms, enzymes, or botanical extracts as an alternative to chemical synthesis, and their subsequent application in herbal drug delivery systems. The objective is to emphasize the rapid, straightforward, and reliable synthesis of nanoparticles using a novel, preferably eco-friendly process. Herbal drugs are gaining prominence due to their ability to treat chronic diseases, such as arthritis and hypertension. However, several constraints, such as poor solubility, poor bioavailability, and low oral absorption, have restricted their use. Nanoparticle-loaded phytochemicals disperse conveniently in liquid and thus perforate easily. Merging nanotechnology with herbal medicine is required to produce better therapeutics with improved activity in the fight against long-term chronic disorders. Tissue engineering is another significant application of nanotechnology.

Keywords: Drug delivery, Gold nanoparticles, Green synthesis of Nanoparticles, Herbal nanoparticles, Microbial synthesis of nanoparticles, Nanotechnology in tissue engineering, Nanoparticles synthesis, Plant mediated nanoparticles. Therapeutic efficacy of Medicinal plants using nanoparticles, Synthesis of Nanoparticles of plants extracts, Viral nanotechnology.

INTRODUCTION

The chemical and physical methods (non-biological) used in the production of nanoparticles, show explicit health hazards and have high toxicity for living organisms. However, the biological production of nanoparticles is one step, low-cost, and eco-friendly method. There are several techniques for developing nano-

* **Corresponding Author Akhlesh K. Jain**: School of Pharmaceutical Sciences, Guru Ghasidas Central University, Bilaspur- 495 009 (C.G.), India, Tel: +91-8871211758; E-mail: **akjain.ie@gmail.com**

Akhlesh K. Jain & Keerti Mishra (Eds.)

particles using environmentally friendly methods. Recently, phyto-nano synthesis has emerged as a major area of nanoscience, encompassing green approaches to synthesis [1]. Instead of using chemical reducing agents, biological methods for nanomaterial synthesis uses microbial enzymes or phytochemicals as reducing and capping agents. The advantages of synthesizing nanoparticles in this way are that the method is enviormental friendly (green synthesis), economical (not using any costly chemical), plants or microbes are readily available, and it is easy to tailor the size, shape and nature of the produced nanoparticles by simply modifying the culture conditions like pH, temperature or the nutrient media. We can further purify and characterize nanoparticles for their size, shape, and morphology by using techniques of optical spectroscopy, Fourier transforms infrared spectroscopy (FTIR), X-ray diffraction (XRD) analysis, transmission electron microscopy (TEM), and various other methods. Once these nanoparticles have been characterized, we can bio-functionalize them (by adding a moiety to these nanoparticles) and thus broaden their applications [1].

Synthesis of Nanoparticles using Microbes

The bacteria are potential biofactories for the synthesis of gold, silver, and other metal nanoparticles and can produce the nanoparticles either intracellularly or extracellularly. In the periplasmic space of bacteria, the pseudomonas bacteria isolated from silver mines have the ability to convert silver nitrate into silver nanoparticles. Similarly, bacteria in soil samples can convert copper into copper nanoparticles. Morganella species bacteria isolated from the midgut of an insect are proficient in secreting nanoparticles extracellularly. Magnetotactic bacteria are a heterogeneous class of prokaryotes. They lack flagella; they move in accordance with the geomagnetic field, and their migration is based on the intracellular magnetic structure (magnetosomes). When Fe^{3+} is added to this bacteria's culture, it converts into iron oxide nanoparticles.

Yeast (Candida) can be used to synthesize cadmium sulphide nanoparticles, and recently the yeast strains have been identified for making gold nanoparticles and other metal nanoparticles. We can manipulate the size and shape of nanoparticles by using yeast. The yeast is widely available and simple to cultivate, and the production of nanoparticles is inexpensive. Fungi (Verticillium spices) can be used to produce gold nanoparticles with elevated monodispersity. Furthermore, fungi are known to secrete a much higher amount of proteins, allowing for greater productivity of nanoparticles [1].

The Mechanism of Synthesis of the Nanoparticle by Microbes

The broadly acknowledged mechanism of synthesis of silver nanoparticles in the presence of nitrate reductase is well studied in the bacillus microbes. Nitrate reductase (An enzyme present in the nitrogen cycle) is accountable for the conversion of nitrate to nitrate. The nitrate is converted to nitrate, and an electron is released, which is accepted by the incoming silver irons. The bacillus microbe secretes cofactors like NADH and NADH-dependent enzymes and converts Ag^{+} to Ag^{0}, and the production of silver nanoparticles takes place. Fig. **(15.1)** depicts the mechanism of nanoparticle synthesis by microbes.

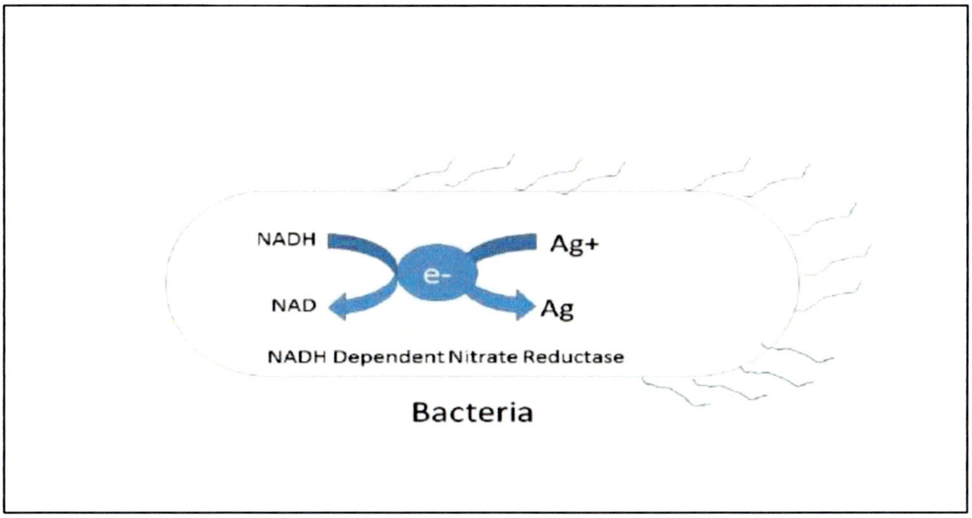

Fig. (15.1). Mechanism of nanoparticle production by bacteria.

Viral Nanotechnology

It entails the use of viruses and their nanostructure for a variety of applications. The attachment of the virus to the cells is the first step in the virus's life cycle. Once attached, their nucleic acid is injected into the host cell, where it uses the host machinery to integrate with the host cell's genome and replicate the viral genetic material multiple times. The viral genetic material, whether DNA or RNA, produces the proteins required for virus and replication in millions, and eventually destroys the entire cell. If the nucleic acid of the virus is removed, the virus's protein cage architecture can be used for a variety of purposes. Fig. **(15.2)** depicts several applications of the virus cage structure. Protein cage architecture can be used in the following ways.

The interior of the capsid can be loaded with a therapeutic agent, such as an anti-cancer drug, and thus used for therapeutic purposes.

The addition of gadolinium metal ions to the capsid wall makes it suitable for cancer imaging. We can target specific cells by adding RGD peptides (three amino acid peptides) to the surface of protein cage architecture.

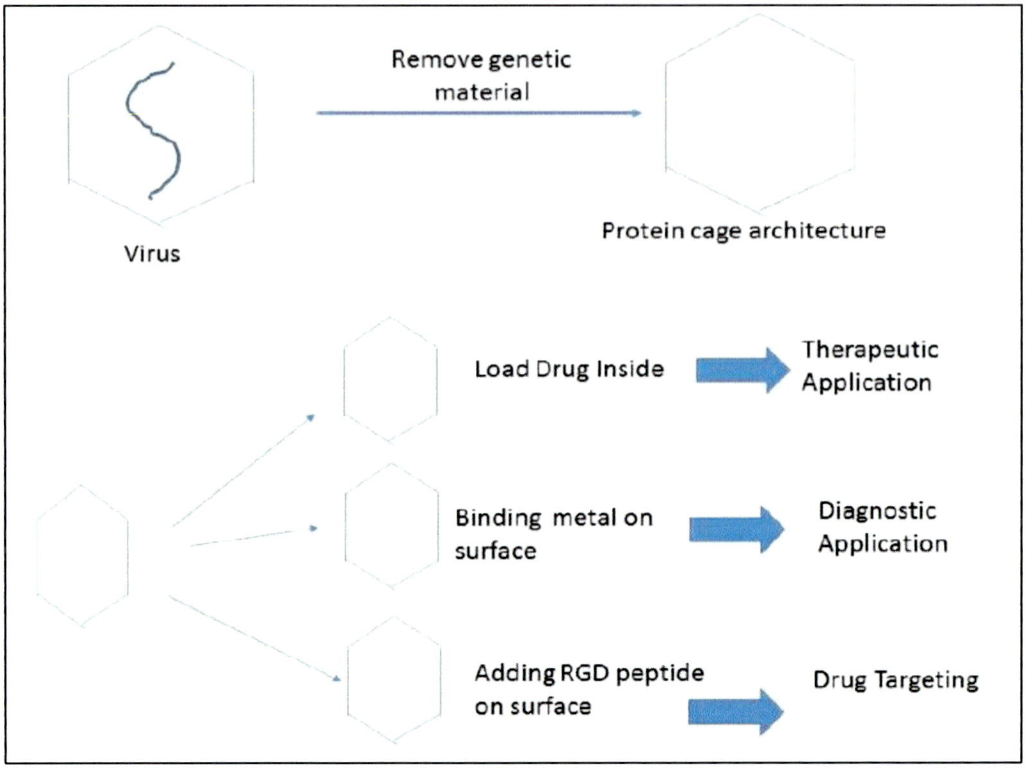

Fig. (15.2). Viral Protein cage architecture and its applications.

As a result, it behaves similarly to multi-functional Nanoparticles derived from plants, animals, and insect viruses. Human viruses are not employed because of chances of interaction of viral cage with human proteins and the likelihood of immune response generation and other toxic effects. The preferred choice is a plant virus as they have different shapes and sizes and according to the desired application, we can use plant viruses of any suitable size and shape. The larger surface area allows for greater drug loading. Furthermore, by using a small plant tissue (leaf), we can economically produce millions of viruses. The use of animal viruses necessitates the use of an animal for virus generation and the subsequent killing of the animal for virus collection, which adds to the cost [2].

Virus can also be used as a scaffold for 3D cell culture. We add RGD surface ligated viral magnetic nanoparticles to the cell to create 3D cell culture. Magnetic nanoparticles attach to cells as a result of RGD. When cells are incorporated into culture vessels, they settle to the bottom and cover the bottom. Apply a magnetic field to the top of the culture, which will cause cells to elevate due to the presence of magnetic nanoparticles. Allowing cells to grow in 3D conditions results in a 3D cell culture.3D culture better mimics body organs to study drug efficiency [2].

Green Synthesis - Nanoparticles from Plants Extracts

The establishment of dependable and environment-friendly techniques for the production of metal nanoparticles is very much required. Plants have emerged as an efficient living factory for the Green synthesis of metal nanoparticles as a solution. This is non-toxic, quick, occurs at room temperature, and economical. Metal nanoparticles have been successfully synthesized using a variety of plants and their parts, including bark, leaves, and plant enzymes.

Plant biomolecules serve as both capping agents for stabilization and reducing agents in the synthesis of plant-mediated nanoparticles. As a result, plant-derived nano drugs have a promising future, with elevated bioactivity overshadowing the usual drawbacks of low solubility and lower bioavailability associated with herbal drugs. Fig. **(15.3)** represents one possible method of producing nanoparticles.

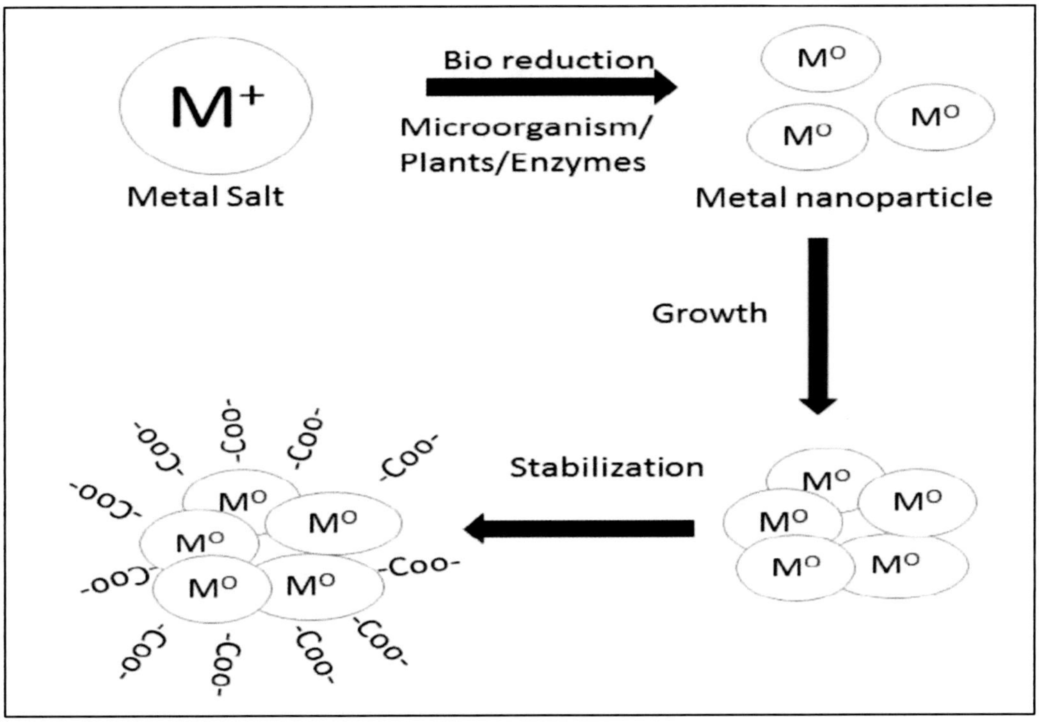

Fig. (15.3). Mechanism of biological synthesis of nanoparticle.

Although leaves are the most commonly used material for obtaining plant extract for nanoparticle synthesis, other parts such as fruit, seed, bark, root, flower, and rhizome have also been exploited. The reaction of plant extract with metal salt in an aqueous medium at room temperature is considered necessary for plant-based biosynthesis. This technique has been used to synthesise various metal nanoparticles (such as Ag, Au, and others).

Phyto-constituents and proteins are the principal biological molecules responsible for the reaction and carry out the dual role of capping as well as reducing agents. The secondary metabolites also intervene as stabilizing agents after the production of plant derived nanoparticles. This technique is simple and can be performed in a room. The properties of produced nanoparticles, as well as their rate of production and amount produced, are influenced by phytoconstituent concentration, temperature, pH, and metal salt type [3].

Preparation of Silver Nanoparticles using Leaf Extract

Silver nanoparticles are the most extensively used nanoparticles due to their wide range of applications and unique properties. The Ag^+ ion can form a strong bond with nitrogen; oxygen and Sulphur containing groups (electron donating groups) are present in biomolecules and thus have antimicrobial properties. The silver-based nanoparticles act more efficiently and have many advantages over nanoparticles produced by larger metal molecules.The silver salt is biologically reduced from Ag^+ to Ag^0, followed by self-assembling and, finally, colloidal aggregation. The silver nanoparticles have high applicability (in the biomedical as well as medical fields) [3].

Fresh leaves from any suitable plant are taken and chopped into small pieces after being thoroughly washed. Leaf pieces are mixed with deionized water and heated for 15 minutes at 80-90 degrees Celsius. When the water turned green, it was filtered out, and the resulting plant leaf extract can be used as a reducing and capping agent in the synthesis of nanoparticles. Silver Nitrate is heated in deionized water until the temperature reaches 60-70°C. Now leaf extract is added dropwise until the color of the Silver Nitrate solution turns light yellow. The light-Yellow color indicated the formation of Silver Nanoparticles. The nanoparticles synthesis can be confirmed using UV-Vis spectroscopy (absorption peak around 420 nm).

Preparation of Gold Nanoparticles using Leaf Extract

First plant leaf extract was developed. Tetrachloroauric acid in deionized water was kept on a hot plate with a magnetic stirrer and allowed to reach a temperature of 80°C. Now, leaf extract was added dropwise with continuous agitation until the tetrachloroauric acid solution turned red or violet in colour. The formation of gold nanoparticles in water is indicated by the red or violet colour. The absorption peak of 530 nm in UV-Vis spectroscopy confirms nanoparticle synthesis [4].

Synthesis of Nickel Nanoparticles using Leaf Extract

The first plant leaf extract is developed. In a conical flask, nickel chloride was added to deionized water, and the flask was kept on a hot plate with a magnetic stirrer at an 80°C temperature. Drop by drop, leaf extract was added to the solution until the colour changed to grey, indicating the formation of nickel nanoparticles. The absorption peak in UV spectroscopy around 270nm confirms their synthesis.

The composition and concentration of secondary metabolites (reducing agents in plant extracts) influence various properties of synthesized nanoparticles such as size, shape, and morphology. Researchers have also demonstrated that changing parameters such as pH and temperature have an effect on the size, shape, and morphology of nanoparticles.

Synthesis of Iron Nanoparticles

Green tea extract is used in the facile, inexpensive, and eco-friendly synthesis of iron nanoparticles (FeNP). So far, the majority of the data show green tea leaves being used for FeNP synthesis. Limited information about the exploitation of other plants that contain a significant amount of antioxidants, though the antioxidant potential of some tree leaves has recently been evaluated to determine their feasibility [4].

Mechanism of Nanoparticle Synthesis by using Plant Extract

To control the size and prevent aggregation of nanoparticles, a metal salt (silver nitrate), a reducing agent (sodium borohydride), and a capping or stabilising agent (polyvinyl alcohol) are used in the chemical synthesis of silver nanoparticles. However, in biosynthesis, the plant extract serves as both a reducing agent and a capping agent.Various plants, as well as their parts, are utilized in the synthesis of nanoparticles. Plant extracts are rich in phytochemicals like flavonoids, proteins, alkaloids, polysaccharides, and phenolic compounds and secondary metabolites. When plant extracts react with metal ions, their monovalent/divalent oxidation status is transformed to zero valent status. Afterward, nucleation (of the reduced metals atoms) takes place. Finally, nanoparticle aggregates in a variety of shapes such as a sphere, wires or other. Capping is done to control the size and stabilize nanoparticles [4].

Characterization of Nanoparticles

The first qualitative indication for nanoparticle synthesis is a change in the colour of the reaction solution. Surface plasmon vibration causes the characteristic colour change. The morphology, size, and shape of nanoparticles are essential aspects of their applications. Various techniques used for the purpose of nanoparticle characterizations are ultraviolet-visible spectroscopy (UV), scanning electron microscopy (SEM), transmission electron microscopy (TEM), dynamic light scattering (DLS), X-ray powder diffraction (XRD), Fourier transform infrared spectroscopy (FT-IR), and others. UV-vis spectroscopy in the range of 300 and 800 is prevalently applied for nanoparticle characterization, which is in the size range of 2 to 100 nm. Dynamic light scattering is employed to obtain size distribution and surface charges of nanoparticles dispersed in a liquid. Electron microscopy (SEM/TEM) and atomic force microscopy are broadly used to envisage the size, shape, and morphology of synthesized nanoparticles. The zeta potential analysis reveals the surface charges on nanoparticles, which influence their stability.

Electron Probe Micro Analysis (EPMA)

EPMA is a predictable technique employed in the characterization of Nanosized substances. It aids by producing the images of the surface by probing and scanning the sample physically. Elemental analysis of metal nanoparticles is also possible if Energy dispersive spectroscopy is coupled with EPMA.

X-Ray Diffraction (XRD)

XRD is a technique used to identify crystalline materials as well as analyse unit cell dimensions.XRD is frequently used to analyse the crystal structure of nanoparticles.X-rays has the ability to penetrate nanoparticle and the diffraction pattern so generated is matched to standards in order to derive structural data. Each crystalline solid has a unique XRPD pattern that serves as a “fingerprint” for identification.

Fourier Transform Infrared Spectroscopy (FTIR)

It can be employed for the identification of functional groups present in phyto-constituents which are responsible for the bioreduction of metal ions into nanoparticles. FTIR is capable not only of detecting probable biomolecules responsible for conversion but also of their ability for capping. FTIR spectra also deliver data about chemical transformations in the bio-reduced functional group.

Laser- Induced Breakdown Spectroscopy (LIBS)

LIBS can identify any matter, solid, liquid or gaseous, irrespective of its state. Based on the principle that all elements generate light encompassing distinct frequencies on arriving excitation state at appropriate temperatures, elemental identification of nanoparticles can be done through LIBS.

Use of Nanoparticles in the Development of Herbal Formulations

Herbal medicines have been used to treat various ailments for several years worldwide.Particularly in the developing world, herbals preparation is gaining popularity. World Health Organization estimated that eighty percent of the world population relies on herbal medicines for primary healthcare. The increasing incidences of unwanted side effects and costly therapy with the existing formulations have resulted in considering the conventional drugs as an alternative therapy, with the hope to treat patients with safe and effective herbal medicines. Several medicinal plants have been reported in ethno medicinal data and are still unknown to the scientific fraternity [5].

The application of herbal medicines is on the surge owing to their ability to treat diseases without significant side effects.Although plants have always been a prototypical source of potent medicines for ages, herbals exhibit low absorption, poor membrane permeability, high molecular weight, poor bioavailability and efficacy over the biological system. To address these issues, nano-carriers are being used as an alternative approach. A lot of research work is going on in the field of novel herbal formulations, and these researches have exhibited remarkable advantages of novel herbal formulations over respective crude drug preparations or extracts by improving their solubility, bioavailability, and pharmacological activity, stability, and improved tissue distribution. Furthermore, sustained delivery and shield from degradation (physical and chemical) are other advantages offered by novel formulations. Thus, the study of the synergistic efficacy of plant products and nanoparticles is of vital importance.

Nanoparticles are the drug carriers having at least one of the dimensions in the size range of 1 to 100 nanometers (nm) [6]. As contrasted micro and macro material, nanomaterials demonstrate distinctive biological, physical, and chemical properties owing to their small size, shape, morphology composition and distribution.

With the accession of the twenty-first century, modern medicinal science has undergone a rapid and novel transformation, particularly in the use of nanocarriers for drug delivery.However, the use of nano- particles in the form of 'Bhasma' was first described in Ayurveda (the traditional Indian system of medicine) some 5,000 years back [7].

With nanoparticles targeting of herbal drug to specific organ can be achieved which improves the selectivity, effectiveness and safety of drug.Herbal drug solubility can be increased by using nanoparticles, which can then localize the drug in a specific site, resulting in improved efficacy. Because of their nano size and high drug loading nanoparticles can deliver high concentrations of drugs to site of action. Nanoparticle ensures quicker dissolution in the blood due to enhanced surface to volume ratio of nanoparticles. Nanoparticles based herbal formulations exhibit enhanced permeation through membranes as of the small size and good retention due to poor lymphatic drainage. Lastly, passive targeting of herbal drug can also be achieved without the need for ligand.

Herbal drugs are used since ages in both developing and developed world to treat and cure diseases. The advances in analytical techniques have it possible to detect and elucidate the structure of phyto-constituents present in herbal medicines. Some phytoconstituents in herbals (like tannins, terpenoids, flavonoids) tannins, exhibit sufficient aqueous solubility, but are poorly absorbed upon administration as their inability to penetrate biological membranes of the cells.

Moreover, they also have high molecular weight.All of this contributes to their low bioavailability and overall efficacy when administered.Certain phyto-constituents, on the other hand, have low water solubility and poor pharmacokinetics.These obvious problems have held back the use of many phytopharmaceuticals in clinics. To circumvent these limitations, nanotech-nology-based approaches for delivery of herbal drugs have been used. Nanoparticles can be utilized to adapt and improve the pharmacokinetic and pharmacodynamic properties of herbals.Nanocarriers can also be used to deliver bioactive phytoconstituents of herbal drugs to specific targets like cells or tissue. Nanocarriers holds a great possibility of delivering herbal drugs. Long-term safety, economy needs to be further investigated. Nano formulation of herbal drugs were tested for their suitability to deliver the phytoconstituents in sufficient concentration to target sites during the course of therapy. Conventional herbal formulations cannot fulfill these needs. With conventional herbals, only a small portion of administered dose of active phytoconstituents reaches target site [8].

Impact of Plant Mediated Nanoparticles on Therapeutic Efficacy of Medicinal plants

Plant extracts play dual role of both reducing agents as well as stabilizing/and or capping agents in the nanoparticle's synthesis. Since different plants contains different phyto-constitutes and that too in varied concentrations, plant origin markedly affects the properties (like size) of the synthesized nanoparticle and their yield. These nanoparticles synthesized using plant or other biological approach when combined with phyto-constituents can be promising approach for the development of value-added herbal formulations [9].

Phyto synthesized Nanoparticles presents suitability with bioactive phyto molecules [10]. Since nanoparticles are primary source of soluble metal therefore, drug loaded nanoparticles have been shown to increase the bioavailability, half-life, water solubility, and absorption of herbal drugs *vis* a *vis* their extract or powders. Syzygiumcumini seeds derived silver nanoparticles demonstrated enhanced antioxidant activity as compare to the original plant extract due absorption of antioxidant on nanoparticle surface.

Silver nanoparticles synthesized biologically from the Ocimum sanctum leave extract, demonstrated antimicrobial activity against both Streptococcus aureus (a gram positive) and *E. coli* (a gram-negative bacteria) [11].Gold nanoparticles synthesised using a biological approach using Cassia fistula aqueous extract demonstrated enhanced hypoglycemic activity when compared to the whole plant and its bark.This augmented efficacy was due to the aggregation of extract derived hypoglycemic on the surface of the metal nanoparticles. Copper nanoparticles produced employing Magnolia leaf extract showed enhanced antibacterial efficacy against *E. coli.* Plant synthesized Iron nanoparticle displayed better free radical scavenging ability and stability due to the existence of polyphenols or antioxidants (in green tea extract).

The potent antimalarial artemisinin has a short half-life and poor pharmacokinetic properties, minimizing its clinical application.The nano-coated artemisinin solubilized well in aqueous solutions and its hydrophilicity was also enhanced [12]. Centellaasiatica extract (CAE) possesses high physical instability and the powder shows high hygroscopicity. The. Chitosan- alginate nanoparticles encapsulating Centellaasiatica extract prepared by ionic gelation method exhibited higher physical stability as compared to its extract.

Curcumin, derived from turmeric, is a highly effective phytomolecule.But its application was limited due to its short biological half-life, poor aqueous solubility, rapid rate of metabolism and rapid elimination rate, and hence poor bioavailability upon oral administration. Nanoparticles of curcumin are freely dispersible in water [13].

Danshen used for cerebrovascular diseases and hyperlipidemia is reported to have slow pharmacological action. Nano-coated drug showed stronger antioxidant property and fast release of drug compared to powered samples. Moreover, nanoparticles also enhanced oral bioavailability. Dodder obtained from Cuscut-tachinensis Lam. (Family: Convolvulaceae) contains flavanoids and lignans is primarily used as anti-cancer agent has poor aqueous solubility. Cuscuttachinensis coated nanoparticles outperformed ethanolic seed extract in terms of hepatoprotective and antioxidant activity (at lower concentrations) [14].

Genistein, aisoflavone, which is an active component of soybean, has poor aqueous solubility. The genistein nanoparticles improve its solubility and bioavailability. Study exhibited that genistein loaded nanoparticles showed two-fold higher relative bioavailability compared to genistein alone.

Paclitaxel (anticancer drug) has limited aqueous solubility (0.7- 30 ug/ml-1) which limits its efficacy. However, paclitaxel encapsulated nanoparticles not only enhanced its anti- tumor activity but also drug stability and bioavailability. Table **15.1** showcase various examples of plant extract mediated bio reduction of metal ion to produce nanoparticle.

Table 15.1. Summarizes examples of plant extract mediated bio reduction of metal ion to produce nanoparticle.

S. No.	Plant extract	Reduction of	Attributed to the Presence of	References
1	*C. camphora* (Leaf extract)	Ag & Au ions	terpenoids, polysaccharides	[15]
2	*D. metel* (Leaf extract)	Ag ions	Alkaloids & polysaccharides	[16]
3	*indica* (Leaf extract)	Ag & Au ions	activity than plant reducing sugars	[17]
4	*Sorghum bran* (aq extract)	Ag & Fe ions	reducing agents	[18]
5	Green Tea (Leaf extract)	Fe ions	polyphenols	[19]

Nano Technology in Tissue Engineering

Tissue engineering inculcates the principles of engineering and life science and involves development of biological substitutes, which helps in restoring maintaining or improving the tissue function. tissue engineering is done to replace the diseased or damage tissue. Tissue engineering is a method to treat patients who require a new organ or tissue with the human made organ or tissues.

Tissue engineering is accomplished by obtaining patents own cells and growing them on polymer scaffolds, which act as extracellular matrix in laboratory conditions.The three-dimensional Polymer scaffolds act as a support structure, allowing nutrients to permeate through the porous structure. We replaced the damaged tissue with engineered tissue. A three-dimensional scaffold mimics the *in vivo* state while also acting as a support for cell growth, making it useful for creating artificial tissue to replace damaged tissue [20].

Tissue engineering is required because the donor tissues and organs are scarce secondly, the availability of sufficient donors to get tissue is limited and lastly, foreign organs attract immune response and present a threat of rejection. Therefore, patient's own cells are used to prevent immune response and thus, human-made tissue is engineered.

Three tools are needed for tissue engineering the cells, the scaffold and cell signaling [21]. We procure cells as embryonic stem cells or adult stem cells because stem cells can differentiate into any kind of cells. The stem cells can give rise to many different types of cells depending upon suitable conditions or signals. Scaffolds should be properly biodegradable and biocompatible. Scaffolds can be made from metal, ceramics, or they can be synthesized from synthetic and natural polymers, depending on the tissue that needs to be grown.Cell signaling may be like a growth factor or hormone, which causes cell differentiation. For example, with a suitable growth factor, the stem cells can be allowed to differentiate into liver cells or kidney cells.

Scaffolds are artificial structures that can support to accomplish three-dimensional tissue generation. Scaffolds allow the cells to attach them. They also retain the cells and growth factors, and allow the diffusion of vital cell nutrients. Scaffolds are available in various structures and materials depending on the tissue to be grown. When a micropores scaffold is used, the cells cannot attach properly but with microporous scaffolds with fibers in nanometer range, ensuring better cell attachment and nanofibers-based scaffold exactly resembles extracellular matrix [21].

Production of Nanofibers by Electrospinning Technique

Electrospinning is a technique where fibers and particles are produced from a polymer solution. It is a voltage-dependent methodology that is guided by electrical phenomena. The instrument includes a pump, a reservoir for polymer solution (typically a syringe with a blunt-tipped needle), a high voltage source, and a collector (usually in the form of a rotating drug). Voltage is applied to create an electric field between needle tip and collector, and polymer solution is pumped at a constant rate with the help of a pump; this marks the starting of the spinning process. A typical electrospinning setup is shown in Fig. (**15.4**). Charge accumulates at the liquid surface, and the meniscus of the liquid is distorted when the electrostatic repulsion is greater than surface tension; it assumes the shape of a cone which is called the Taylor cone (Fig. **15.5**).

As soon as the Taylor cone is formed, the liquid jet is thrown towards the collector. In the course of its time of flight, from cone to the collector, the solvent evaporates, resulting in the production of a non-woven fiber, which is collected on the collector [22]. Plants crude extracts are prepared by extraction of fresh or dried plants with the help of organic solvents. These extracts can be loaded/ or encapsulated in electro-spun fibers as Centellaasiatica extract is encapsulated in cellulose acetate fibers, which can be spun into a matt and thereafter can be used for wound dressing application [23]. Baicalein extract [24], green tea extract [25], Garcinia mangostana extract [26], Tecomellaundulata extract [27], aloe vera extract [28], grape seed extract [29], and Azadirachtaindica extract [30] have also been successfully uploaded in nano spun fibres for various applications. Table **15.2** illustrates plant extract-loaded nanowire and its various applications.

Table 15.2. Summarizes various drug-loaded nanofibers, their scaffold construction material and applications.

Electrospun Fiber Material	Plant extract	Use	Reference
Ultra-fine cellulose acetate	*CentellaAsiatica*	Wound Dressing	[31]
Chitosan	Green Tea	Wound Dresing	[32]
Polyvinyl alcohol-Chitosan	Curcumin	Tissue enginering	[33]
Polyurethane	Aloe Vera	Bone regeneration	[34]
Silk fibroin (SF)	Grape Seed Extract	Wound Healing	[35]
PCL/PVP Nanofiber mat	Bark Extract of *Tecomella Undulata*	wound healing	[36]

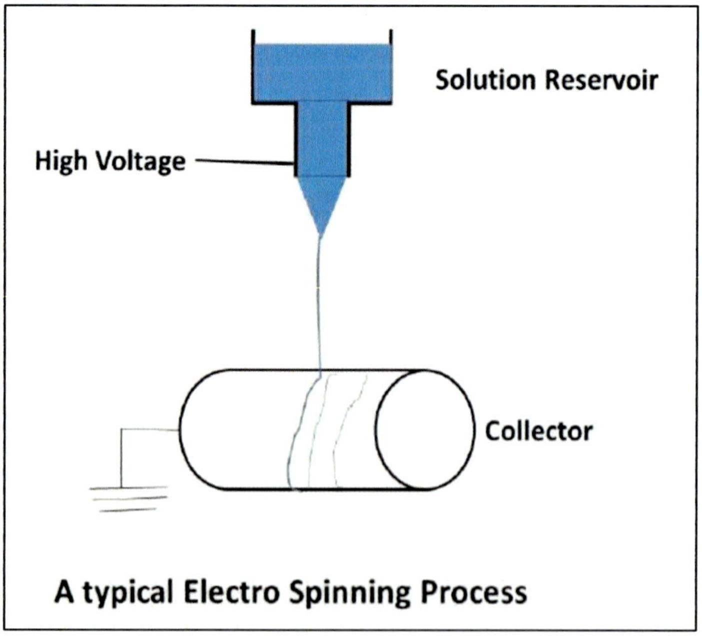

Fig. (15.4). Electrospinning process for nanowire production.

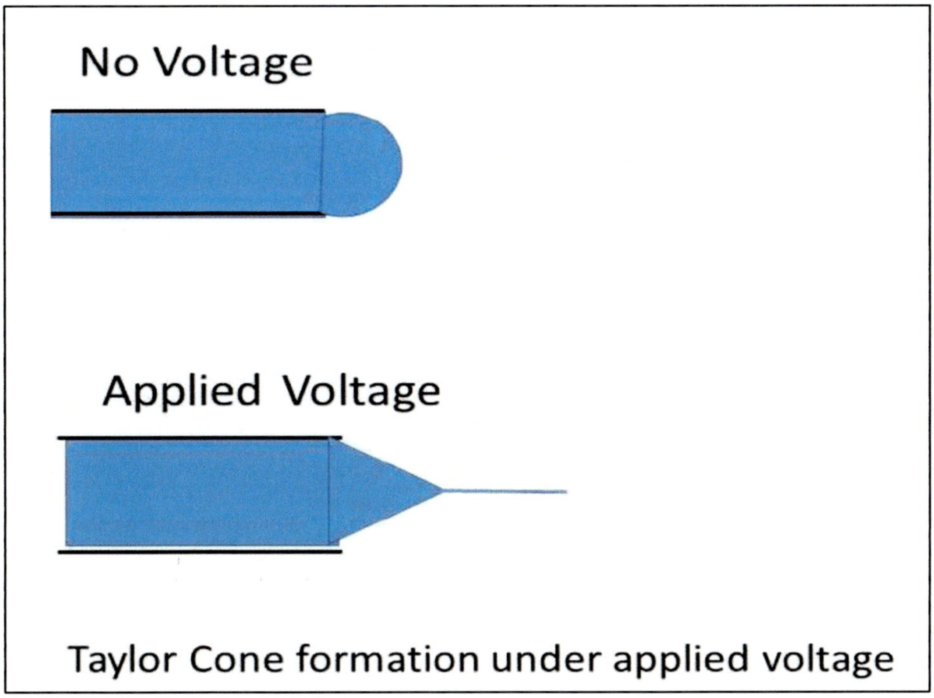

Fig. (15.5). Diagram of Taylor cone formation.

CONCLUSION

The current need to develop better drugs with superior activity is to integrate nanotechnology and traditional herbal medicine systems. A lot of research has recently been executed on the biological synthesis of nanoparticles and their applications in the delivery of herbal drugs. Development of herbal formulations containing antimicrobial agents, novel drug delivery systems, lab and disease diagnostics, different cell labelling, use of isolated biomarkers, tagging of biologic materials, environmental factors, and the pharmaceutical industry are examples of these areas of research. Globally, research and development in this field are advancing rapidly.

Metal nanoparticles have gained much attention due to their biomedical applications. Due to their numerous applications, silver (Ag) and iron (Fe) nanoparticles have received considerable attention. With the rising demand for metal nanoparticles, efforts have been made to synthesize these nanoparticles by easy, safe and quick methods. The oxidation-reduction and cellular respiration occurring in plants and animals use iron at the active site of many redox enzymes. It also plays a role as a structural component as well as a cofactor for different enzymes.

Many steps are involved in the physical and chemical methods of nanoparticle synthesis, require high-energy, pose difficulty in refining and require the use of harmful chemicals. As a result, developing a cost-effective, commercially reproducible, and environmentally friendly method of synthesizing nanoparticles remain a challenge.

The biological production of nanoparticles is advantageous over physical and chemical methods, as it is inexpensive, eco-friendly, commercially viable and does not require the use of harmful chemicals. Biological approach to synthesize nanoparticles using microorganisms, enzymes or plant extracts has been established as an alternative to chemical synthesis. More research needs to be carried out to further understand the mechanism of nanoparticle formation. Once the mechanism of nanoparticles formation is thoroughly established, we can fine-tune the size and shape of nanoparticles by simply changing the critical synthesis parameters.

Further investigations are required to review the role of different natural products during the synthesis of nanoparticles. The fruit tree leaves, in particular, contain high levels of natural antioxidants (polyphenols). As a result, these phyto-antioxidants not only have pharmacological benefits, but can also act as better reducing agents in the synthesis of nanoparticles. Biological methods of nanoparticle synthesis are eco-friendly, easy, non-toxic, safe, and economically viable green approaches that employ enzymes, plant and microorganisms as reducing agents. Therefore, various nanoparticles (polymeric nanoparticles, liposomes, solid lipid nanoparticles and Nanoemulsions) have potential utilization to deliver herbal medicines with enhanced therapy.

CONSENT FOR PUBLICATION

Not applicable.

CONFLICT OF INTEREST

The authors declare no conflict of interest, financial or otherwise.

ACKNOWLEDGEMENT

Declared none.

REFERENCES

[1] Elzoghby AO, Samy WM, Elgindy NA. Protein-based nanocarriers as promising drug and gene delivery systems. J Control Release 2012; 161(1): 38-49. [http://dx.doi.org/10.1016/j.jconrel.2012.04.036] [PMID: 22564368]

[2] Fang R, Hao R, Wu X, Li Q, Leng X, Jing H. Bovine serum albumin nanoparticles promotes the

stability of quercetin in simulated intestinal fluid. J Agric Food Chem 2011; 59(11): 6292-8. [http://dx.doi.org/10.1021/jf200718j]

[3] Fessi H, Puisieux F, Devissaguet JP, Ammoury N, Benita S. Nanocapsule formation by interfacial polymer deposition following solvent displacement. Int J Pharm 1989; 55(1): R1-4. [http://dx.doi.org/10.1016/0378-5173(89)90281-0]

[4] Formica JV, Regelson W. Review of the biology of quercetin and related bioflavonoids. Food Chem Toxicol 1995; 33(12): 1061-80. [http://dx.doi.org/10.1016/0278-6915(95)00077-1] [PMID: 8847003]

[5] Fukuda K, Hibiya Y, Mutoh M, Koshiji M, Akao S, Fujiwara H. Inhibition of activator protein 1 activity by berberine in human hepatoma cells. Planta Med 1999; 65(4): 381-3. [http://dx.doi.org/10.1055/s-2006-960795] [PMID: 10364850]

[6] Gleave M, Bruchovsky N, Goldenberg SL, Rennie P. Intermittent androgen suppression for prostate cancer: Rationale and clinical experience. Eur Urol 1998; 34 (Suppl. 3): 37-41. [http://dx.doi.org/10.1159/000052297] [PMID: 9854195]

[7] Goyal A, Kumar S, Nagpal M, Singh I, Arora S. Potential of novel drug delivery system for herbal system for herbal drugs. Indian journal of pharmaceutical education and research 2011; 45: 225-35.

[8] Gupta VK, Karar PK, Ramesh S, Misra SP, Gupta A. Nanoparticle formulation for hydrophilic and hydrophobic drugs. International journal of research in pharmaceutical sciences 2010; 1: 163-9.

[9] Hua-Yan , Li , Dng-Peng , *et al.* JNanosciNanotechnology 2010; 10(4): 2325-31.

[10] Kang DG, Oh H, Sohn EJ, *et al.* Lithospermic acid B isolated from Salvia miltiorrhiza ameliorates ischemia/reperfusion-induced renal injury in rats. Life Sci 2004; 75(15): 1801-16. [http://dx.doi.org/10.1016/j.lfs.2004.02.034] [PMID: 15302225]

[11] Kiuchi F, Goto Y, Sugimoto N, Akao N, Kondo K, Tsuda Y. Nematocidal activity of turmeric: Synergistic action of curcuminoids. Chem Pharm Bull (Tokyo) 1993; 41(9): 1640-3. [http://dx.doi.org/10.1248/cpb.41.1640] [PMID: 8221978]

[12] Kumari A, Yadav SK, Pakade YB, Singh B, Yadav SC. Development of biodegradable nanoparticles for delivery of quercetin. Colloids Surf B Biointerfaces 2010; 80(2): 184-92. [http://dx.doi.org/10.1016/j.colsurfb.2010.06.002] [PMID: 20598513]

[13] Kumar K, Rai AK. Miraculous therapeutic effects of herbal drugs using novel drug delivery systems. International Research Journal of Pharmacy 2012; 3: 2733.

[14] Vollath D. Nanomaterials – An introduction to synthesis, properties and application. Environ Eng Manag J 2008; 78: 65-70.

[15] Huang J, Li Q, Sun D, *et al.* Biosynthesis of silver and gold nanoparticles by novel sundried *Cinnamomum camphora* leaf. Nanotechnology 2007; 18(10): 105104. [http://dx.doi.org/10.1088/0957-4484/18/10/105104]

[16] Kesharwani J, Yoon KY, Hwang J, Rai M. Phytofabrication of silver nanoparticles by leaf extract of Datura metel: Hypothetical mechanism involved in synthesis. Journal of Bionanoscience 2009; 3(1): 39-44. [http://dx.doi.org/10.1166/jbns.2009.1008]

[17] Tripathy A, Raichur AM, Chandrasekaran N, Prathna TC, Mukherjee A. Process variables in biomimetic synthesis of silver nanoparticles by aqueous extract of Azadirachta indica (Neem) leaves. J Nanopart Res 2010; 12(1): 237-46. [http://dx.doi.org/10.1007/s11051-009-9602-5]

[18] Njagi EC, Huang H, Stafford L, *et al.* Biosynthesis of iron and silver nanoparticles at room temperature using aqueous sorghum bran extracts. Langmuir 2011; 27(1): 264-71. [http://dx.doi.org/10.1021/la103190n] [PMID: 21133391]

[19] Weng X, Huang L, Chen Z, Megharaj M, Naidu R. Synthesis of iron-based nanoparticles by green tea

extract and their degradation of malachite. Ind Crops Prod 2013; 51: 342-7.
[http://dx.doi.org/10.1016/j.indcrop.2013.09.024]

[20] Kingsley JD, Ranjan S, Dasgupta N, Saha P. Nanotechnology for tissue engineering: Need, techniques and applications. Journal of pharmacy research 2013; 7: 200-4.

[21] Coutinho D, Costa P, Neves N, Gomes ME, Reis RL. Micro-and nanotechnology in tissue engineering. Tissue Engineering. 2011; pp. 3-29.
[http://dx.doi.org/10.1007/978-3-642-02824-3_1]

[22] Li WJ, Laurencin CT, Caterson EJ, Tuan RS, Ko FK. Electrospun nanofibrous structure: A novel scaffold for tissue engineering. J Biomed Mater Res 2002; 60(4): 613-21.
[http://dx.doi.org/10.1002/jbm.10167] [PMID: 11948520]

[23] Yao CH, Yeh JY, Chen YS, Li MH, Huang CH. Wound-healing effect of electrospun gelatin nanofibres containing *Centella asiatica* extract in a rat model. J Tissue Eng Regen Med 2017; 11(3): 905-15.
[http://dx.doi.org/10.1002/term.1992] [PMID: 25711743]

[24] Chan WP, Huang KC, Bai MY. Silk fibroin protein-based nonwoven mats incorporating baicalein Chinese herbal extract: Preparation, characterizations, and *in vivo* evaluation. J Biomed Mater Res B Appl Biomater 2017; 105(2): 420-30.
[http://dx.doi.org/10.1002/jbm.b.33560] [PMID: 26540289]

[25] Sadri M, Arab-Sorkhi S, Vatani H, Bagheri-Pebdeni A. New wound dressing polymeric nanofiber containing green tea extract prepared by electrospinning method. Fibers Polym 2015; 16(8): 1742-50.
[http://dx.doi.org/10.1007/s12221-015-5297-7]

[26] Suwantong O, Pankongadisak P, Deachathai S, Supaphol P. Electrospun poly(l-lactic acid) fiber mats containing crude Garcinia mangostana extracts for use as wound dressings. Polym Bull 2014; 71(4): 925-49.
[http://dx.doi.org/10.1007/s00289-014-1102-9]

[27] Suganya S, Senthil Ram T, Lakshmi BS, Giridev VR. Herbal drug incorporated antibacterial nanofibrous mat fabricated by electrospinning: An excellent matrix for wound dressings. J Appl Polym Sci 2011; 121(5): 2893-9.
[http://dx.doi.org/10.1002/app.33915]

[28] Agnes Mary S, Giri Dev VR. Electrospun herbal nanofibrous wound dressings for skin tissue engineering. J Textil Inst 2015; 106(8): 886-95.
[http://dx.doi.org/10.1080/00405000.2014.951247]

[29] Lin S, Chen M, Jiang H, *et al.* Green electrospun grape seed extract-loaded silk fibroin nanofibrous mats with excellent cytocompatibility and antioxidant effect. Colloids Surf B Biointerfaces 2016; 139: 156-63.
[http://dx.doi.org/10.1016/j.colsurfb.2015.12.001] [PMID: 26707696]

[30] Jin G, Prabhakaran MP, Kai D, Annamalai SK, Arunachalam KD, Ramakrishna S. Tissue engineered plant extracts as nanofibrous wound dressing. Biomaterials 2013; 34(3): 724-34.
[http://dx.doi.org/10.1016/j.biomaterials.2012.10.026] [PMID: 23111334]

[31] Suwantong O, Ruktanonchai U, Supaphol P. Electrospun cellulose acetate fiber mats containing asiaticoside or Centella asiatica crude extract and the release characteristics of asiaticoside. Polymer (Guildf) 2008; 49(19): 4239-47.
[http://dx.doi.org/10.1016/j.polymer.2008.07.020]

[32] Selvakumar M, Pawar HS, Francis NK, Das B, Dhara S, Chattopadhyay S. Excavating the role of aloe vera wrapped mesoporous hydroxyapatite frame ornamentation in newly architectured polyurethane scaffolds for osteogenesis and guided bone regeneration with microbial protection. ACS Appl Mater Interfaces 2016; 8(9): 5941-60.
[http://dx.doi.org/10.1021/acsami.6b01014] [PMID: 26889707]

[32] Sadri M, Arab-Sorkhi S, Vatani H, Bagheri-Pebdeni A. New wound dressing polymeric nanofiber containing green tea extract prepared by electrospinning method. Fibers Polym 2015; 16(8): 1742-50. [http://dx.doi.org/10.1007/s12221-015-5297-7]

[33] Abbas M, Hussain T, Arshad M, *et al.* Wound healing potential of curcumin cross-linked chitosan/polyvinyl alcohol. Int J Biol Macromol 2019; 140: 871-6. [http://dx.doi.org/10.1016/j.ijbiomac.2019.08.153] [PMID: 31437503]

[34] Selvakumar M, Pawar HS, Francis NK, Das B, Dhara S, Chattopadhyay S. Excavating the role of aloe vera wrapped mesoporous hydroxyapatite frame ornamentation in newly architectured polyurethane scaffolds for osteogenesis and guided bone regeneration with microbial protection. ACS Appl Mater Interfaces 2016; 8(9): 5941-60. [http://dx.doi.org/10.1021/acsami.6b01014] [PMID: 26889707]

[35] Bacakova L, Pajorova J, Zikmundova M, *et al.* Nanofibrous scaffolds for skin tissue engineering and wound healing based on nature-derived polymers.Current and future aspects of nanomedicine. 2019; pp. 69-80.

[36] Suganya S, Senthil Ram T, Lakshmi BS, Giridev VR. Herbal drug incorporated antibacterial nanofibrous mat fabricated by electrospinning: An excellent matrix for wound dressings. J Appl Polym Sci 2011; 121(5): 2893-9. [http://dx.doi.org/10.1002/app.33915]

SUBJECT INDEX

A

Akhlesh K. Jain & Keerti Mishra (Eds.)

B

D

E

F

H

I

K

L

M

N

O

P

Q

R

S

U

V

W

X

Made in the USA
Las Vegas, NV
22 August 2025

276344bf-381e-4b7b-84e9-a37225484fdaR06